VOLUME V
Current advances in
oral and maxillofacial surgery:
orthognathic surgery

VOLUME V

Current advances in oral and maxillofacial surgery: orthognathic surgery

Edited by

DAVID W. SHELTON, B.S., D.M.D., F.I.C.D.

Professor, Department of Oral and Maxillofacial Surgery,
School of Dentistry; Professor, Department of Surgery,
School of Medicine, Medical College of Georgia;
Attending Staff: Eugene Talmadge Memorial Hospital and
U.S. Veterans Administration Hospital,
Augusta, Georgia

WILLIAM B. IRBY, D.D.S., M.S., F.A.C.D.

Professor Emeritus, Medical University of South Carolina;
Director, William B. Irby Craniofacial Pain Center,
Charleston, South Carolina

With 692 illustrations

The C.V. Mosby Company

ST. LOUIS • TORONTO • PRINCETON   1986

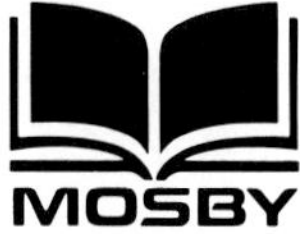

Editor: Darlene Barela Warfel
Assistant editor: Melba Steube
Manuscript editor: George B. Stericker, Jr.
Production: Jeanne A. Gulledge, Ginny Douglas

VOLUME V

The C.V. Mosby Company
11830 Westline Industrial Drive, St. Louis, Missouri 63146

AC/MV/MV 9 8 7 6 5 4 3 2 1   01/D/034

Contributors

Robert A. Bays, D.D.S.

Associate Clinical Professor of Oral and Maxillofacial Surgery and Anatomy, Medical College of Georgia; Private Practice of Oral and Maxillofacial Surgery, Augusta, Georgia; Diplomate, American Board of Oral and Maxillofacial Surgery

Lewis A. Coveler, M.D.

Associate Professor and Chief, Department of Anesthesiology, Ben Taub General Hospital, Houston, Texas; Diplomate, American Board of Anesthesiology

John J. Dann, D.M.D., M.D.

Surgical Director, Center for Correction of Dentofacial Deformities; Associate Clinical Professor, University of California, San Francisco, Schools of Medicine and Dentistry; Adjunct Assistant Professor, University of the Pacific School of Dentistry, San Francisco, California; Diplomate, American Board of Oral and Maxillofacial Surgery

Bruce N. Epker, D.D.S., Ph.D.

Director, Oral and Maxillofacial Surgery, and Director of Residency Training, John Peter Smith Hospital; Director, Fort Worth Cleft Palate Program; Director, Center for Correction of Dentofacial Deformities, Fort Worth, Texas; Diplomate, American Board of Oral and Maxillofacial Surgery

Carla Evans, D.D.S.

Assistant Professor of Orthodontics, Harvard School of Dental Medicine, Boston, Massachusetts

James B. Getz, Jr., D.D.S.

Co-Director, Preprosthetic Surgery Clinic, John Peter Smith Hospital, Fort Worth, Texas

Leonard B. Kaban, D.M.D., M.D.

Associate Professor of Oral and Maxillofacial Surgery, Harvard School of Dental Medicine; Surgeon, Brigham and Women's Hospital; Associate in Surgery, Children's Hospital, Boston, Massachusetts; Diplomate, American Board of Oral and Maxillofacial Surgery

Michael E. Lessin, D.D.S.

Colonel, United States Army Dental Corps; Chief, Oral and Maxillofacial Surgery, and Director of Residency Training, Brooke Army Medical Center, San Antonio, Texas; Diplomate, American Board of Oral and Maxillofacial Surgery

John B. Mulliken, M.D.

Associate Professor of Surgery, Harvard Medical School; Surgeon, Brigham and Women's Hospital; Associate in Surgery, Children's Hospital, Boston, Massachusetts

Joseph E. Murray, M.D.

Professor of Surgery, Harvard Medical School; Chief, Division of Plastic and Maxillofacial Surgery, Brigham and Women's Hospital and Children's Hospital, Boston, Massachusetts

H. Anthony Neal, D.D.S.

Assistant Professor of Oral and Maxillofacial Surgery, Medical College of Georgia; Private Practice of Oral and Maxillofacial Surgery, Augusta, Georgia; Diplomate, American Board of Oral and Maxillofacial Surgery

Lloyd E. Pearson, D.D.S., M.S.D.

Private Practice of Orthodontics, Minneapolis, Minnesota; Diplomate, American Board of Orthodontics

Sterling R. Schow, D.M.D.

Colonel, United States Army Dental Corps; Chief, Oral and Maxillofacial Surgery, and Director of Residency Training, Madigan Army Medical Center, Tacoma, Washington; Diplomate, American Board of Oral and Maxillofacial Surgery

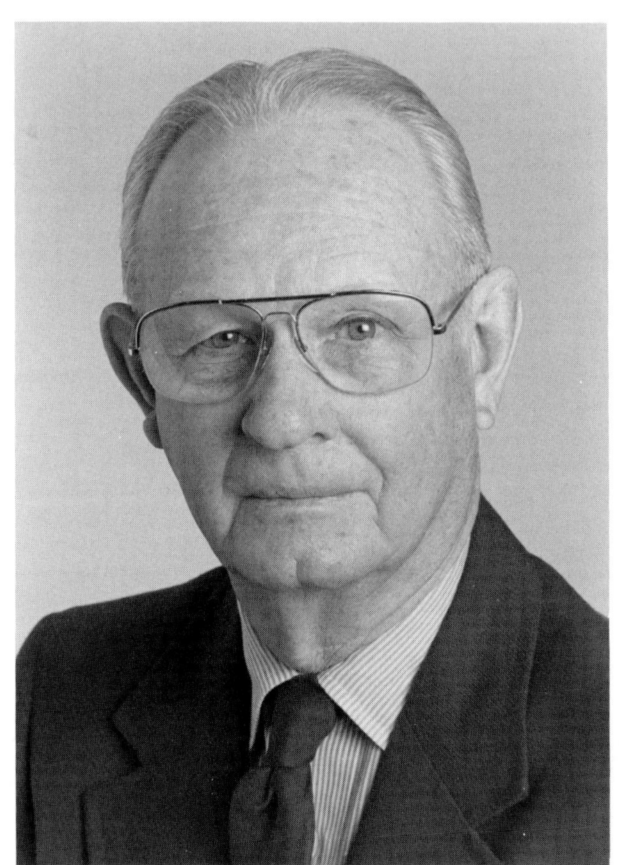

William B. Irby, D.D.S., M.S., F.A.C.D.

The first volume, entitled *Current Advances in Oral Surgery,* appeared in 1974. Its preface contained the statement, "This book has been developed with the intention of presenting current information, in detail, on a variety of subjects applicable to oral and maxillofacial surgery as this specialty is practiced." Throughout its publication history (one issue every 3 years) the authors and editors have striven to keep faith with those expressed goals. With the appearance of Volume V of *Current Advances in Oral and Maxillofacial Surgery,* Dr. Irby, the originator and guiding influence of these volumes, ends his active participation in this endeavor.

Dr. Irby received his Doctor of Dental Surgery degree from the Medical College of Virginia. His completion of residency training in oral surgery at the University of Pittsburgh, where he also earned the degree of Master of Science, virtually coincided with the beginning of World War II. He remained on continuous active duty in the United States Army following the conclusion of hostilities, and by the time of his retirement from military service during the Vietnam War era his long and distinguished military career included involvement with the management of maxillofacial combat casualties of three wars. In addition, he served as Chief of Oral and Maxillofacial Surgery at several U.S. Army medical centers and as Chief of Service and Director of Residency Training at Fitzsimons General Hospital, Denver, Colorado, and Letterman General Hospital, San Francisco, California.

Upon retirement from military service Dr. Irby then became associated with the Medical University of South Carolina at Charleston, where he initiated the training program in oral and maxillofacial surgery. He is now retired from that position and is Emeritus Professor.

Dr. Irby's contributions to the literature are nationally and internationally recognized—ten textbooks as author contributor and editor or coeditor, six other textbooks as author contributor, and numerous contributions to the periodical oral and maxillofacial surgery literature as author or coauthor. He has long been recognized for his expertise and contribution to the management of maxillofacial trauma and for his pioneering interest and work in the diagnosis and treatment of surgical diseases of the temporomandibular joint. His interests in reconstructive, preprosthetic, and orthognathic surgery as well as the surgical management of pathologic lesions of the jaws and infectious processes of the head and neck are reflected in his many publications and in his teaching and training of residents during a lifetime of dedication to the specialty of oral and maxillofacial surgery.

The history of oral and maxillofacial surgery is a reflection of what one age of practitioners finds worthy of note in another. There is much in the contributions of this consummate oral and maxillofacial surgeon, scholar, and gentleman of which we take note, and it is to him that this volume is gratefully and affectionately dedicated.

David W. Shelton, D.M.D.

Preface

Volume V of *Current Advances in Oral and Maxillofacial Surgery: Orthognathic Surgery,* has been compiled for the purpose of presenting information in a comprehensive manner relative to the diagnosis and management of hereditary, congenital, and certain acquired deformities of the oral and maxillofacial region. It reflects the knowledge, experience, and expertise of thirteen contributors, each specifically chosen on the basis of their recognized ingenious and resourceful mastery of the subjects about which they have written. Every attempt has been made to assure that the information presented is current.

It is abundantly clear that in the vast majority of cases the very finest results obtainable are achieved with orthodontic assistance. *Chapter 1* addresses this subject. The author is an orthodontist who has for many years devoted a large share of his practice to the treatment of orthognathic surgical patients and makes an interesting case for the value of the Harvold analysis in conjunction with surgical management.

There is sometimes a tendency on the part of the oral and maxillofacial surgeon to become so intent upon the surgical procedure as to lose sight of the ongoing anesthetic process. *Chapter 2,* written by a superb anesthesiologist, reviews some basic and important anesthetic considerations and discusses useful and unique measures to counter emergencies which may arise during the procedure. Additionally, a brief discussion of deliberate hypotension is presented with mention of new agents that may hold promise for the future.

As are the remaining chapters of this book, *Chapter 3* is written by an oral and maxillofacial surgeon. It covers the role of total alveolar maxillary osteotomy in the surgical management of dentofacial deformities. The author has had vast experience in the field and especially with this particular procedure. Indications, planning, and technique are covered extensively.

Evaluation, timing, and technique—including grafting procedures—as well as other important considerations are lucidly presented in *Chapter 4,* which discusses genioplasty and its use alone or in conjunction with other orthognathic surgical manipulations.

Chapter 5 contains important and highly interesting information concerning the critical and perhaps incompletely understood issues of temporomandibular joint function related to orthognathic surgical manipulations, timing of surgery in patients who manifest temporomandibular joint symptoms, and condylar positioning at the time of surgery. Also presented in this chapter are superb discussions of treatment planning and technique of the maxillary LeFort I and mandibular sagittal split osteotomies.

Chapter 6 contains specific information regarding evaluation, treatment planning, and surgical management of dentofacial deformities that are complicated by the loss of teeth and alveolar bone. The discussion is characterized by a thorough, analytical, and systematic approach to this difficult facet of orthognathic surgery and is yet another excellent example of the many outstanding contributions of its author.

The multiple and diverse implications and functional and esthetic ramifications of the alveolar cleft palate are expertly covered in *Chapter 7.* The author is a surgeon whose experience and expertise with this problem are extensive. Valuable information is provided relative to diagnosis, timing, technique, and (importantly) long-term results.

Chapter 8 and *Chapter 9,* written by nationally and internationally recognized authorities on the subjects, address the problems of, first, hemifacial microsomia and, second, high midface procedures in the management of dentofacial deformities. Each chapter approaches its subject in a logical and analytical fashion; and each is expertly constructed, highly informative, and masterfully written.

A careful examination of this volume will provide the reader with enhanced understanding, expanded knowledge, and valuable guidance in his or her approach to the diagnosis and treatment of dentofacial deformities.

David W. Shelton
William B. Irby

Contents

CHAPTER 1

Orthodontic considerations in orthognathic surgery

LLOYD E. PEARSON

There has been considerable evaluation and improvement in orthognathic procedures in the past several years. This has given the practitioner many options to consider during treatment planning and it has provided improved results together with greater stability for the patient. Previously, during my training period, the only significant orthognathic procedure commonly used was an external body procedure[12] for the mandibular excess patient. Currently there are many procedures from which to choose, and this has been accompanied by a large increase in the number of well-trained orthodontists and oral and maxillofacial surgeons. With this progress has developed a growing awareness of the tremendous benefit of the multidiscipline or team approach in orthognathic treatment.

DIAGNOSIS AND TREATMENT PLANNING

Typically the potential orthognathic patient is examined and records are obtained in the orthodontic office. These may include, but are not limited to, the following:

Orthodontic models
    May need mounting on an adjustable articulator with a facebow transfer,[5] especially in cases involving a maxillary impaction or simultaneous surgery involving both jaws
Radiographs
    Cephalometric, lateral, PA, and submento-vertex[13]
Orthopantomograph or Panorex
Intraoral
Transcranial or tomographic TMJ
Hand
Photographs
    Intraoral
    Oriented lateral and full face

It is most helpful in a growing patient to learn the maturation level. In the mandibular excess patient it is usually best to do the surgery when the major portion of the growth is completed. This prevents additional mandibular growth from bringing the mandible forward again and necessitating a second surgical procedure. Helm et al.[19] have shown that a hand radiograph is a helpful guide in determining the level of maturation. There is also preliminary evidence presented by Huang and Ross[20] in mandibular deficiency cases that some attenuation of growth may occur if the surgical advancement is performed prior to the completion of mandibular growth.

Prediction of the remaining body height growth is very important because the long bones and mandibular growth are fairly well coordinated. Charting the patient's growth will give the clinician a good idea of how much additional growth will occur and should also tell where the patient fits in relation to the expected peak velocity of growth (Figs. 1-1 and 1-2). In boys the peak velocity of growth would be expected to occur just after 14 years of age and the growth would typically continue until age 17 on a declining gradient or fractions of an inch per

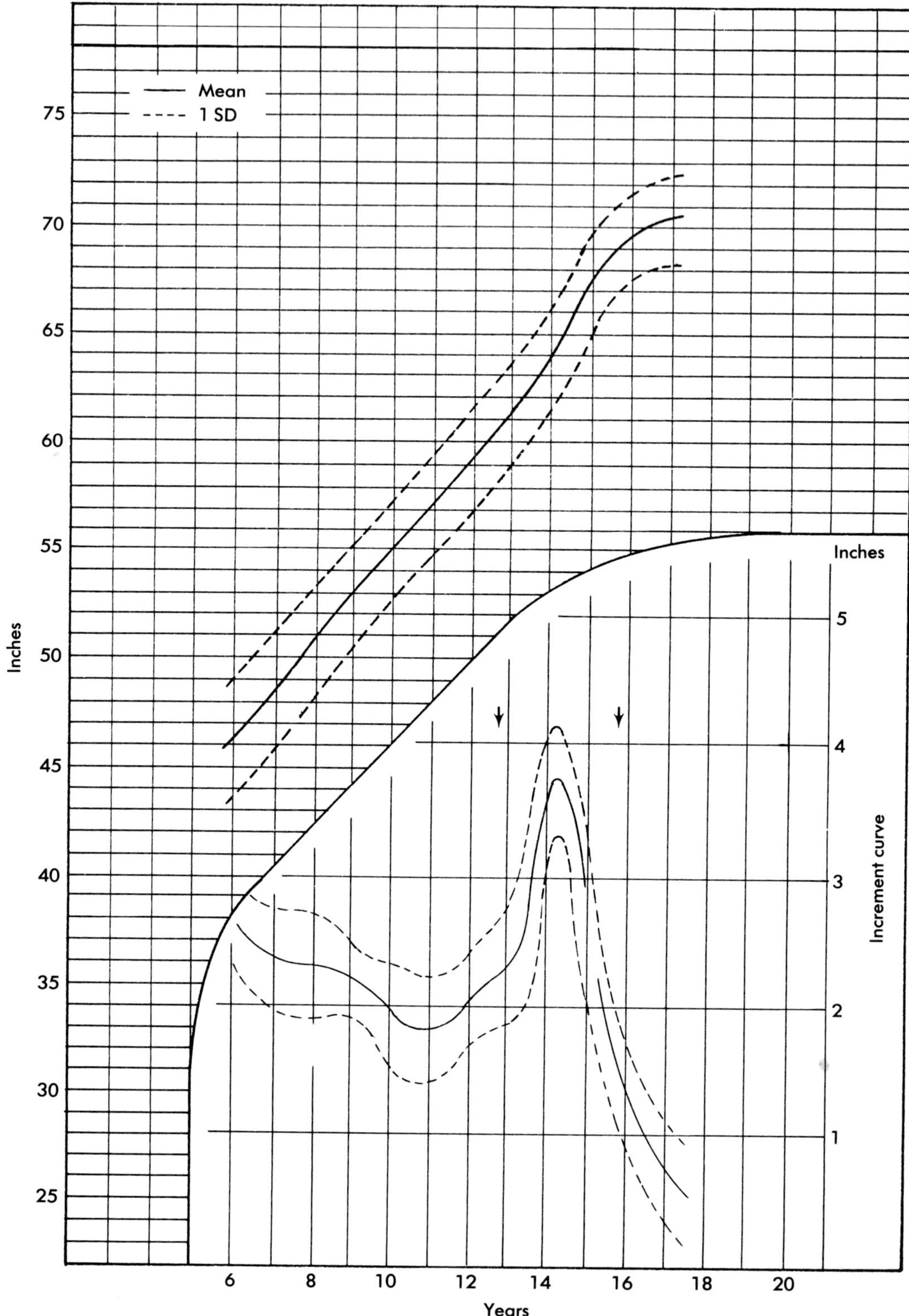

Fig. 1-1.

Male growth curve. Notice that the peak velocity of growth usually occurs just after 14 years of age and by age 17 the major portion of growth is essentially complete.
Courtesy University of Indiana.

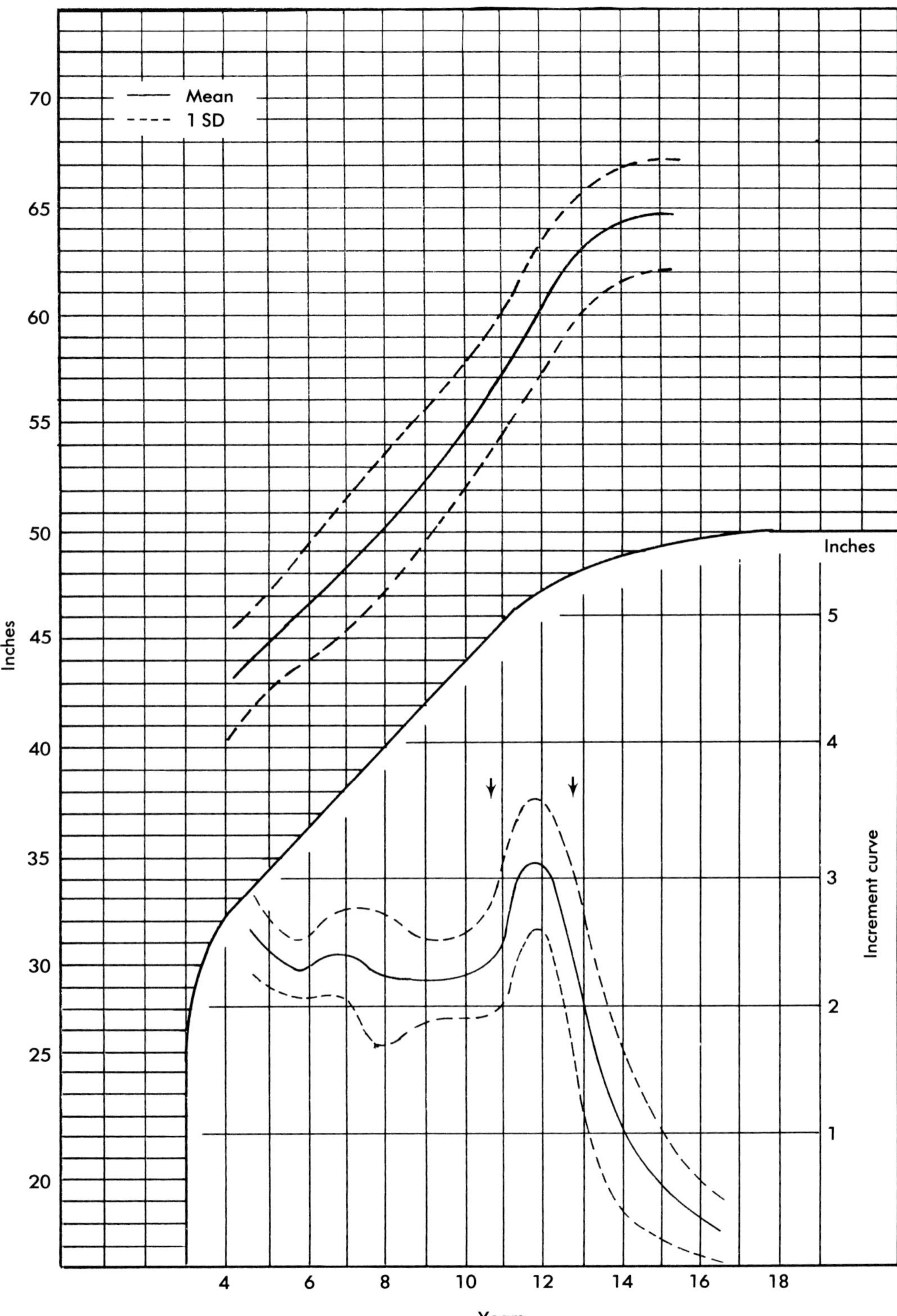

Fig. 1-2.

Female growth curve. Notice that the peak velocity of growth occurs just before 12 years of age and that growth is essentially complete by age 15.

Courtesy University of Indiana.

year. For girls the peak velocity of growth typically occurs at age 11 years 9 months and the growth is essentially completed at 15 years. The implications in treatment timing of a mandibular excess case are very significant. A boy would commonly be in his senior year of high school (age 17) before the clinician might want to have the surgery performed. A girl's surgery might often be performed earlier than the boy's, perhaps in the tenth grade of high school or at age 15. These are, of course, generalizations and each patient must be analyzed and observed on an individual basis. It is not uncommon for boys to have a postpuberal growth spurt between the ages of 16 and 22 that may carry the mandible forward 2 or 3 mm. This could be anticipated and planned for in the amount of the surgical retraction.

It is beneficial to learn the time of menarche to help predict the amount of remaining growth.[7,36] The onset of menstruation occurs after the peak velocity of growth and when growth rates are beginning to decelerate. Typically one might expect a girl to grow 2½ to 3 inches in body height after the menarche.[36] It appears that some Class III–type patients grow even more, as did the mandibular osteotomy patient in (Fig. 1-11), who grew 4½ inches after the menarche (age 12). The development of secondary sex characteristics suggests that the peak velocity of growth has been passed in both boys and girls. For the orthodontist this evaluation is not definitive but is only a guide to knowing that the peak of velocity has been passed.

Family height studies can be helpful, since it has been demonstrated[1] that a similar tendency in the rate of maturation exists between siblings and between the parent and child of the same sex.

An adult mandibular excess patient (*M.B.,* Fig. 1-3) is a useful case to illustrate some important points in treatment planning. She was 24 years 10 months old when she came for treatment. Her mandible appeared very strong and her maxilla was only slightly deficient. Her lower first molars had been extracted, and there was a normal range of movement with no TMJ symptoms. The cephalometric analysis revealed

an A-N-B difference of −7 degrees (S-N-A 82° −S-N-B 89°).[31] When the pretreatment analysis was performed and the oral and maxillofacial surgeon consulted, it was found that the teeth articulated fairly well without any orthodontic preparation. The teeth were equilibrated presurgically to good solid centric stops in a postsurgical occlusion. A Harvold[17] cephalometric analysis (Fig. 1-4) proved to be very valuable in this case, enabling the clinician to compare the maxillary unit length with the mandibular unit length to help determine the location of the discrepancy. The analysis incorporates a lower facial height measurement, which is useful in determining where an excess or deficiency in the mandibular length might be masked by an unusual amount of lower facial height. It is quite simple to use and is helpful in communicating with parents and patients.

The patient's maxillary unit length (from ANS to condylion) measured 90 mm. The mean value for women is 93 mm ± 3.45 SD (Fig. 1-3, *L*). Therefore this length was relatively normal. Her mandibular unit length measured 132 mm, which was 13 mm greater than the mean of 119 ± 4.44 SD for women. Her lower facial height measured 66 mm (as compared to the mean of 65 ± 4.67 SD for women). This excellent analysis demonstrated that the maxillary length was relatively normal, the lower face height was normal, and the discrepancy was clearly in the oversized mandible. The patient was operated upon without any orthodontic appliances; a sagittal ramus osteotomy was done. The teeth were equilibrated again after removal of fixation, and two lower bridges were constructed. The teeth were again equilibrated during the retention period, and the patient remained stable and asymptomatic during the 9 years of postsurgical observation. A final analysis showed that her original mandibular unit length changed from 132 to 124 mm (Fig. 1-3, *M*). Subtracting the maxillary unit length from the mandibular unit length gave the unit difference (mm):

Presurgical	*Postsurgical*
132 Mandibular unit length	124 Mandibular unit length
90 Maxillary unit length	91 Maxillary unit length
42 Unit difference	33 Unit difference

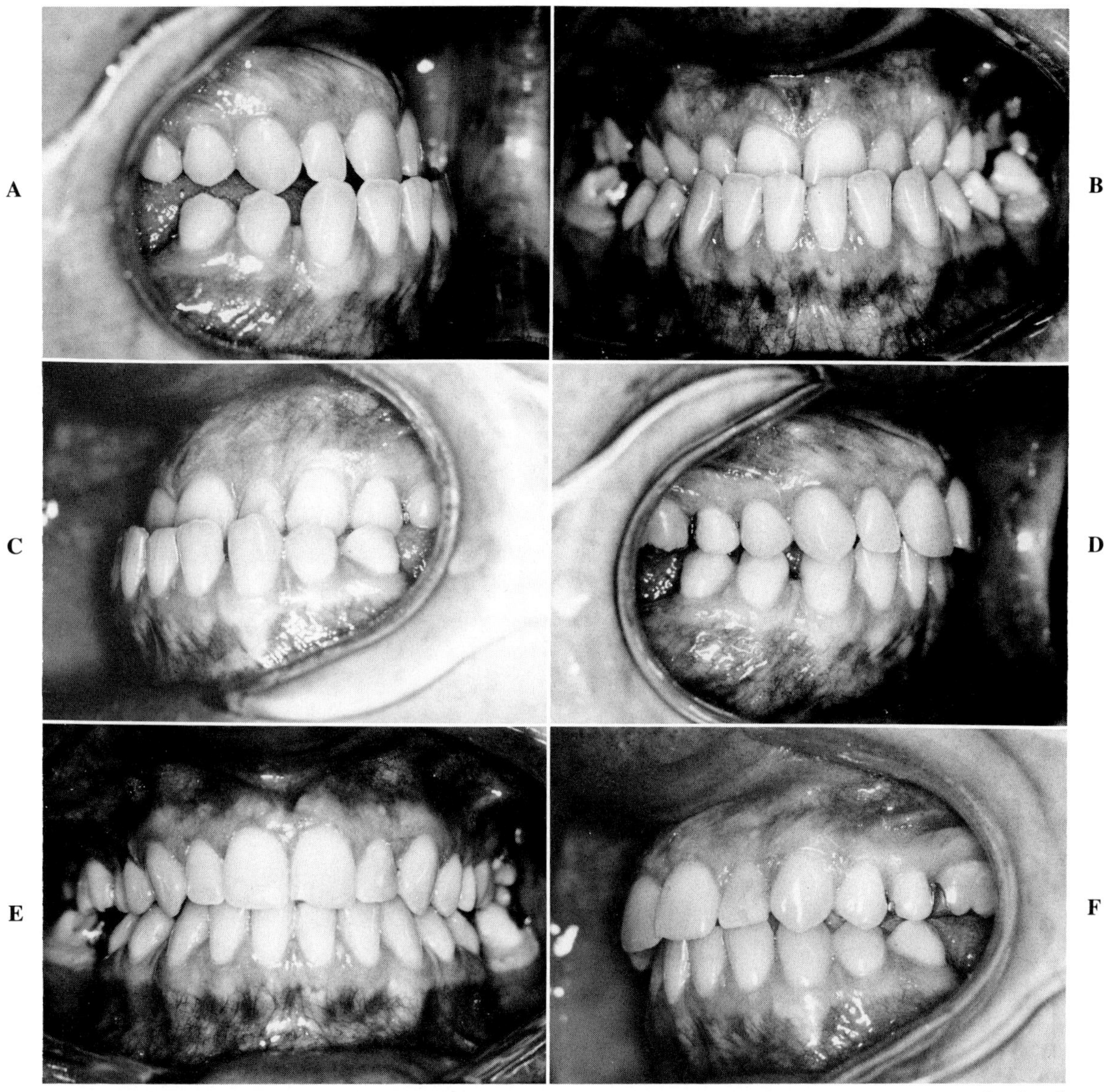

Continued.

Fig. 1-3.
Patient M.B. A woman treated with a sagittal ramus osteotomy without orthodontic appliances. **A** to
C, Pretreatment and, **D** to **F,** posttreatment intraoral views.

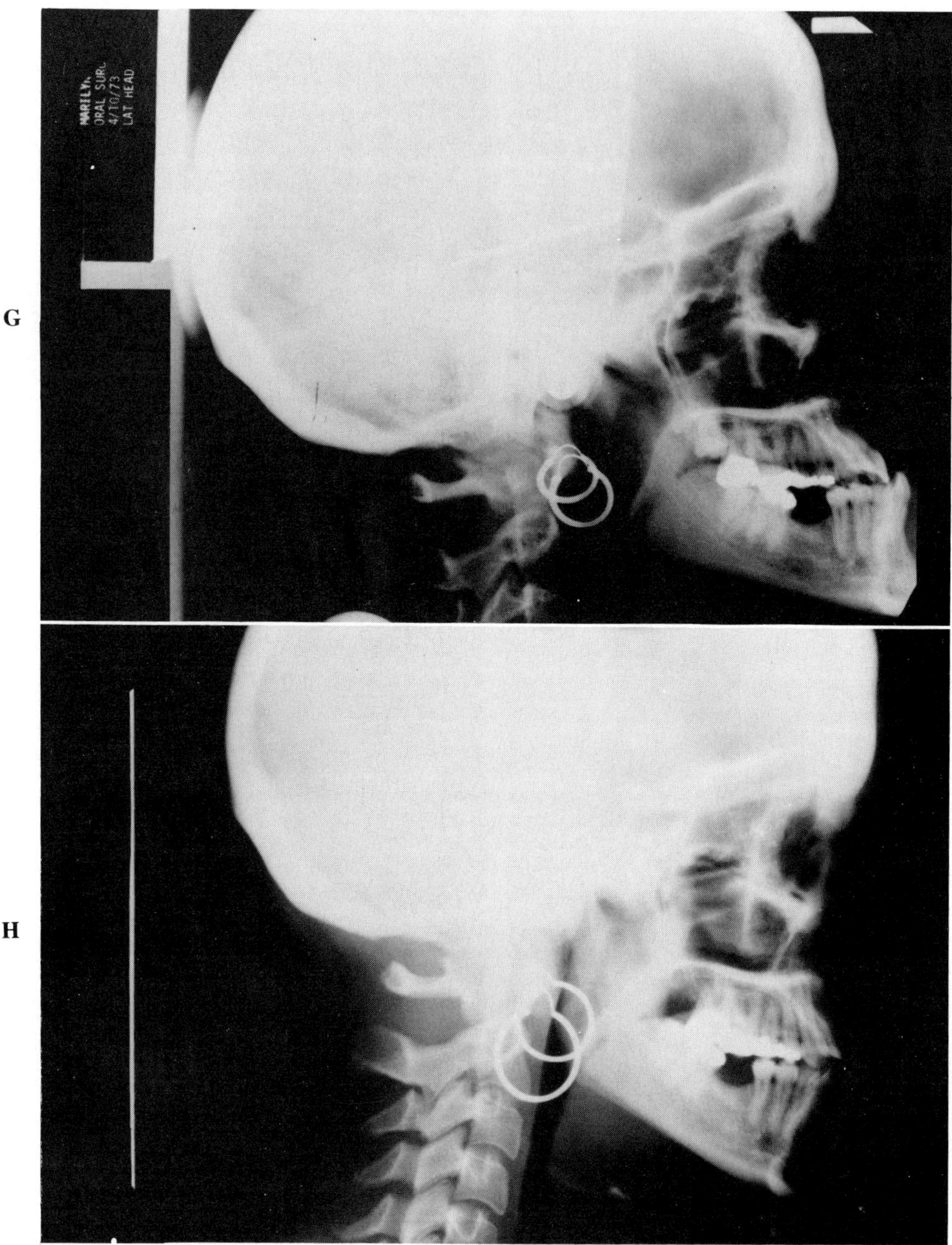

Fig. 1-3—cont'd.
G, Pretreatment and, **H,** posttreatment cephalometric radiographs.

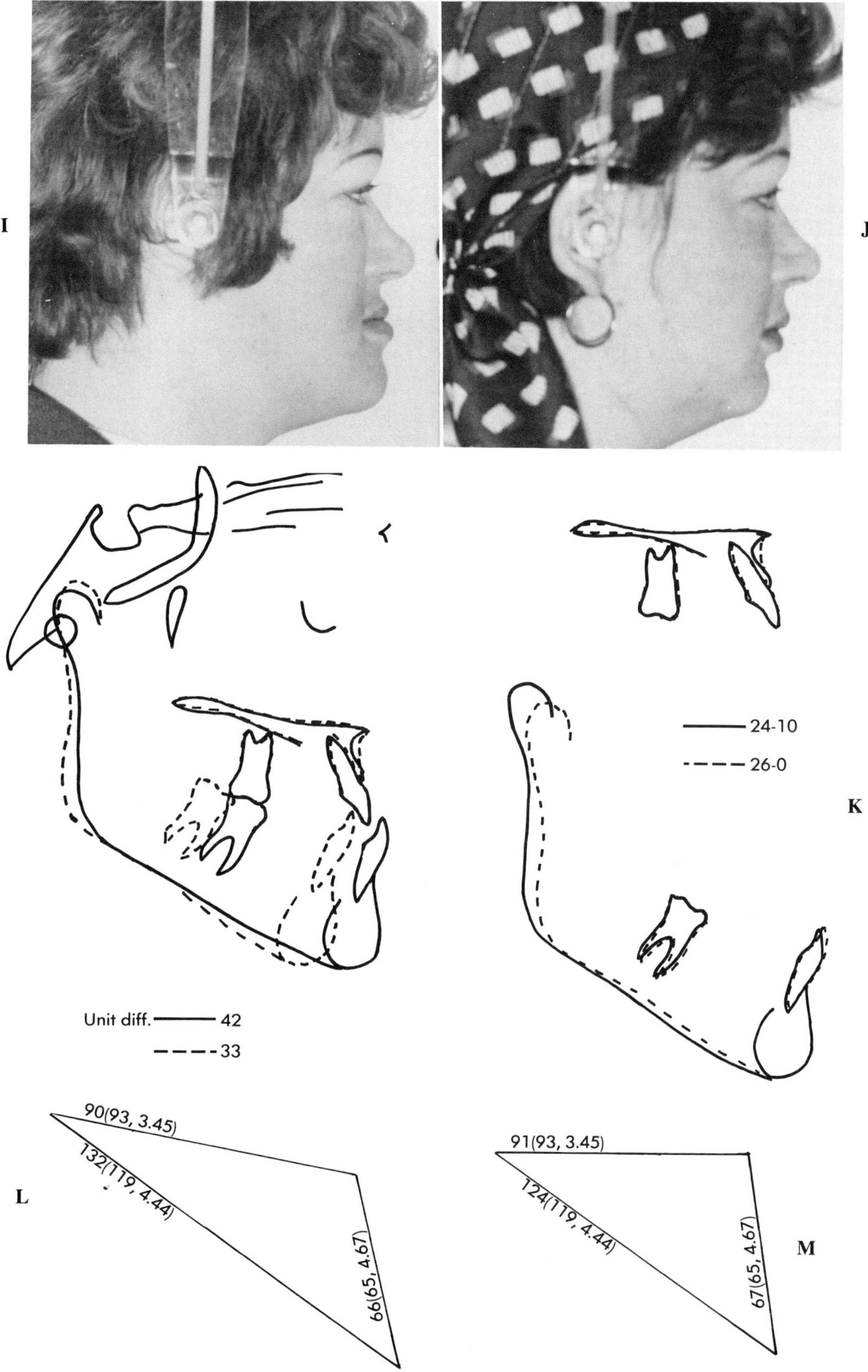

Fig. 1-3—cont'd.
I, Pretreatment and, **J,** posttreatment lateral views. **K,** Lateral cephalometric tracing illustrating the amount of mandibular retraction. **L** and **M,** Harvold's unit difference analysis, pre- and posttreatment.

Sample Size and Characteristics : a random sample of male and female children with serial cephalometric records from the Burlington Orthodontic Research Centre

Illustration

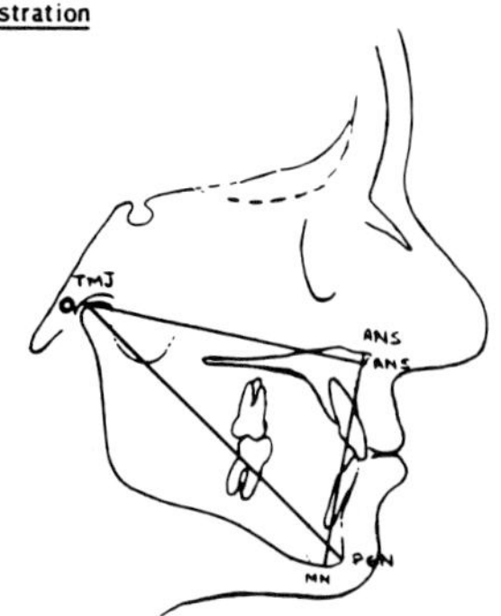

Landmarks

ANS — (anterior nasal spine) — a point on the lower contour of the anterior nasal spine, where the vertical thickness is 3 mm, is used for horizontal measurements. A point on the superior contour of the anterior nasal spine, where the vertical thickness is 3 mm, is employed for vertical measurements.

MN — (menton) — the most inferior point on the contour of the chin.

PGN — (prognathion) — a point on the contour of the bony chin indicating maximum mandibular length measured from the temporomandibular joint. (close to pogonion)

TMJ — (temporomandibular joint) — a point on the contour of glenoid fossa where the line indicating maximum mandibular length intercepts the contour of the fossa. The midpoint between right and left sides is marked

Technique : the following measurements are made in millimeters and compared to standards derived from the above Burlington sample.

Maxillary unit length — the measurement from TMJ to ANS (inferior point where ANS is 3mm thick)

Mandibular unit length — the measurement from TMJ to PGN

Maxillary — mandibular unit length difference — mandibular unit length minus maxillary unit length

Lower anterior face height — measurement from ANS (superior point where ANS is 3mm thick) to menton

Interpretation

Maxillary-mandibular unit length difference is a significant indicator of the degree of matching of maxillary and mandibular unit lengths. Differences toward either end of the sample range indicate unfavorable matching of maxillary and mandibular lengths (dysplasia). Differences at the extremes of the range may not mean that a malocclusion exists, for there may be masking of the skeletal dysplasia through variation in the vertical position of the mandible and dentoalveolar compensation.

Lower anterior face height is an indicator of mandibular vertical position. Extreme values of the range for a particular age group have to be viewed in the light of individual stature and development.

Standards

1 — Temporo-mandibular point (tm) * - Anterior nasal spine (ans) ** Mx. unit length ( )

♂ Age	No.	Min.	Mean Value	Max.	Standard Deviation	♀ Age	No.	Min.	Mean Value	Max.	Standard Deviation
6 yrs.	118	76	82	90	3.19	6 yrs.	89	73	80	89	2.96
9 yrs.	102	80	87	97	3.43	9 yrs.	79	78	85	93	3.43
12 yrs.	96	85	92	101	3.73	12 yrs.	71	80	90	102	4.07
14 yrs.	66	88	96	108	4.52	14 yrs.	49	81	92	104	3.69
16 yrs.	72	93	100	111	4.17	16 yrs.	53	86	93	105	3.45

2 — Temporo-mandibular point (tm) - Prognathion (pgn) Md. unit length ( )

♂ Age	No.	Min.	Mean Value	Max.	Standard Deviation	♀ Age	No.	Min.	Mean Value	Max.	Standard Deviation
6yrs.	118	90	99	108	3.85	6 yrs.	88	88	97	105	3.55
9 yrs.	102	98	107	117	4.40	9 yrs.	79	94	105	113	3.88
12 yrs.	96	102	114	127	4.90	12 yrs.	71	102	113	124	5.20
14 yrs.	66	107	121	137	6.05	14 yrs.	49	104	117	128	4.60
16 yrs.	72	116	127	139	5.25	16 yrs.	53	109	119	128	4.44

3 — The lower face height: Anterior nasal spine (ans) - gnathion (gn) ( )

♂ Age	No.	Min.	Mean Value	Max.	Standard Deviation	♀ Age	No.	Min.	Mean Value	Max.	Standard Deviation
6 yrs.	118	52	59	72	3.55	6 yrs.	88	49	57	65	3.22
9 yrs.	102	53	62	74	4.25	9 yrs.	79	50	60	70	3.62
12 yrs.	96	53	64	76	4.62	12 yrs.	71	53	62	74	4.36
14 yrs.	66	56	68	82	5.23	14 yrs.	49	54	64	72	4.39
16 yrs.	72	57	71	86	5.73	16 yrs.	53	55	65	74	4.67

Difference between (tm - pgn) and (tm - ans) (2 - 1)

♂ Age	No.	Min.	Mean Value	Max.	♀ Age	No.	Min.	Mean Value	Max.
6 yrs.	118	10	17	27	6 yrs.	88	10	17	24
9 yrs.	102	13	20	28	9 yrs.	79	13	20	28
12 yrs.	96	12	22	30	12 yrs.	71	16	23	36
14 yrs.	66	14	25	38	14 yrs.	49	18	26	39
16 yrs.	72	17	27	39	16 yrs.	53	19	26	39

Fig. 1-4.

Harvold's standards.

From Harvold, E.: The activator in interceptive orthodontics, St. Louis, 1974, The C.V. Mosby Co.

In a 12-year old child it is usually possible to treat nonsurgically when the unit differences are between 15 mm in Class II and 30 mm in Class III cases.[38] As the differences rise toward 30, it becomes increasingly difficult to treat with a nonsurgical approach. The mean unit difference for women is 26 mm, and for men 27 mm[17] (Fig. 1-4).

LIMITS OF FIXED ORTHODONTIC APPLIANCES

If we apply the Harvold analysis[17] to a young boy approximately 12 years of age with a developing Class III malocclusion, it becomes apparent how useful this analysis can be. *R.E.* (Fig. 1-5) had an end-to-end incisor relationship, and the mandible moved forward into an anterior crossbite upon closure. He was treated by widening the maxilla with sutural expansion and use of a protraction face mask. The face mask was attached to the sutural expander's buccal arms with elastics to move the maxilla forward.[11,28] When the cephalometric tracings were evaluated by using Harvold's analysis, some significant changes became apparent:

	Mandibular length	*Maxillary length*	*Unit difference*
Age 12	116 mm (114 ± 4.90 SD)	88 mm (92 ± 3.73 SD)	28 mm (22 mean)
Age 14	118 mm (121 ± 6.65 SD)	89 mm (96 ± 4.52 SD)	29 mm (25 mean)

These measurements illustrate a most significant factor: This is really a maxillary deficiency problem rather than a Class III mandibular excess problem.

In spite of the widening and protraction of the maxilla, the unit difference worsened by 1 mm. The mandible measurement increased 2 mm, but the maxillary length increased only 1 mm. Prolonged wearing of the protraction face mask to a partial upper appliance may guide the growth sufficiently to prevent this case from becoming surgical.[35] The Harvold analysis (Fig. 1-4) is helpful in predicting which patients may be treated in the preceding manner. If the unit difference were larger, this patient would likely have been a candidate for orthognathic surgery. The best treatment then might be to observe on a yearly basis until ready for appliance placement to prepare for surgery. Such surgery could be considered as the patient neared the end of his growth.

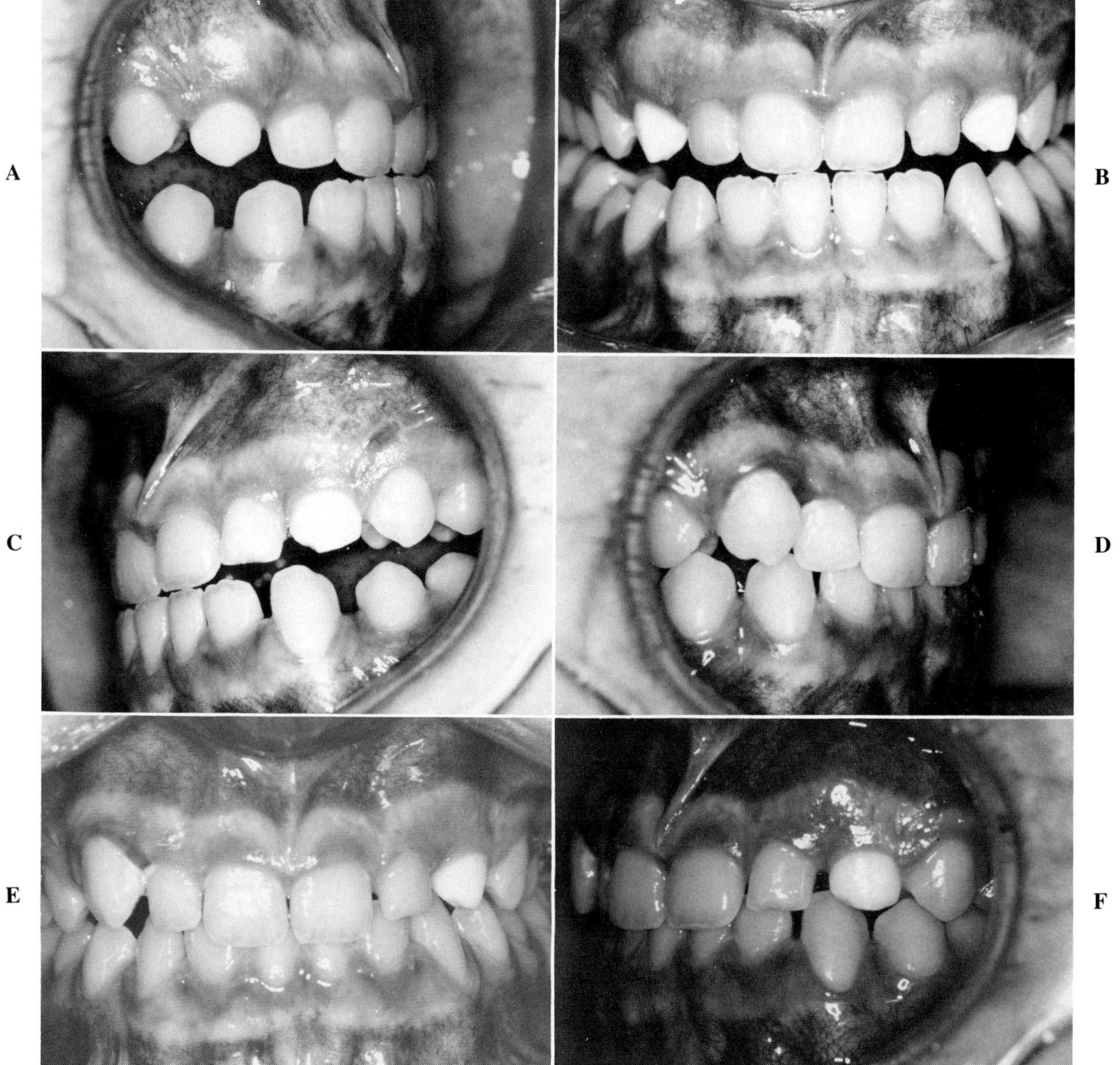

Fig. 1-5.
Patient R.E. A young man with a maxillary deficiency that was treated by sutural expansion and a protraction face mask to advance the maxilla. **A** to **C**, Pretreatment and, **D** to **F**, posttreatment intraoral views.

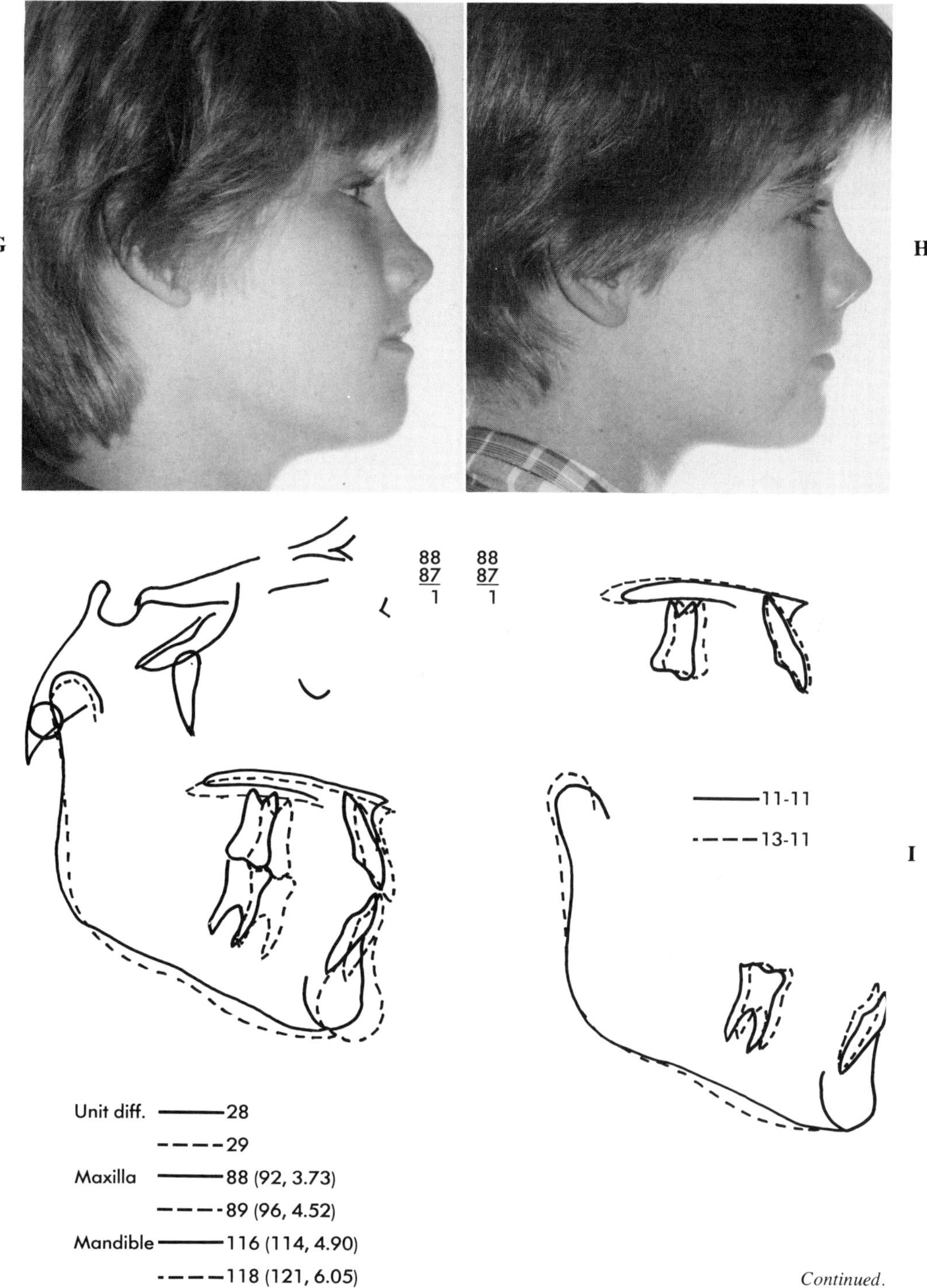

Continued.

Fig. 1-5—cont'd.
G, Pretreatment and, **H,** posttreatment lateral views. **I,** Pre- and posttreatment lateral cephalometric tracings.

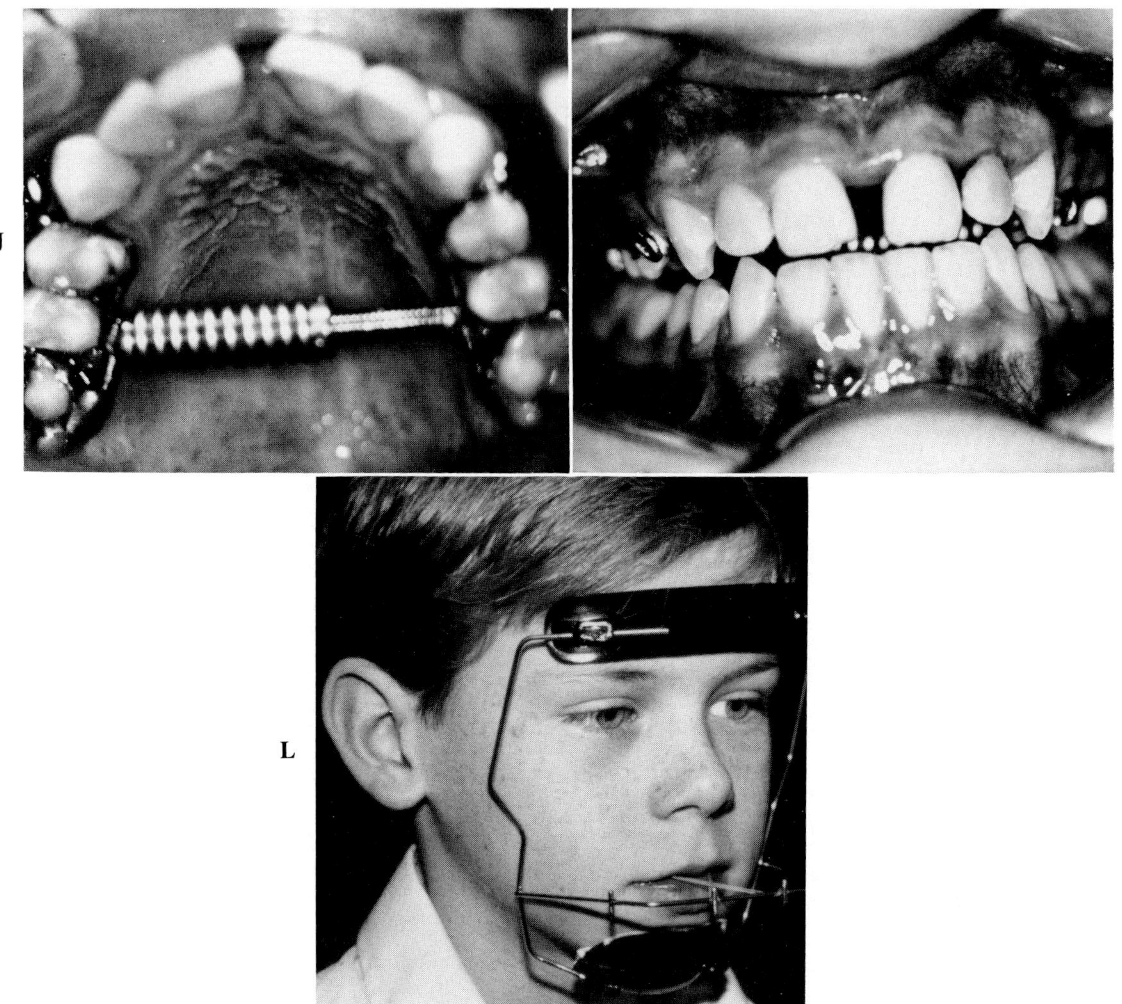

Fig. 1-5—cont'd.
J and **K,** Sutural expansion appliance with buccal arms for attaching elastics to the protraction face mask. **L,** Maxillary protraction face mask.

LIMITS AND POTENTIALS OF FUNCTIONAL APPLIANCES

There is considerable interest and discussion among orthodontists on how functional appliances work and whether or not condylar stimulation of growth does actually occur in retrognathic mandibular deficiency cases. It may eventually be shown that functional appliances can be effective even if significant amounts of condylar stimulation cannot be demonstrated.

A clinical example can illustrate what might be the outer limits for functional appliance therapy in a mandibular deficiency case. A young patient (*A.J.*, Fig. 1-6) who was almost 10 years old presented with an extremely retrognathic mandible. Cephalometrically she had an A-N-B difference of 12 degrees, an overjet of 11 mm, and a Harvold unit difference of 9. The parents were informed that she might eventually require a mandibular surgical advancement but treatment would be started with a functional appliance to determine how much improvement could be accomplished. If sufficient improvement were achieved, a surgical advancement might not be necessary or if needed the amount might be reduced. There is some evidence that

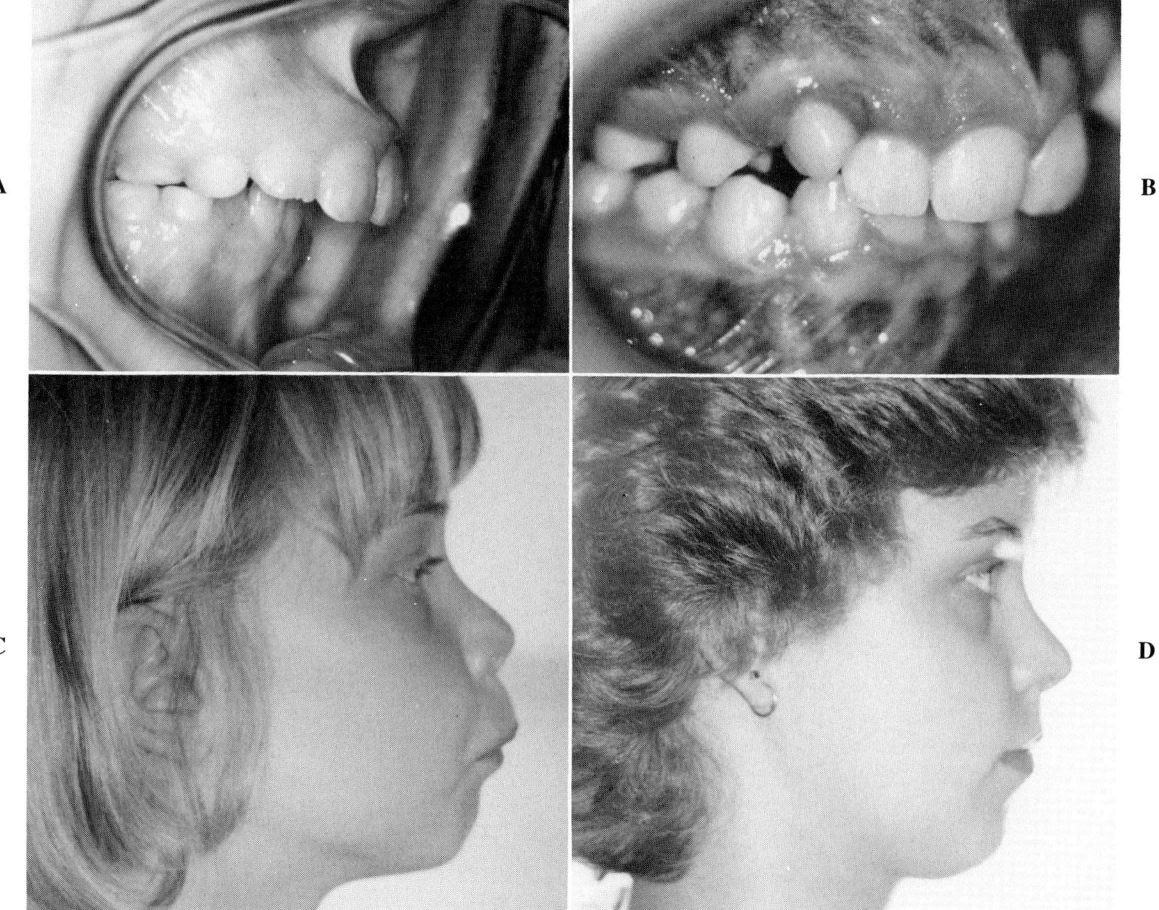

Continued.

Fig. 1-6.
Patient A.J. A 10-year-old girl treated with functional appliances while waiting for the eruption of her permanent teeth. She illustrates what might be considered the outer limit of feasible therapy in a growing child without surgery. Lateral intraoral views taken, **A** and **C,** pretreatment and, **B** and **D,** just prior to banding.

E

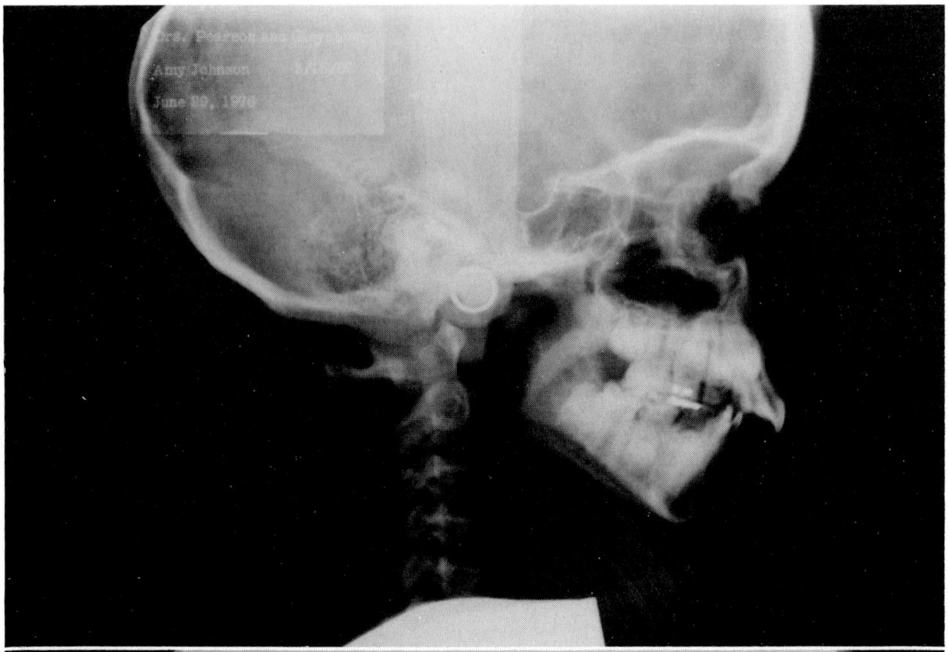

F

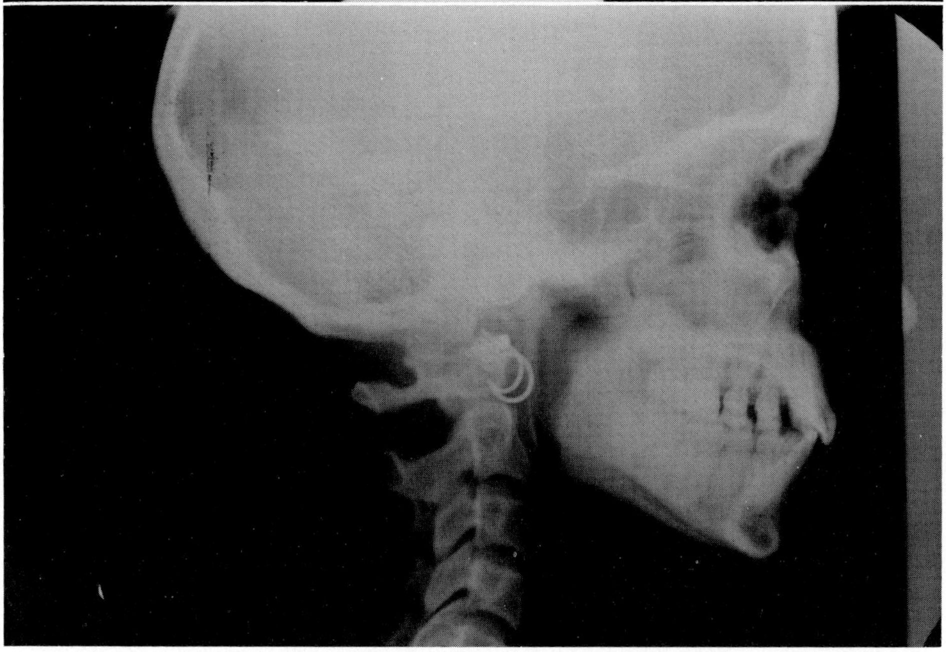

Fig. 1-6—cont'd.
E, Pretreatment and, **F,** posttreatment lateral cephalometric radiographs.

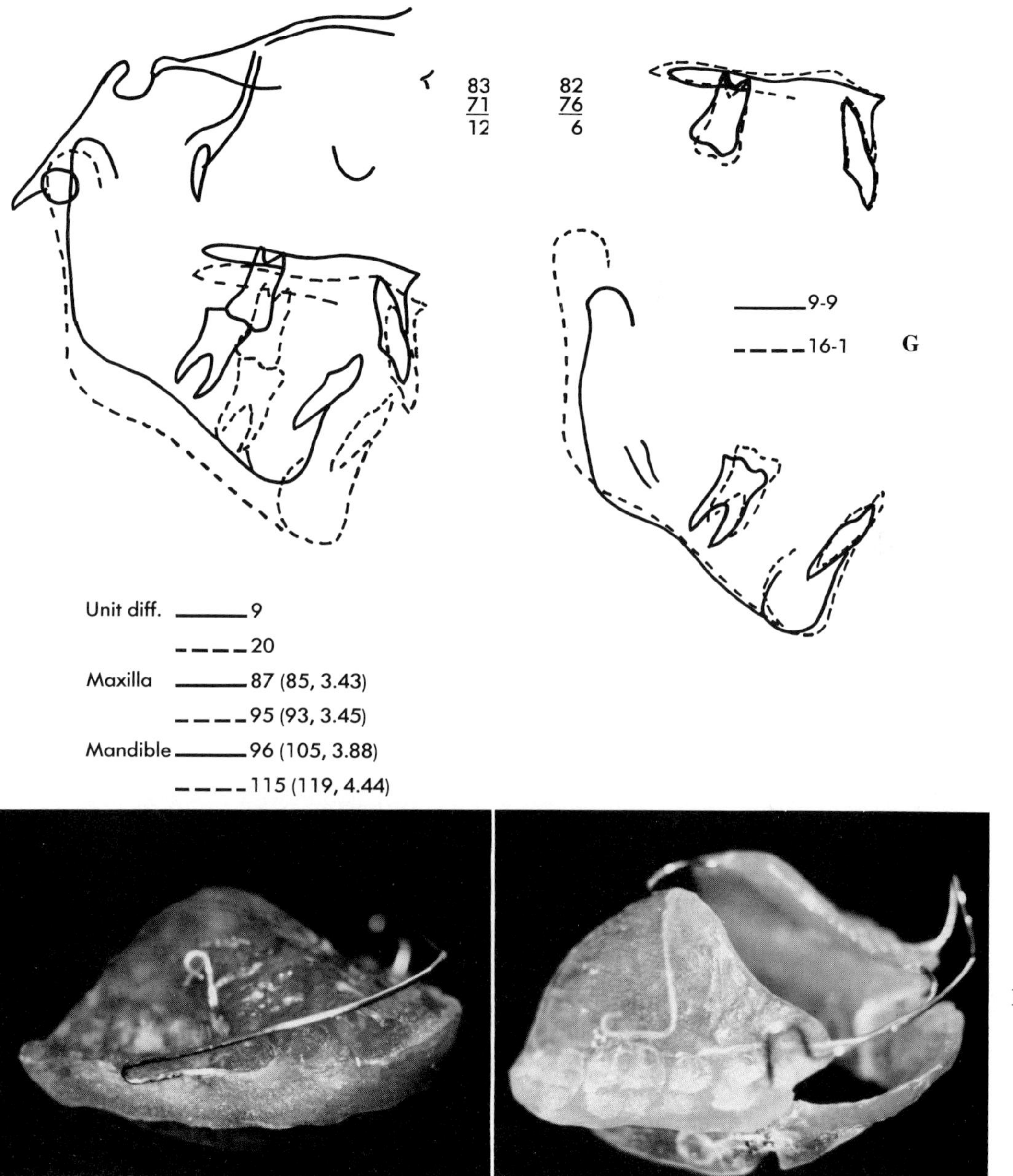

Fig. 1-6—cont'd.
G, Illustrating the change that occurred in chin position during this 6-year period. **H,** Activator monobloc. **I,** Bionator Orthopedic Corrector.

Fig. 1-6—cont'd.
Laminagraphs of the right TMJ illustrating, **J,** the posterior joint space and, **K,** the condyle evenly centered in the fossa.

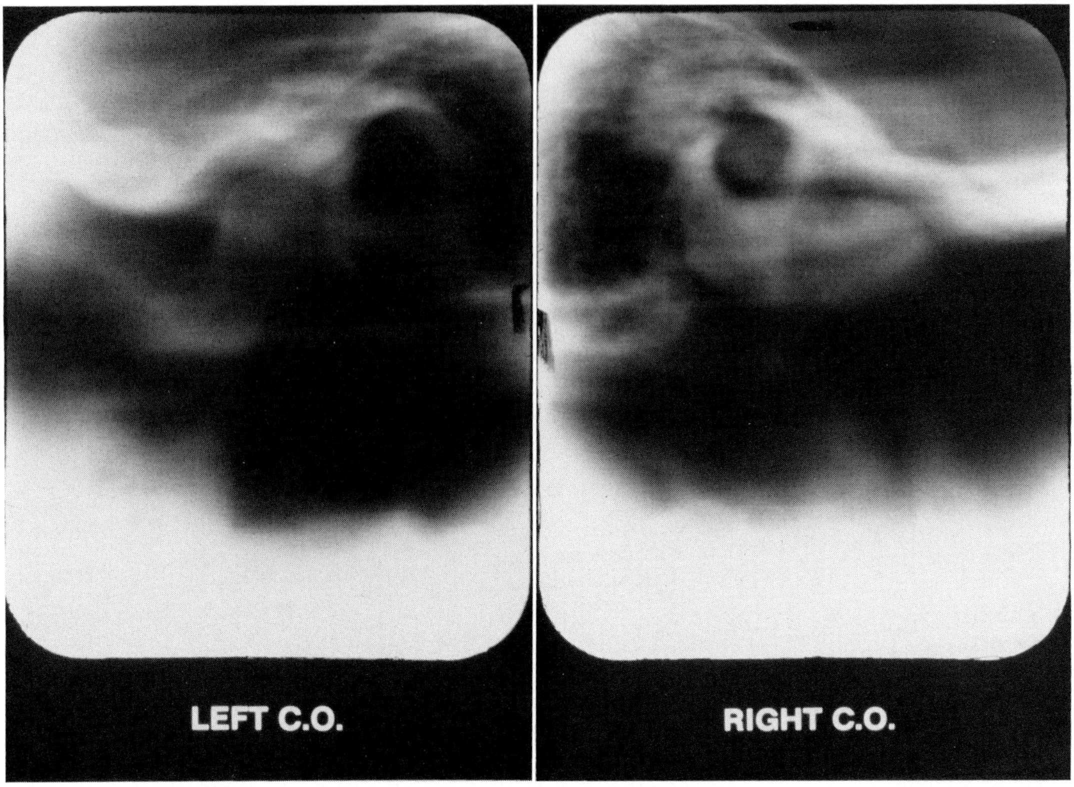

smaller mandibular advancements have fewer deleterious side effects than do larger ones.[20] She was treated for 4¼ years first with an activator monobloc and then with an orthopedic corrector (Bionator) type of appliance. A maxillary headgear and a lower lip bumper were then used for 1¼ years. During this time (6 years) the patient grew 13¾ inches and had slow eruption of her permanent teeth.

If the slow eruption of her teeth had been anticipated, it is unlikely that the patient, the family, or the orthodontist would have agreed to 6 years of treatment prior to the placement of the fixed appliances. If the clinician inquires about the timing of eruption of permanent teeth in siblings and parents, some valuable predictive information may be obtained and there appears to be a correlation. This girl was an ex-

tremely cooperative patient, and her response to treatment was rather remarkable. Her A-N-B difference was reduced from 12 to 6 degrees, and her overjet changed from 11 to 5 mm. The Harvold analysis showed a maxillary unit change of 87 (85 ± 3.43) to 95 mm (93 ± 3.45) while the maxillary unit length remained 2 mm greater than the mean throughout this period, which is very close to the amount of increase one would expect without treatment.[24] The mandibular unit length changed from 96 (105 ± 3.88) to 115 mm (119 ± 4.44), a 19 mm increase, which also is close to what one would expect without treatment. McNamara[24] has reported approximately 3 mm of mandibular growth per year, and Woodside[38] 2.7 mm per year, as what one can usually expect. The lower face height (ANS-Gn) increased only 2 mm during the 6 years of therapy. Usually the lower face height in an average skeletal pattern increases at the rate of 1 mm/year.[24] This patient had 4 mm less than the usual amount of vertical increase, so one might conclude that the functional appliances achieved at least part of their effect by inhibiting vertical development.

Both the monobloc activator and the Orthopedic Corrector (Bionator) have acrylic between the posterior teeth to retard vertical facial development or eruption of teeth. This permits the major portion of the condylar growth to express itself in a more forward direction and thereby bring the chin into a more anterior position. Laminagraphs of her temporomandibular joints showed that the right condyle was evenly centered in the fossa and the left condyle had diminished joint space posteriorly in the fossa (Fig. 1-6, *J* and *K*). Class II elastics were used during the appliance stage of treatment to center the condyle in the fossa. Not all young patients will respond as favorably as this one did, and the orthodontist must evaluate the skeletal pattern as well as make a growth prediction.[6,7] Patients who have a less favorable prediction, or are unwilling to cooperate by the wearing of a functional appliance, should be observed on a yearly basis until ready for placement of appliances and preparation for advancement surgery.

SURGICAL ADVANCEMENT FOR MANDIBULAR DEFICIENCY IN AN ADOLESCENT

To illustrate the details of growth prediction and skeletal pattern evaluation during the late stages of growth, it is beneficial to examine a patient with a less favorable pattern and less growth potential.

A young boy (*K.L.*, Fig. 1-7) age 14 years 3 months had a severe Class II, Division 2, malocclusion with 12 mm of overjet, an A-N-B difference of 9 degrees, and a steep mandibular plane angle (43° Sn-Go-Gn). His lower facial height was excessive by 10 mm (78 mm, 68 ± 5.23), and the unit difference was 23 mm (mean 25) (Harvold[17]). The excessive vertical dimension exaggerated the discrepancy by rotating the mandible down and back. Analysis of his initial cephalogram using Björk's[6] method demonstrated that this was a true "backward rotater" with very little potential for forward growth rotation. The men in his family were short, and thus the conclusion was drawn that this patient possessed an unfavorable skeletal pattern with limited growth potential. There was considerable crowding in both arches, and the decision was made to utilize orthognathic surgical advancement combined with orthodontic extraction therapy.

It was an ideal time to consult the other related professionals who would be needed for treatment. This is best done before presenting the treatment plan to the patient and family. Experience has shown that the patient is better served and there is less need for changes during treatment if there has been adequate and continual consultation between the different professionals on the orthognathic team—an oral and maxillofacial surgeon, a periodontist, a restorative or general dentist, the family physician, a psychologist, and an orthodontist. Each of those professionals, and perhaps some others, may have special insights and experience that will contribute to the specific treatment plan.

After the consultations, primarily with the oral and maxillofacial surgeon, it was decided to treat by removal of both upper first premolars, both lower second premolars, a mandibular surgical advancement, and a sliding horizontal genioplasty. Full appliances were planned and special efforts were made to intrude the upper anteriors to shorten the amount of exposed upper anterior gingival tissue.[8] The patient had excessive lower facial height, so intrusive forces were used on the posterior segments during space closure to prevent any extrusion of the posterior teeth.[27] To increase the prominence of the chin, it was decided to supplement the mandibular surgical advancement with a sliding horizontal genioplasty. Maxillary impaction[4] might have been a treatment alternative, however.

Before surgery the upper and lower incisors were retracted and the upper incisors were intruded. The cephalometric tracings revealed that there was no extrusion of the posterior teeth in either arch. The patient wore occipital-type

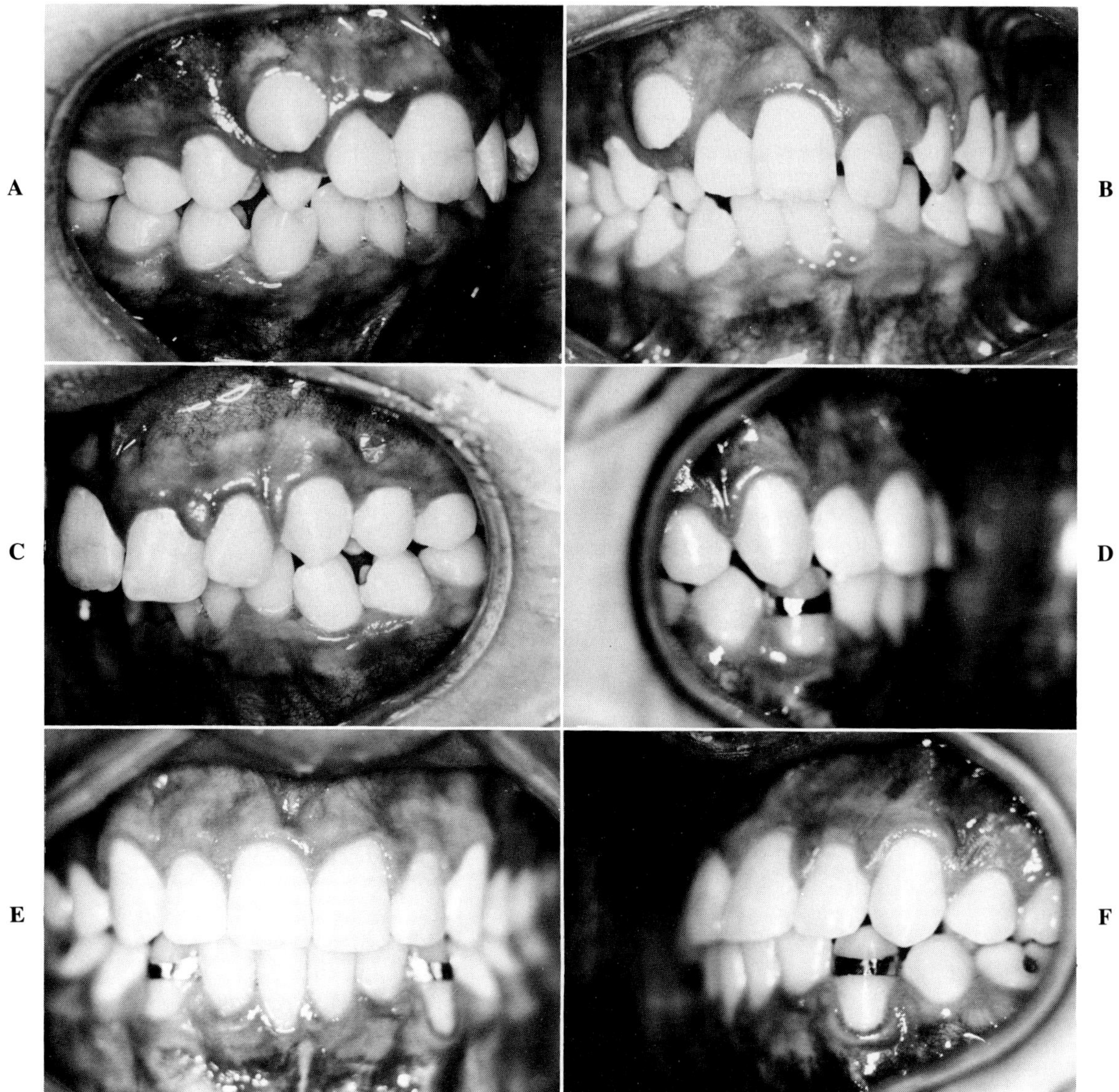

Fig. 1-7.
Patient K.L. An unfavorable skeletal pattern with limited growth potential. The case was planned from the beginning as one that would require a mandibular advancement. **A** to **C,** Pretreatment and, **D** to **F,** posttreatment views.

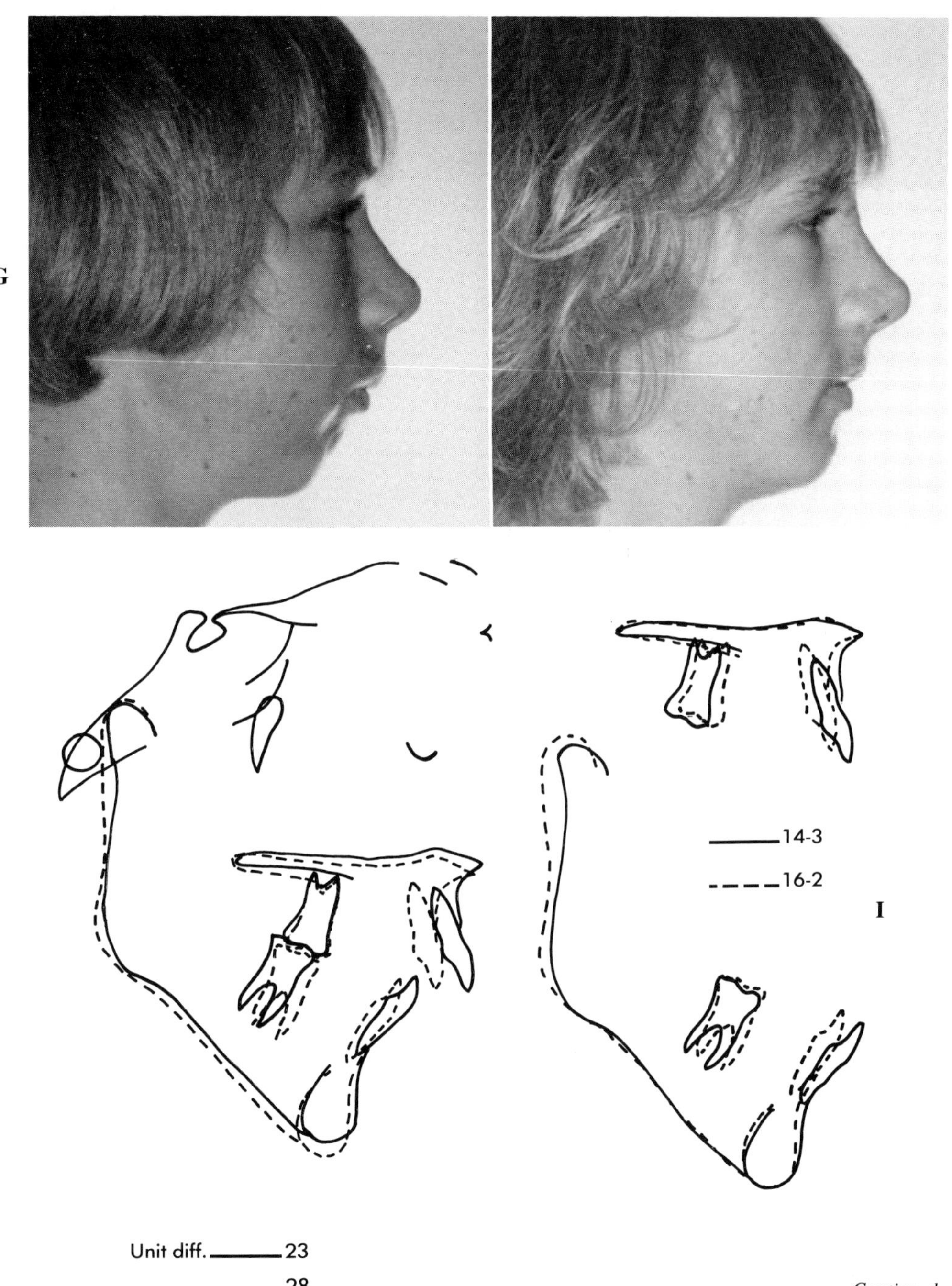

Fig. 1-7—cont'd.
G, Pretreatment and, **H,** posttreatment. **I,** Cephalometric tracing of a patient treated with premolar extraction therapy, full appliances, and intrusion of the upper anterior teeth preparatory to surgical advancement of the mandible and a sliding genioplasty. *Solid line,* original tracing; *dotted line,* movements accomplished in preparation for the surgery.

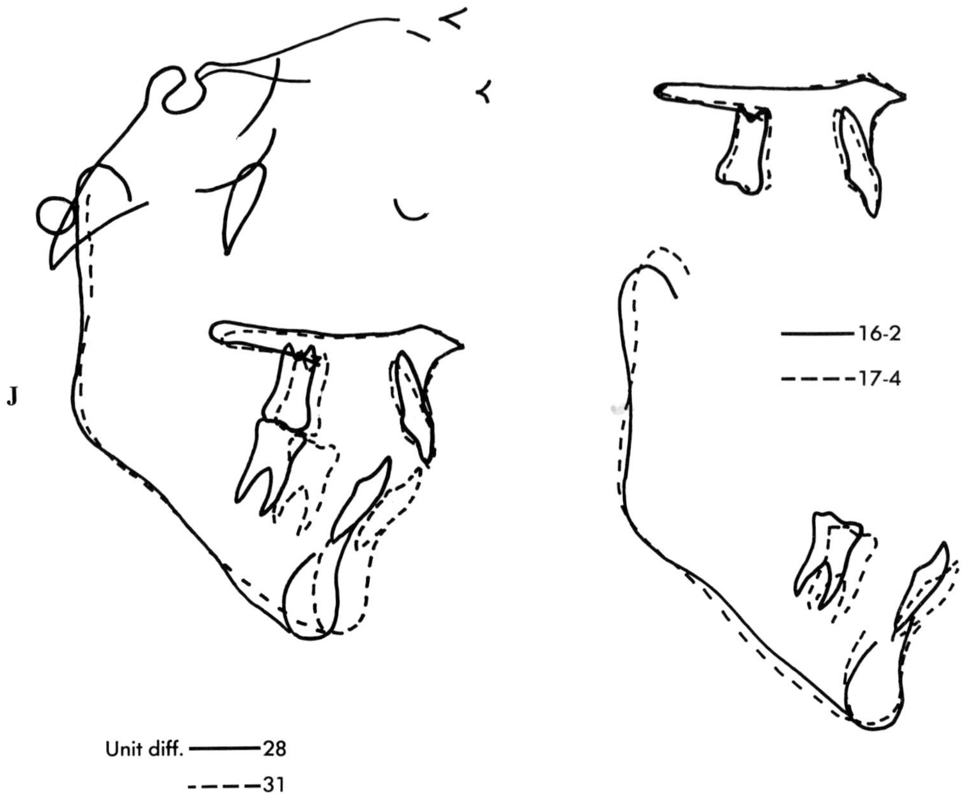

Fig. 1-7—cont'd.
J *(left),* At age 16 years 2 months, just prior to surgery; *(right),* at age 17 years 4 months (3 months after appliance removal), illustrating the surgical and orthodontic changes that were achieved.

maxillary headgear and a vertical-pull chin cup to gain this vertical control.

It is traditional in orthodontics to preserve anchorage of the posterior teeth so the anterior teeth can be retracted into the extraction sites. In mandibular advancement cases the orthodontist must monitor the use of maxillary headgear carefully, because if too much anchorage is preserved the upper anterior teeth might be retracted excessively. This would then reduce the available overjet needed for adequate advancement of the mandible. McNamara's[24] and Burstone's[9] cephalometric analyses are useful in planning this portion of treatment.

Progress records were taken after the extraction spaces were closed. The models were useful in coordinating arch widths and helping to achieve the postsurgical occlusion that was desired. It may be necessary in some cases to make the adjustments and repeat the progress models even three or four times before proper interdigitation and arch coordination are achieved. A better occlusion and excellent posterior interdigitation seem to promote bone healing and a faster adjustment to normal functioning after the surgery. It is also important to analyze incisor inclinations and root paralleling at this time by taking a progress Panorex-type radiograph.

When the orthodontist is satisfied with the presurgical preparation, another meeting is scheduled with the oral and maxillofacial surgeon to finalize the surgical procedure. New full orthodontic records are necessary for this final preparation. It is important to analyze the growth changes and the treatment changes that have occurred and to verify the fulfillment of the pretreatment goals. It may also be desirable to alter the original plan at this time or to add an additional procedure to improve the final result.

In this case the occlusal splint was constructed on articulator-mounted models (Bell[4]). The two surgical procedures were then performed and the patient was followed during the fixation. It may be desirable for the orthodontist to obtain lateral cephalometric and TMJ radiographs at this time to evaluate the mandibular position as well as the condylar positions within the fossae. When the fixation is removed, the patient should return to the orthodontic office because there may be bands to recement or brackets to rebond. When the occlusion and condylar positions within the fossae are both satisfactory, the bands can be removed and retainers placed.

Evaluation of this advancement patient *(K.L.)* revealed a much-improved profile with good occlusion. He had grown only 2¼ inches during the preceding 3 years, so our original analysis and prediction were fairly accurate. His mandibular plane angle had closed 3 degrees, and his unit difference (Harvold[17]) had changed from 23 to 31 mm. His lower facial height increased from 78 (68 ± 5.23) to 74 mm (71 ± 5.73). Because of this patient's poor skeletal pattern and limited growth, it would not have been possible to treat him well without the orthognathic procedures.

SURGICAL ADVANCEMENT FOR MANDIBULAR DEFICIENCY IN AN ADULT

Treatment of the adult (nongrowing) patient frequently involves some compromises because of missing teeth and often periodontal problems.

An example is patient *M.R.*, who was almost 40 years old when she came for treatment (Fig. 1-8). She was missing both lower first molars, and the upper left first molar had been replaced with a fixed bridge. She had some periodontal problems and was referred to the periodontist for evaluation and treatment prior to the placement of her appliances. Throughout her orth-

odontic treatment she was seen every 3 months by the periodontist, and the pocketing on the upper left central was kept under excellent control by her good oral hygiene and the periodontist's treatment. The cephalometric analysis revealed an A-N-B difference of 12 degrees (82° − 70°) and a steep mandibular plane angle (47° Sn-Go-Gn) with a retrognathic mandible. Her unit difference was 17 mm (mean 26), and the discrepancy was largely in the mandible. The mandibular unit length measured 105 mm (mean 119 ± 4.44), which is 14 mm less than the mean for women. Her treatment involved removal of an upper right third molar as well as removal of the upper left first molar bridge. The plan was to close the space of the three missing first molars by moving the second and third molars mesially. After this preliminary orthodontic preparation there was to be a mandibular advancement followed by a horizontal advancement genioplasty. It took 15 months of orthodontic treatment to close the spaces and to level and align the teeth before she was ready for orthognathic surgery.

Placement of the orthodontic appliance is an absolutely critical step to improving the final result and minimizing treatment time. It is beneficial to place a full appliance with all the teeth banded or bracketed. This will enable the orthodontist to gain full control over the position of each tooth. In a recent study Rinchuse and Sassouni[32] reported that 97% of orthodontically treated patients had balancing interferences. These were found especially on the distal aspects of the second molars. Accurate placement of each bracket or band helps in leveling the teeth and can eliminate the necessity of many up and down bends in the archwire. It also may enable the oral and maxillofacial surgeon to slide the archwire through posterior brackets when doing a procedure such as premaxillary surgical retraction. A full appliance is also desirable for intermaxillary fixation for orthognathic procedures.

Many orthodontists have found that in cases such as this indirect bonding improves the accuracy of bracket placement over what might be obtained with direct bonding. The indirect method enables the orthodontist to measure each bracket carefully for the most accurate

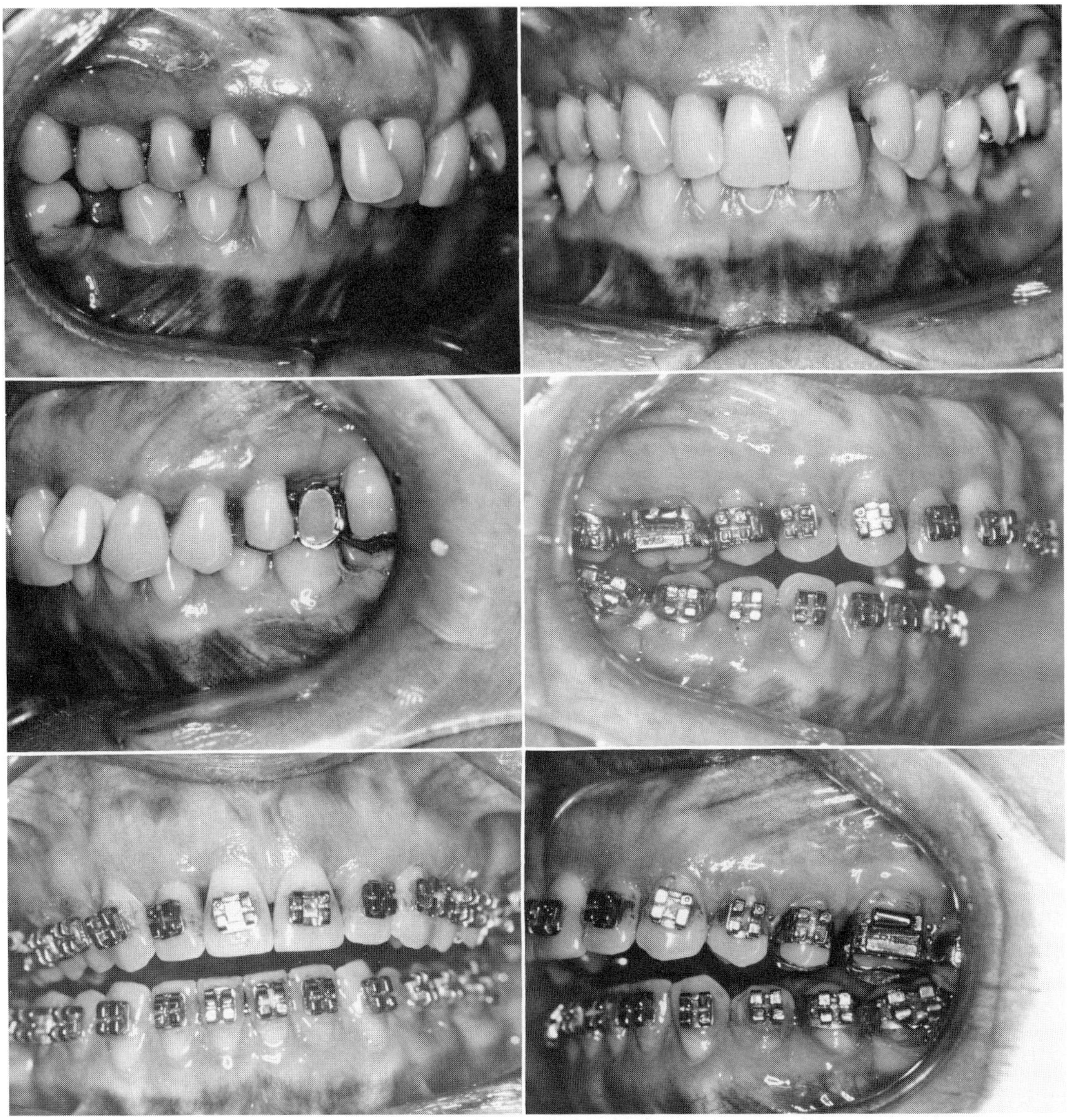

Fig. 1-8.
Patient M.R. Periodontal problems and three missing first molar teeth. The upper left first molar bridge was removed, and the second and third molars were moved mesially in three quadrants. **A** to **C,** Pretreatment and, **D** to **F,** presurgical views illustrating closure of the three missing first permanent molars.

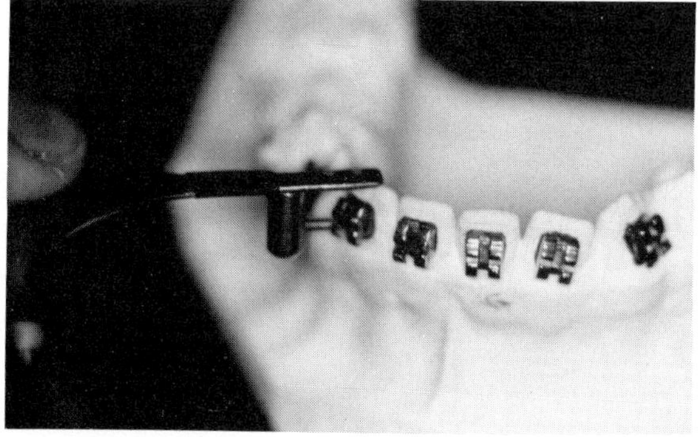

G

OPTIMUM CRITERIA OF GOOD OCCLUSION

Avoid cross arch and cross tooth interferences in lateral excusive movements

Strive for cuspid protection in lateral excursive movements

Strive for anterior guidance in protrusion for posterior protection

Centric relation equal to or very close to centric occlusion

Good neuro-muscular release

Cuspid protection

Anterior guidance

No balancing interferences

No working interferences

Neuro-muscular release

H

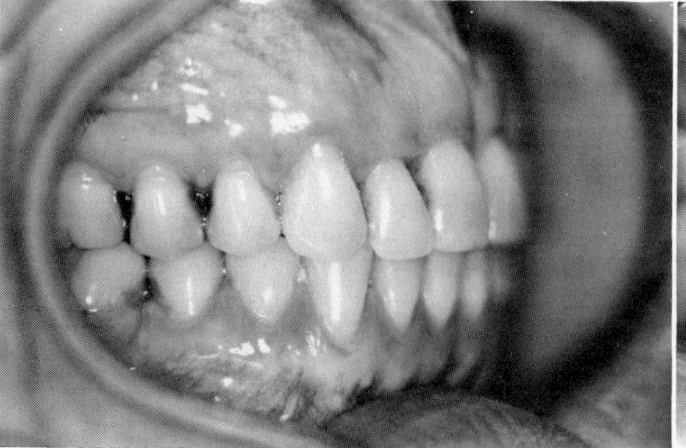

I

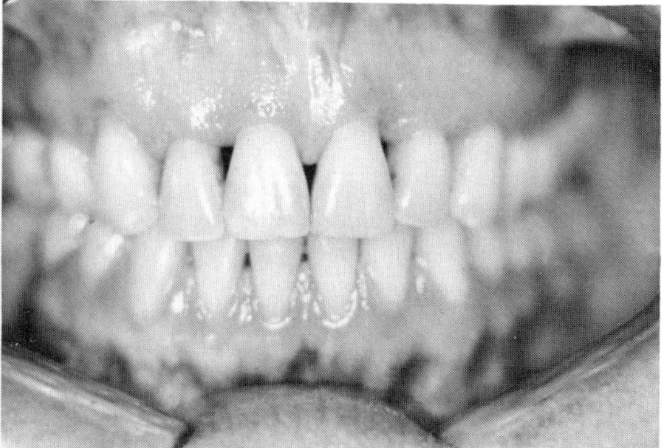

J

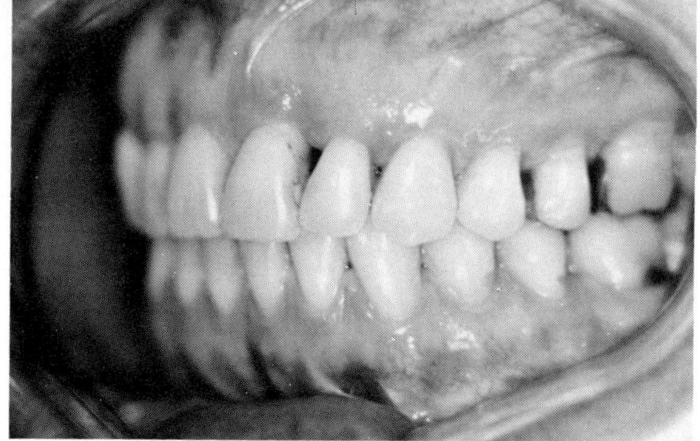

K

Continued.

Fig. 1-8—cont'd.
G, The indirect method of bonding permits precise placement of the appliance. **H,** Goals of optimum occlusion. **I** to **K,** Posttreatment views. The first molar spaces were closed and the periodontal health has improved.

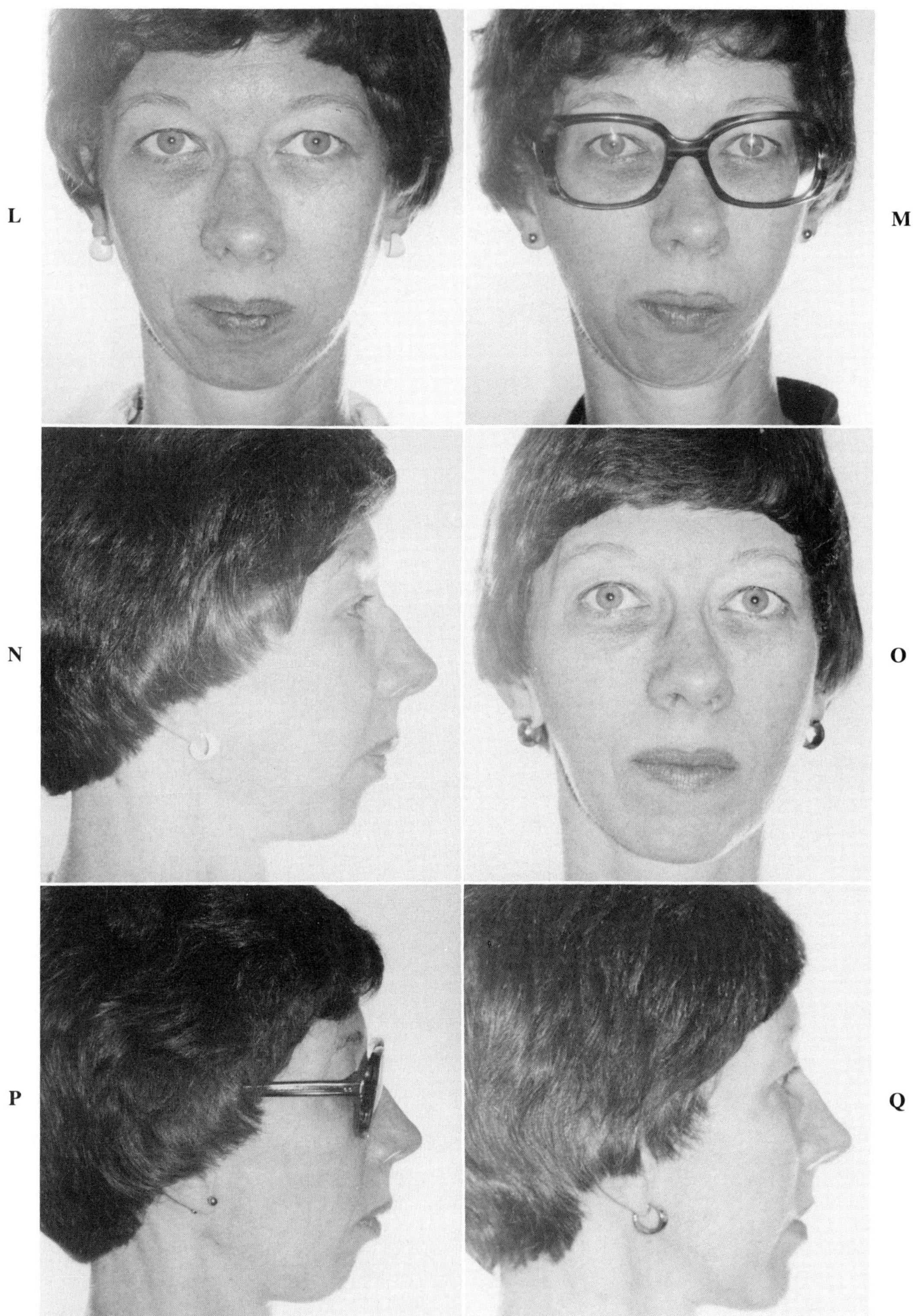

Fig. 1-8—cont'd.
L, Pretreatment, **M,** presurgical, and, **N,** posttreatment views. **O,** Pretreatment, **P,** presurgical, and, **Q,** posttreatment.

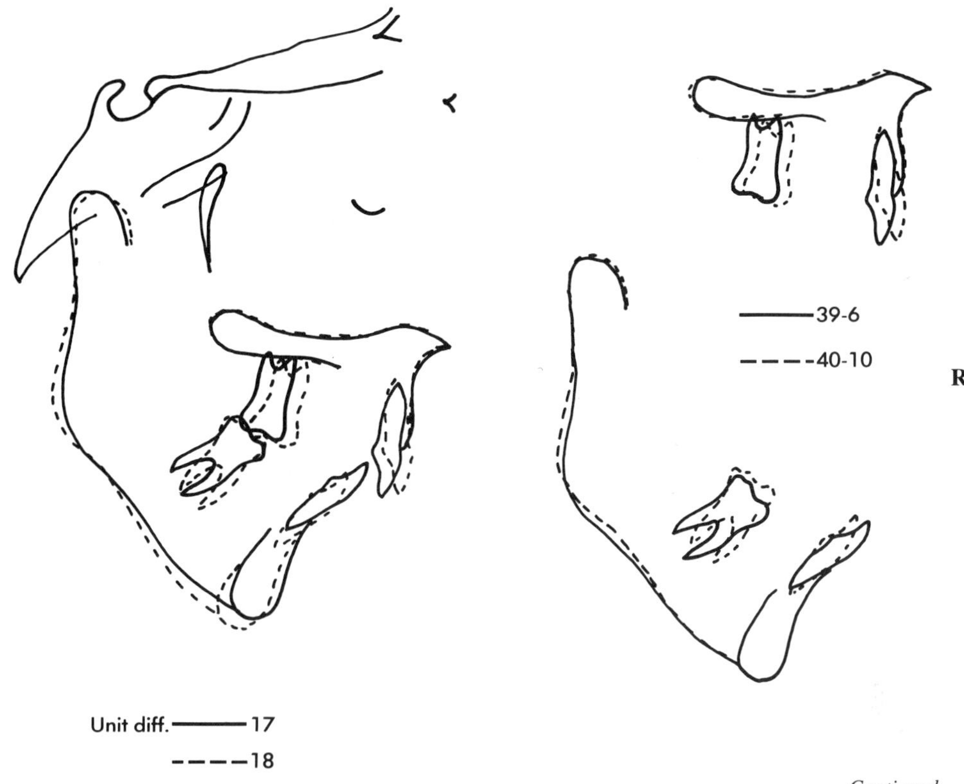

Fig. 1-8—cont'd.

R, Cephalometric tracings. *Solid line,* pretreatment tooth positions; *dotted line,* presurgical positions after removal of the dental compensations.

positioning (Fig. 1-8, *G*). Modern-day brackets are usually pretorqued, and the orthodontist can have at least two sets readily available for selection with different degrees of torque built into the slot. In the case being considered, Class II, Division 2, upper anterior brackets with built-in lingual root torque were used and then a relatively flat archwire was placed to achieve the desired lingual movement of the upper anterior roots. In a Class III case the upper anteriors would usually be inclined in the opposite direction or the teeth would already be labially inclined, and a bracket without any built-in root torque or with but slight labial torque would be most desirable.

The presurgical intraoral photographs of patient *M.R.* (Fig. 1-8, *D* to *F*) illustrate the change in the anterior inclinations as well as the space closure of the three missing permanent first molars. At this time she could occlude on only two teeth, the upper and lower left second molars. The upper left posterior teeth were still in complete buccal cross-bite. After her surgery the unit difference changed from 17 (26) to 28 mm (26) and her A-N-B difference was reduced from 12 to 7 degrees. It took 12 months of treatment, including the period of fixation, to detail her occlusion and to finish her treatment. She was occlusally quite sensitive; and as the occlusion improved, the difference was very apparent to her. The teeth were marked with typewriter ribbon, and it was attempted to get each lower buccal cusp to occlude evenly in the central fossa of each upper posterior tooth.[15,30] It was also attempted to get each upper posterior lingual cusp to occlude evenly in the central fossa of the opposing lower tooth. Strong efforts were made to achieve the goals of occlusion[15] (Fig. 1-8, *H*). Splint therapy, to establish her true centric occlusion, was not used in this

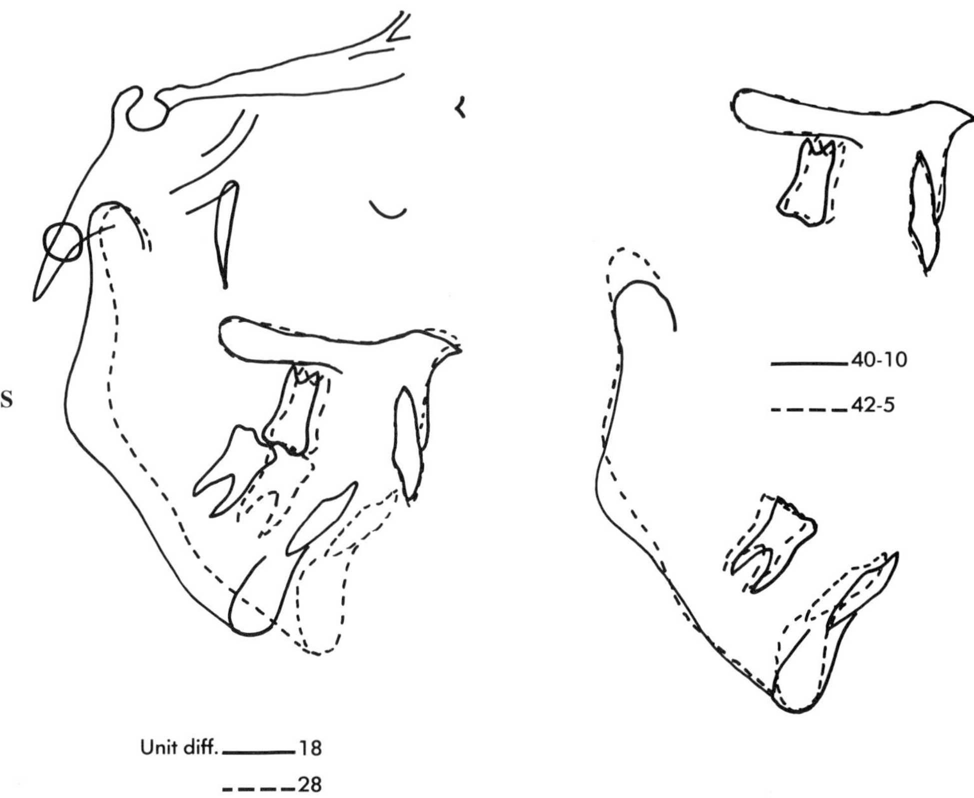

Fig. 1-8—cont'd.
S, *Solid line,* presurgical; *dotted line,* postsurgical. The unit difference changed from 18 to 28 mm.

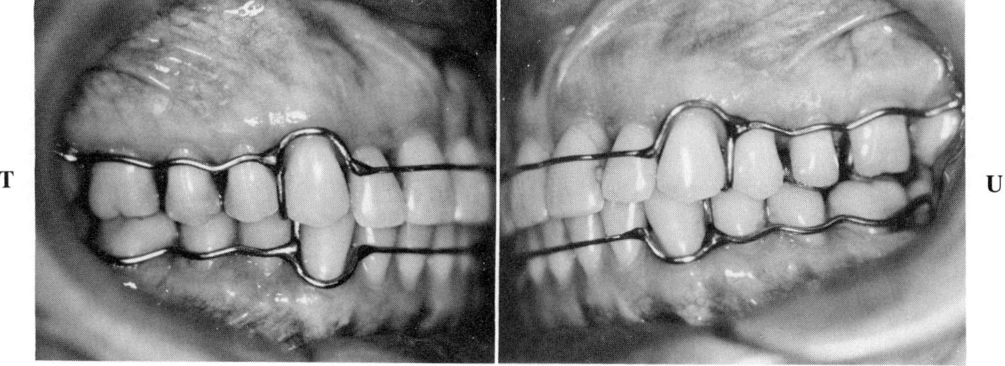

Fig. 1-8—cont'd.
T and **U,** Buccal arm wraparound retainers. This design is excellent for holding detailed positions of individual teeth.

particular case, although it might have merit in similar finishing procedures.[33] When her occlusion was stable and she was comfortable, her appliances were removed and full wraparound buccal arm retainers were employed (Fig. 1-8, *T* and *U*). It would seem logical that if the orthodontist is to go to significant effort to establish a careful and detailed occlusion the teeth should be carefully retained so as not to lose this detail. Patient *M.R.* has retained well, and only a slight amount of equilibration has been necessary.

Widening of the adult maxilla

There are several indications for widening the adult maxilla as a first step in orthognathic treatment:

1. The patient may have a vertical maxillary excess, and a one-piece impaction is desired because of a nonextraction treatment plan.
2. There may be a malocclusion in which the maxillary width deficiency is the only aspect requiring surgical treatment.
3. There may be a mandibular deficiency with a narrow maxilla, and it then becomes desirable to widen the maxilla using a combination of surgical freeing of the maxillary sutures and sutural expansion.*

In patient *B.B.* (Fig. 1-9), age 42 years, a sutural expansion appliance was placed and the sutures were then freed. The oral and maxillofacial surgeon activated the appliance, and the patient continued to reactivate it daily. The maxilla was expanded approximately 5 mm, but a large diastema opened between the upper central incisors. Although in young patients a diastema usually closes by itself after sutural expansion, in adults it is usually necessary to close the space orthodontically and to retain the maxillary expansion for a few months while bone remodeling and deposition occur.

Mandibular excess treatment for the nonextraction patient

Occasionally a young patient will have such a strong mandible and unusual growth potential that mandibular surgery appears to be the eventual necessity.

In patient *P.W.* (Fig. 1-10), a strong Class III malocclusion existed at age 11 years 9 months.

---

*References 3, 16, 22, 23, 34, 37.

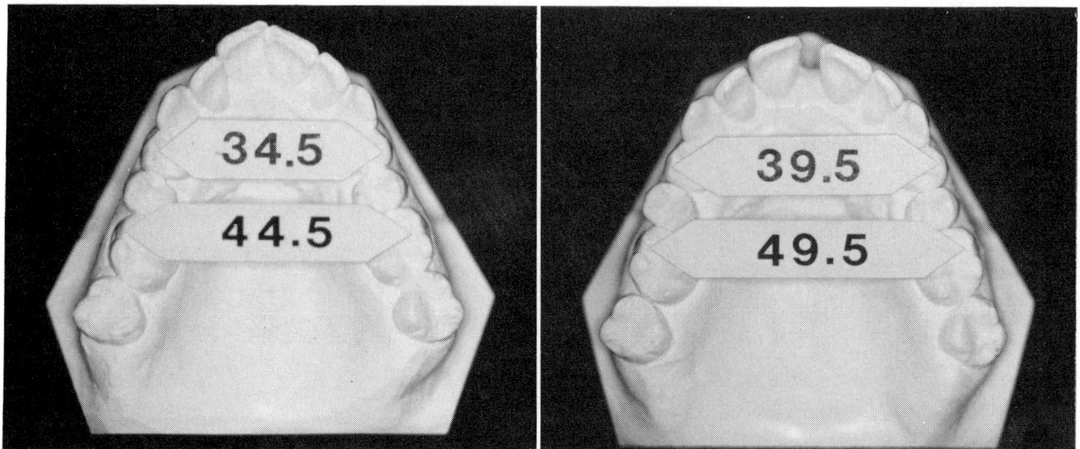

Fig. 1-9.
Patient B.B. A 42-year-old woman. **A,** Pretreatment and, **B,** posttreatment views following sutural expansion and surgical freeing of the maxillary sutures.

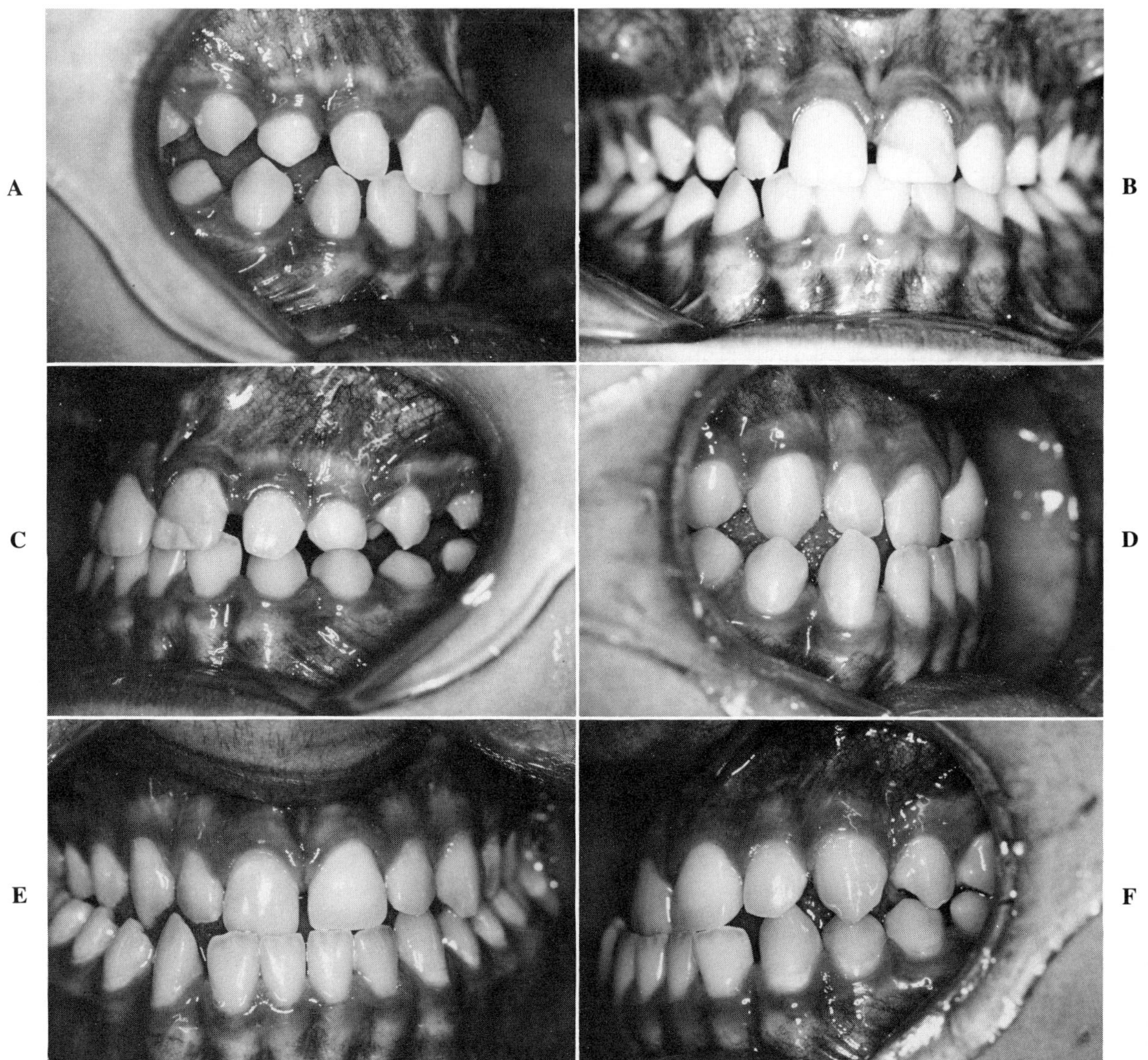

Fig. 1-10.
Patient P.W. At age 12 years he had a strong Class III growth tendency. **A** to **C,** The original malocclusion and, **D** to **F,** the increased severity of prognathism that occurred in 3 years 5 months.

His maxillary unit length of 88 mm was 4 mm less than the mean for his age (92 ± 3.73) (Harvold[17]). His mandibular unit length (122 mm) was 8 mm longer than the mean (114 ± 4.80). The unit difference (mm) was found by subtracting the maxillary from the mandibular unit lengths:

$$\begin{array}{r} 122 \\ \underline{88} \\ 34 \end{array}$$

At the age of 12 years it is usually possible to treat without surgery when the unit differences are between 15 and 30 mm, but it becomes increasingly difficult to do so as the differences get into the high 20s and approach 30. *P.W.*'s unit difference (at 34) was definitely in the expected surgical area at age 12 years. Cephalometric radiographs were obtained on a yearly schedule, and four tracings (Fig. 1-10, *G*) illustrated the progressive increase that had occurred in the severity of his malocclusion. His maxillary unit length increased 15 mm, from 88 to 103 (mean 96 ± 4.52), during this 4-year observation period. His mandibular unit length increased 23 mm, from 122 to 145 (mean 121 ± 6.05). His unit difference was as follows:

$$\begin{array}{l} 145 \ (121 \pm 6.05) \\ \underline{103 \ (\ 96 \pm 4.52)} \\ 42 \ (\text{mean } 27) \end{array}$$

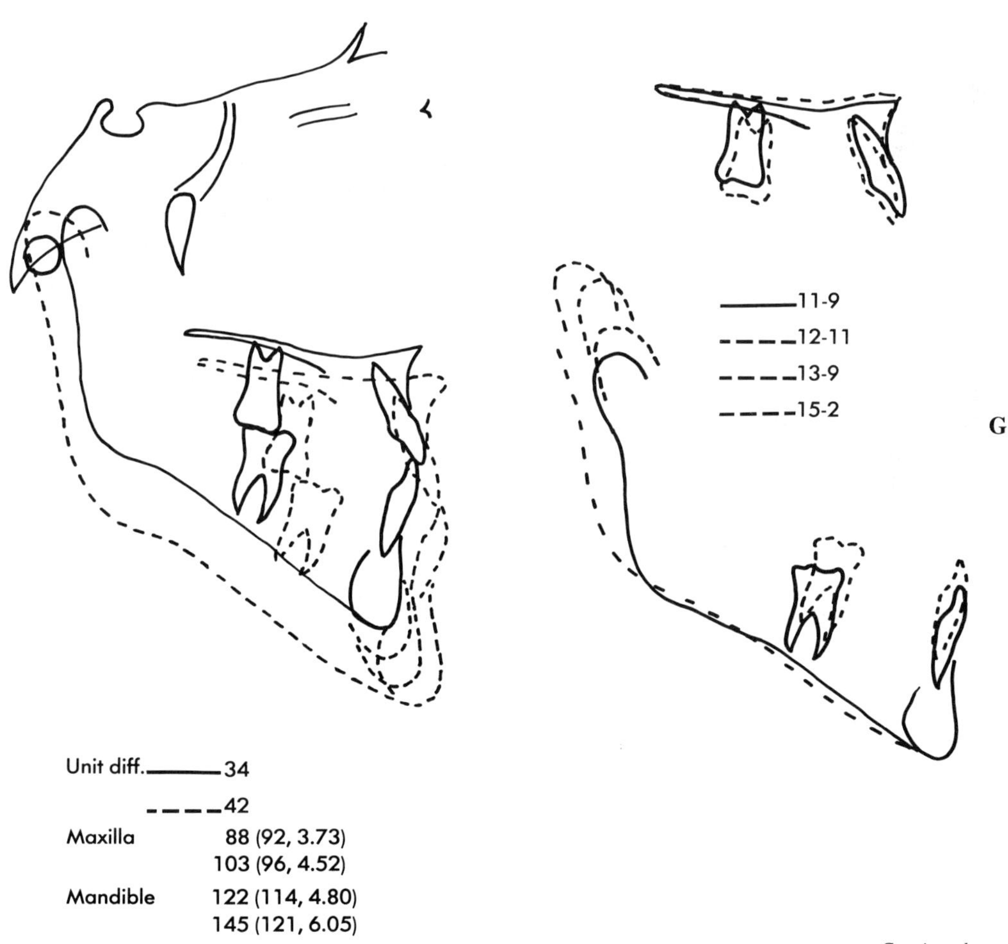

Continued.

Fig. 1-10—cont'd.
G, Serial cephalometric tracings demonstrating the strong Class III growth pattern exhibited over the 3 year 5 month observation period.

The patient's family had been advised that at about the time his growth stopped (12 years of age) orthognathic surgery would be necessary. He had worn a Class III chin cup between the ages of 12 and 14 years but had not been consistent with it. Full orthodontic appliances were placed at age 15 years 6 months, and his teeth were moved into the desired presurgical positions. The upper anteriors were tipped labially, and the lower anteriors lingually. Class II elastics were used to remove these dental compensations along with labial root torque on the upper and lingual root torque on the lower anterior teeth. This combination of forces further increased the negative overjet. Fig. 1-10, *H,* illustrates the uprighting of the upper anterior

teeth that occurred over a 6-month period. During this time his unit difference increased further, from 46 to 49 mm.

Progress records were taken when it appeared clinically that the teeth might be prepared for the surgery. The models were articulated in their postsurgical position so the intercuspation and arch coordination could be evaluated. Incisor inclinations were measured and a growth evaluation was also made on the new cephalometric tracings. It is sometimes necessary to change arch widths or tooth positions after this evaluation has been completed. Then the progress models are repeated and another evaluation is performed. This is repeated until an excellent occlusion and intercuspation are ob-

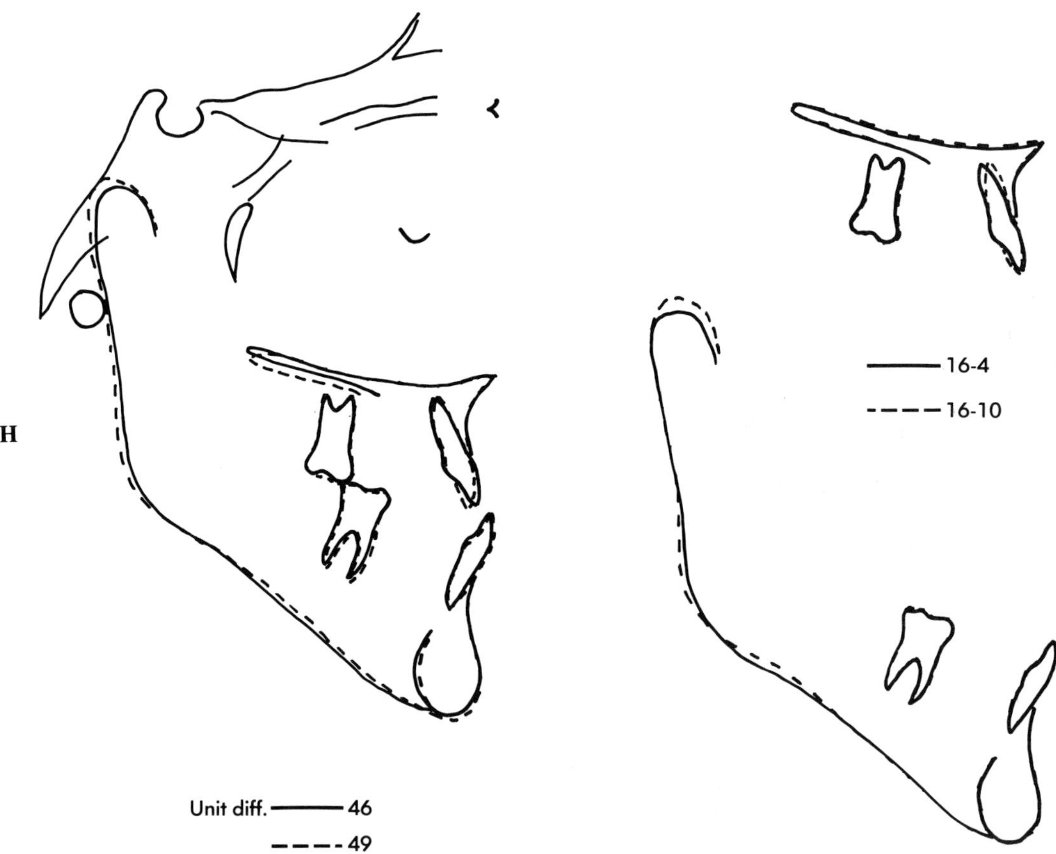

Fig. 1-10—cont'd.
H, Removal of the dental compensations by Class II elastics. Notice that the upper anteriors were uprighted and the crowns were moved lingually. The lower anteriors were tipped labially to a small extent.

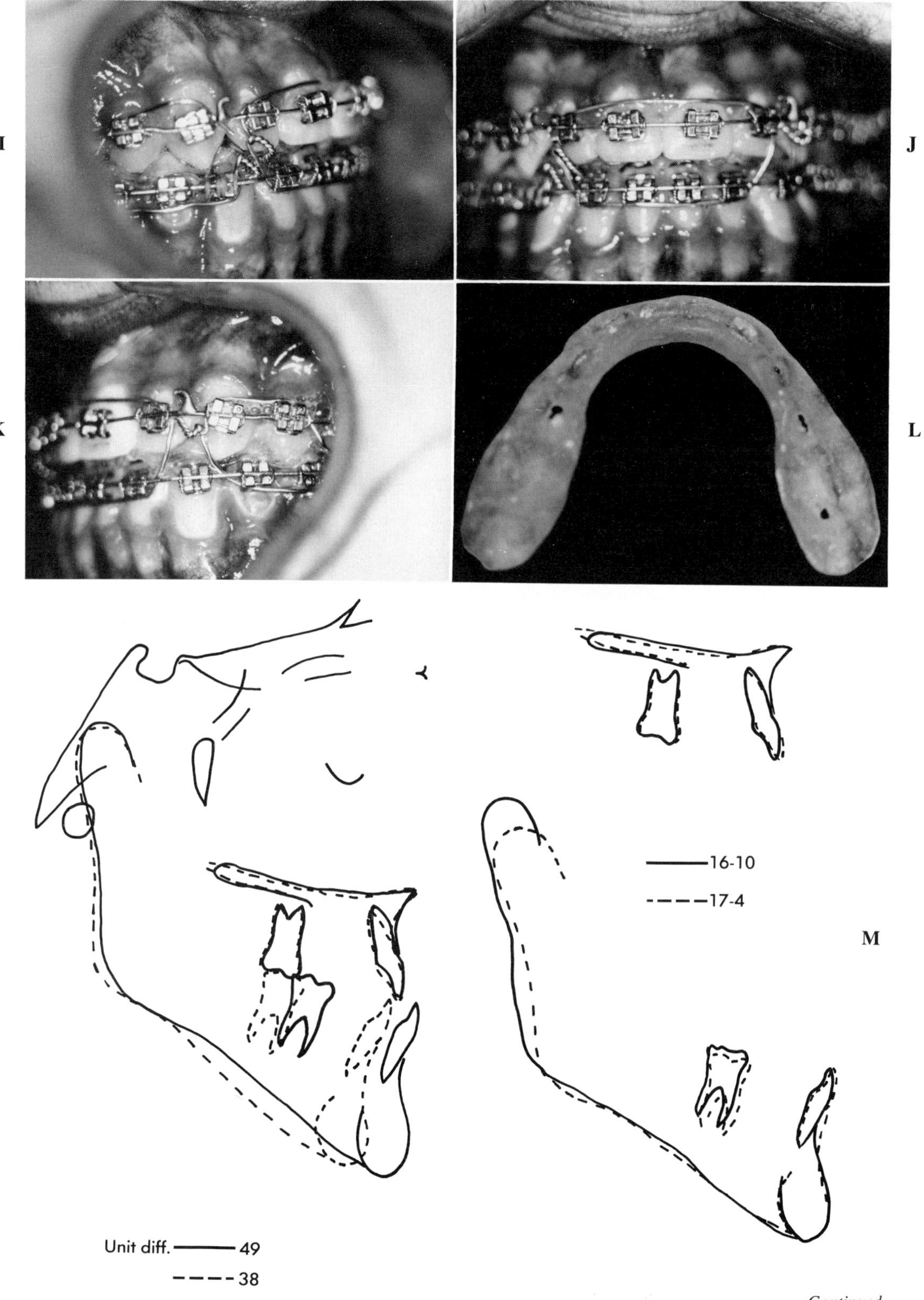

Fig. 1-10—cont'd.
I to **K,** Method of fixation used by the maxillofacial surgeon with the occlusal splint in place. **L,** Typical splint used during fixation. **M,** Cephalometric tracing illustrating the amount of mandibular retraction that was accomplished.

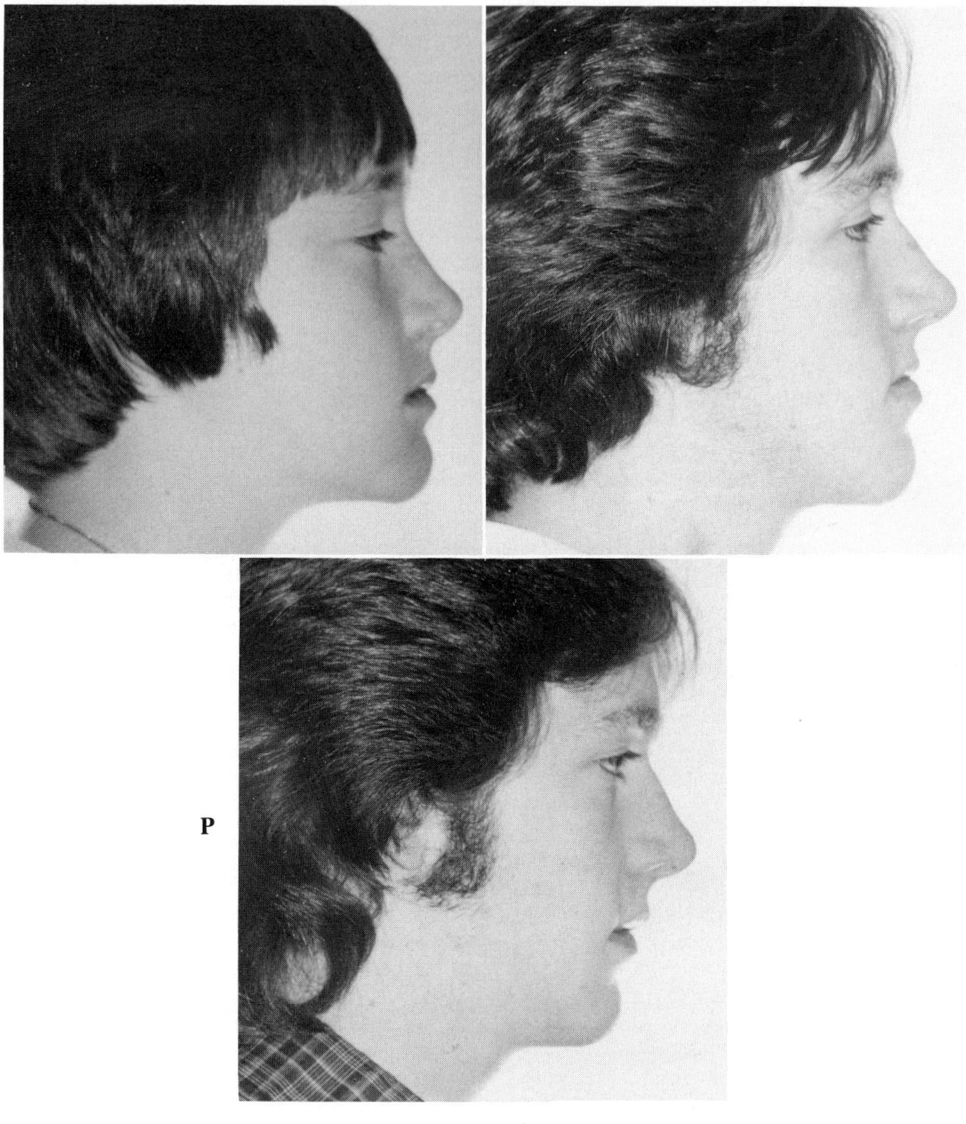

Fig. 1-10—cont'd.
N to **P,** Facial changes—age 12 (beginning of observation), presurgical, and postsurgical.

tained. A good solid postsurgical occlusion promotes healing and an earlier return of normal function. The patient probably appreciates it also because it shortens the time that appliances must be worn following the surgery. Heldt et al.[18] reported in a recent article that several patients in their study were discouraged with the amount of time required to complete orthodontic treatment after the surgery.

When all appears ready and well prepared, the case can be reviewed with the oral and maxillofacial surgeon. The splint is now constructed on models mounted on an articulator.[4] Where an anterior overbite increase is desired, the articulator can be opened posteriorly. This will thicken the posterior portion of the splint. Usually it is not necessary, however. If no change is needed in the vertical dimension, it is

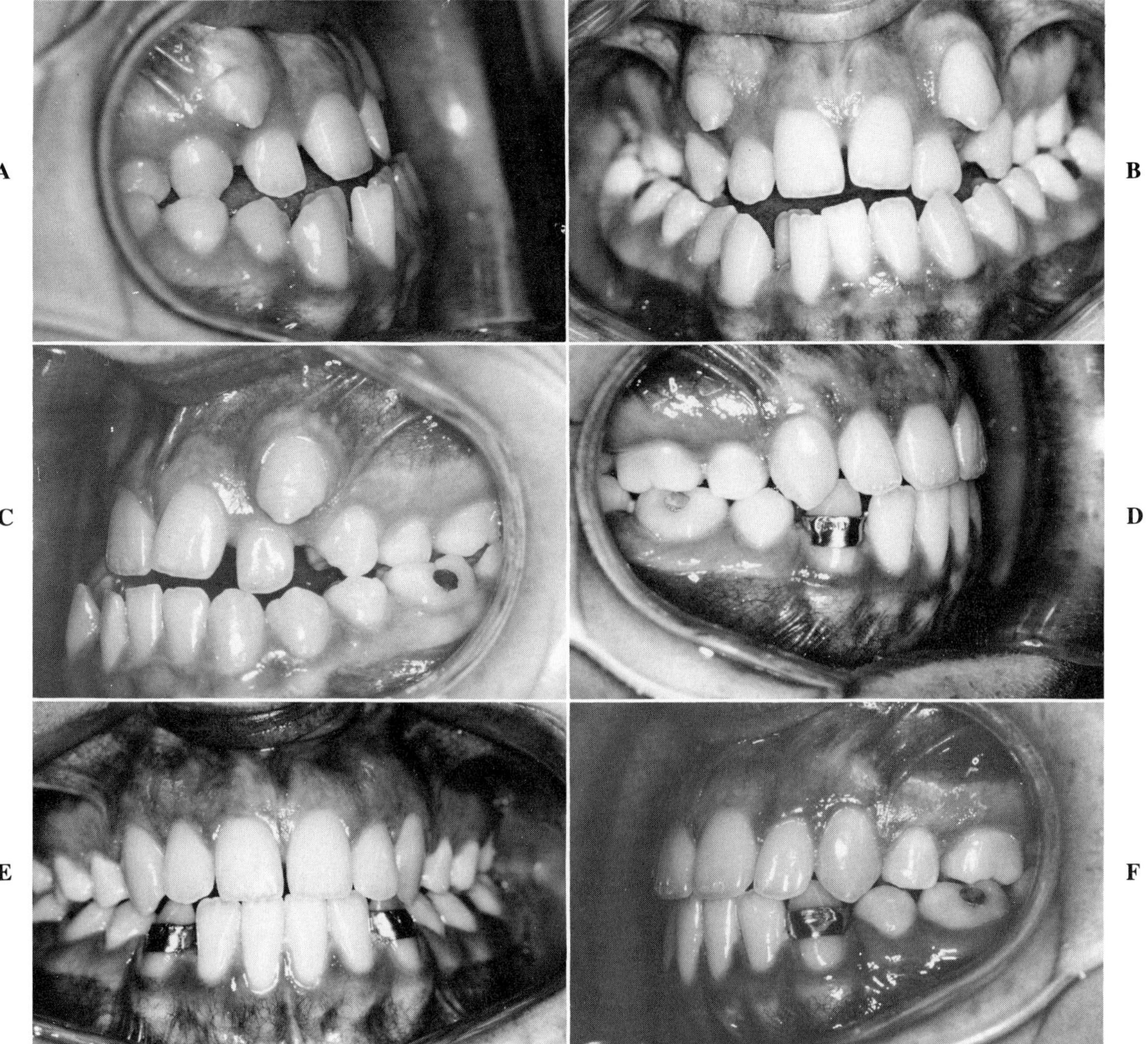

Continued.

Fig. 1-11.
Patient V.E. Class III open-bite with crowding. **A** to **C,** Pretreatment and, **D** to **F,** posttreatment views.

often possible not to use any splint. *When the case is well prepared and the teeth intercuspate properly, fixation without the use of a splint works well.*

Patient *P.W.* underwent mandibular surgical retraction at age 17 years, and the unit difference was changed from 49 to 38 mm. Fig. 1-10, *J* to *K,* illustrates the intermaxillary fixation with splint in place. His occlusion was detailed an then retained. In cases such as this it may be desirable to use a Class III chin cup during re-

tention, since boys sometimes have an additional postpuberal growth spurt during the late teen years or in the early 20s.[39]

Mandibular excess surgery combined with premolar extraction therapy

The etiology of some rather extreme Class III cases can often be traced to genetic influences and then can be further impacted by environmental influences. Patient *V.E.* (Fig. 1-11) at age 8 years 9 months had an obvious Class III

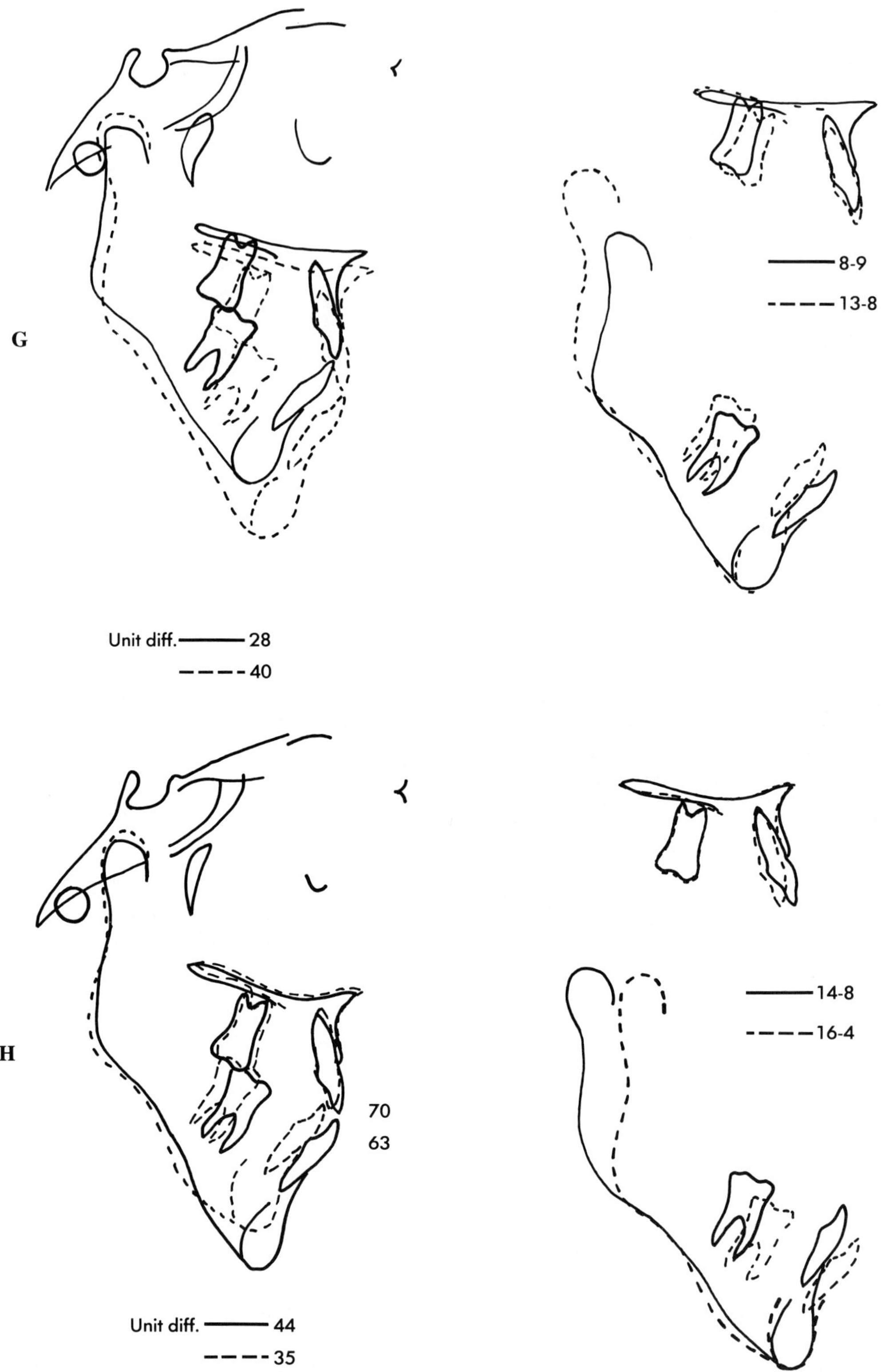

Fig. 1-11—cont'd.
G, Cephalometric tracing illustrating significant vertical growth prior to surgery. **H,** Illustrating the amount of mandibular retraction and vertical reduction that was achieved.

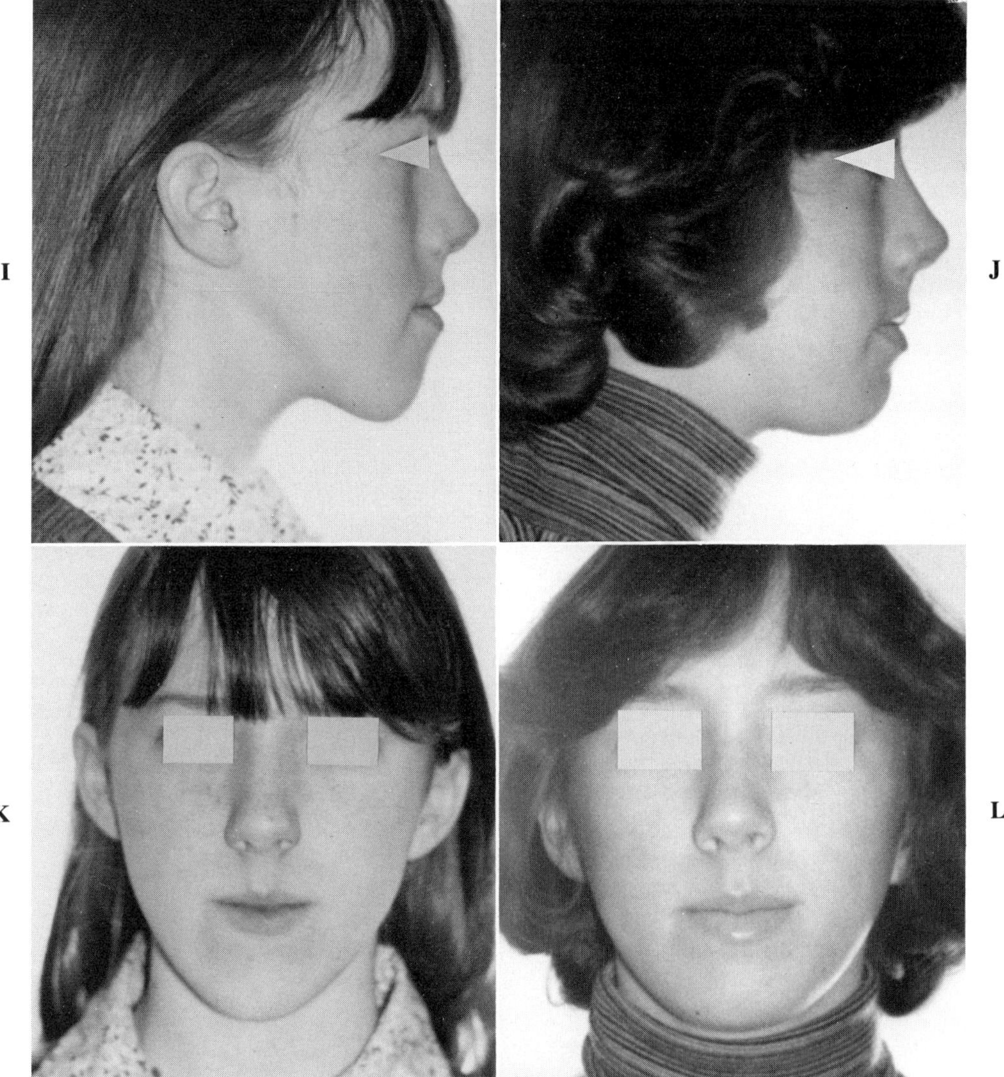

Fig. 1-11—cont'd.
I and **J,** Presurgical and postsurgical and, **K** and **L,** presurgical and postsurgical views.

steep pattern. Her mandibular plane angle was 53 degrees (Sn-Go-Gn), and there was an anterior open-bite with considerable crowding. A history of prognathism existed on both sides of her family. She was also very allergic, and her physician advised that no surgery should be performed in the spring or fall of the year. The patient was observed until age 14, when all four first premolars were removed and full appliances were placed. Her menarche occurred at age 12, and she grew more than usual (4½ inches) following the onset of menstruation. Her unit difference (Harvold[17]) was 28 mm at age 8 years 9 months and it changed to 44 mm just prior to her surgery. The mandibular plane angle increased from 53 to 58 degrees, and facial height increased from 67 to 76 mm. Her teeth were prepared and the mandible was operated upon with a ramus body procedure. A vertical reduction genioplasty was also performed. Her unit difference changed from 44 to 35 mm, and the lower facial height was reduced from 76 mm presurgically to 70 mm postsurgically (Harvold[17]). Fig. 1-11 shows the differences that were achieved dentally and facially.

SUMMARY AND CONCLUSIONS

One of the most important decisions in treatment planning is to decide whether or not an orthognathic procedure is to be part of the treatment. The teeth are usually positioned differently in a surgical plan and the dental compensations are usually removed during the initial stages of orthodontic therapy. Harvold's unit difference analysis has proved to be a most helpful guide in this decision-making process. The mandibular unit length as measured from condylion to gnathion is compared with the mean for the particular age and sex of the patient. The maxillary unit length is determined and, again, is compared with the mean for the age and sex of the patient. The maxillary unit length is then subtracted from the mandibular unit length for the unit difference.

If the unit difference (prognathic-type malocclusion) is in the high 20s and approaching 30 at age 12, it is believed that it will become increasingly more difficult to treat nonsurgically. At the other end of the spectrum (i.e., with a recessive mandible), if the unit difference is much below 15 at age 12 it too will become increasingly difficult to treat with a nonsurgical method. The clinician must also measure the lower facial height and include this measurement in the total assessment. If the lower facial height is excessive, it will have the effect of rocking the mandible open or shortening its length. This can aggravate the problems in a Class II malocclusion.

Retention of an orthognathic case really begins in the diagnosis and treatment planning stage. The correct choice of treatment procedures, properly executed and based on a carefully considered diagnosis, will give the best assurance of success and minimal retention problems. There is such a wide range of orthognathic procedures available that it is difficult to find an orthodontist who is well experienced in all of these.[2,5] Usually there are certain specific procedures that are well developed by the oral and maxillofacial surgeon with whom each orthodontist usually treats his patients. Consequently individuals in different practice areas may choose one procedure over another based partly on their previous experiences and partly on the skills and expertise of the available surgeon. It is beneficial if these specialists can attend courses and symposia together so newer techniques can be studied. This tremendous progress makes the future of orthognathic surgery quite promising for the patient as well as stimulating for the participating professionals.

REFERENCES

1. Acheson, R.M., and Dupertuis, C.S.: The relationships between physique and rate of skeletal maturation in boys, Human Biol. **269:**167, 1957.
2. Bell, W.H.: Increasing mandibular arch length by subapical osteotomy, Am. J. Orthod. **74:**276, 1978.
3. Bell, W.H., and Epker, B.N.: Surgical-orthodontic expansion of the maxilla, Am. J. Orthod. **70:**517, 1976.
4. Bell, W.H., et al.: Surgical correction of dentofacial deformities, Philadelphia, 1980, W.B. Saunders Co.
5. Bell, W.H., et al.: Treatment of Class II deep bite by orthodontic and surgical means, Am. J. Orthod. **85:**1, 1984.
6. Björk, A.: Prediction of mandibular growth rotation, Am. J. Orthod. **55:**585, 1969.
7. Burstone, C.J.: Process of maturation and growth prediction, Am. J. Orthod. **49:**907, 1963.
8. Burstone, C.J.: Deep overbite correction by intrusion, Am. J. Orthod. **72:**1, 1977.
9. Burstone, C.J.: Cephalometrics for orthognathic surgery, J. Oral Surg. **36:**264, 1978.
10. Cehbib, F.S., and Chamma, A.M.: Indices of craniofacial asymmetry, Angle Orthod. **51:**214, 1981.
11. Delaire, J., and Salagnac, J.M.: Anatomie et physiologie du pilier antérieur maxillaire et architecturale faciale, Rev. Stomatol. 447, 1978.
12. Dingman, R.O.: Surgical correction of developmental deformities of the mandible, Plast. Reconst. Surg. **3:**124, 1948.
13. Forsberg, C.T., et al.: Diagnosis and treatment planning of skeletal asymmetry with the submental-vertical radiograph, Am. J. Orthod. **85:**224, 1984.
14. Grayson, B.H., et al.: Analysis of craniofacial asymmetry by multiplane cephalometry, Am. J. Orthod. **84:**217, 1983.
15. Guichet, N.F.: Occlusion in everyday dentistry, Anaheim, Calif., 1977, Niles F. Guichet.
16. Haas, A.J.: Rapid expansion of the maxillary dental arch and nasal cavity by opening the midpalatal suture, Angle Orthod. **31:**73, 1961.
17. Harvold, E.: Morphogenetic response to activator treatment, Am. J. Orthod. **60:**478, 1971.

18. Heldt, L.H., et al.: The physiological and social aspects of orthognathic treatment, Am. J. Orthod. **82:**318, 1982.
19. Helm, S., et al.: Skeletal maturation of the hand in relation to maximum puberal growth in body height, Tandaegebladt **75:**1223, 1971.
20. Huang, C.S., and Ross, R.B.: Surgical advancement of the retrognathic mandible in growing children, Am. J. Orthod. **82:**89, 1982.
21. Isaacson, J.R., et al.: Extreme variation in vertical facial growth and associated variation in skeletal dental relations, Angle Orthod. **41:**219, 1971.
22. Isaacson, R.J., et al.: Forces produced by rapid maxillary expansion, Angle Orthod. **34:**256, 1964.
23. Jacobs, J., et al.: Control of the transverse dimension with surgery and orthodontics, Am. J. Orthod. **77:**284, 1980.
24. McNamara, J.A.: Components of Class II malocclusion in children 8-10 years of age, Angle Orthod. **51:**177, 1981.
25. McNamara, J.A.: Influence of respiratory pattern on craniofacial growth, Angle Orthod. **51:**269, 1981.
26. McNeil, W.R., et al.: Skeletal relapse following intermaxillary fixation, J. Oral Surg. **31:**212, 1972.
27. Pearson, L.E.: Vertical control in treatment of patients having backward rotational growth tendencies, Angle Orthod. **48:**132, 1978.
28. Petit, H.: Adaptation following accelerated facial-mask therapy. In McNamara, J.A., Jr., editor: Clinical alteration of the growing face. Monograph 14, Craniofacial growth series, pp. 253-289, Ann Arbor, 1983, Center for Human Growth and Development, University of Michigan.
29. Popovich, F., and Thompson, G.W.: Craniofacial templates for orthodontic case analysis, Am. J. Orthod. **71:**406, 1977.
30. Ramfjord, S.P., and Ash, M.M.: Occlusion, pp. 275-286, Philadelphia, 1966, W.B. Saunders Co.
31. Riedel, R.R.: The relation of maxillary structures to the cranium in malocclusion and in normal occlusion, Angle Orthod. **22:**142, 1952.
32. Rinchuse, D.J., and Sassouni, V.: An evaluation of functional occlusal interferences in orthodontically treated and untreated subjects, Angle Orthod. **53:**2, 1983.
33. Serrano, P.T., et al.: Centric relation change during therapy with a corrective occlusal prosthesis, J. Prosthet. Dent. **51:**97, 1984.
34. Steinhauser, E.W.: Midline splitting of the maxilla for correction of malocclusion, J. Oral Surg. **30:**413, 1972.
35. Subtelny, J.D.: Personal communication, 1984.
36. Tanner, J.M.: Growth at adolescense, chaps. 1 and 7, Springfield, Ill., 1955, Charles C Thomas, Publisher.
37. Wertz, R.A.: Skeletal and dental changes accompanying rapid mid palatal suture opening, Am. J. Orthod. **58:**41, 1970.
38. Woodside, D.: Personal communication, 1984.
39. Worms, F.W., et al. Posttreatment stability and esthetics of orthognathic surgery, Angle Orthod. **50:**251, 1980.

CHAPTER 2

Anesthetic considerations in orthognathic surgery

Lewis A. Coveler

Orthognathic surgery is being performed with increasing frequency as the number of surgeons trained in these techniques grows and patient awareness of the availability of these operative procedures increases. Perioral surgical procedures provide the anesthesiologist with a unique set of problems, some of which require inventive solutions. These include the shared airway and remote positioning of the anesthesiologist, as well as the surgeon's frequent requests to avoid muscle relaxants and provide controlled intraoperative hypotension. These considerations as well as the topics of preoperative and often prehospital patient evaluation and preparation and early postoperative management will be discussed in the context of orthognathic surgery.

PREOPERATIVE ASSESSMENT AND PREPARATION
History and physical examination

A comprehensive medical history and a thorough physical examination are mandatory for any patient scheduled for elective surgery. The usual investigation of current and past illnesses is supplemented by a careful review of patient and familial experiences with prior anesthetics. Patient responses to sedatives, tranquilizers, and analgesics are carefully recorded. Idiosyncratic reactions associated with the administration of anesthetic drugs or adjuvants are particularly noteworthy. A familial history of malignant hyperpyrexia, for example, would not contraindicate elective surgery. Preopera-

tive preparation of the patient with orally administered dantrolene sodium (Dantrium) can help avoid an incident. This drug, in addition to its role in prophylaxis, has reduced the mortality rate of a full-blown episode from 70% to almost zero.

Prolonged paralysis after succinylcholine chloride (Anectine) can be a hindrance to safe perioperative management.[16] The associated pseudocholinesterase deficiency can often be diagnosed from a positive family history or a previous anesthesia during which the patient experienced "delayed awakening" or a prolonged recovery-room stay.

If necessary, surgery is delayed and old records are obtained for review. It is desirable, however, to anticipate in advance of scheduling operating room time whether the surgery will be delayed because of a need for old records and to initiate the search for these records prior to hospital admission.

During the physical examination, in addition to the usual features, special attention should be paid to vascular access sites; and because perioral surgery is frequently facilitated by nasotracheal intubation, assessment of nasopharyngeal anatomy and a determination of the patency of the nares are necessary.

Laboratory testing
HEALTHY PATIENTS

The minimum laboratory testing necessary for young healthy patients is a spun hematocrit. Although individual preference and local regulation may require additional evaluation, more extensive laboratory workup should be undertaken only if dictated by history or current patient condition. This will become increasingly important as greater emphasis is placed on the cost/benefit analysis of preoperative testing.[17]

DIAGNOSIS-BASED SCREENING

Certain patient diagnoses appear frequently in the surgical population. For hypertensive patients or those with suspected or documented ischemic heart disease, electrolytes and BUN should be measured and a urinalysis performed in addition to the spun hematocrit. Laboratory evaluation of a diabetic patient would include electrolytes, BUN, urinalysis, and a fasting blood glucose determination. The last, done immediately preoperatively, will facilitate the smooth intraoperative control of this critical parameter.

Other laboratory studies, such as liver function tests, are not routinely ordered unless indicated by the clinical condition of the patient. A carefully elicited bleeding history is more valuable than the routine ordering of clotting studies,[17] but a positive history demands a complete coagulation workup prior to the surgical procedure.

Additional preoperative studies should be approached in a similarly conservative way. Radiographic examination of the chest should be performed per indication, one of which is chronologic age greater than 40. An electrocardiogram should also be recorded for patients whose age is greater than 40, or for those with a suggestive history or physical examination.[17] For example, a patient with underlying lung disease should have a chest x-ray and ECG examination as well as an arterial blood gas measurement while breathing room air.

CONTROLLED HYPOTENSION

Patients for whom controlled hypotension is contemplated require more extensive preoperative screening. The chest radiograph and ECG are obtained regardless of patient age or apparent good health. Laboratory evaluation of renal and hepatic function should also be routine, along with the measurement of electrolytes, blood glucose, and room air arterial blood gases. The last can be done in the operating room when the arterial catheter is placed preoperatively.

• • •

A summary of the suggested preoperative laboratory workup is found in Table 2-1. With few exceptions, it and the patient examination can be performed before the actual hospitalization. Any additional studies suggested by abnormal laboratory results or positive findings in the history or physical examination also can be performed. If necessary, medical consultation is obtained and, if possible, the patient's condition optimized prior to hospitalization. After preoperative assessments and preparation are

Table 2-1.
Preoperative patient assessment

	Patient condition				
	Healthy		*Hypertension*	*Diabetes*	*Controlled hypotension*
Study	*(<40 yr)*	*(>40 yr)*	*(any age)*	*(any age)*	*(any age)*
Hematocrit	x	x	x	x	x
Urinalysis			x	x	x
Electrolytes			x	x	x
BUN			x	x	x
Blood glucose				x	x
Liver functions					x
ECG		x	x	x	x
Chest x-ray		x	x		x
Blood gas					x

completed, surgery is scheduled and the patient can be hospitalized.

PREANESTHETIC VISIT
Interview

The preanesthetic interview is typically accomplished the evening before surgery. During this visit the anesthesiologist reviews the patient data base and conducts a directed history and physical examination. Particular attention is focused on the emotional preparation of the patient.

Patient cooperation is essential during orofacial surgical procedures. The prospect of awake-sedate nasal intubation, if this technique is chosen, can be extremely frightening, and an adequate explanation must be given so the patient will remain cooperative.

In teaching hospitals, and even in private practice, patients scheduled for elective nasotracheal intubation routinely undergo awake-sedate intubation, providing training and practice for anesthesia residents, nurse anesthesia students, and full-time attending staff. Properly carried out, awake-sedate nasal intubation causes minimal discomfort for the patient, and recall of the event is extremely limited.

Some patients will remain intubated for several hours into the recovery period. This should be anticipated, and again the patient prepared for the eventuality. Ideally, the patient will have been forewarned of this possibility before entering the hospital, when there is less intimidation by the hospital environment. A thoughtful explanation outlining the reasons for choosing awake intubation and the reasons for delayed extubation postoperatively can do much to allay apprehension.

Premedication

Nonpharmacologic premedication begins during the preoperative visit, when patient concerns are often voiced for the first time. These concerns can be dealt with by the anesthesiologist; but if the patient has detailed questions about the operation, the surgeon should be notified.

Pharmacologic premedication also begins the night before surgery. A hypnotic given at bedtime assures a quiet night. I prefer triazolam (Halcion) for this use because of its high frequency of first administration effectiveness and its low incidence of morning hangover.

On the morning of surgery an anticholinergic and any necessary preoperative sedation are administered. Narcotics are useful premedicants, making vascular access procedures and airway topicalization quite tolerable. Orally administered diazepam (Valium) is also an effective sedative and has a high rate of patient acceptance. Additionally, it helps reduce patient recall of preoperative manipulations. Heavy sedation is rarely needed until the patient is under constant observation in the operating room.

Cimetidine (Tagamet) may be administered with the premedication, especially if awake-sedate intubation (facilitated by topical airway anesthesia) is planned. Regurgitation prior to intubation is always a hazard. The patient whose airway reflexes have been obtunded with sedatives and local anesthetics is more likely than most to regurgitate and aspirate secondary to intraoral manipulations. The preoperative administration of a histamine H_2 receptor antagonist can help raise the gastric pH above the critical level, reducing the risk of serious complications if the patient should aspirate. Maximum effectiveness in this regard can be achieved by administering the first dose of cimetidine at bedtime the night before surgery as well as a second dose with the premedication.

ENDOTRACHEAL INTUBATION
Nasal intubation

Nasotracheal intubation is quite desirable for orthognathic surgery and can be quickly accomplished with little patient discomfort. Several techniques are commonly employed, including "blind" intubation (without laryngeal visualization) and intubation under oral or flexible laryngoscopic control. These can be performed with the patient awake-sedate or after the induction of general anesthesia. Other, more elaborate, intubation techniques have been described, usually for the management of difficult intubations but are rarely needed for this group of patients.

For patients in whom awake-sedate intubation is planned, topical anesthesia of the upper airway is essential. This is produced with cocaine or lidocaine (Xylocaine) spray and can be supplemented by superior laryngeal nerve blocks and a transtracheally or translaryngeally administered local anesthetic.

The nasal mucosa is treated with a vasoconstrictor such as cocaine, phenylephrine (Neo-Synephrine) prepared as a 0.25% solution in lidocaine or commercially available agents such as 0.05% oxymetazoline (Afrin). This last is very long acting and can be administered at bedside along with the premedicants.

There are three locations where the nasally inserted endotracheal tube meets obstruction to its passage: (1) the nares and nasal passages, (2) the posterior pharyngeal wall and pharyngeal tubercle, and (3) the glottic opening.

The size of the nares and nasal passages limit the size of the endotracheal tube that can be used. Care must be taken to avoid an oversized tube, for a brisk nasal hemorrhage can result and will require rapid intubation to prevent aspiration of blood. The nasal passages can be progressively and atraumatically dilated by passing a series of graduated, well-lubricated, latex nasal airways. This will lessen the risk of nasal hemorrhage and the possibility of damage to the cuff on the endotracheal tube. It also is helpful in evaluating the quality of topical anesthesia.

Upon passage through the nose the tube impinges on the posterior pharyngeal wall and the bony prominence of the pharyngeal tubercle. It is at this level that submucosal dissection can occur during nasal intubation. The newer round-tipped endotracheal tubes (such as the Rae and Endotrol tubes*) (Fig. 2-1) are less likely to dissect a false passage, and extension of the neck helps to pass this bony obstacle.

In the event of a submucosal dissection, unless major bleeding is encountered surgery is permitted to continue. I have not observed significant sequelae in elective surgical patients during the management of numerous submucosal dissections caused by nasotracheal intubation or the insertion of a nasogastric tube.

---

*National Catheter Corporation, Argyle, New York.

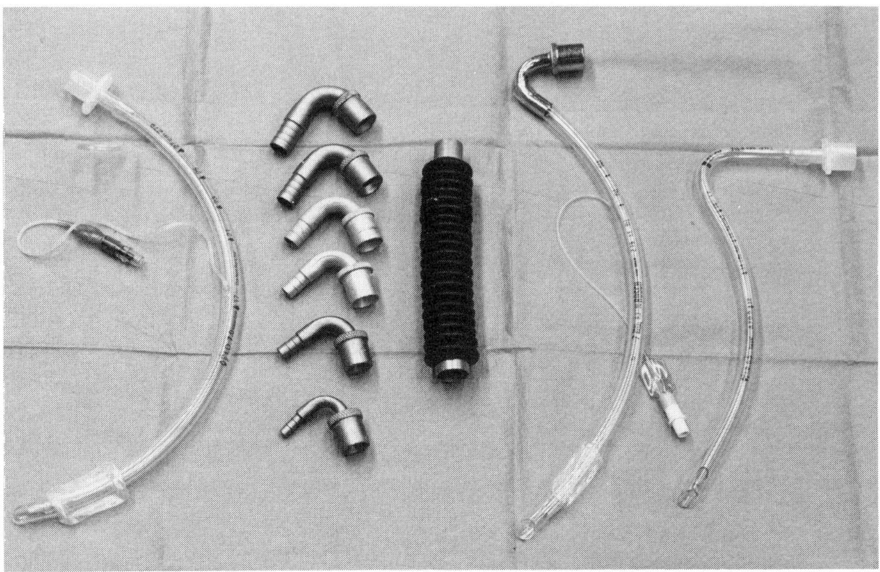

Fig. 2-1.
Left to *right,* An Endotrol tube, a low-profile connector set, an endotracheal tube with low-profile connector inserted, and a nasal Rae tube.

Finally, the tube comes to the glottic opening, where it may be diverted laterally into the piriform sinus, posteriorly into the esophagus, or anteriorly to press on the anterior laryngeal commissure. Passage can be facilitated at this level by direct vision and manipulation of the tube with Magill forceps or by adjusting traction on the guide ring of the Endotrol tube.

Low-profile techniques

After the trachea is intubated, the standard 15 mm endotracheal connector is removed from the tube, the tube is trimmed to length, and a low-profile* curved connector is attached. If an Endotrol tube has been used, the guide ring should be removed at this time. Alternatively, a nasal Rae tube can be used (Fig. 2-1). Both of these arrangements and several others are sufficient to keep the endotracheal tube from intruding upon the surgical workspace. The endotracheal tube itself is generally not fixed to the face, and care must be taken to avoid placing excessive traction on the tube lest the naris be injured.

---

*Dupaco, Inc., San Marcos, California.

BREATHING CIRCUITS

Many anesthesiologists committed to the recently repopularized low-flow or closed-circuit techniques will choose the circle system. Others may find the light weight and reduced bulk of the coaxial circuit advantageous. With either design the circuit must be securely fastened to the patient's head to prevent accidental displacement of the endotracheal tube.

A 2-inch wide band of adhesive tape placed circumferentially about the patient's head and breathing circuit has proved serviceable in our operating rooms. The ears must be padded as well as the forehead, and careful attention to eye protection is required since the patient's head will be covered by the surgical drapes for several hours and not be open to inspection (Fig. 2-2).

POSITIONING OF EQUIPMENT

The anesthesiologist is usually situated adjacent to the patient's right hip, allowing the surgical team free access to the head. A long breathing circuit is a must (Fig. 2-3). Because of this remote positioning relative to the airway and the obscuring of all connectors by the sur-

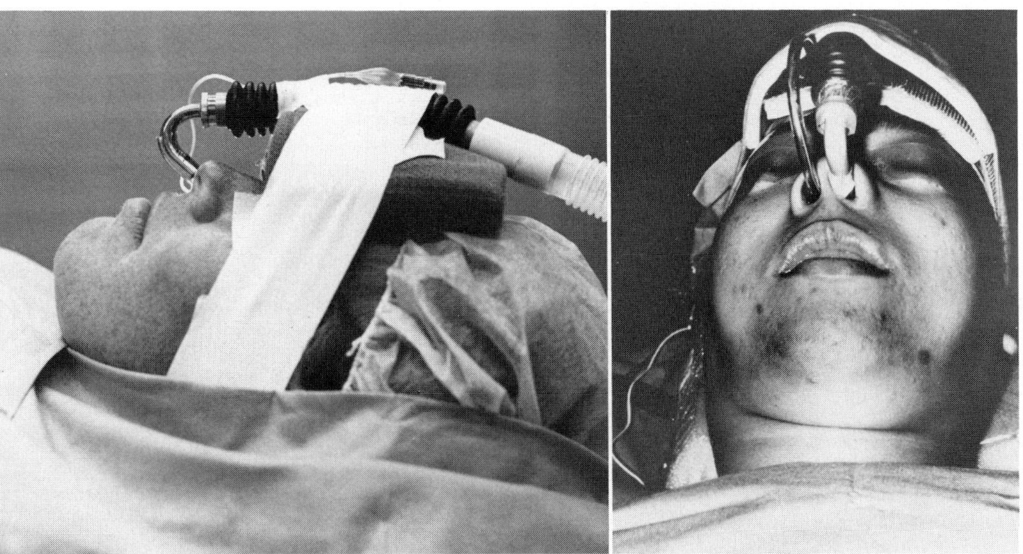

Fig. 2-2.
Low-profile connector in a nasally placed Endotrol tube. The guide ring has been removed. The eyes are lubricated and taped closed. Padding is placed on the forehead and behind the ears before the wide tape band is applied. The head rests on a foam donut to provide greater stability during surgery.

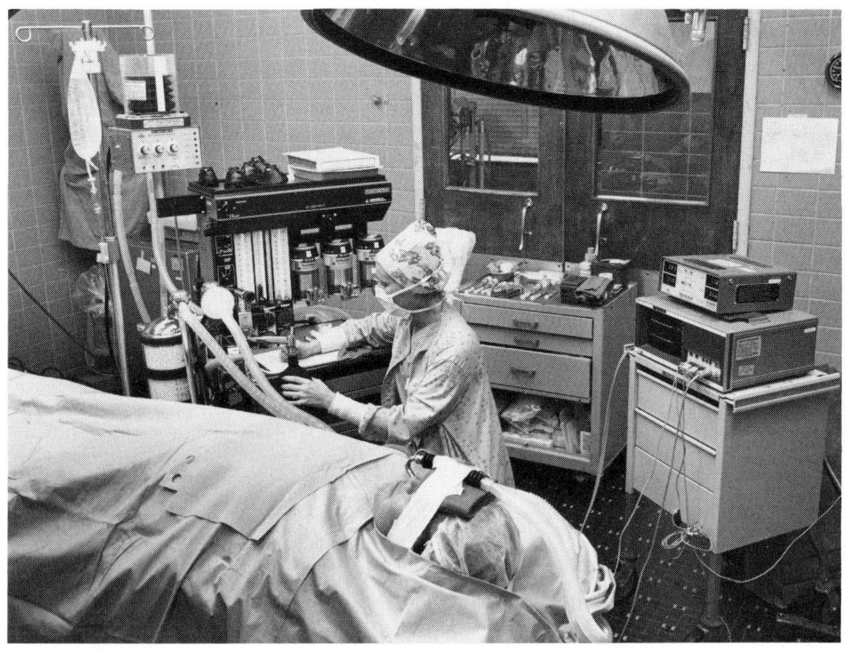

Fig. 2-3.
The anesthesia equipment is situated adjacent to the patient's right hip. The surgical team thus has uncompromised access to the patient's head.

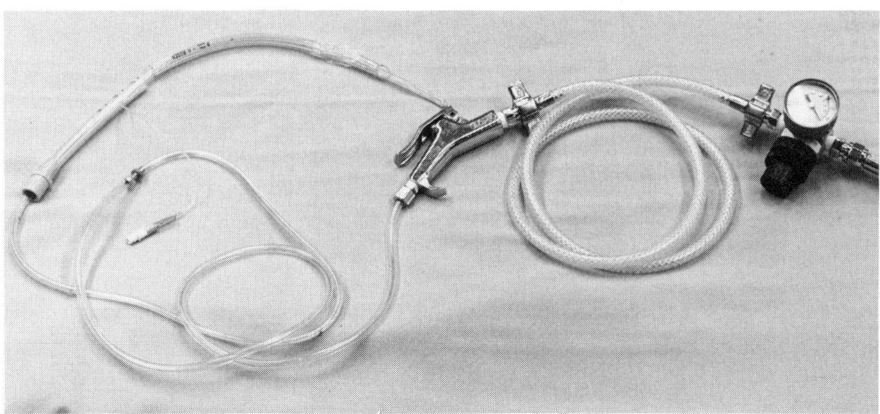

Fig. 2-4.
A nasogastric tube is seen through a partially severed endotracheal tube. An oxygen-powered injector is connected to the proximal end of the nasogastric tube to allow emergency ventilation.

gical drapes, extra vigilance is required to ensure that the endotracheal tube does not become dislodged or the breathing circuit disconnected.

Just as an in-circuit oxygen analyzer can assist the modern anesthesiologist in detecting equipment or gas source failure, an airway pressure alarm can help detect a loss of positive pressure in the breathing circuit of mechanically ventilated patients. Airway disconnects occurring during spontaneous breathing can be detected by the monitoring of exhaled tidal volume or end tidal carbon dioxide. These breathing circuit monitors represent the standard of anesthesia monitoring, and all modern operating rooms are equipped with them.

Because of the proximity of the endotracheal tube to the operative site, it is possible to sever the pilot tube[23] accidentally or, worse yet, the endotracheal tube itself.[9] Reintubation during the operative procedure is not without hazard but will sometimes be required.

An unusual yet functional solution is to insert a well-lubricated nasogastric tube through the severed endotracheal tube into the trachea. The severed tube can then be removed and a new tube placed over the gastric tube, which serves as a guide to facilitate reintubation of the trachea. During the time that the endotracheal tube is not in place, ventilation can be maintained if necessary by an oxygen powered injector connected to the nasogastric tube. This can often be done without a major violation of the surgical field (Fig. 2-4).

If only the pilot tube is severed, a pharyngeal pack can allow completion of the surgery contingent upon minimal bleeding and the adequacy of ventilation. An arterial blood gas determination would be reassuring or, alternatively, exhaled tidal volume or end tidal carbon dioxide should be monitored. Reintubation with an intact endotracheal tube is mandatory, however, prior to intraoral fixation or in the event that the tube itself is damaged.

MONITORING

Intraoperative monitors for routine cases should include an ECG, precordial stethoscope, blood pressure cuff, and temperature probe. When patient condition demands, monitoring is escalated. If controlled hypotension is used, radial arterial and central venous catheters are placed along with an indwelling bladder catheter to allow measurement of urine output. V_5 is monitored on the electrocardiogram to help detect myocardial ischemia.

Serial hematocrits should guide intraoperative transfusion. Blood requirements can be reduced by allowing isovolemic hemodilution to reduce the hematocrit to approximately 30% before beginning transfusion. As indicated, arterial blood gases, electrolytes, and blood sugar are measured as well.

ANESTHETIC MAINTENANCE

Regardless of whether endotracheal intubation is performed awake or asleep, thiopental sodium (Pentothal) is the induction agent most frequently used. Maintenance is with nitrous oxide and oxygen supplemented with narcotics and other intravenous agents, a potent inhalation anesthetic, or a combination of both. If muscle relaxants are to be avoided, the addition of an inhaled agent provides for a smoother intraoperative course.

Frequent dysrhythmias seen during orthognathic surgical procedures are secondary to the intense sympathetic and parasympathetic stimulation associated with surgical procedures on the maxilla.[1] The addition of potent inhaled agents may help avoid some of these by providing a deeper level of anesthesia. Epinephrine injected by the surgeon can often contribute to these dysrhythmias.

Halothane (Fluothane) has been associated with a high frequency of rhythm disturbances during maxillofacial surgery and is best avoided. Enflurane[2,26] (Ethrane) has been widely studied and is less likely to provoke the appearance of rhythm problems. Isoflurane (Forane) has not been as extensively studied for these operations but seems comparable to enflurane.

DELIBERATE HYPOTENSION

In recent years the application of hypotensive anesthetic techniques to patients undergoing orthognathic surgery has been increasing. The objectives of these techniques are to reduce blood pressure and, as a direct effect,[20] to reduce intraoperative blood loss and the need for

Table 2-2.
Development and treatment of cyanide toxicity

Metabolism of nitroprusside → Cyanide
Cytochrome oxidase + Cyanide → Cyanide-oxidase complex
Diagnosis of toxicity = Acidosis or Drug resistance
Intravenous sodium nitrite + Hemoglobin → Methemoglobin
Cyanide oxidase complex + Methemoglobin → Cytochrome oxidase + Cyanmethemoglobin
Cyanmethemoglobin + Intravenous thiosulfate → Thiocyanate (nontoxic) + Methemoglobin

intraoperative transfusion. Additionally, a drier field permits more precise surgical manipulation and results in shorter operating times.[24] Contraindications include preexisting hypertension, ischemic heart disease, and obstructive cerebrovascular disease. Complications have been well described by Edwards.[7]

In separate studies Shaberg et al.[19] and Chan et al.[6] have shown that a blood pressure reduction of 20% from preoperative levels results in a 40% reduction in operative blood loss. Animal studies by Bergman et al.[3] have examined the regional blood flow variations during deep enflurane anesthesia compared with enflurane in combination with an infusion of sodium nitroprusside (SNP) (Nipride) or nitroglycerin (NTG) (Tridil). They found a greater reduction in orofacial blood flows with the combination of enflurane and an infusion of SNP or NTG and suggested that this reduced flow might help reduce blood loss.

Sodium Nitroprusside

Sodium nitroprusside (SNP),[21] a potent arterial and venous vasodilator, has been associated with tachyphylaxis and rebound hypertension after discontinuation of the drug. Tachyphylaxis, if it occurs, is managed by switching to another hypotensive technique. Rebound hypertension[15,22] can be precipitated by rapid termination of the infusion but will usually be avoided by tapering the infusion rate over 30 minutes. Pretreatment with propranolol (Inderal) has also been effective in preventing the rebound hypertension.

SNP infusion has also been associated with cyanide toxicity and sudden death. The drug is metabolized to cyanide, which can interfere with oxidative phosphorylation by binding to cytochrome oxidase and causing diffuse cellular injury. Administration of captopril (Capoten), a converting enzyme inhibitor, prior to the infusion of SNP has been associated with a marked reduction in SNP dose requirements and a parallel reduction in blood cyanide levels.[25] Signs of cyanide toxicity include increasing dose requirements, systemic acidosis, and rising mixed venous oxygen content. In the face of any of these signs the drug infusion should be stopped and cyanide antagonists administered if acidosis or hypotension persist. Cyanide antagonists include sodium nitrite followed by sodium thiosulfate, both administered intravenously. Table 2-2 outlines the steps in development and treatment of cyanide poisoning.

Nitroglycerin

Because nitroglycerin (NTG),[10] a mild arterial and marked venous dilator, has not been associated with any of the aforementioned complications, it may be safer. However, some young patients receiving a narcotic-based anesthetic may be relatively refractory to NTG's hypotensive action, making adequate operating conditions difficult to establish and maintain. Additionally, Todd et al.[22] have shown that the hypotension induced by NTG may persist for some time after the infusion is terminated, a serious disadvantage in surgical procedures in which the identification of bleeding sites is dependent upon the restoration of normal blood pressure.

Adenosine Triphosphate

A more recent addition to the pharmacologic armamentarium is adenosine triphosphate (ATP),[11,18] a potent arterial vasodilator. This naturally occurring adenine nucleotide has been used to induce intraoperative hypotension.[12] Tachyphylaxis does not occur and toxic metabolites are not produced. Blood pressure was easily controlled in the studies reported. A sinus bradycardia is produced, but cardiac output is well maintained. Like SNP and NTG, ATP reduces blood flow in orofacial bony structures.[18] Further clinical trials during procedures in the maxillofacial area will determine its utility in humans.

ISOFLURANE

Recently Bishay et al.[4] described a group of patients undergoing orthognathic surgical procedures utilizing induced hypotension produced by the administration of high concentrations of inhaled isoflurane. They found the technique simple, convenient, and easy to control. Additional studies are necessary to compare this technique to others already mentioned before a single choice can be made.

POSTOPERATIVE CARE

At the completion of the operative procedure a decision is made concerning the length of time the patient will require intubation. If the patient is to be left intubated for a few hours or longer, a narcotic analgesic should be administered before the patient awakens. Intravenous xylocaine 1 to 1.5 mg/kg may help suppress coughing stimulated by the endotracheal tube, but the effect is short lived. Narcotics appear to be more effective antitussives in the awake patient. Nausea should be treated with an antiemetic such as droperidol (Inapsine), a gastric emptying agent such as metoclopramide (Reglan), or a nasogastric tube. If analgesics are required, methadone (Dolophine), a long-acting agent chosen for its lower incidence of nausea, should be administered. Another useful property of methadone is that it causes less sedation than other narcotic analgesics and its use may permit earlier extubation.[13]

Proper timing of extubation is a critical decision, which should be made jointly by the surgeon and the anesthesiologist. Patients must be fully awake and have intact airway reflexes. Care must be exercised in patients who have received a narcotic antagonist since they may renarcotize during the period of reduced observation following extubation. Additionally, the use of narcotic antagonists may result in

hypertension, tachycardia, or even vomiting (a serious problem for the patient in intraoral fixation).

The usual criteria of sustained head lift, a 20 cm H_2O subatmospheric inspiratory pressure, or a vital capacity in excess of 15 ml/kg demonstrate the absence of clinically significant residual muscle relaxant effects. Intraoral bleeding must be minimal. If the patient has been placed in intraoral fixation, a wire cutter must be at the bedside. Finally, a member of the surgical team must be available at the bedside in the event that urgent reintubation is required.

When all these criteria are met, the patient may be safely extubated. After a suitable interval of recovery room observation the patient is returned to the ward bed.

SUMMARY

I have endeavored to review several of the aspects of anesthesia care unique to orthognathic surgery. Prospective payment plans will encourage outpatient evaluation and shorter hospital stays. Continuing advances in pharmacology and noninvasive monitoring will make controlled hypotension easier and safer; but regardless of technologic advance, the patient will continue to be dependent upon a skillful and caring operating team. In the final analysis, successful outcomes will always be based on the tripod of thorough preoperative workup, careful intraoperative management, and attentive postoperative surveillance.

REFERENCES

1. Alexander, J.P., and Murtagh, J.G.: Arrhythmia during oral surgery: fasicular blocks in the cardiac conducting system, Br. J. Anaesthesiol. **51:**149, 1979.
2. Barker, G.L., and Briscoe, C.E.: The Pathfinder high-speed E.C.G. analyser, Br. J. Anaesthesiol. **53:**1079, 1981.
3. Bergman, S., et al.: Blood flow to oral tissues: an experimental study with enflurane, sodium nitroprusside, and nitroglycerin, J. Oral Maxillofac. Surg. **40:**13, 1982.
4. Bishay, E., et al.: Cardiovascular effects of prolonged isoflurane induced hypotension. Presented at the annual meeting of the International Anesthesia Research Society, March 1984.
5. Brunsoman, J.K., et al.: A new endotracheal tube for maxillofacial surgery, J. Oral Surg. **38:**847, 1980.
6. Chan, W., et al.: Effects of hypotensive anesthesia in anterior maxillary osteotomy, J. Oral Surg. **38:**504, 1980.

7. Edwards, M.W., Jr.: Complications of deliberate hypotension. In Orkin, F.K., and Cooperman, L.H., editors: Complications in anesthesia, Philadelphia, 1983, J.B. Lippincott Co.

8. Egbert, L.D., et al.: The value of the preoperative visit by an anesthetist, JAMA **185:**553, 1963.

9. Fagraeus, L., et al.: A serious anesthetic hazard during orthognathic surgery, Anesth. Analg. **59:**150, 1980.

10. Fahmy, N.R.: Nitroglycerin as a hypotensive drug during general anesthesia, Anesthesiology **49:**17, 1978.

11. Fukunaga, A.F., et al.: ATP-induced hypotensive anesthesia during surgery, Anesthesiology **57**(3A):A65, 1982.

12. Fukunaga, A.F., et al.: Hypotensive effects of adenosine and adenosine triphosphate compared with sodium nitroprusside, Anesth. Analg. **61:**273, 1982.

13. Goth, A.: Medical pharmacology: principles and concepts, ed. 9, St. Louis, 1978, The C.V. Mosby Co.

14. Grzesik, L., and Kurek, M.: Nasotracheal general anesthesia in maxillofacial surgery, Anaesth. Resusc. Intensive Ther. **3:**165, 1975.

15. Khambatta, H.J., et al.: Hypertension during anesthesia on discontinuation of sodium nitroprusside-induced hypotension, Anesthesiology **51:**127, 1979.

16. O'Ryan, F., and Epker, B.N.: Prolonged apnea after orthognathic surgery due to atypical cholinesterase, Int. J. Oral Surg. **10:**338, 1981.

17. Roizen, M.F.: Preoperative evaluation of the healthy patient. In Miller, R.D., editor: Anesthesia, New York, 1981, Churchill Livingstone, Inc.

18. Satinover, I.A., et al.: A comparison of the cardiovascular and orofacial blood flow changes resulting from hypotension induced by sodium nitroprusside and adenosine triphosphate in the rat, J. Oral Maxillofac. Surg. **41:**500, 1983.

19. Schaberg, S.J., et al.: Blood loss and hypotensive anesthesia in oral-facial corrective surgery, J. Oral Surg. **34:**147, 1976.

20. Sivarajan, M., et al.: Blood pressure, not cardiac output, determines blood loss during induced hypotension, Anesth. Analg. **59:**203, 1980.

21. Tinker, J.H., and Michenfelder, J.D.: Sodium nitroprusside, Anesthesiology **45:**340, 1976.

22. Todd, M.M., et al.: Hemodynamic consequences of abrupt withdrawal of nitroprusside or nitroglycerin following induced hypotension, Anesth. Analg. **61:**261, 1982.

23. Tsueda, K., et al.: Hazards to anesthetic equipment during maxillary osteotomy: report of cases, J. Oral Surg. **35:**47, 1977.

24. Washburn, M.C., and Hyer, R.L.: Deliberate hypotension for elective major maxillofacial surgery: a balanced halothane and morphine technique, J. Maxillofac. Surg. **10:**50, 1982.

25. Woodside, J., et al.: Captopril reduces the dose requirement for sodium nitroprusside induced hypotension, Anesthesiology **60:**413, 1984.

26. Wright, C.J.: Dysrhythmias during oral surgery: a comparison between halothane and enflurane anaesthesia, Anaesthesia **35:**775, 1980.

CHAPTER 3

Role of the total maxillary alveolar osteotomy in orthognathic surgery

STERLING R. SCHOW

With the large number of patients now being treated for deformities of the midface and maxilla by an ever increasing variety of procedures, degree of expertise, and greater number of surgeons, it is difficult to realize that the first report of maxillary surgery in English for the correction of dentofacial deformities was published in 1959.[20] In 1870 Cheever[11] described operations of the right hemimaxilla and total maxilla, in different patients, for gaining access to nasopharyngeal tumors. In 1921 Cohn-Stock[12] reported a segmental osteotomy of the maxilla, and in 1935 Wassmund[32] described a total maxillary or LeFort I osteotomy for movement of the entire maxilla to a new position.

Obwegeser's visit to the United States in 1966 generated considerable interest and enthusiasm toward investigation and utilization of maxillary surgical procedures in the correction of dentofacial deformities. The concentrated effort devoted to improved recognition, treatment planning, and care of problems in the midface in which we are involved today really began less than 20 years ago. Since the mid-1960s few publications dealing with surgical correction of the masticatory apparatus have failed to devote considerable time to maxillary surgery.

The purpose of this chapter is to review one of the many surgical procedures developed for correction of maxillary deformities—the total maxillary alveolar osteotomy (TMAO) or simultaneous osteotomies of the posterior and anterior maxillary alveolar processes.

HISTORY

In 1969 Paul[25] described his treatment of a patient with midface hypoplasia utilizing a total alveolar procedure based on the experiences of Kole[21] and Mohnac.[23] Other authors[1,2,37] published their experiences with posterior (Schuchardt,[27] Kufner[22]) and anterior segmental maxillary osteotomies, all of which have contributed to the fund of knowledge drawn upon in the design of maxillary surgery in its present form.

In 1972 West and Epker[33] discussed posterior maxillary surgery and its place in the treatment of dentofacial deformities. They also combined operations on the posterior alveoli with anterior maxillary surgery to mobilize the entire alveolar process, and they listed as indications for this surgery the following: (1) correction of posterior maxillary alveolar hyperplasia, (2) correction of total maxillary alveolar hyperplasia, (3) correction of posterior crossbite, and (4) repositioning of the posterior maxillary alveolar fragment to provide space for an impacted tooth.

Subsequent publications by Hall and Roddy,[17] Wolford and Epker,[36] West and McNeill,[34] and Hall and West[18] further described the total maxillary alveolar osteotomy, in single or multiple segments, and expanded upon the indications, intricacies, and methods of achieving the desired surgical results. Considerable emphasis was placed upon treatment planning and stability of the surgical result in these papers. In addition, the recognition and diagnostic evaluation of maxillary alveolar hyperplasia and vertical facial excess was described in detail.

Few truly new contributions or findings concerning the total maxillary alveolar osteotomy have been published since 1976. Maloney et al.[24] reviewed the procedure in 1982 and (surprisingly, based upon their experience and review of two patients) concluded the TMAO a "good technique in its time" but one now rarely of use. However, they did comment on the stability of results obtained and generally gave a favorable accounting of the versatility of this alveolar surgery, basing their objections to the operation upon its difficulty of accomplishment compared to other surgical procedures.

By contrast, we find several conditions existing in the maxilla that lend themselves well to correction with the TMAO and other deformities that may be approached equally well with the TMAO or the LeFort I down-fracture osteotomy. Nevertheless, there are times when the TMAO is not indicated and the LeFort I osteotomy is the procedure of choice.

INDICATIONS

Our experience with the total maxillary alveolar osteotomy (TMAO), in single or multiple segments, has been accumulated through its use on more than 150 patients over 8 years. Although it may require more exacting and time-consuming surgery than other operations used to achieve similar results, we have never been impressed with its difficulty to the point of avoiding it when we felt there was an advantage in doing so. As would be expected with any surgical technique, familiarity, repeated use, and adaptation of the method to a well-defined set of problems all enhance the surgeon's skill, ability, and speed.

The TMAO is used to best advantage in the intrusion of a hyperplastic maxillary alveolus to correct posterior or total alveolar hyperplasia with or without anterior open-bite. This is particularly true when impaction of the segments will be 5 mm or more. We have observed significant obstruction of the nasal airway when a large amount of vertical impaction was done with the LeFort I osteotomy, particularly in the posterior maxilla. Other authors[7,13,30] have also commented on the potential for obstruction

when the palate is elevated to excess. Deliberate correction of vertical maxillary excess with a procedure such as the LeFort I osteotomy unquestionably will violate the integrity of the nasal airway. This does not seem advisable, especially when one considers that a compromised airway may have been the cause of the problem from the beginning.[10,19] With the TMAO, impaction of the posterior maxillary segments is done at the expense of the maxillary sinus. Anteriorly the hyperplastic alveolar process may frequently be sectioned for intrusion below the level of the piriform rim of the nose (in the alveolar process itself), and the dentoalveolar segment elevated with no obstruction of the anterior nares. When an adequate amount of alveolar process is not available between the tooth apices and the piriform rims to allow the desired amount of vertical repositioning subnasally, the difference must be made up by a degree of anterior impingement into the nasal cavity. However, this is modified somewhat by grooving the superior surface of the alveolar segment to accommodate the nasal septum and by removing a portion of the cartilaginous nasal septum if needed. Seldom if ever, despite the amount of vertical alveolar repositioning, does the TMAO result in compromise of the nasal airway. Because the horizontal hard palate and the floor of the nose are not mobilized, the inferior turbinates do not become an obstruction to the repositioned segments as they may with impaction of the total maxilla. Bothersome procedures such as turbinectomy or fracturing of the nasal turbinates[8,30] are thus avoided.

The deep, highly arched, palatal vault frequently seen with maxillary alveolar hyperplasia is used to advantage in completion of the TMAO. The tall vertical palatal shelves make osteotomies at the junction of the vertical and horizontal portions of the palate easy to accomplish into the nasal cavity anteriorly and into the maxillary sinus posteriorly. This is the case when the surgery on the palatal portion of the alveolus is done with either facial (transantral) or palatal access. The methods of approaching the palatal osteotomies will be reviewed later in the chapter. It is mentioned here only to point out the potential surgical advantage of the TMAO in patients with vertical alveolar excess.

After impaction of the alveolar segments the highly arched palate is somewhat flattened and assumes a more normal contour.

The TMAO may also be used to advantage, even in the absence of vertical maxillary excess, when multiple alveolar segments are to be used to expand, contract, or recontour the constricted, excessively wide, or malformed alveolar process. In these instances it provides an alternative to the LeFort I down-fracturing procedure and offers the advantage of retaining a stable virtually untouched horizontal hard palate, an intact nasal airway, and the ability to address many maxillary deformities where they exist (in the alveolar process itself).

The TMAO is not the procedure of choice in two instances—when the maxilla is to be significantly advanced to correct horizontal maxillary deficiency and when the maxilla is to be down-grafted in the treatment of a short face. Close approximation of the intact horizontal hard palate and the mobilized alveolar segment is lost when these movements are accomplished. As a result, not only is intraoperative and postoperative stability somewhat compromised but a very real possibility of oronasal fistula development on the palate is created. If the objective of surgery is advancement or inferior positioning of the maxilla, the LeFort I osteotomy is better suited.

TREATMENT PLANNING

A detailed and carefully completed evaluation of the patient to include clinical examination, photographs, cephalometric studies of both soft and hard tissue, and study models properly transferred to a semiadjustable articulator will provide the necessary information to make a choice of the surgery to be performed. Preoperative diagnosis, clinical evaluation, cephalometric norms, and the formulation of data-based patient problem lists and surgical planning with cephalometric templates and model surgery have been well detailed by many authors* and will not be reviewed in this chapter.

The surgical changes and effects on facial

____
*References 6, 14-16, 18, 31, 33, 36.

soft tissues and postoperative stability with the TMAO are no different from those expected with the LeFort I osteotomy. For example, when planning maxillary impaction to correct vertical excess and overexposure of the anterior teeth, we may predict that the upper lip will move superiorly 20% as far as the upper anterior teeth are moved by the operation.

Model surgery, however, must be varied from that done when planning a LeFort I procedure. The palatal osteotomies with the TMAO are placed at the junction of the horizontal and vertical processes of the hard palate. The planning osteotomies on the surgical models should be made in the same location as the osseous incisions will be done at surgery. The horizontal palate on the models is not moved from its preoperative position. After the alveolar processes on the models have been repositioned to their desired location, the osteotomy sites are slightly overwaxed to provide soft tissue relief from the acrylic palatal surgical stent that will be constructed on the surgical models. Appliances so constructed will have little chance of exerting excessive pressure on the palatal mucosa when used at surgery (Fig. 3-1).

If the mandible will autorotate to the repositioned maxillary dentition in satisfactory occlusion, a final interocclusal acrylic wafer is fabricated to be used in positioning the maxilla accurately during surgery and during the period of intermaxillary fixation. If the mandible will not autorotate to a satisfactory occlusion, an intermediate acrylic interocclusal appliance is constructed between the repositioned maxillary dentition and the nonrepositioned mandibular model. This appliance will be used intraoperatively, after the maxillary alveolus has been mobilized, to ensure proper repositioning and stabilization of the alveolus in its new position while the mandible remains intact. The intermediate interocclusal appliance is retained for the surgical procedure and the mandibular model is repositioned to the desired occlusal relationship. A final interocclusal acrylic appliance is then fabricated on the surgical models and retained for use at surgery (Fig. 3-2).

Accurate dimensional recording of the planned surgery is made on both the surgical models and in the patient's record to be readily available in the operating room. The availability of the appliances and measurements of the proposed changes will ensure accurate and rewarding surgical results with an absence of confusion and minimal error or delay when the osteotomies are completed.

Of particular advantage with the TMAO is the ability to utilize the stable, unoperated, horizontal hard palate for vertical stability with the application of an acrylic palatal appliance. Positioning of the mobilized maxillary alveolus by use of an intermediate acrylic interocclusal appliance with the intact mandible and suspension or fixation of the alveolus by transosseous wiring, circumzygomatic suspension, piriform rim suspension, or inferior orbital rim suspension, in combination with a palatal appliance

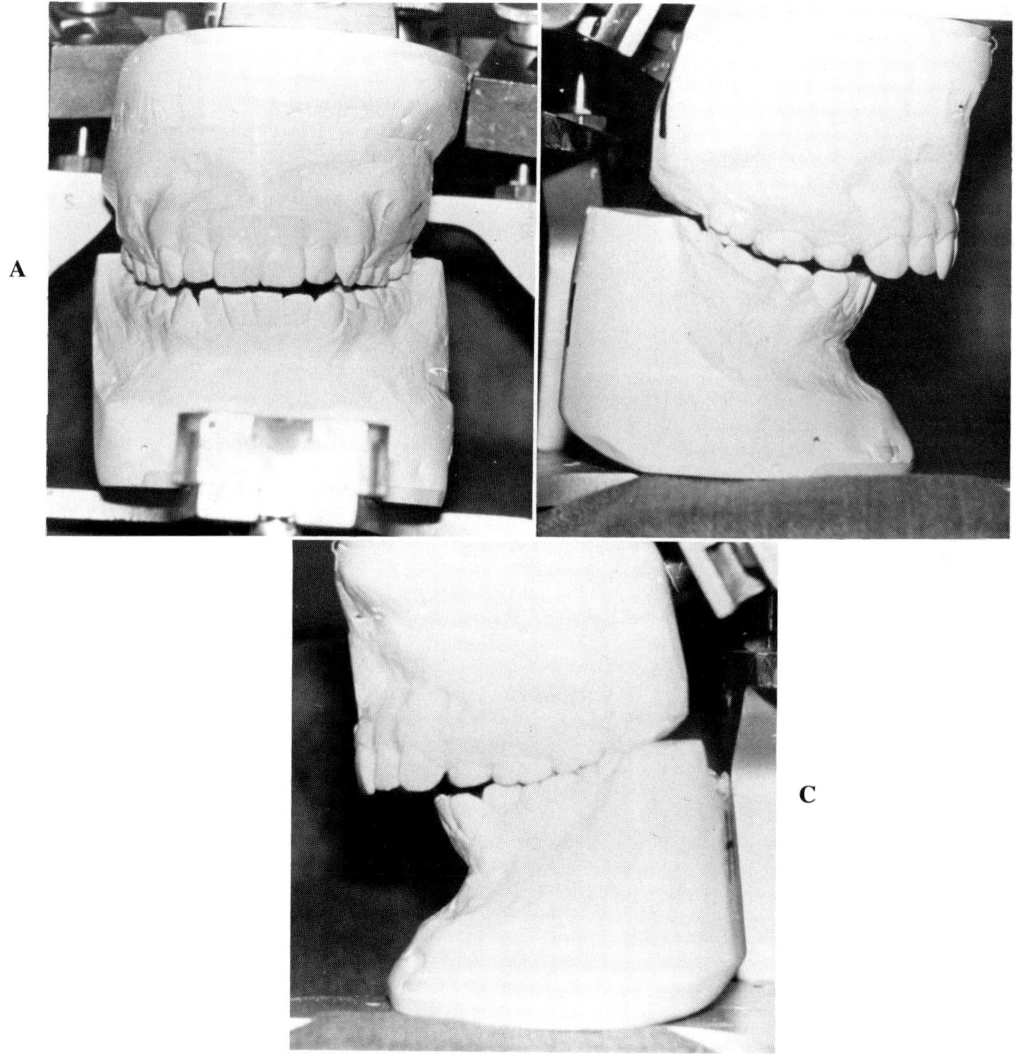

Continued.

Fig. 3-1.
A to **C,** Preoperative models mounted on a semiadjustable anatomic articulator with a facebow transfer. There is facial asymmetry, vertical maxillary excess, and a retrognathic mandible.

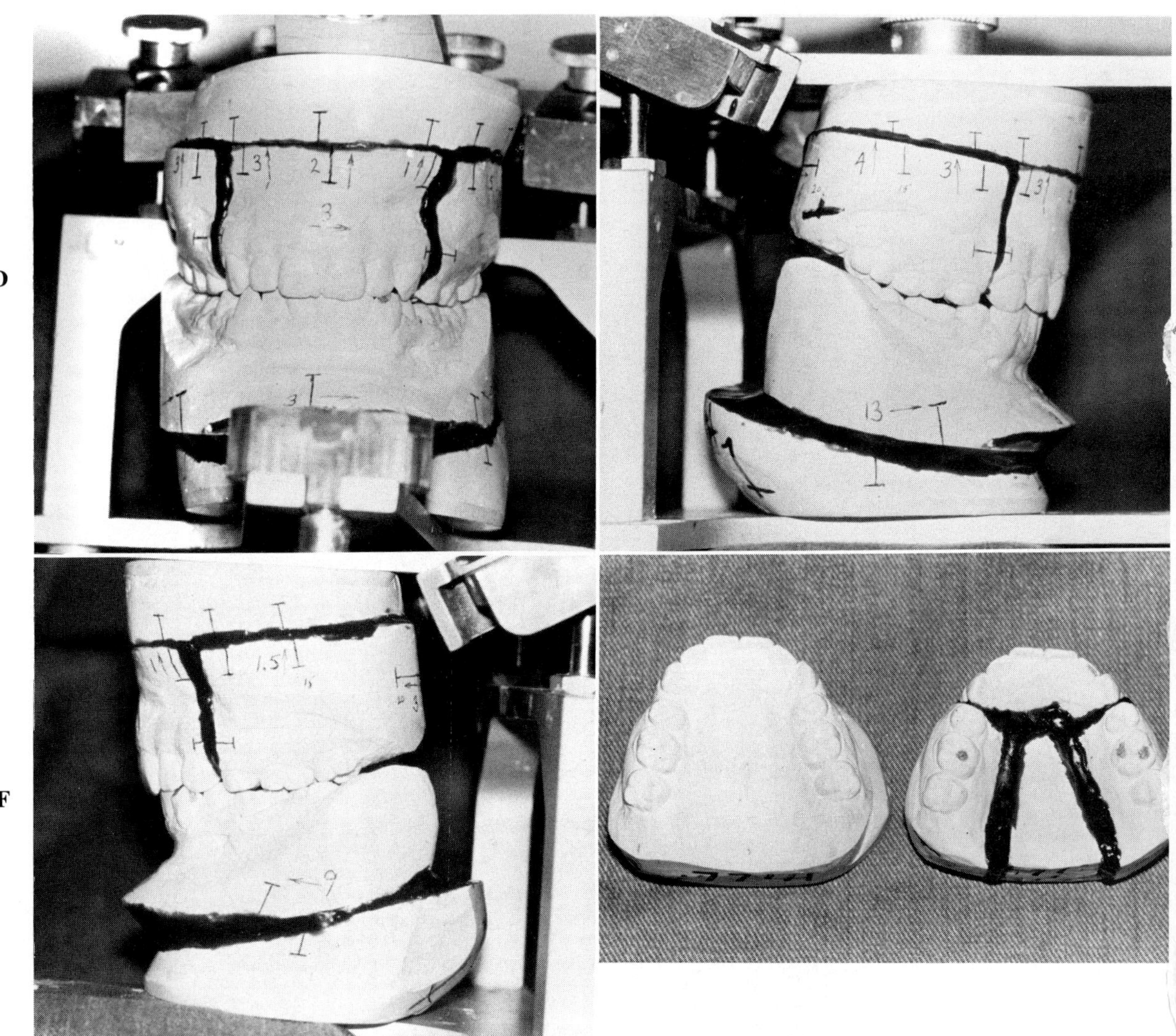

Fig. 3-1—cont'd.
D to **F,** "Operated" models with the dimensions of the osteotomies and segmental movements marked. Interocclusal intermediate and final acrylic appliances will be constructed to these models to assist the positioning and stabilization of the mobilized segments at surgery. **G,** Palatal views of preoperative and postoperative models. Note the position of the palatal osteotomy sites at the junction of the vertical and horizontal palatal osseous walls.

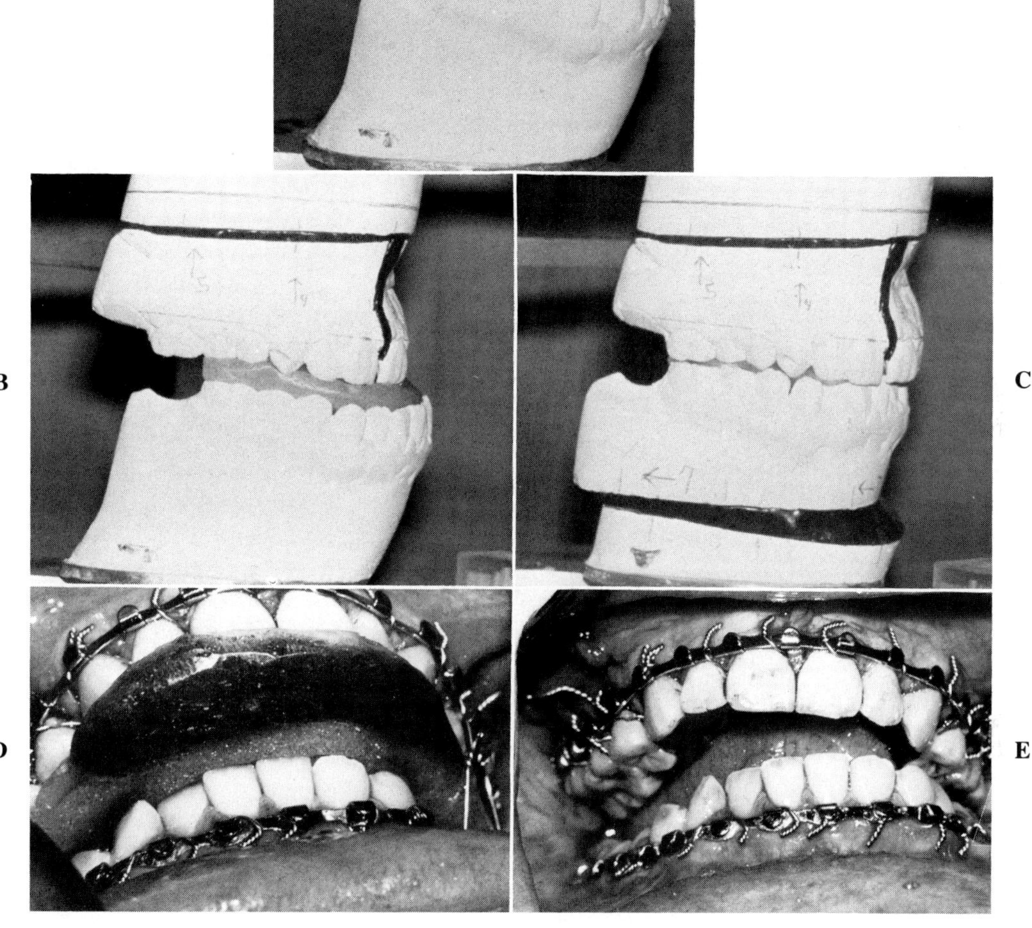

Fig. 3-2.
A, Models of a patient with vertical maxillary excess, maxillary constriction, and mandibular prognathism. The planned maxillary surgery has been completed on the models. **B,** An interocclusal intermediate wafer has been constructed between the "operated" maxilla and the intact mandible. This appliance will be used at surgery to position and stabilize the mobilized maxilla. **C,** Surgery has been planned for the mandible, and the ultimate occlusal relationship determined. A final occlusal wafer, to be used during the period of intermaxillary fixation, has been constructed. **D,** At surgery for a patient with vertical maxillary excess and asymmetry, the mobilized maxillary alveolus is being repositioned and stabilized by means of the intermediate wafer. The intact mandible, fully retruded in the condylar fossae, ensures accurate positioning. **E,** The maxillary alveolus has been stabilized, and the intermediate wafer removed. Mandibular surgery will now be completed. Note the alveolus repositioned superiorly more on the right than on the left to correct the facial asymmetry.

stabilizing the alveolus against the intact hard palate, ensure positive fixation of the maxilla. The intraoperative stability of a maxillary alveolus so immobilized is very reassuring when the surgeon proceeds to any subsequent mandibular osteotomy.

SEGMENT VITALITY

In studies on bone healing and revascularization after anterior, posterior, and total maxillary osteotomy, Bell,[2] Bell and Levy,[5] and Bell et al.[9] demonstrated the viability of large or small segments of the maxilla when vascular pedicles from palatal, facial, or both mucosal surfaces were not detached from the osteotomized segments. These authors further determined that ligation of the greater palatine arteries bilaterally did not adversely affect the outcome of maxillary surgery when adequate palatal mucosa and labiobuccal gingival pedicles were maintained, and they concluded that the transosseous and soft tissue collateral circulation as well as the numerous vascular anastomoses of the maxilla allowed for considerable variation of osteotomy techniques without jeopardizing the periosteal blood supply to the dentoalveolar segments.

As pointed out by Azaz and Shteyer[1] and Westwood and Tilson,[35] the most common complication in surgery with multiple segments is loss or devitalization of an occasional tooth adjacent to an interradicular osteotomy site. This has occurred infrequently in our practice and is rarely a problem in properly planned surgery.

On the basis of these studies, well-designed maxillary alveolar osteotomies, in single or multiple segments, are comfortably within the realm of most maxillofacial surgeons' capabilities.

STABILITY

The postoperative stability of the healed osteotomized maxilla, in particular the maxilla that has been superiorly repositioned, has been well documented for both the LeFort I osteotomy* and the total maxillary alveolar osteotomy.† In our series of patients we have also

---

been impressed with the absence of long-term relapse toward the preoperative condition.

However, it must be stressed that this stability is secondary to proper treatment planning, adequate mobilization of the segments during surgery, adequate stabilization and fixation during the healing period, and provision for a long-term stable and functional occlusion after the jaws have been mobilized.

We have been particularly impressed with the intraoperative stability after fixation and suspension of the TMAO. If the occlusion is satisfactory, intermaxillary fixation may not be necessary after a surgical procedure in the maxilla alone. Instead, the patient is allowed to function, is prescribed a soft diet for the initial 3 to 4 postoperative weeks, and wears light training elastics to the mandibular appliances if they are required for minor repositioning of the maxillary segments during the first few weeks.

The intact horizontal hard palate, bridged to a surgical stent attached to the dentition by circumdental wires, provides outstanding vertical maxillary stability and helps prevent additional vertical impaction of the posterior maxilla if craniofacial suspension must be maintained or function is allowed. Lateral stability is provided by the suspension used, transosseous wiring, and the lateral and anterior osteotomized shelves of the intact horizontal hard palate and their relationship to the impacted alveolar segments. There need be little concern for inadvertent mobilization of a maxillary alveolus so stabilized when attention is directed to the osteotomies and mobilization of the mandible in two-jaw surgical procedures.

SURGICAL TECHNIQUE

The total maxillary alveolar osteotomy may be accomplished with surgical access obtained solely through horizontal mucoperiosteal incisions near the depth of the labial vestibule,[13,33,36] similar to those described for the LeFort I down-fracture, or through multiple vertical facial incisions with tunneling beneath the alveolar mucosa and palatal access through incision and elevation of a palatal "horseshoe" mucoperiosteal flap.[7,17,18,34]

Either procedure can be expected to be readily accomplished when vertical positioning of the maxillary alveolus is planned. Both pro-

---

*References 14, 24, 26, 29.
†References 13, 24, 26, 28, 36.

cedures are easily adapted to mobilizing the alveolus in single or multiple segments. In these instances selection of the procedure to be used depends upon the experience or whim of the surgeon. However, it is our opinion that significant intrusion (beyond 5 mm) of the alveolus is somewhat more cumbersome if the palate is not exposed and osteotomized directly. This is because of the relative inelasticity of the dense mucoperiosteum of the palate. When significant vertical repositioning is planned, adequate mobility of the alveolar segment or segments is more readily obtained when the palatal mucosa is properly incised, reflected, and repositioned after intrusion of the segments.

In addition, transantral and transalveolar access to complete the osteotomies on the palatal side of the alveolus is difficult when only a facial approach is used and the TMAO is being done for recontouring of the alveolus and not for vertical repositioning. The narrow facial osteotomies needed here make visualization of the medial wall of the sinus and direction of instruments transantrally to complete the palatal osteotomies difficult to accomplish. We therefore prefer to perform the TMAO on these occasions with both facial and direct palatal access.

The most difficult area to osteotomize and mobilize adequately is the posterior portion of the maxillary tuberosity. Accomplishing the TMAO via horizontal incisions from the facial allows better visibility and access than when the procedure is performed with both facial and palatal access. However, this rarely presents a significant problem with either approach. Furthermore, if the maxillary tuberosity is of adequate length proximal to the last molar or if maxillary third molars have been recently removed, the osteotomies do not need to be carried to the pterygomaxillary junction to mobilize the alveolar segments. Instead, the horizontal subapical osteotomies on both facial and palatal surfaces, regardless of the technique being used, may be directed to either the tuberosity or the third molar extraction socket and then continued vertically to the alveolar crest, avoiding the necessity of osteotomizing or fracturing the posterior wall of the tuberosity.

We most frequently approach the TMAO from both the facial and the palatal surfaces.

These will be described in the next several paragraphs, and the reader's choice of technique should be based on personal experience and on individual objectives. Either the buccal or the palatal soft tissue alone is capable of providing adequate blood supply to the richly anastomosing vessels in the anterior and posterior osseous segments,[18] and these procedures generally retain a blood supply to the segments from both mucosal surfaces.

TMAO through horizontal labial incisions[13,33,36] (Fig. 3-3)

1. A circumvestibular incision, similar to that performed for the LeFort I osteotomy, is made at or slightly above the root apices from the right to the left zygomaticoalveolar crest.

2. The mucoperiosteum is elevated minimally inferiorly, leaving as much alveolar mucosa and gingiva attached to the dentoalveolus as possible.

3. Superior to the incision the mucoperiosteum is elevated to expose the lateral maxillary walls and, in the anterior maxilla, the piriform rims and anterior nasal spine. Posterior to the zygomaticoalveolar crests the mucoperiosteum is tunneled and undermined to reach the pterygomaxillary junctions. Anteriorly the nasal mucoperiosteum is elevated from the lateral nasal walls, nasal floor, and inferior nasal septum extending 10 to 15 mm into the nasal cavity. This exposes the anterior floor of the nose.

4. The proposed horizontal osteotomy line is identified 4 to 5 mm above the apices of the teeth and vertical reference lines are etched on the lateral maxillary walls to cross the proposed horizontal osteotomy. After insertion of a nasal freer or other protective instrument along the lateral nasal wall beneath the nasal mucoperiosteum (to protect it from being cut by a bur), the horizontal osteotomy through the lateral maxillary wall is made and extended from the nasal cavity to the pterygomaxillary junction. The anterior 10 to 15 mm of the osseous lateral nasal wall is also transected.

5. If an ostectomy with alveolar impaction is planned, the inferior osteotomy is completed initially 4 to 5 mm above the tooth apices and is followed by the superior osteotomy to remove the measured amount of bone from the lateral

Text continued on p. 60.

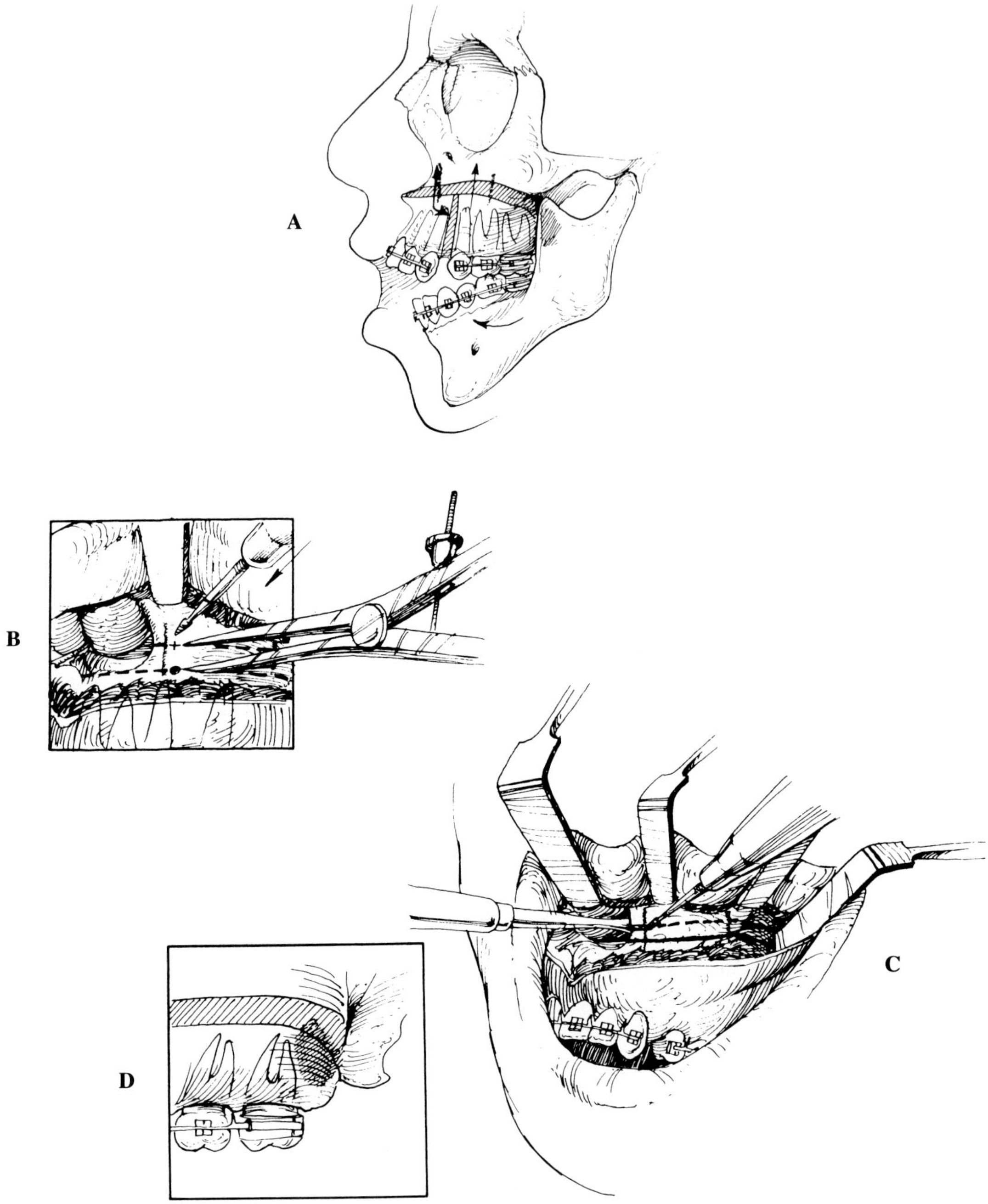

Fig. 3-3.
A, Planned total maxillary alveolar surgery in three segments to be accomplished from a facial approach. **B,** After exposure of the piriform aperture and lateral maxillary walls, the planned horizontal ostectomy and vertical reference lines are marked and begun. **C,** The nasal mucosa is elevated from the floor and lateral nasal walls and is protected with a retractor while the horizontal osteotomies are completed. **D,** Posterior to the second molar the ostectomy is directed inferiorly through the tuberosity and into the pterygomaxillary fissure.

A to **P** from Epker, B.N., and Wolford, L.M.: Dentofacial deformities: surgical-orthodontic correction, St. Louis, 1980, The C.V. Mosby Co.

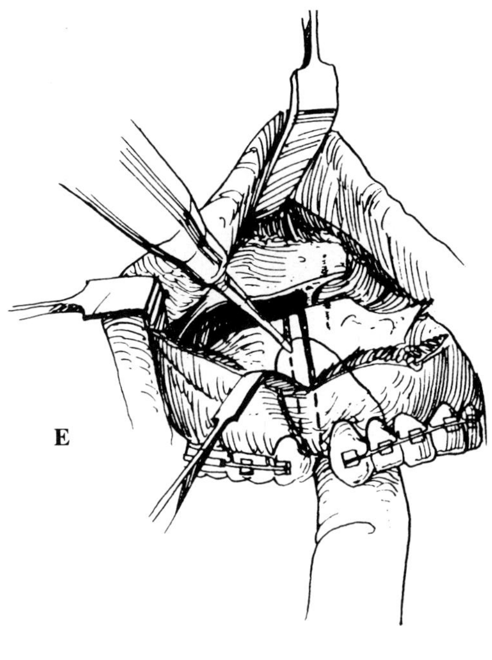

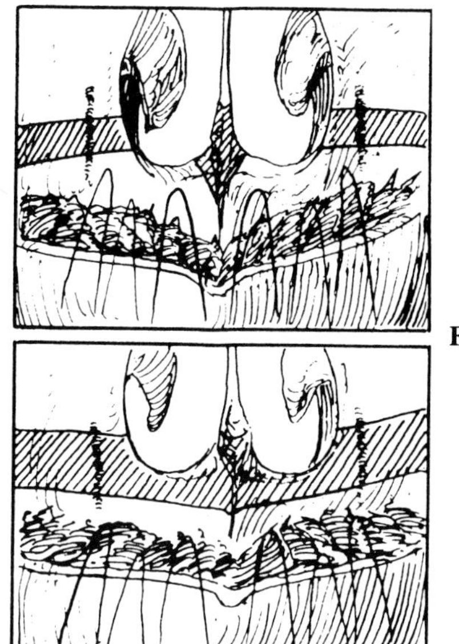

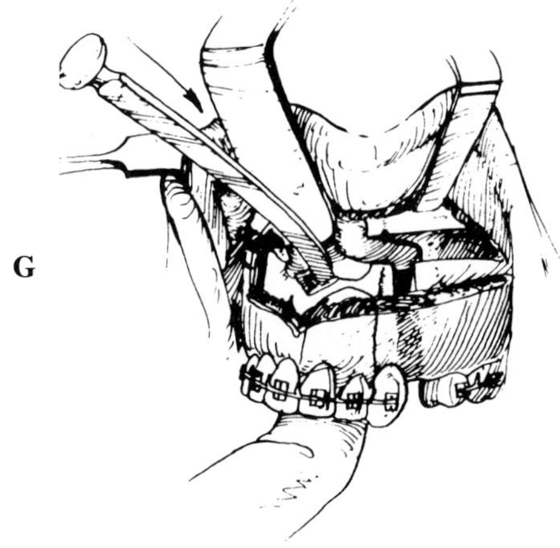

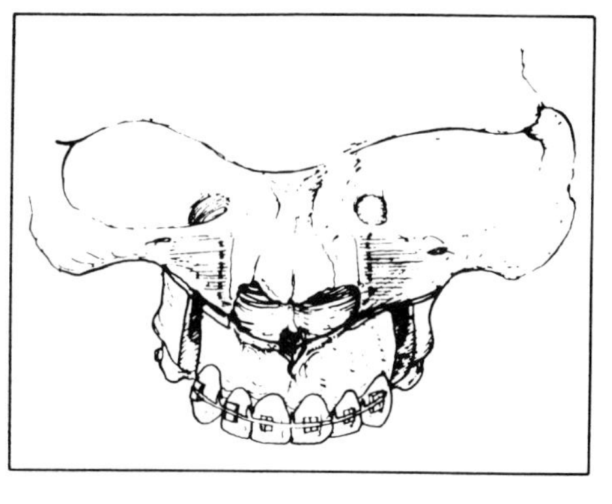

Continued.

Fig. 3-3—cont'd.

E, The vertical ostectomy to segment the dentoalveolus is made from facial to palatal. The palpating finger on the palate confirms completion of the osteotomy and helps prevent injury of the palatal mucosa from overpenetration of the cutting instrument. **F,** Anteriorly the planned ostectomy is carried either into or below the piriform aperture depending on whether sufficient alveolus is available between the root apices and the nasal floor. **G,** The cartilaginous nasal septum has been separated from the superior surface of the maxilla. An osteotome or fissure bur is used to begin the transnasal osteotomy through the palate. A finger is kept on the palate to detect penetration of the instrument through the bone. **H,** Posteriorly and laterally the palatal osteotomy enters the maxillary sinus. It continues posteriorly toward the tuberosity through the medial sinus wall to the junction of the vertical and horizontal osseous palatal walls. More medial direction of the osteotome would create an osteotomy into the nose and should be avoided.

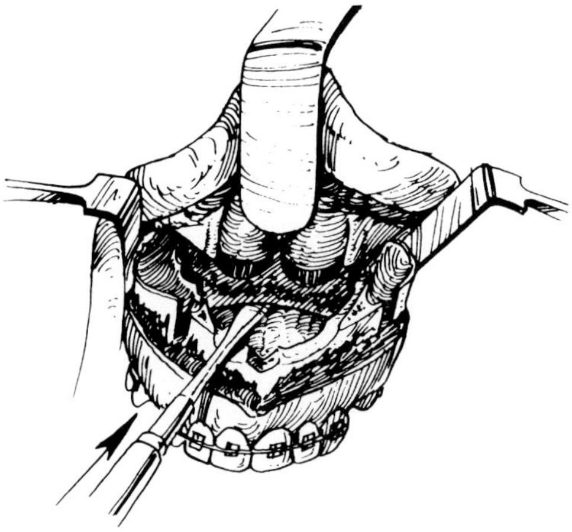

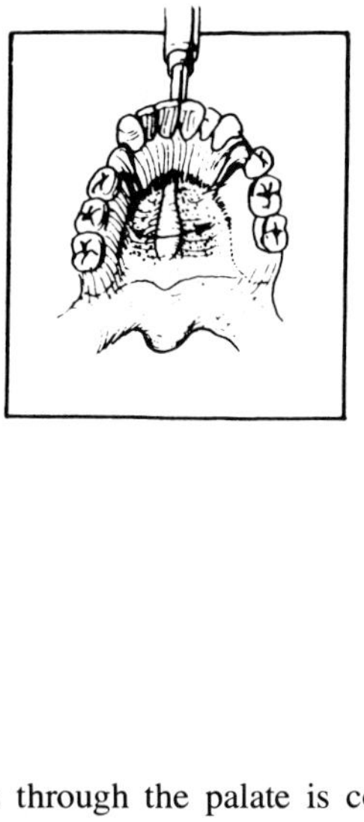

Fig. 3-3—cont'd.
I, The osteotomy on the medial wall of the sinus through the palate is continued transantrally posterior to the first molar. Posterior to this, the thin palatal bone from here to the pterygomaxillary suture will be fractured when the alveolus is mobilized. **J,** The alveolar segments are down-fractured with digital pressure and torquing instruments, in this instance as individual segments. A rotating instrument or an osteotome is then used to relieve the superior maxillary surface, thereby preventing distortion of the nasal septum when the segments are superiorly repositioned. If necessary, a portion of the cartilaginous nasal septum may also be removed. **K,** If the posterior segments are not readily mobilized by down-fracturing, the pterygoid plates are separated from the maxillary tuberosity by means of a small curved osteotome directed medially and slightly anteriorly. **L,** The palatal mucoperiosteum is widely undermined to allow the segments to be more easily repositioned without tearing or otherwise injuring the palatal mucoperiosteum.

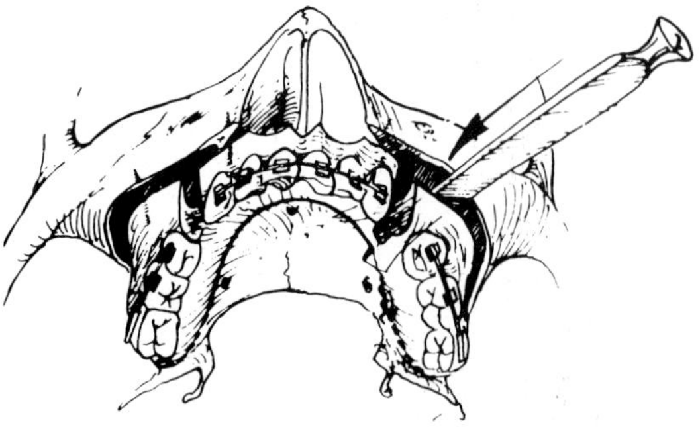

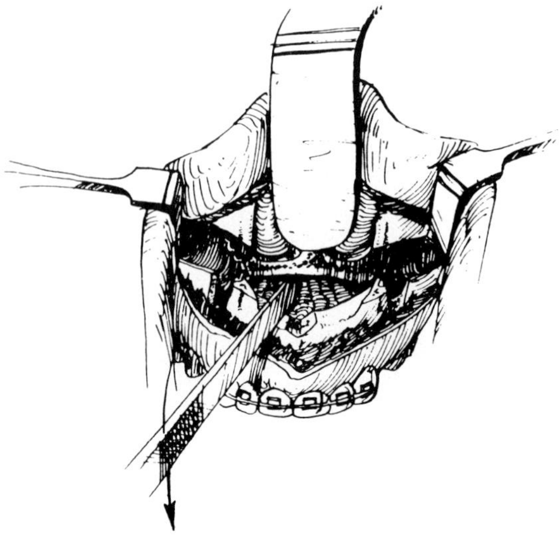

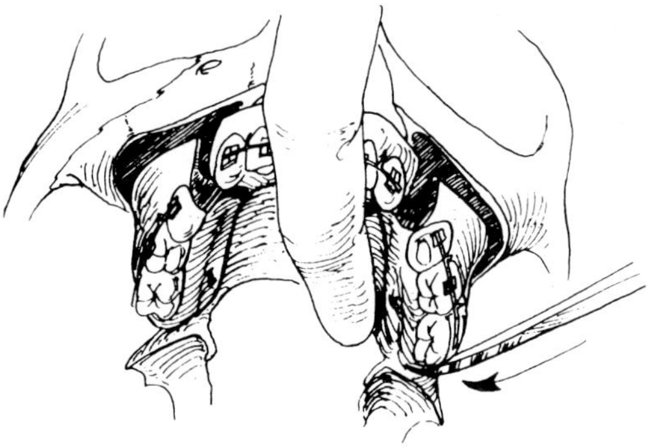

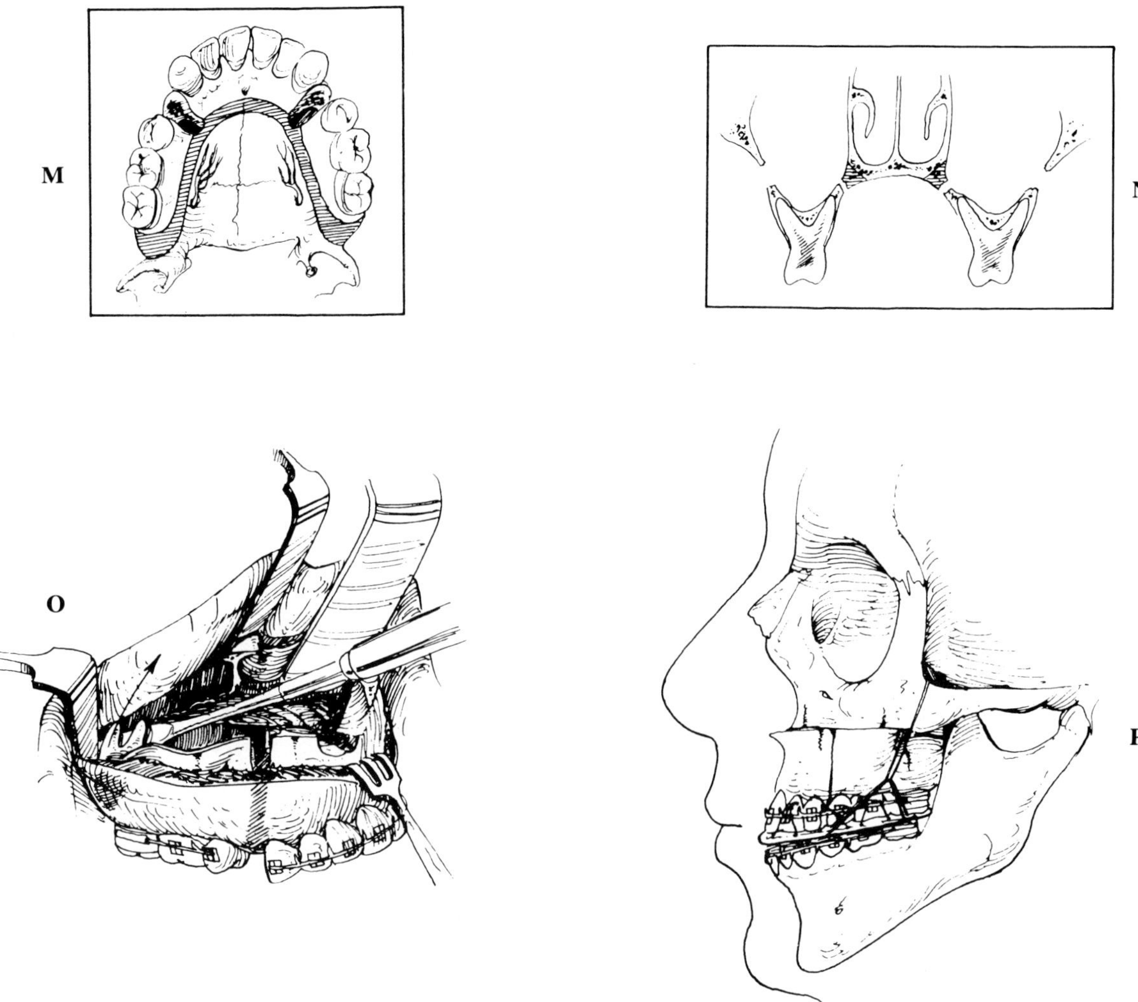

Fig. 3-3—cont'd.

M and **N,** Bone is selectively removed from the shaded areas to allow repositioning of the dento-alveolar segments to their planned position. This may be accomplished with rotating instruments, rongeurs, or small osteotomes. **O,** If an impacted third molar is in place, it is removed superiorly through the floor of the maxillary sinus. Bone is then removed in the posterior tuberosity–vertical plate areas of the palatine bone to allow repositioning of the segments. Care must be taken to avoid injury to the soft tissue vascular pedicles. **P,** The dentoalveolar segments are stabilized against each other by means of orthodontic appliances, palatal splints, occlusal indices, or combinations of these; the occlusion is then established with the mandibular condyles rotating in the fossae, and the maxilla is repositioned superiorly and stabilized. The vertical reference lines on the lateral maxillary walls are checked to verify the final position of the dentoalveolar segment.

maxillary wall. Posteriorly the osteomy or ostectomy may be extended to the pterygomaxillary junction, directed inferiorly toward the inferior aspect of the pterygomaxillary junction if a large ostectomy is planned, or directed into the third molar extraction site if this tooth has been removed 4 to 6 weeks prior to surgery.

6. The same procedure is completed on the opposite side of the maxilla.

7. If the dentoalveolus is to be divided into multiple segments, the mucoperiosteum overlying the alveolus at the site where it is to be divided is gently elevated from the initial mucoperiosteal incision to the alveolar crest. If a tooth must be removed where the alveolus is to be sectioned, it is removed at this time. Elevation of this mucoperiosteal tunnel is minimal, to allow adequate bone removal while retaining the maximum periosteal attachment to the segments and still provide an adequate vascular pedicle.

8. A finger is placed against the intact palatal mucosa at the proposed vertical osteotomy site and a bur or osteotome is used to complete the vertical alveolar osteotomy or ostectomy. The finger palpates the transsection of bone on the palatal side of the alveolus to prevent injury to the palatal mucosa.

9. The cartilaginous nasal septum is separated from the maxillary nasal crest approximately 15 mm into the nasal cavity by means of a double-guarded osteotome. The septum is retracted superiorly and laterally and protected while the anterior portion of the nasal crest of the maxilla is grooved with a vulcanite bur to a depth equal to the distance the maxilla is to be impacted. If this distance is excessive and the groove would approach closer than 4 mm to the apices of the central incisors, the inferior portion of the cartilaginous septum is removed to make up the difference. These maneuvers will prevent displacement or deviation of the nasal septum when the maxilla is elevated.

10. When there is a large amount of alveolar bone anteriorly between the floor of the nose and the apices of the teeth, an ostectomy may be performed below the level of the floor. Removal of this bone will further minimize any reduction of the anterior nasal airway when the maxilla is repositioned superiorly.

11. With a small osteotome or fissure bur a transnasal osteotomy is completed from right to left across the palate approximately 10 to 15 mm into the nasal cavity. A palpating finger is kept on the palatal mucosa to detect completion of it and to prevent damage to the palatal mucosa. Laterally the osteotomy enters the anterior maxillary sinuses. Posteriorly it extends along the medial wall of the floor of the maxillary sinuses and below the level of the nasal floor. It then enters the oral cavity and not the floor of the nose. The palpating finger on the palatal mucosa ensures penetration of the bur or osteotome through the palatal bone. The osteotomy is carried posteriorly, lateral to the greater palatine foramen, to the medial side of the pterygomaxillary junction or to the palatal wall of the third molar extraction site.

12. The maxillary alveolus is mobilized manually. If it is segmented, the anterior dentoalveolus is mobilized first followed by down-fracturing of the posterior segments. If difficulty is encountered in mobilizing the posterior segments, the pterygomaxillary junction is separated with a small curved osteotome aimed from lateral to medial in a slightly anterior direction.

13. When all the segments are mobilized, the palatal mucoperiosteum is elevated from the stable horizontal hard palate with an instrument passed transantrally. This provides the mobility of the palatal mucosa to allow the dentoalveolar segments to be superiorly or laterally repositioned without crimping or tearing of the mucosa and preserves a palatal blood supply to the segments.

14. The palatal acrylic surgical splint, constructed on the surgical models, is placed and ligated to the teeth to stabilize the segmented dentoalveolus. The intermediate occlusal index (if the mandible is to be osteotomized later) or the final occlusal index (if the mandible is to be autorotated) is placed between the maxillary and mandibular teeth and temporary intermaxillary fixation is applied. With the mandible retruded and rotating about the condyles, the maxillary dentoalveolus is superiorly repositioned. Any interference along the osteotomy and ostectomy sites is noted and relieved until the dentoalveolus can be freely rotated into its planned position. If interference is present, it

must be addressed in the region of the posterior tuberosity or anterior palatal osteotomy.

15. Stabilization of the repositioned dentoalveolus is accomplished with transosseous wiring at the zygomaticoalveolar crests and piriform rims; circumzygomatic, piriform rim, or infraorbital rim suspension; or any combination of these methods. The lateral reference lines on the maxilla are checked to verify accurate positioning of the segments.

16. The temporary intermaxillary fixation is removed and the stability of the maxillary dentoalveolus is checked. When satisfied with the stability of the segments, the surgeon may proceed to completion of the mandibular osteotomies if they have been planned.

17. If no mandibular surgery is needed, intermaxillary fixation is reapplied and the mucoperiosteal incisions are closed with continuous horizontal mattress 4-0 chromic gut sutures.

If the occlusion is stable, the fixation may be removed in about 1 week and the patient allowed to function and consume a soft diet. Interarch training elastics may be used for several weeks to ensure continued accurate positioning of the segments. If the occlusion is not stable and additional orthodontic treatment or restorative dentistry is needed to finalize the occlusion, fixation is left in place from 4 to 6 weeks.

TMAO through vertical labial and palatal incisions[7,17,18,34]

In contrast to the preceding technique, access to the posterior and anterior maxilla with a combined facial and palatal approach is obtained by using multiple vertical incisions through the alveolar mucosa superior to the attached gingiva. These are placed bilaterally at the height of the zygomaticomaxillary crests, just distal to the canines and anteriorly over the nasal spine. If the alveolus is to be mobilized as a single segment, no further extension of these incisions is necessary (Fig. 3-4, *A*). However, if multiple (three or four) segments are planned, the incisions distal to the canines are extended through attached gingiva to the alveolar crest to allow up-fracturing of the premaxillary segment upon completion of the osteotomies (Fig. 3-4, *B*).

1. Mucoperiosteal tunnels are elevated between the vertical incisions beneath the alveolar mucosa. The attached gingiva is not elevated and reflected from the alveolar segments except minimally in areas where the alveolus is to be segmented.

2. Elevation of the mucoperiosteum exposes the maxillary wall from the pterygomaxillary junction to the lateral piriform rims. Anteriorly the mucosa of the lateral nasal wall, floor of the nose, and nasal septum is elevated from the osseous walls of the nasal cavity and septum posteriorly approximately 15 mm.

3. After vertical reference lines have been etched in the lateral maxillary walls, and with the mucosa of the lateral nasal wall elevated and protected, a horizontal osteotomy is made in the lateral maxilla 4 to 5 mm above the apices of the teeth. It extends from the lateral piriform rim to the pterygomaxillary junction or to the socket of the third molar if available (Fig. 3-4, *C*).

4. If a large ostectomy is planned, the osteotomy is directed to the inferior portion of the pterygomaxillary junction distal to the second molar to facilitate bone removal in this area. Anteriorly the osteotomy extends through the anterior 15 mm of the lateral nasal wall as well as the lateral maxillary wall. If there is sufficient alveolar height between the apices of the anterior teeth and the floor of the nose to carry the osteotomy through alveolar bone beneath the nasal floor, this is done (Fig. 3-4, *C*). Removing alveolar bone beneath the nasal floor will prevent impingement on the anterior nasal airway when the segment is repositioned superiorly.

5. A second osteotomy, superior to the first, is measured and cut to allow bone removal from the lateral maxillary wall equal in width to the planned amount of alveolar intrusion. It likewise extends from the lateral piriform rim posteriorly to the pterygomaxillary junction or third molar socket. The bone between the osteotomy lines is removed.

6. If the alveolus is to be divided into multiple segments, the vertical osteotomies are completed from the horizontal ostectomy to the alveolar crest. When a tooth is to be removed from the site of segmentalization, this is completed and then the osteotomy or ostectomy is

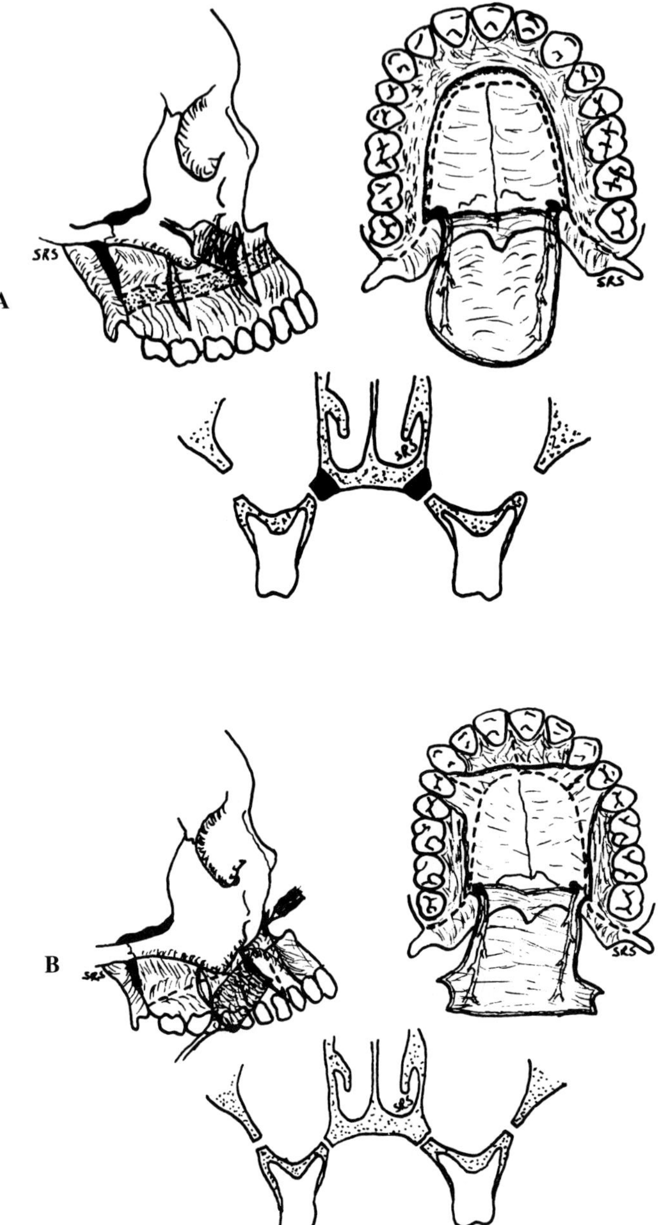

Fig. 3-4.
A, Total maxillary alveolar osteotomy in one segment for vertical impaction, accomplished from facial and palatal access. The vertical facial incisions are placed in the freely movable alveolar mucosa from the depth of the vestibule to the attached gingiva. The palatal incision is approximately 1 cm from the dentogingival margin. *Shaded areas,* Potential osseous impingement when the segment is repositioned superiorly. These locations may require additional bone removal if interference is noted. **B,** Total maxillary alveolar osteotomy in multiple segments for expansion or contraction of the dentoalveolus. Both facial and palatal mucoperiosteal incisions may be altered to allow direct access to complete the vertical alveolar osteotomies. These osteotomies, however, may also be accomplished with osteotomes or burs through mucogingival tunnels elevated beneath the attached gingiva at the site of the area to be segmented.

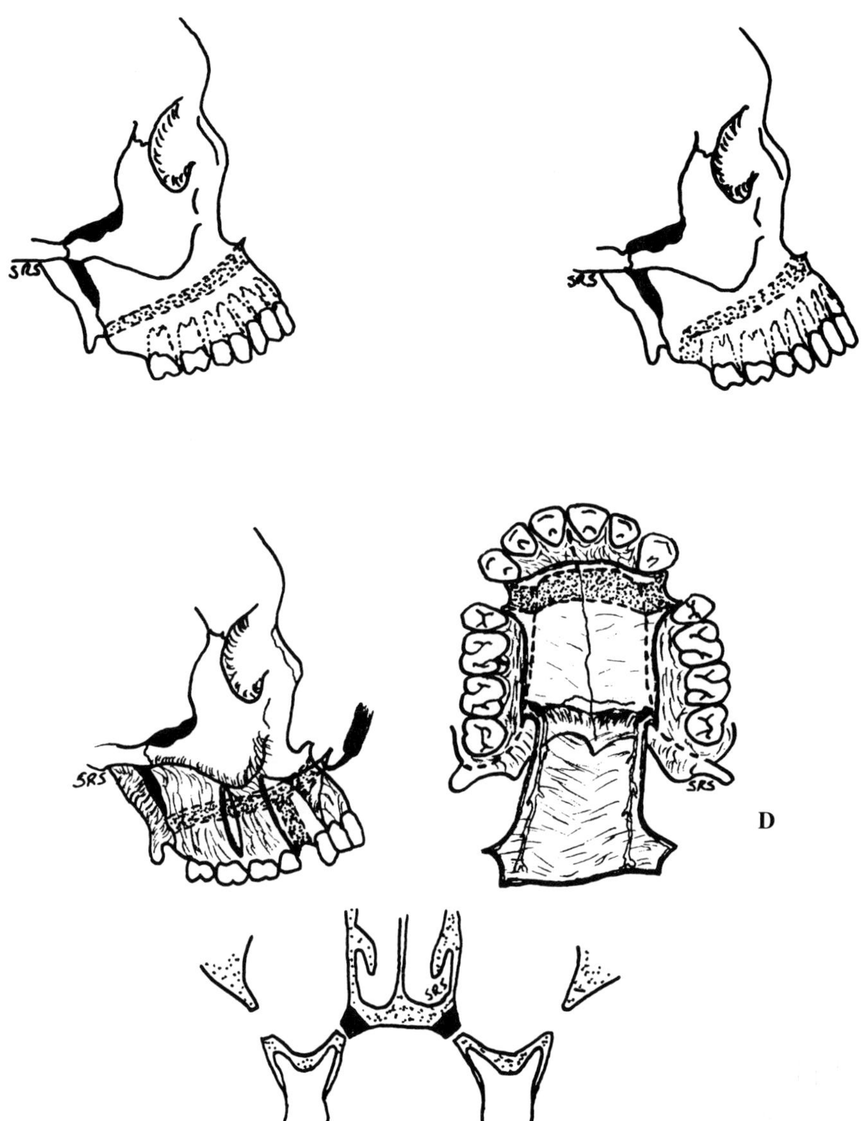

Fig. 3-4—cont'd.

C, Lateral maxilla in a total maxillary alveolar osteotomy. The osteotomy may extend posteriorly to the tuberosity, third molar socket, or pterygomaxillary junction. Anteriorly, if sufficient alveolar height exists to prevent injury to the dentition, the bone that is removed to allow vertical repositioning may be taken between the nasal floor and the apices of the teeth. **D,** Total maxillary alveolar osteotomy in segments for vertical repositioning and reconfiguration of the dental arch. Soft tissue incisions may be designed to provide direct access to the sites of bone removal, especially areas where troublesome osseous impingement is likely to be found. Palatal osteotomies enter the maxillary sinus lateral to the greater palatine foramen.

performed through the labial cortical plate of bone (Fig. 3-4, *D*).

7. The same procedures are completed on the opposite side of the maxilla.

8. Anteriorly, through the vertical incision over the nasal spine, the cartilaginous nasal septum is separated from the maxillary crest approximately 15 mm into the nose with a double-guarded osteotome. It is then retracted superiorly and laterally to facilitate removal of a measured amount of alveolus between the apices of the teeth and the nasal floor, grooving of the area of the nasal septum on the maxillary crest, or both, and to prevent its buckling or displacement when the alveolus is intruded. If necessary, a portion of the septum can be trimmed to allow an even greater amount of vertical repositioning.

9. With the measured facial osteotomies completed, the palatal mucosa is incised approximately 1 cm from the necks of the teeth, lateral to the greater palatine foramen on the vertical portion of the hard palate, in a U shape extending from the distal of the second molars and anteriorly passing just palatal to the nasopalatine papilla (Fig. 3-4, *A*). If the alveolus is to be segmented, the palatal incision is designed to provide access to the planned interdental osteotomy sites (Fig. 3-4, *B* and *D*).

10. A full-thickness mucoperiosteal flap containing the greater palatine vessels is elevated to expose the horizontal hard palate and its junction with the vertical walls of the dentoalveolus. Posteriorly the flap is elevated to expose either the palatal wall of the third molar socket or the palatal surface of the pterygomaxillary junction depending upon the site of planned osteotomy.

11. Osteotomies are completed with a fissure bur from the junction of the horizontal and vertical palatal shelves laterally into the maxillary sinuses, extending from the third molar socket or pterygomaxillary junction to the anterior extent of the maxillary sinus. Anteriorly lateral osteotomies are joined horizontally across the palate into the nasal cavity at the level of the front of the maxillary sinus (Fig. 3-4, *A*). These are not completed into the nasal cavity at this time but are deepened sufficiently to allow completion easily with a small sharp osteotome. Finally, if the alveolus is being segmented, vertical osteotomies on the palatal surface of the dentoalveolar segment are completed from the alveolar crest to the palatal osteotomy (Fig. 3-4, *B* and *D*).

12. If the alveolus is being mobilized in segments, the premaxillary portion is freed by an up-fracturing maneuver with digital pressure while the palatal osteotomy is being completed with an osteotome. The posterior segments are mobilized by up-fracturing with digital pressure and torquing of instruments placed in the osteotomy lines. If the posterior segments are not readily mobilized, the pterygomaxillary junction is separated with a small curved osteotome directed from lateral to medial and slightly anteriorly.

13. If the alveolus is being mobilized as a single segment, digital pressure, an osteotome on the anterior palatal osteotomy, and torquing of instruments in the osteotomy sites should readily produce the desired mobility. The pterygomaxillary junction may require separation with an osteotome.

14. When the dentoalveolar segment has been mobilized sufficiently to be digitally repositioned, the palatal surgical appliance is ligated to the teeth to solidify the segmented alveolus and to reposition the palatal mucoperiosteal flap.

15. The intermediate or final interocclusal appliances are placed as was done with the previous procedure, and temporary intermaxillary fixation is applied. The intact mandible, rotating about the condyles, is then used to reposition and intrude the maxillary dentoalveolar seg-

ment to its predetermined position. Any areas of osseous impingement are located and relieved as needed.

16. The intruded or recontoured dentoalveolar segment is stabilized by means of transosseous wiring, circumzygomatic suspension, piriform rim suspension, or any combination of these.

17. After the temporary intermaxillary fixation is removed, the stability of the dentoalveolar segment is checked. The surgeon may now proceed with any planned mandibular surgery or, if the mandible does not require surgery, place final intermaxillary fixation and close the vertical maxillary mucoperiosteal incisions.

Length of immobilization and time of return to function are judged according to stability of the segments, adequacy of the occlusion after surgery, and the need for postoperative orthodontic or restorative dental care.

POSTOPERATIVE CARE

For the past 7 years we have used the regimen of corticosteroid therapy to be described here in a total of over 700 patients and have been quite impressed with the apparent reduction of postoperative edema and morbidity. On the rare occasion when we have not used corticosteroids the resultant edema and increased patient discomfort have been obvious.

At present we administer dexamethasone sodium 8 to 10 mg every 6 hours, the first dose being given in the operating room immediately after the intravenous infusion is started. This is continued for 48 hours, after which 80 mg of methylprednisolone acetate (Depo-Medrol) is given IM each 24 hours for 2 days. Corticosteroid administration is then discontinued.

Even after more extensive or difficult surgical procedures, we have seen little or no early or delayed (rebound) edema when this program of corticosteroid administration is followed.

We are unaware of any absolute contraindications to the administration of corticosteroids on such a short-term basis and have had no postoperative complications that could be attributed to these medications.

Prophylactic antibiotics are used in patients undergoing maxillary surgery, because of oral and nasal wound contamination, hematoma accumulation (especially in the maxillary sinuses), and anticipated early reduction in blood flow to the osteotomized segments. We give 2 million units of aqueous potassium penicillin intravenously every 4 to 6 hours, beginning with the starting of the IV in the operating room. When the IV is discontinued, the patient is changed to oral penicillin V suspension, which is continued at 500 mg every 6 hours for another week. We have had no instance of postoperative wound infection when this program has been followed. In patients with an allergy to penicillin, erythromycin, clindamycin, or one of the cephalosporins has proved to be a satisfactory substitute.

Finally, after maxillary surgery, we recommend elevating the head of the bed 15 to 20 degrees and using a face tent with humidified room air for a minimum of 24 hours. This promotes the drainage of nasal secretions and hemorrhage and minimizes the accumulation and crusting of debris in the nasal passage. Retention of the nasal endotracheal tube or the use of nasopharyngeal airways is not recommended beyond the time any patient with intermaxillary fixation would be extubated—hopefully, shortly after completion of surgery, in the operating room. Afrin nasal spray or 0.25% phenylephrine nasal preparation is used every 8 hours for 48 hours postoperatively to shrink the nasal mucous membranes and reduce secretions. The nasal passages are inspected and cleaned daily by means of a speculum, suction and direct vision until there is no accumulation of crusted blood or mucus.

CASE PRESENTATIONS
CASE 1 (Fig. 3-5)

J.V., an 18-year-old white woman, was seen on referral from her general dentist for removal of four third molars and evaluation of a "gummy" smile. The patient was not happy with her inability to approximate her lips or with the amount of gingival tissue exposed when she smiled.

Problem list
Esthetics

> Frontal: Exposure of 7 mm of maxillary incisors with the lips at rest and 5 mm of gingival tissue with a full smile; 7 mm of interlabial gap with the lips at rest; lip approximation accomplished with considerable mentalis strain
>
> Profile: Long lower third of the face with a retrusive chin and no labiomental groove; convex appearance

Cephalometric analysis

> Facial convexity (S-N-A, 80 degrees; S-N-B, 75; A-N-B, 5; $\underline{1}$ to N-A, 18; $\overline{1}$ N-B, 25)
>
> Deficient mandible (S-N-B, 75 degrees; angle of facial convexity, 27 degrees)
>
> High-angle growth pattern (mandibular plane to S-N, 49 degrees; vertical maxillary excess)

Occlusion

> Dental arch form: Symmetric and well coordinated
>
> Dental alignment: Satisfactory; no crowding, tipping, or displacement
>
> Dental occlusion: Class I molar and canine relationships bilaterally

Treatment plan

Total maxillary alveolar osteotomy to
> Vertically impact the maxilla 7 mm to reduce tooth exposure
>
> Reduce interlabial gap
>
> Allow mandibular autorotation to help correct the appearance of mandibular deficiency

Advancement genioplasty with vertical reduction to
> Correct further the interlabial gap
>
> Increase chin prominence
>
> Decrease vertical height of the chin

Follow-up

Surgery was accomplished as a one-stage procedure, and the desired amount of maxillary impaction was obtained. Postoperative intermaxillary fixation was retained for 2 weeks, after which the patient was allowed to function and to consume a soft diet for the next 4 weeks. Stability of the maxillary dentoalveolus was excellent, and training elastics were not required. All appliances were removed 6 weeks after surgery. Twenty months postoperatively there was no evidence of relapse of the maxillary repositioning and the osteotomized anterior mandible had recontoured as expected.

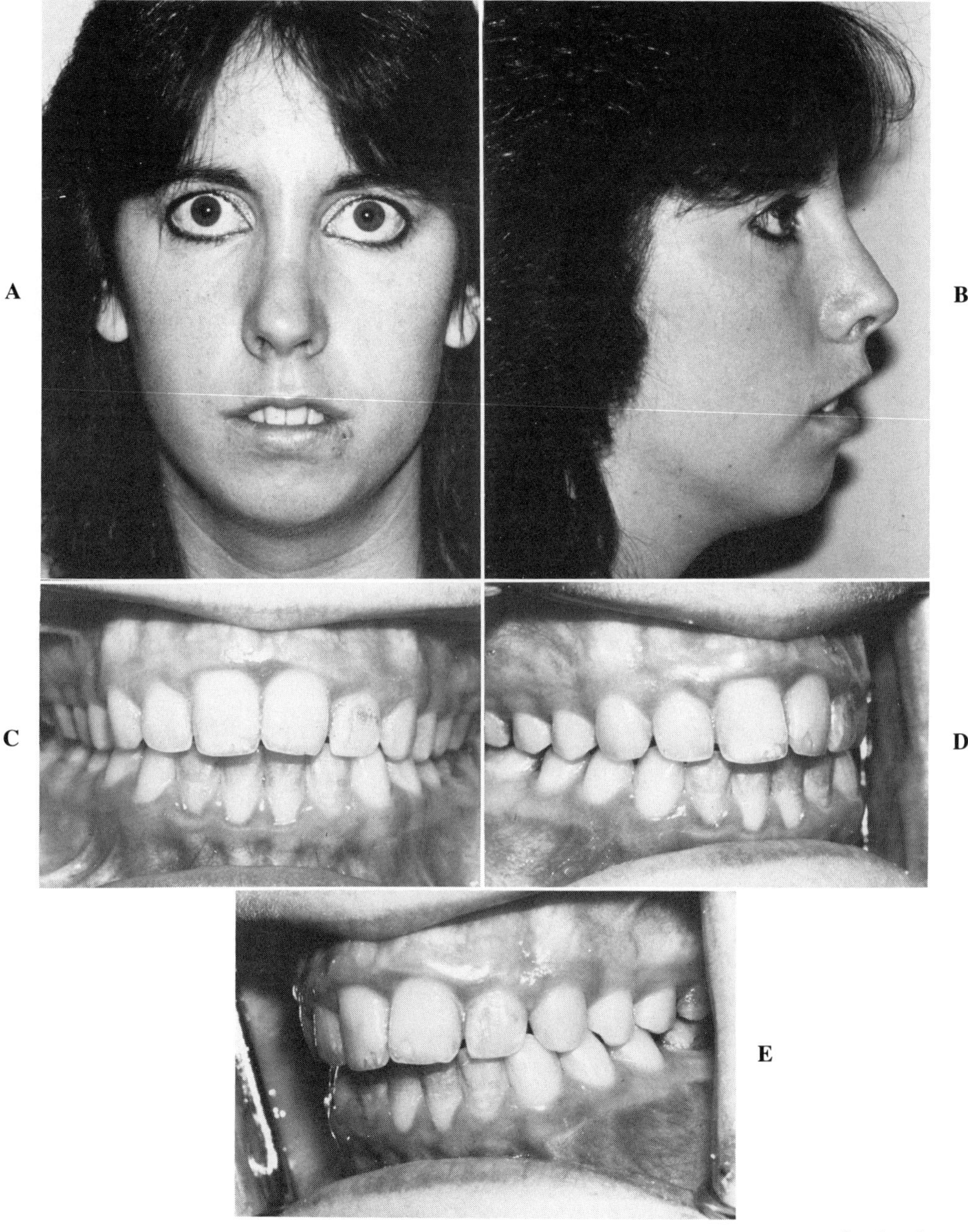

Continued.

Fig. 3-5.
Case 1. **A** to **E,** Preoperative views showing vertical maxillary excess and mandibular retrognathism with lip incompetence, a retrusive chin, excessive dental exposure, and a long lower facial third. Satisfactory Class I molar and canine interdental relationship preoperatively.

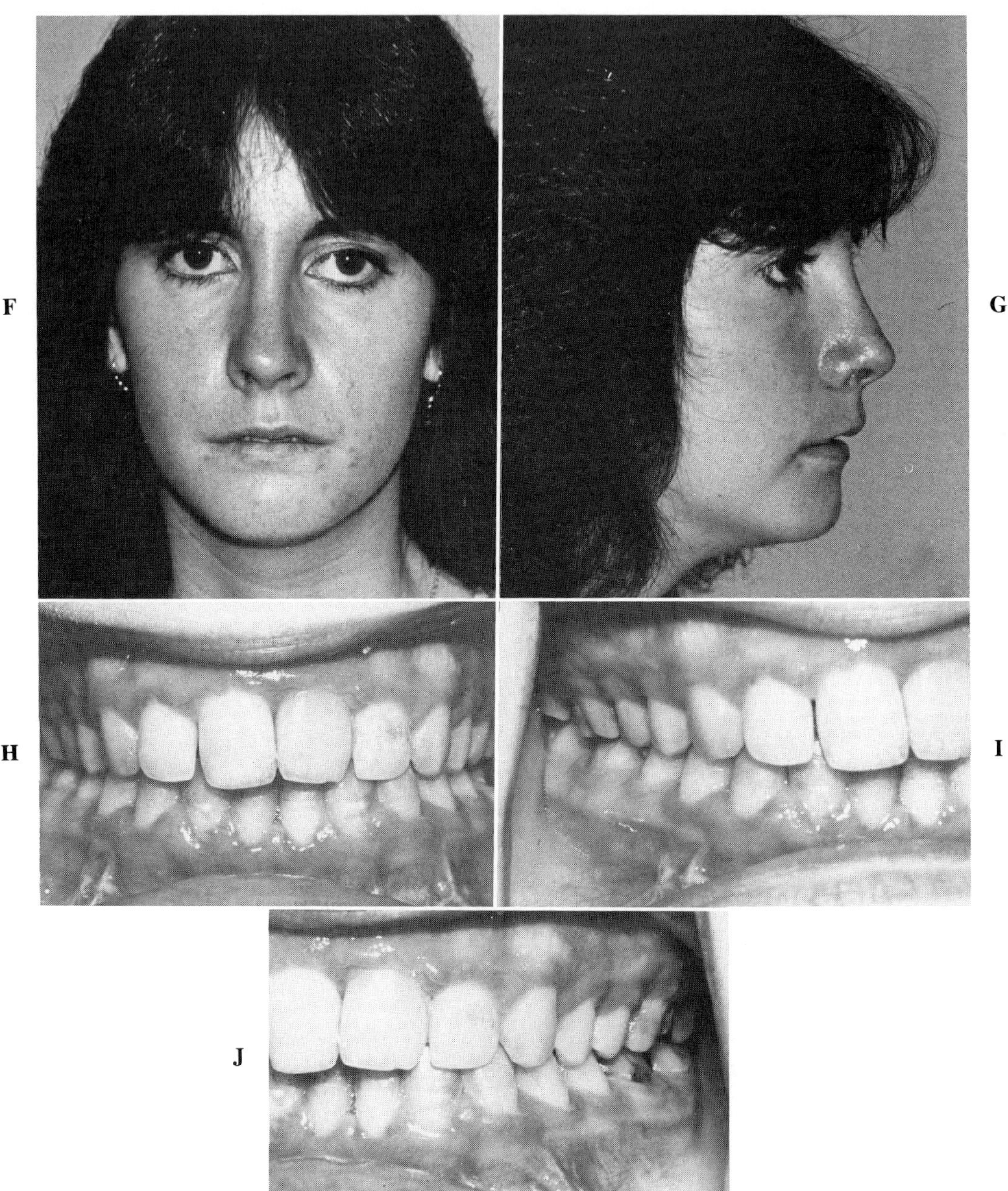

Fig. 3-5—cont'd.
F to **J,** Postoperative views. After correction of vertical maxillary excess with 7 mm of anterior maxillary impaction, mandibular autorotation, and advancement genioplasty. The occlusion is essentially unchanged since the maxillary dentoalveolus was impacted as a single unit and the mandible allowed to autorotate.

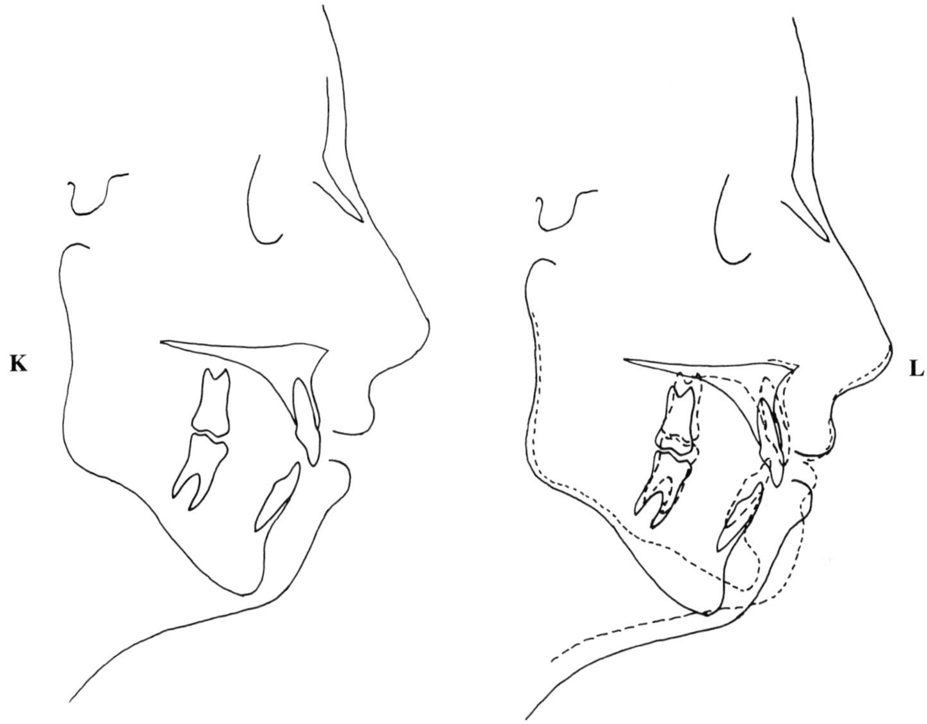

Fig. 3-5—cont'd.
K, Preoperative cephalometric tracing. Vertical maxillary excess, lip incompetence, and a vertically excessive horizontally deficient chin. **L,** Composite preoperative and 6-month postoperative tracings. Results of vertical repositioning of the maxilla and advancement genioplasty with mandibular autorotation.

CASE 2 (Fig. 3-6)

D.L., a 31-year-old white woman, was seen with a chief complaint of excessive exposure of her maxillary dentition and gingival tissues and an anterior open-bite relationship with an inability to incise foods.

Problem list

Esthetics

Frontal: Exposure of 5 mm of the maxillary incisors with lips at rest; lip incompetence
Profile: Lip incompetence, with slight elongation of the lower facial third

Cephalometric analysis

Anterior open-bite secondary to a posterior maxillary vertical excess
Steep mandibular plane (S-N, 44 degrees)
A-N-B difference, 4 degrees
Angle of facial convexity, 16 degrees
1 to N-A, 35 degrees

Occlusion

Dental arch form: Maxilla and mandible symmetric
Dental alignment: Satisfactory; anterior open-bite secondary to excessive height of the posterior maxillary alveolus
Dental occlusion: Class I molar and canine relationships bilaterally; 3 mm anterior open-bite with 7 mm overjet

Treatment plan

Total maxillary alveolar osteotomy in three segments with ostectomies between the first premolars and canines to
Upright and vertically reposition the maxillary anterior teeth 3 mm
Impact the posterior maxillary dentoalveolar segments 4.5 mm
Level and coordinate the maxillary dental arch to the mandibular arch
Mandibular autorotation

Follow-up

The surgery determined on the basis of this treatment plan was accomplished. A palatal acrylic appliance and labial arch bar were placed, and intermaxillary fixation was maintained for 6 weeks. A satisfactory Class I molar and canine relationship was retained. The lip incompetence and excessive dental exposure were eliminated. The anterior open-bite was corrected, and an overjet of 3 mm with an overbite of 2 mm resulted. Two years 4 months postoperatively there was good stability and retention of the surgical result with a satisfactory periodontal status and no apparent interradicular bone loss at the site of the vertical osteotomies between the canines and first premolars.

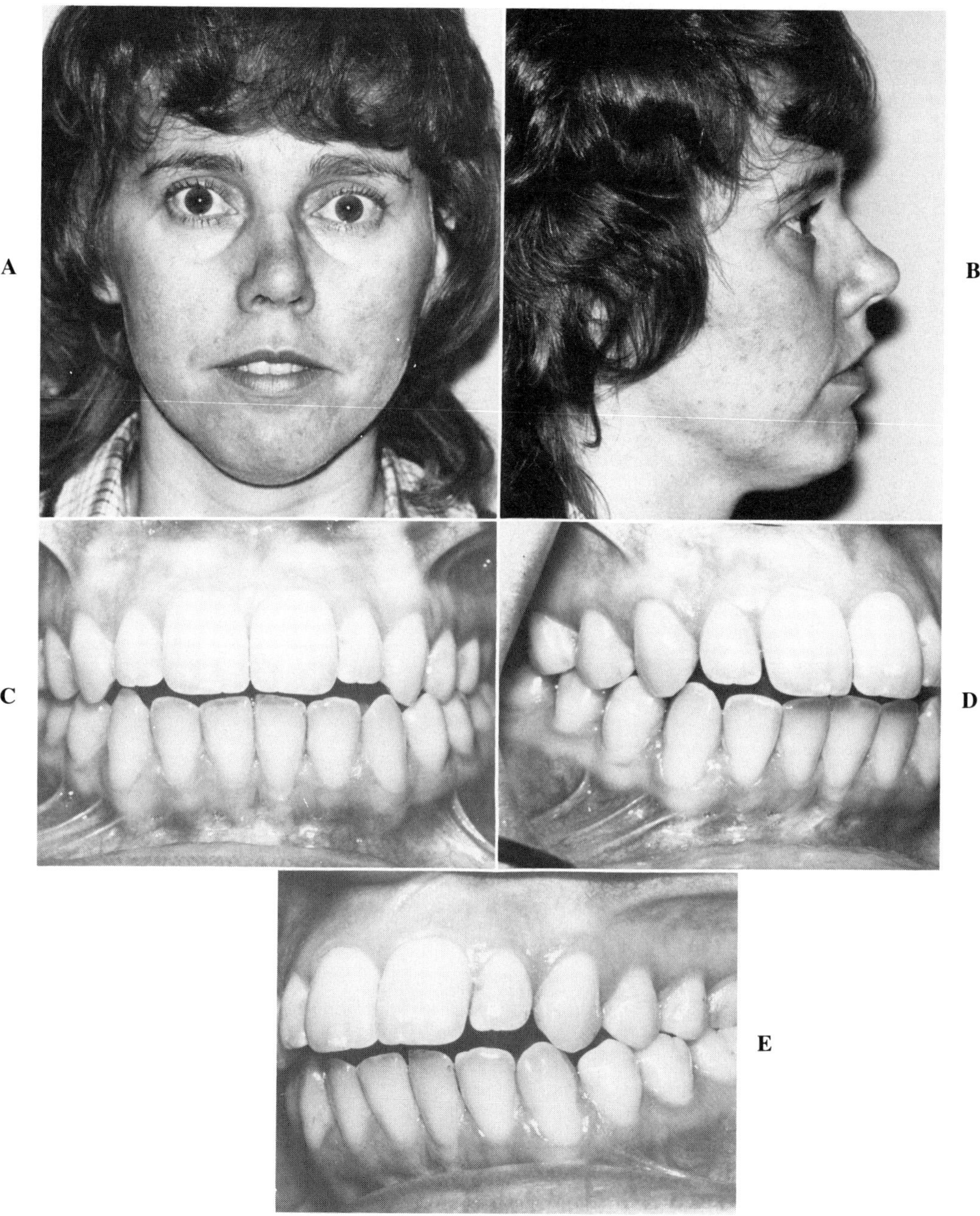

Continued.

Fig. 3-6.

Case 2. **A** to **E,** Preoperative views. Mild vertical maxillary excess and lip incompetence with anterior open-bite. There is a satisfactory Class I molar and canine relationship with anterior open-bite and excessive overjet preoperatively.

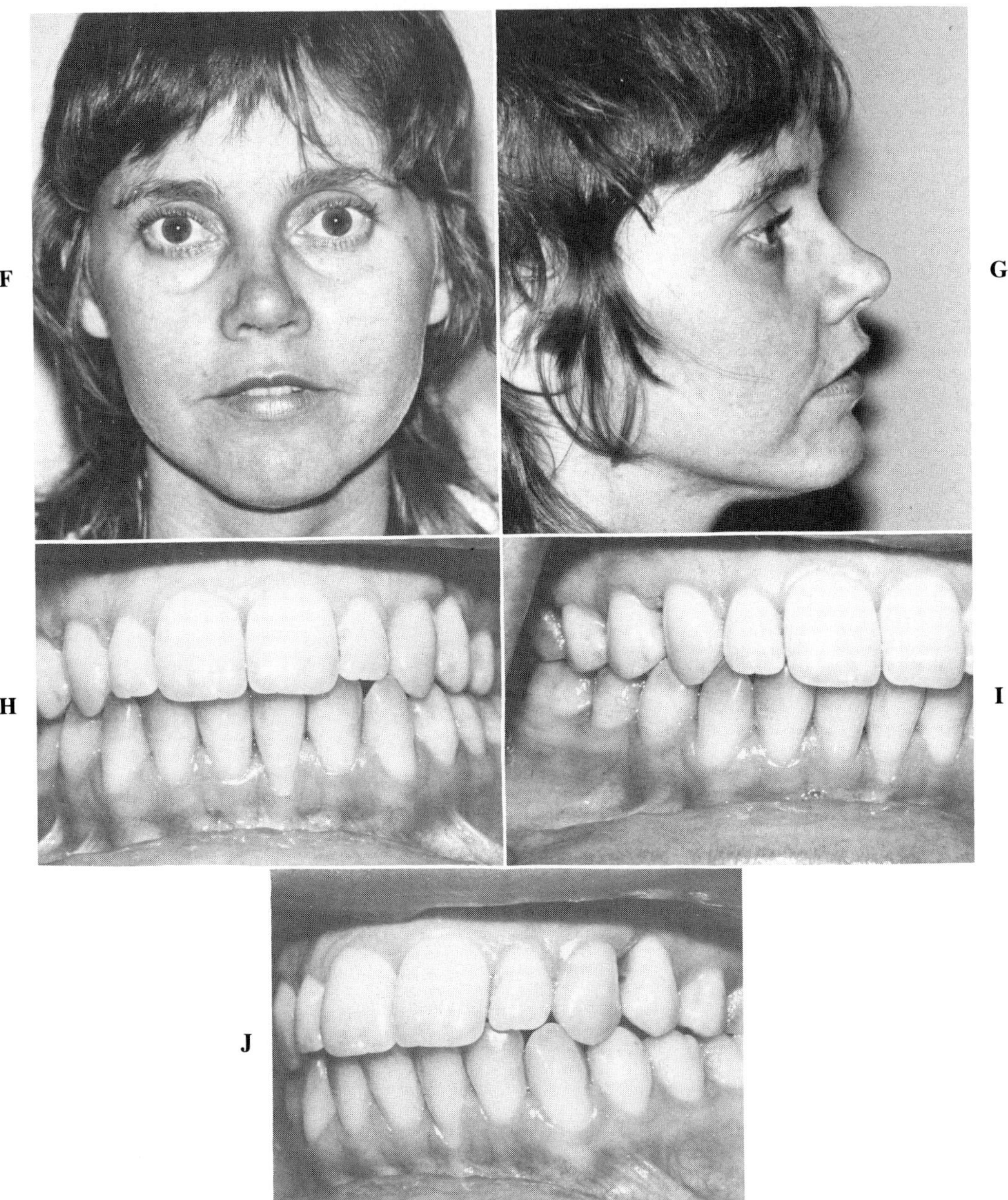

Fig. 3-6—cont'd
F to **J,** Postoperative views. After correction of the vertical maxillary excess and open-bite with a three-segment total maxillary alveolar osteotomy and mandibular autorotation. The open-bite has been corrected, with 3 mm of overjet and 2 mm of overbite resulting. The interdental osteotomy sites for the three-segment total maxillary alveolar osteotomy were between the canine and first premolar teeth.

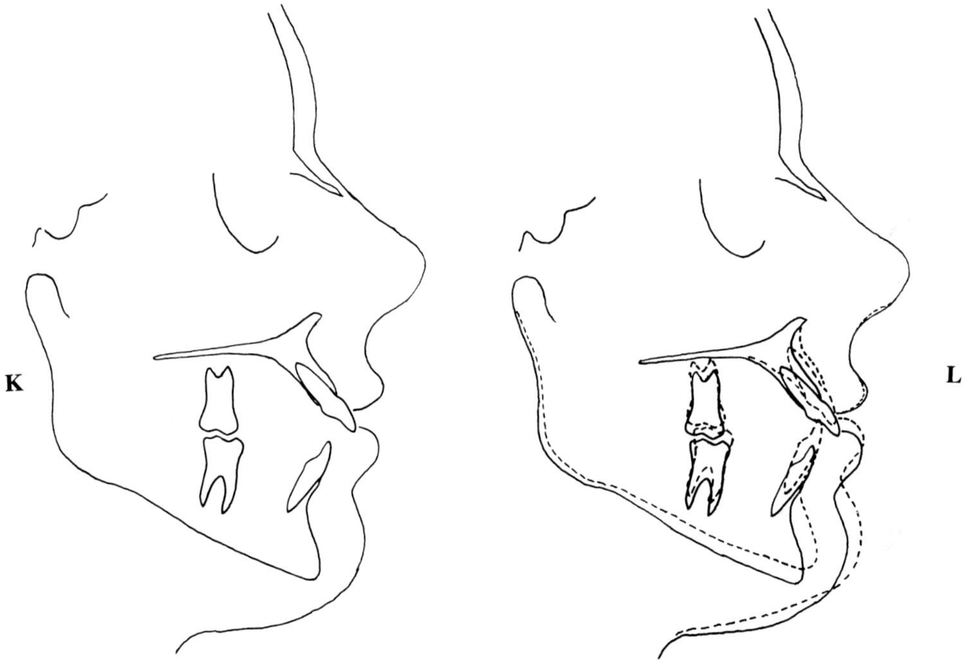

Fig. 3-6—cont'd.
K, Preoperative cephalometric tracing. Mild vertical maxillary alveolar excess, lip incompetence, and anterior open-bite. **L,** Composite preoperative and postoperative tracings. Closure of the anterior open-bite and the results of mandibular autorotation.

CASE 3 (Fig. 3-7)

P.S., a 32-year-old white woman, had been undergoing orthodontic therapy for 20 months prior to her referral for orthognathic surgery. She was unhappy with the amount of gingival tissue exposed when she smiled and with the receding appearance of her lower jaw.

Problem list

Esthetics

Frontal: No facial asymmetry; exposure of 5 to 6 mm of maxillary anterior teeth with the lips in repose and 5 mm of gingiva when smiling; 7 mm interlabial gap; lack of chin prominence
Profile: Retrusive mandible and chin

Cephalometric analysis

Facial convexity (S-N-A, 80 degrees; S-N-B, 74; A-N-B, 6; $\underline{1}$ to N-A, 28; $\overline{1}$ to N-B, 29)
Deficient mandible (S-N-B, 74 degrees; angle of facial convexity, 24 degrees)
High-angle growth pattern (mandibular plane to S-N, 41 degrees; vertical maxillary excess)

Occlusion

Dental arch form: Maxilla and mandible symmetric
Dental alignment: Satisfactory after orthodontic treatment
Dental occlusion: Class II bilaterally; midlines in the mandible and maxilla correct; 4 mm overbite with 8 mm overjet

Treatment plan

Total maxillary alveolar osteotomy with vertical repositioning of the maxilla 4 mm to
Reduce the interlabial gap
Decrease the vertical exposure of teeth and gingiva
Allow mandibular autorotation and partially correct the mandibular deficiency
Sagittal osteotomies of the mandibular rami bilaterally to advance the mandible to a Class I canine and molar occlusion and further correct the mandibular deficiency
Advancement and vertical reduction genioplasty to
Further correct the interlabial gap
Increase the chin prominence
Finishing orthodontics to refine and stabilize the occlusion

Follow-up

Surgery was scheduled and completed expeditiously since the presurgical orthodontics had already been completed. After 8 weeks of intermaxillary fixation, active orthodontic therapy was resumed and completed 6 months later. After 1 year of follow-up there was minimal positional change of the maxilla and mandible. The patient, her orthodontist, and her family are pleased with the esthetic and occlusal results of combined surgical and orthodontic treatment.

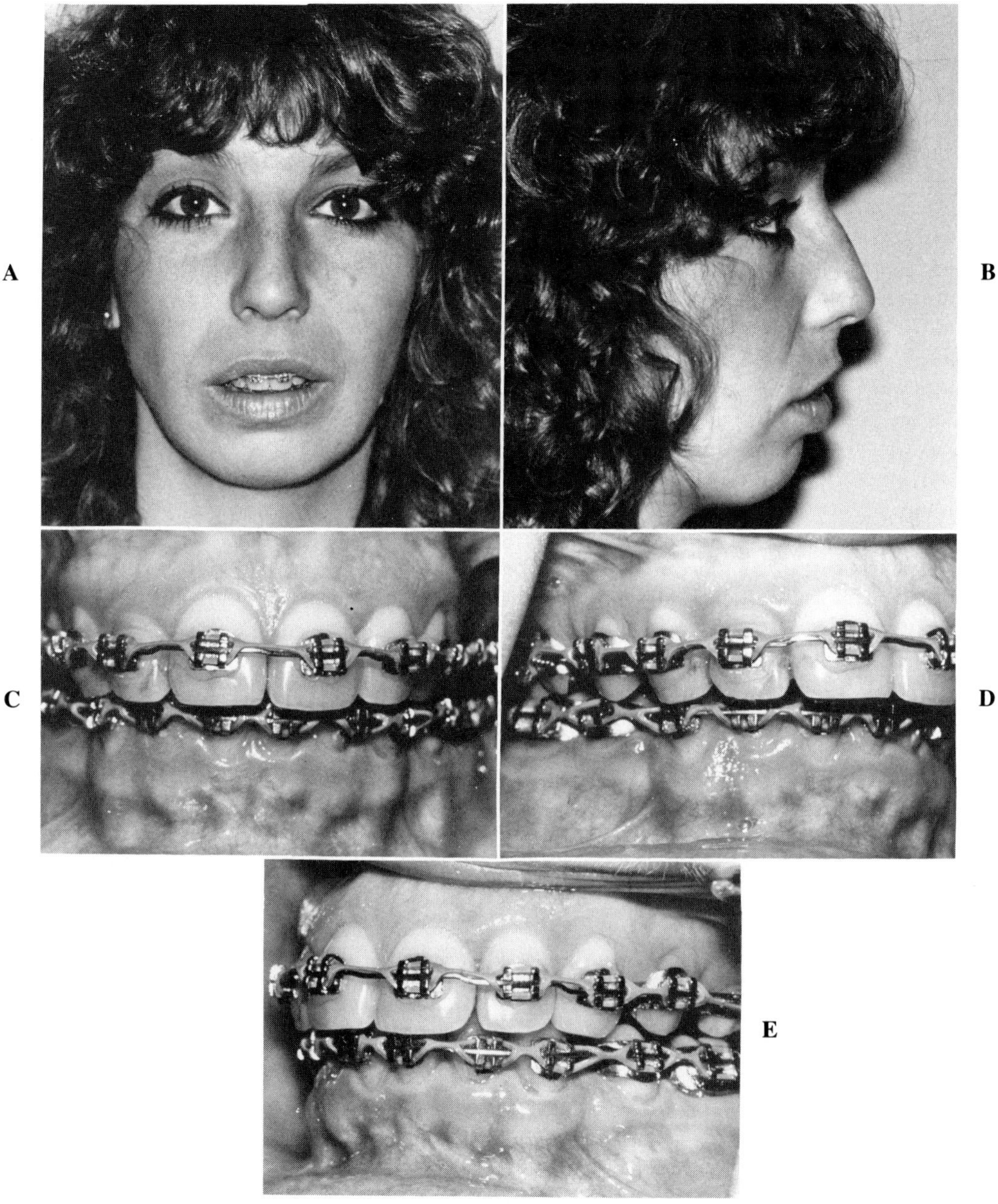

Continued.

Fig. 3-7.
Case 3. **A** to **E**, Preoperative views. The patient received orthodontic care in preparation for surgery to correct a vertical maxillary excess, mandibular retrognathism, and microgenia. She had an orthodontically coordinated occlusion and was ready for correction with total maxillary alveolar osteotomy, sagittal osteotomies of the mandibular rami, and advancement genioplasty.

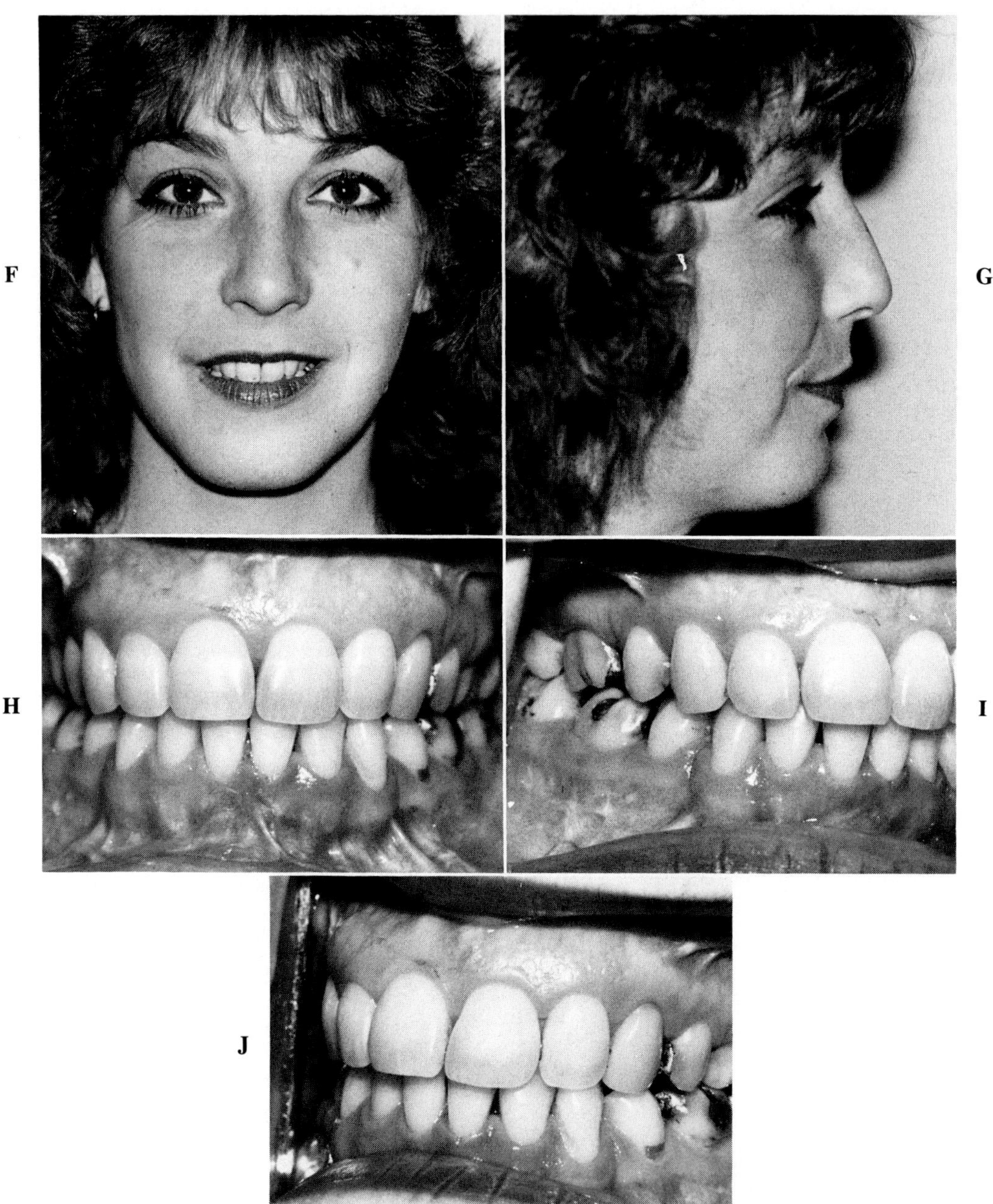

Fig. 3-7—cont'd.
F to **J,** Surgery and orthodontics completed. Lip competence, tooth exposure, and facial profile were significantly improved with maxillary vertical repositioning and advancement of the mandible and chin.

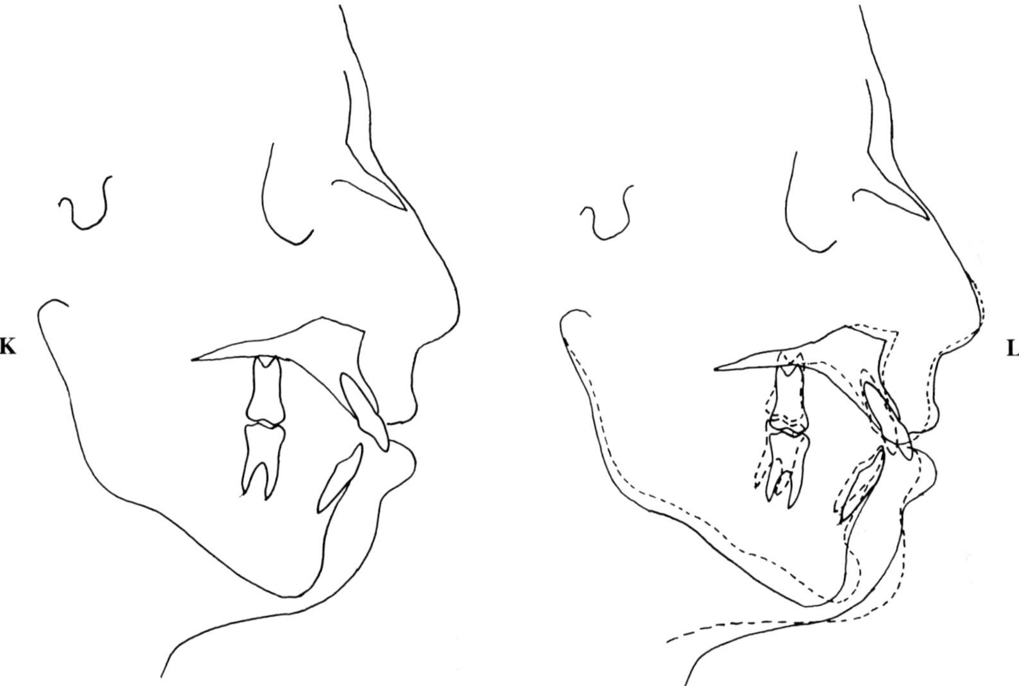

Fig. 3-7—cont'd.
K, Preoperative cephalometric tracing. Vertical maxillary excess, mandibular retrognathism, and microgenia. **L,** Composite preoperative and posttreatment tracings demonstrating the corrective procedures.

CASE 4 (Fig. 3-8)

D.H., a 25-year-old white woman referred by her friends for evaluation and treatment of a dentofacial deformity, was concerned with the long "horsey" appearance of her face, the excessive exposure of her teeth and gingiva, and the inability to close her mouth.

Problem list

Esthetics

Frontal: Exposure of 10 mm of the maxillary anterior teeth with lip incompetence, dry hyperplastic maxillary gingival tissue secondary to the inability to approximate the lips

Profile: Long face with lip incompetence, tooth exposure, a retrusive mandible, and a long retrusive chin; everted lower lip

Cephalometric analysis

Steep mandibular plane (S-N angle, 57 degrees)

Convex facial profile (S-N-A, 82 degrees; S-N-B, 71; A-N-B, 11; angle of facial convexity 29)

Mandibular retrognathism (S-N-B, 71 degrees; overjet, 12 mm)

Vertical maxillary excess

Occlusion

Dental arch form: Symmetric

Dental alignment: Satisfactory, with no crowding or malpositioning

Dental occlusion: Class II of molars and canines; 12 mm overjet

Treatment plan

Total maxillary alveolar osteotomy with 10 mm impaction to

Reduce tooth and gingival exposure

Correct the lip incompetence

Allow mandibular autorotation to partially correct the mandibular retrusion

Sagittal osteotomies of the mandibular rami for advancement and further correction of the retrognathic appearance

Secondary genioplasty to reduce the chin vertically and horizontally advance it

Follow-up

The total maxillary dentoalveolar impaction and mandibular advancement were accomplished, and the patient was retained in intermaxillary fixation for 8 weeks. These procedures achieved the desired goals of reducing exposure of the dentition, reducing the lip incompetence, and advancing the mandible. Occlusion and function were satisfactory. The patient was followed for 6 months, with no evidence of relapse of the surgical results. Then her husband was transferred from the area, and we were unable to complete the genioplasty procedure. Now, several years later, with more experience in predicting treatment results, we would have accomplished the genioplasty as a simultaneous procedure, which would have resulted in a further correction of the patient's lip incompetence and a marked improvement in facial profile.

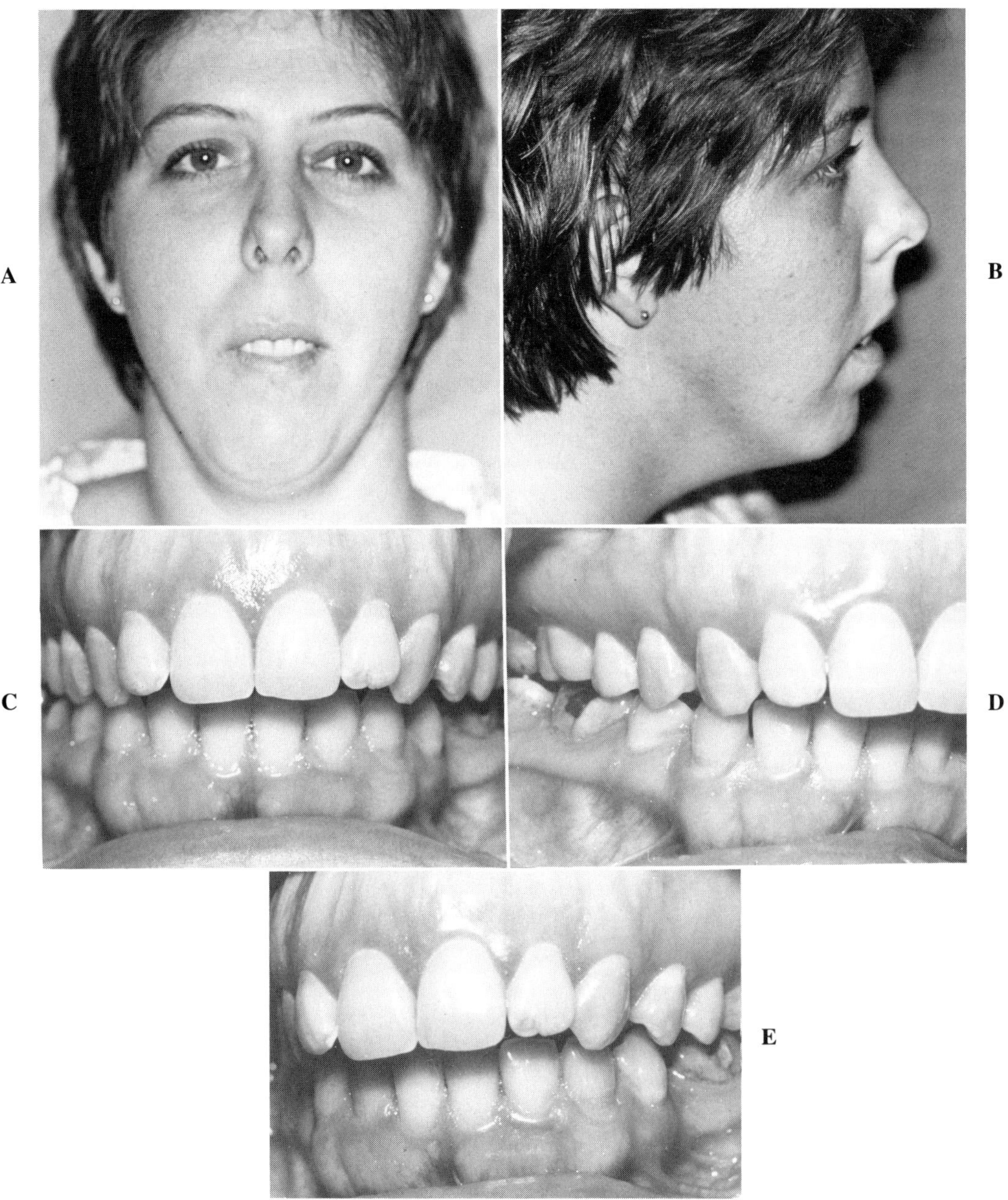

Continued.

Fig. 3-8.
Case 4. **A** to **E,** Preoperative views. Severe vertical maxillary excess and mandibular retrognathism. There is excessive exposure of the maxillary dentition, lip incompetence, and an elongated face with retrognathic mandible. A Class II canine relationship exists bilaterally preoperatively. The mandibular premolars have been removed, and there has been mesial drift of the molar teeth. Maxillary alveolar hyperplasia is evident.

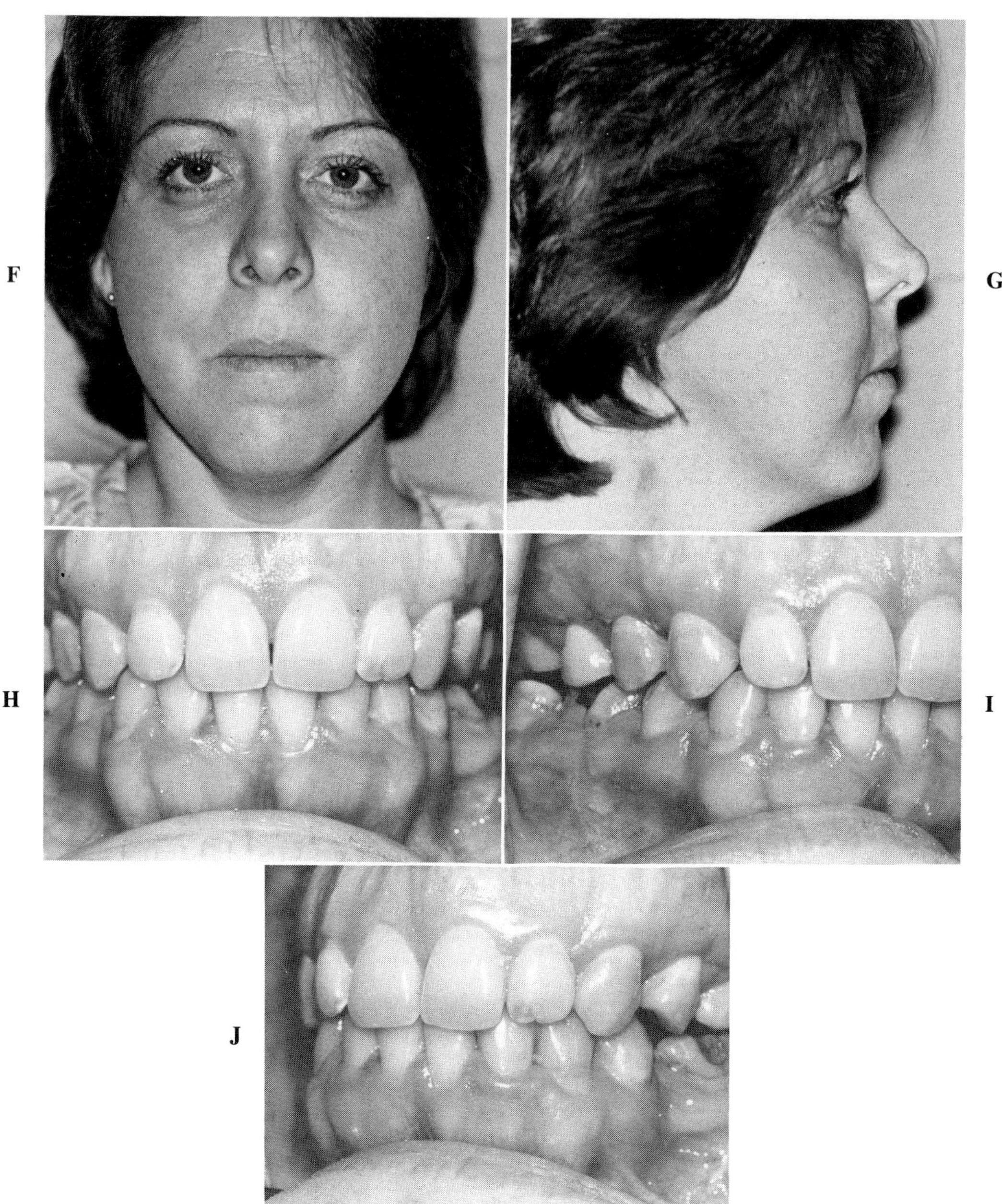

Fig. 3-8—cont'd.

F to **J,** Postoperative views. After correction of the vertical maxillary excess with 10 mm of dentoalveolar impaction and correction of the retrognathic mandible with autorotation and advancement via sagittal osteotomies of the rami. A Class I canine relationship exists postoperatively. The 10 mm impaction of the maxilla was accomplished entirely in the alveolus, below the level of the nasal floor.

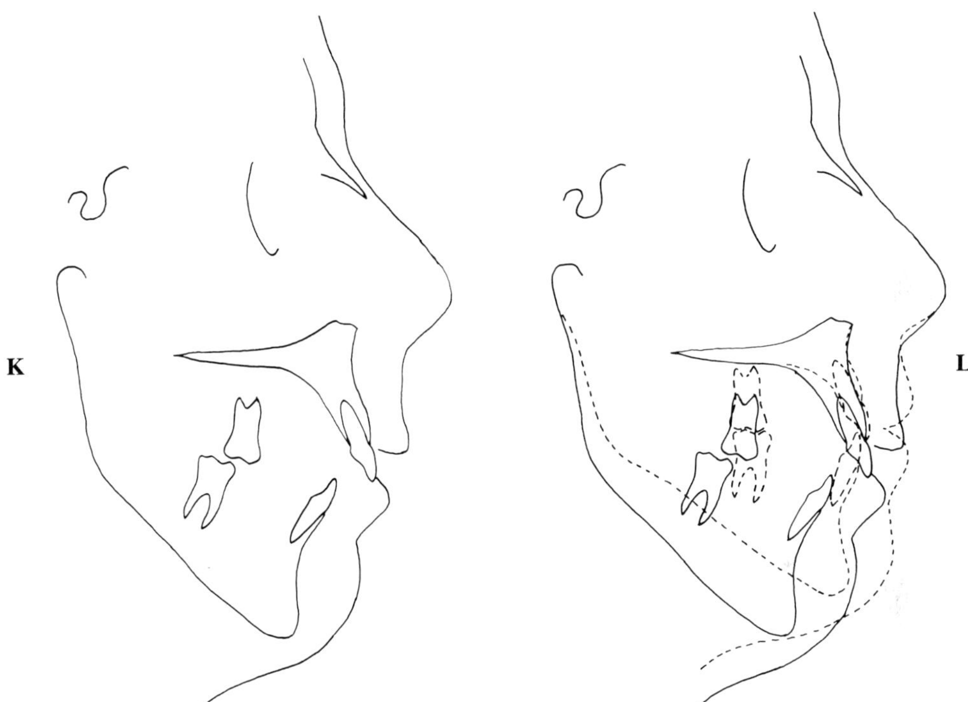

Fig. 3-8—cont'd.
K, Preoperative cephalometric tracing. Vertical maxillary excess, lip incompetence, and mandibular retrusion. **L,** Composite preoperative and postoperative tracings. A genioplasty, planned as a secondary procedure but not accomplished, would have resulted in an even more satisfactory correction of the patient's deformity.

CASE 5 (Fig. 3-9)

K.H., a 24-year-old white woman seeking correction of a severe malocclusion with overbite and facial asymmetry, had undergone 4 years of orthodontic therapy including removal of the first premolars and did not want further orthodontic care. She preferred instead to be treated by surgery alone.

Problem list

Esthetics

Frontal: Asymmetric facial outlines with shift of the mandibular and maxillary dental midlines to the right; maxillary asymmetry with a cant from left to right; lack of chin prominence

Profile: Upper face and nasal contour acceptable; retrusive mandible

Cephalometric analysis

Moderate to severe facial convexity (S-N-A, 80 degrees; S-N-B, 72; A-N-B, 8; $\underline{1}$ to N-A, 25; $\overline{1}$ to N-B, 27)

Deficient mandible (with S-N-B, 72 degrees; angle of facial convexity, 23 degrees)

Occlusion

Dental arch form: Mandibular arch satisfactory; maxillary arch canted (4 mm lower at second molar and 3 mm at canine on right than on left); horizontal constriction of the alveoli with a V-shaped arch form

Dental alignment: No crowding; diastemas between the canine and second premolar; arch width discrepancy (maxillary narrower than mandibular)

Dental occlusion: Class II bilaterally (2 mm anterior open bite, 9 mm overjet)

Treatment plan

Total maxillary alveolar osteotomy in three segments to

Impact the right maxilla 4 mm at the second molar and 3 mm at the canine to level the arch

Shift the dental midline 3 mm to the left

Expand and recontour the arch to accommodate the mandibular dentition

Sagittal osteotomies of the mandibular rami bilaterally to

Achieve a Class I canine and molar relationship

Correct the mandibular deficiency

Horizontal sliding osteotomy of the inferior border of the mandible to increase chin prominence

Follow-up

Surgery was completed uneventfully, with the desired esthetic and occlusal changes achieved. Intermaxillary fixation was removed after 8 weeks, and the patient returned to function immediately. She was available for follow-up for a period of only 6 months, however, during which time no appreciable changes of the surgical result were noted.

Comment

This patient would most likely have benefited from presurgical orthodontic alignment as a nonextraction case, although her preorthodontic records were not available for us to evaluate. Nevertheless, a very satisfactory occlusal and esthetic result was obtained with surgical leveling and rounding of the maxillary arch in segments using spaces left between the maxillary canines and second premolars as osteotomy sites. Her orthodontic treatment time and result would have been considerably improved if her treatment had been initially planned to combine surgery and orthodontics.

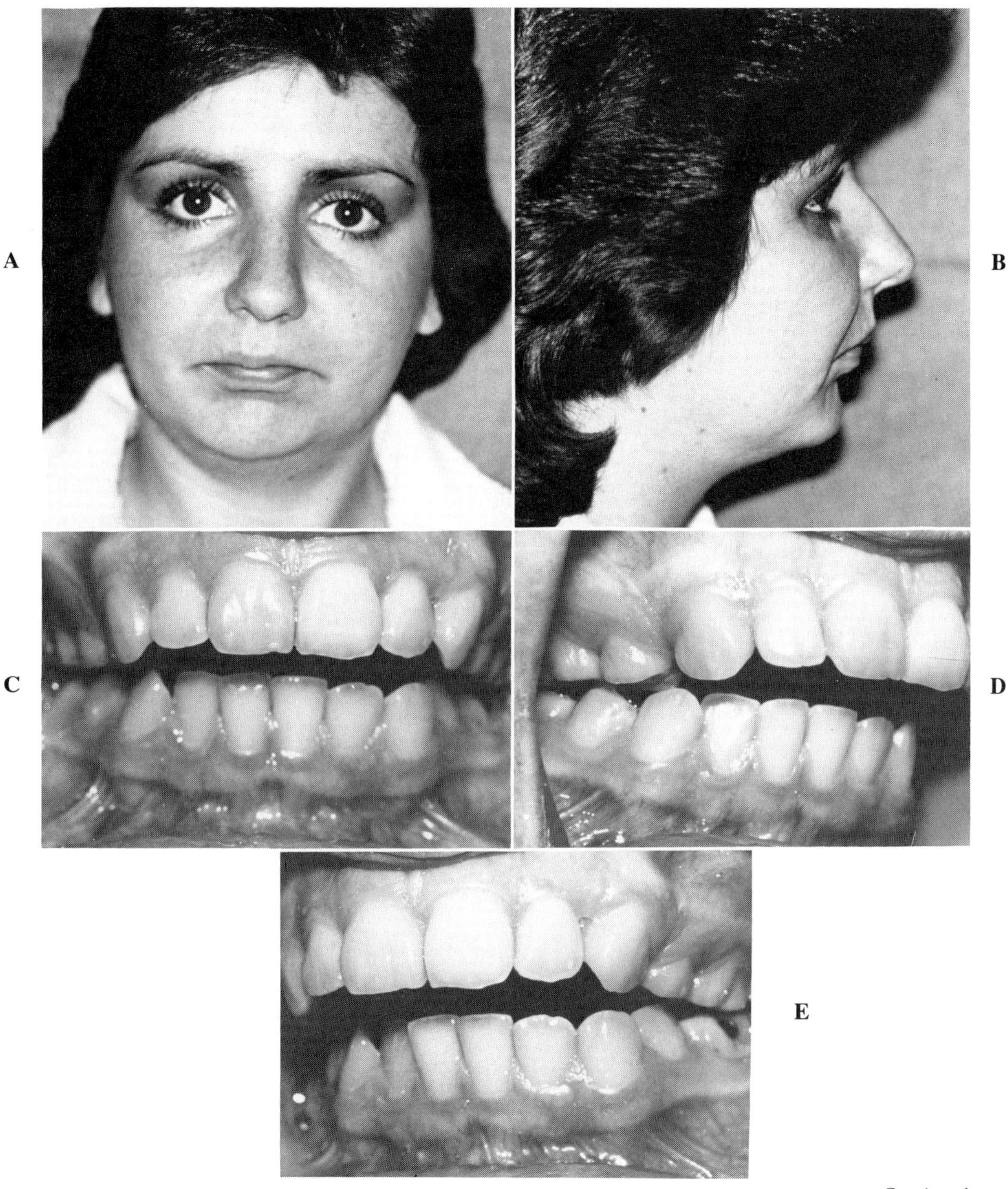

Continued.

Fig. 3-9.

Case 5. **A** to **E,** Preoperative views. Facial asymmetry, arch width discrepancy, and mandibular retrognathism with microgenia. The patient had undergone removal of her first premolar teeth and 4 years of unsuccessful orthodontic therapy preoperatively.

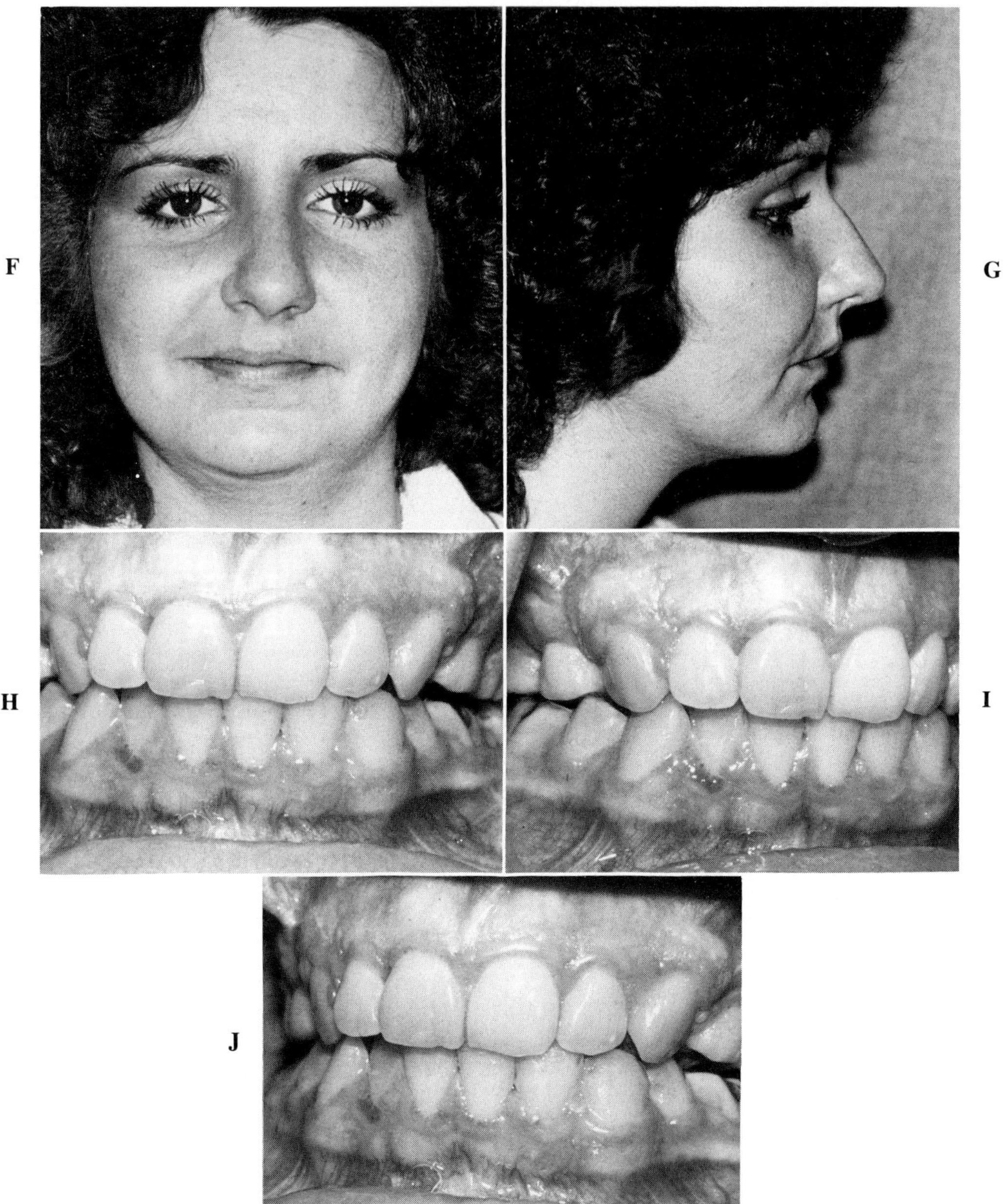

Fig. 3-9—cont'd.
F to **J,** Postoperative views. The facial asymmetry, mandibular retrognathism, and microgenia have been treated; and the occlusal cant, arch width discrepancy, and Class II discrepancy were all remedied with surgery.

CASE 6 (Fig. 3-10)

D.S., a 17-year-old white girl, came to us complaining of facial asymmetry of long duration with deviation of her anterior mandible to the left. She reported that there had been no increase in her deformity for the past several years. Radiographs revealed a right mandibular condylar hyperplasia with resultant facial deviation and downward canting of the occlusal plane on the right side.

Problem list

Esthetics

Frontal: Mandible deviated to the left at the midline with distortion of the lip line as well; height of the right mandible increased; occlusal plane of the maxillary and mandibular posterior teeth 6 mm lower on the right than on the left

Profile: Pleasing, with no evidence of the asymmetry from the front

Cephalometric analysis

Lateral: Good relationships, with little evidence of deformity

PA

Deviation of the mandibular midline 5 mm to the left

Plane of the inferior mandibular border 6 to 7 mm lower on the right than on the left

Mandibular dental midline deviated 3 mm to the left with tipping of the anterior teeth to the right

Posterior plane of occlusion 6 mm lower on the right than on the left

Occlusion

Dental arch form: Well coordinated with compensation to the canted occlusal plane and right mandibular hyperplasia

Dental alignment: Minimal crowding and tipping of the mandibular anterior teeth

Dental occlusion: Class I molar and canine relationship; satisfactory overbite and overjet; canting of the occlusal plane downward 6 mm on the right; mandibular midline deviation 3 mm to the left with tipping of the lower incisors to the right

Treatment plan

The patient reported no increase of her facial asymmetry over the preceding several years. Radiographs were taken and compared over 18 months and revealed no increase in the right mandibular condylar hyperplasia or in the cant of the occlusal plane. Nuclear scanning revealed no increase in activity in the right condyle as opposed to the left. The following treatment plan was devised and completed:

1. Total maxillary alveolar osteotomy with 7 mm impaction of the dentoalveolus on the right and an osteotomy cut on the left to level the maxillary dental arch
2. Left mandibular sagittal splitting osteotomy of the ramus
3. Right oblique subcondylar osteotomy to allow leveling and a shift in position of the mandible to correspond to the repositioned maxilla

Follow-up

A one-stage surgical procedure achieved leveling of the dental occlusal plane and correction of the mandibular asymmetry. The dental occlusion remained unchanged, with a deviation of the mandibular dental midline to the left. The maxillary dental midline was accurately positioned. The patient was available for postoperative follow-up for 4 years, and there was no return of the condylar hyperplasia or facial asymmetry.

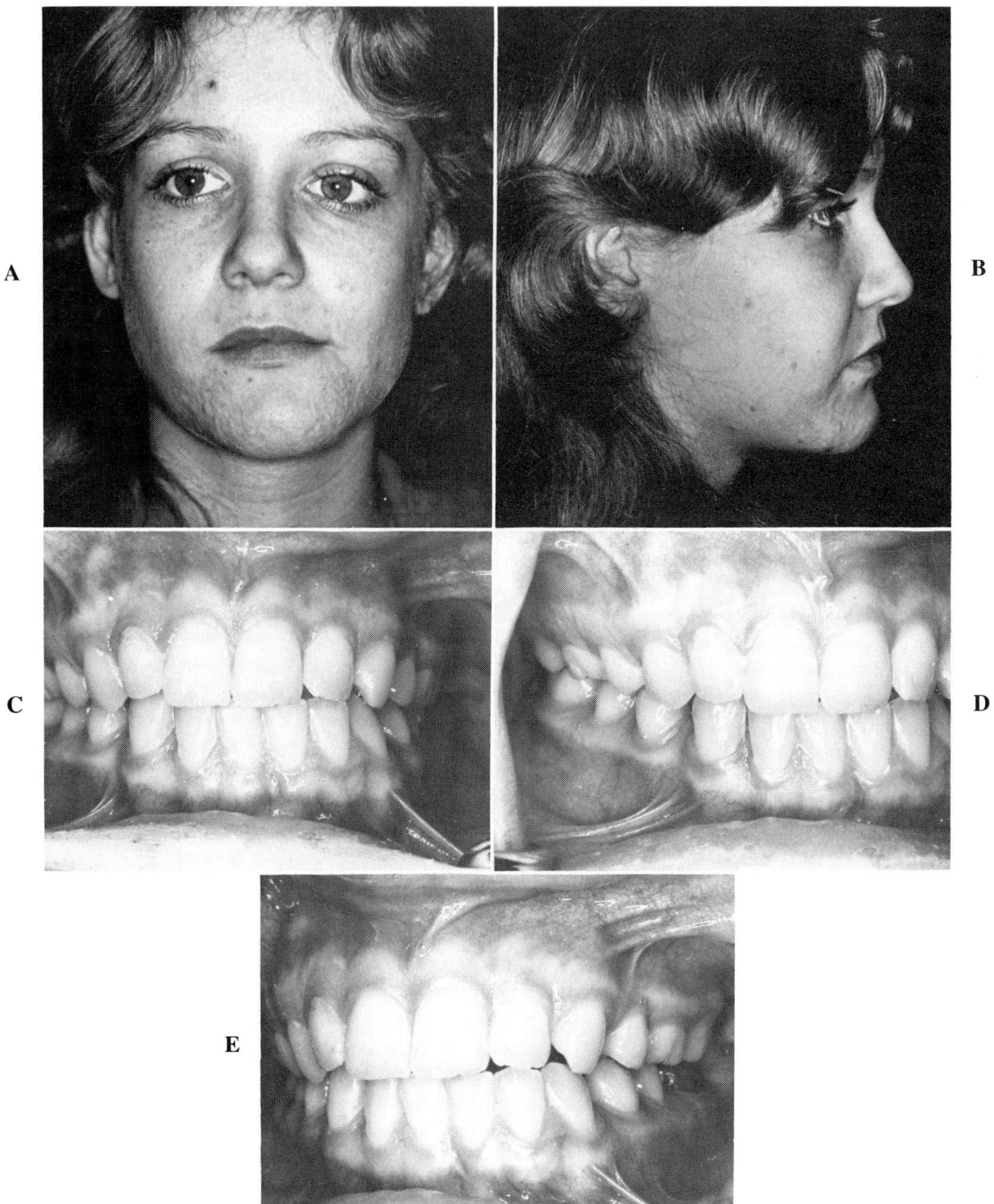

Fig. 3-10.
Case 6. **A** to **E,** Preoperative views. Right condylar hyperplasia causing mandibular and maxillary asymmetry with a canted occlusal plane on the right and mandibular midline deviation to the left. The occlusal plane on the right posterior is 6 mm lower than on the left preoperatively. The mandibular dental midline is shifted to the left. There is a Class I molar and canine occlusion.

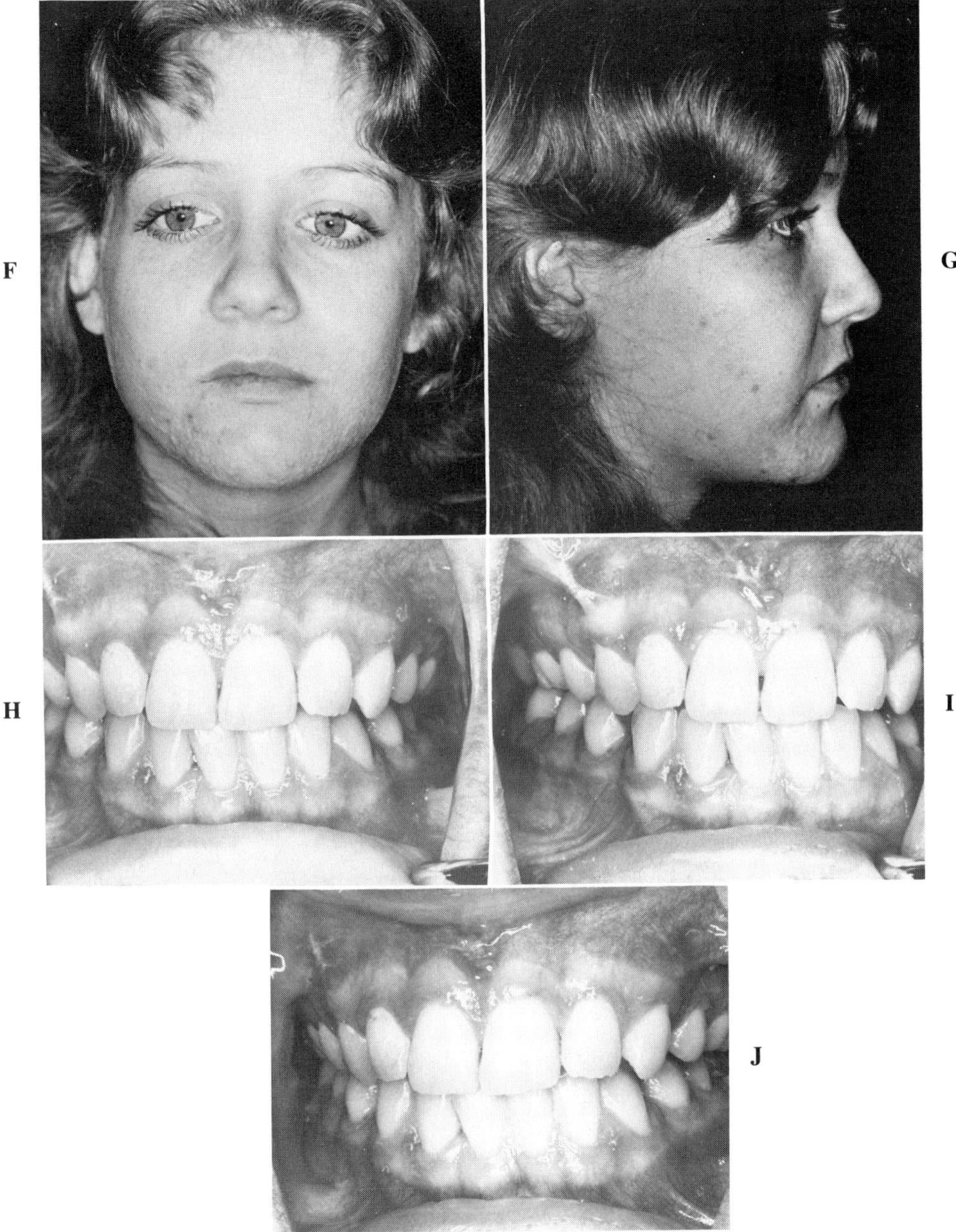

Continued.

Fig. 3-10—cont'd.

F to **J,** Postoperative views 8 months after leveling of the maxillary dentoalveolus with a total maxillary alveolar osteotomy and impaction 7 mm in the right posterior maxilla. The mandible was shifted and leveled with the maxilla by means of left sagittal and right oblique subcondylar osteotomies. The occlusion is essentially unchanged postoperatively. The occlusal plane has been leveled, and the Class I occlusion and deviation of the mandibular midline are the same as preoperatively.

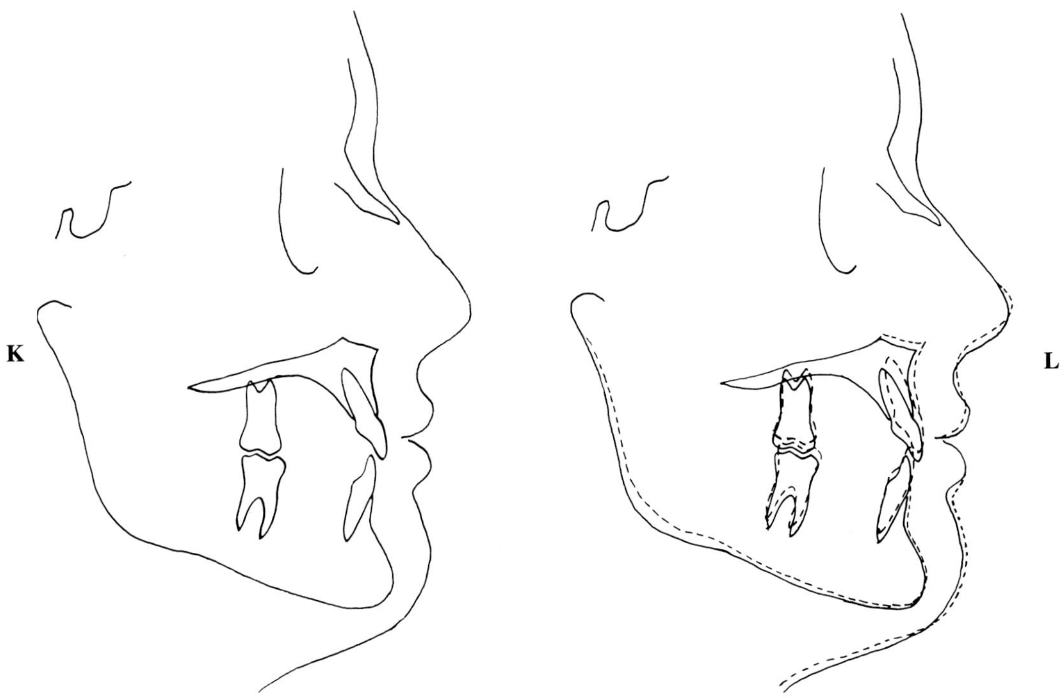

Fig. 3-10—cont'd.
Case 6. **K,** Preoperative cephalometric tracing. Satisfactory facial profile and occlusion, with little evidence of facial asymmetry. **L,** Composite preoperative and postoperative tracings. Little change in the lateral profile, with correction of the asymmetry.

CASE 7 (Fig. 3-11)

J.M., a 22-year-old white man, was referred to the clinic by his orthodontist after an unsuccessful attempt to treat a Class I malocclusion with asymmetry for which the patient had initially sought care. The patient was examined and baseline data obtained.

Problem list

Esthetics

Frontal: Mandibular asymmetry with a shift of the midline to the left; lip line canted inferiorly to the right

Lateral: Satisfactory

Cephalometric analysis

Lateral: Slight Class III molar and canine relationship; other features normal

PA

Mandibular asymmetry with 7 mm shift of the midline to the left

Dental occlusal plane 4 mm lower on the right than on the left

Occlusion

Dental arch form: Symmetric and well coordinated; slight cant inferiorly on the right

Dental alignment: Mandibular midline deviated to the left; left posterior maxillary dentoalveolar constriction

Dental occlusion: Class III molar and canine relationships

Treatment plan

Total maxillary alveolar ostectomy with impaction of the right posterior dentoalveolus 4 mm to level the maxillary occlusal plane

Oblique subcondylar osteotomies of the mandibular rami with retrusion of the mandible asymmetrically to correct the Class III malocclusion and facial asymmetry

Genioplasty with a wedge of bone 4 mm thick on the right to level the anterior mandible and correct the midline of the chin

Follow-up

The surgery was done as a one-stage procedure and the patient was placed in intermaxillary fixation for 6 weeks. After mobilization a satisfactory facial profile and occlusion had been obtained. Eight months' follow-up has revealed no significant change in these results.

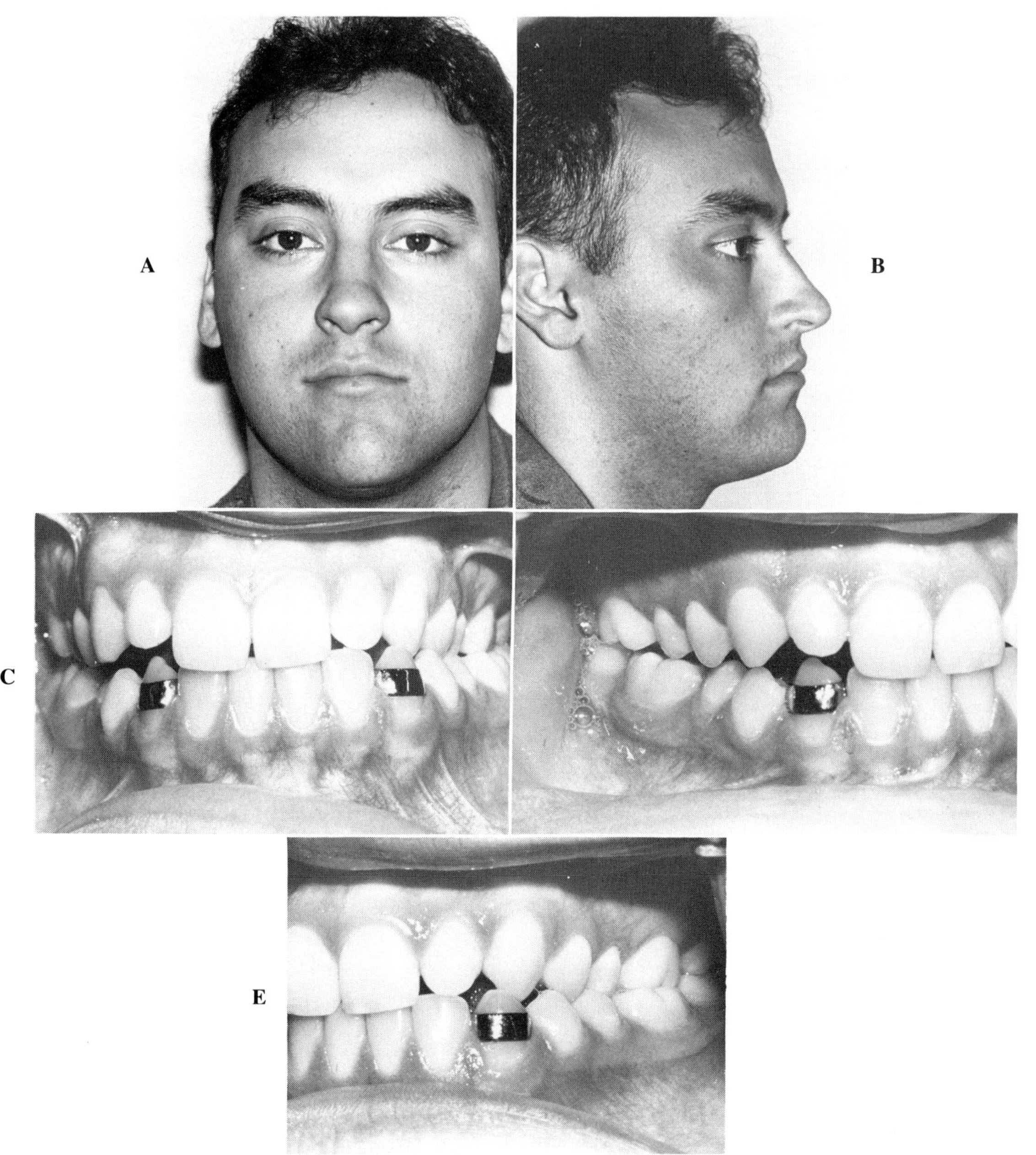

Fig. 3-11.
Case 7. **A** to **E,** Preoperative views showing mandibular asymmetry with deviation to the left. This patient received orthodontic care in preparation for surgery. Note the deviation of the mandibular midline, the cant of the occlusal plane down on the right, and the Class III molar and canine relationship. There is also a left posterior cross-bite.

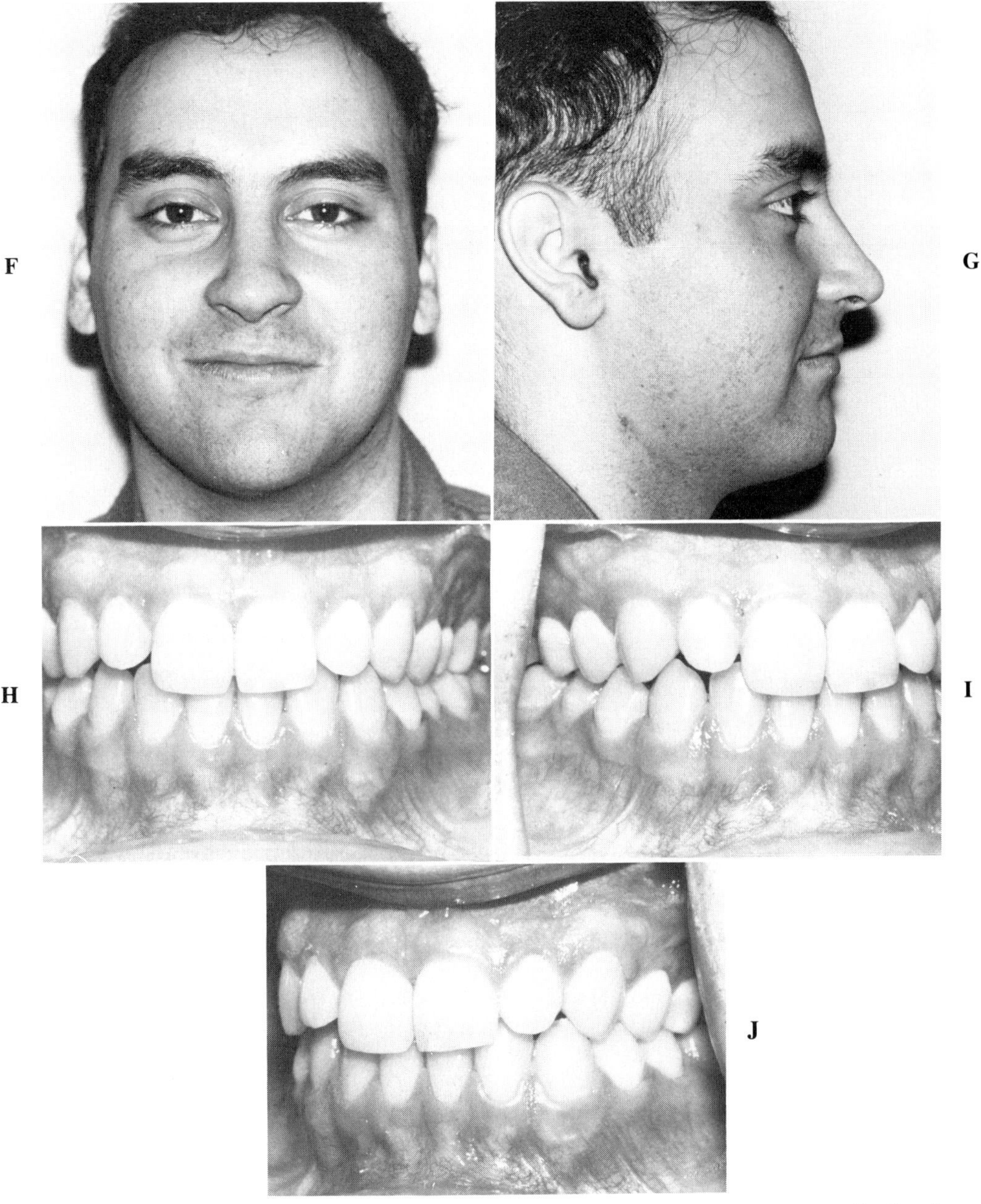

Continued.

Fig. 3-11—cont'd.
F to **J,** Postoperative views after correction of the asymmetry and malocclusion with a total maxillary alveolar osteotomy and 4 mm of right posterior maxillary impaction, mandibular retrusion, and leveling genioplasty. The occlusal plane has been leveled, the dental midlines are approximated, there is a Class I molar and canine occlusion, and the left posterior cross-bite has been corrected postoperatively.

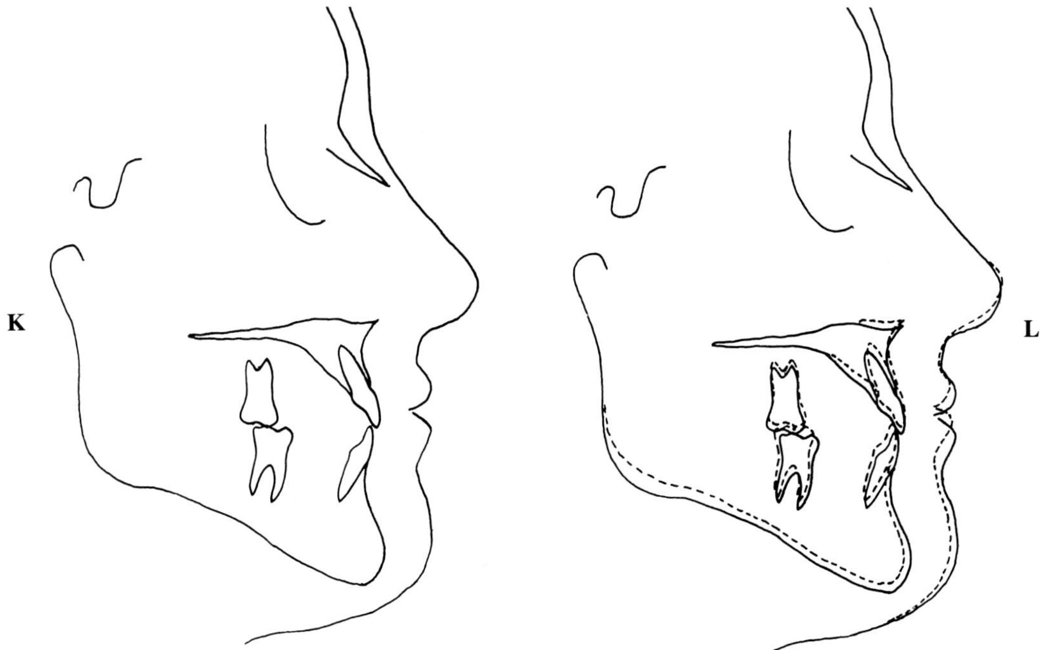

Fig. 3-11—cont'd.
Case 7. **K,** Preoperative cephalometric tracing. Little evidence of facial asymmetry. **L,** Composite preoperative and postoperative tracings. Little change in the lateral profile after leveling of the maxilla, mandible, and chin and minimal mandibular retrusion to correct the Class III malocclusion.

CASE 8 (Fig. 3-12)

J.S., a 19-year-old white man referred for evaluation of his malocclusion by his general dentist, was not unhappy with his facial appearance but complained of difficulty in masticating and of trauma to his palatal soft tissues from the lower anterior teeth.

Problem list

Esthetics

Frontal: Symmetric appearance; good lip competence and no excessive exposure of the dentition on smiling

Profile: Slight retrognathism

Cephalometric analysis

Facial convexity (S-N-A, 88 degrees; S-N-B, 80; A-N-B, 8; 1 to N-A, 18; 1 to N-B, 28)

Deficient mandible, protrusive maxilla, and microgenia; angle of facial convexity, 22 degrees

Occlusion

Dental arch form: Total maxillary and mandibular arch width discrepancy; excessive maxillary and insufficient mandibular dentoalveolar dimensions

Dental alignment: Unsatisfactory because of the arch width discrepancy

Dental occlusion: Complete buccal cross-bite relationship, midlines satisfactory; Class II positional relationship, 7 mm overbite and 8 mm overjet

Treatment plan

Total maxillary alveolar osteotomy in four segments to

Constrict the maxillary dentoalveolus

Vertically reposition the maxilla

Allow mandibular autorotation to partially correct the mandibular deficiency

Bilateral mandibular posterior subapical osteotomies to expand the posterior dentoalveolus to accommodate the now-reduced maxillary arch width

Bilateral intraoral sagittal osteotomies of the mandibular rami to advance the mandible to a Class I canine and molar occlusion and to correct the relative mandibular deficiency

Follow-up fixed prosthetic restorations to replace the first premolars, which were to be removed to allow segmentalization of the dentoalveoli

Follow-up

Surgery was completed in two separate procedures. Initially the planned maxillary vertical repositioning and arch constriction and the mandibular posterior subapical osteotomies for expansion were completed. Four weeks later the mandible was advanced and the patient placed in his final occlusal relationship. After 6 weeks of intermaxillary fixation, the patient was returned to his general dentist and fixed prosthetic restorations to replace the first premolars were constructed. One year postoperatively the occlusion has been well maintained in good function.   *Text continued on p. 99.*

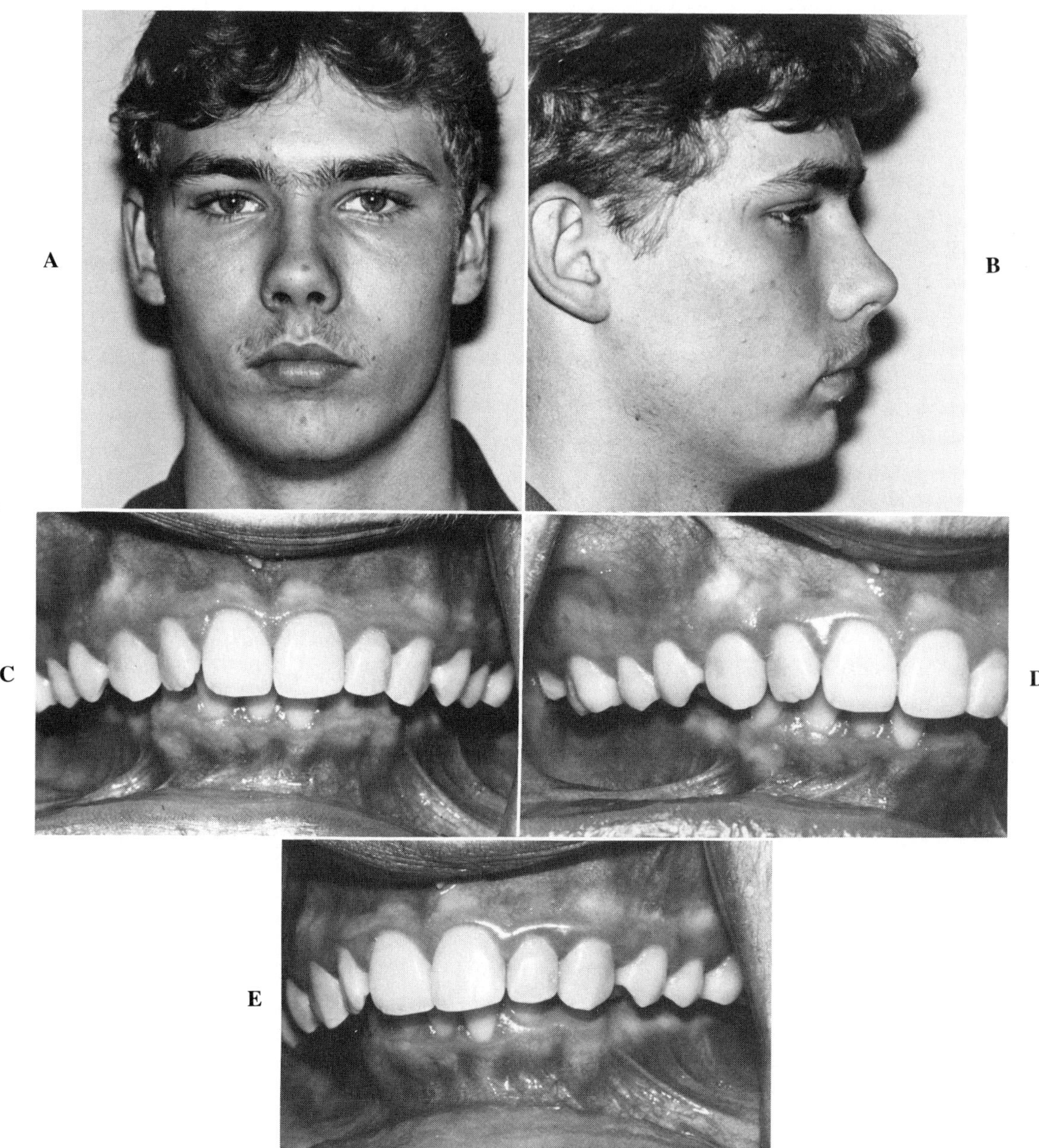

Fig. 3-12.
Case 8. **A** to **E,** Preoperative views of a Class II malocclusion, mandibular retrognathism, and complete arch width discrepancy with total buccal cross-bite.

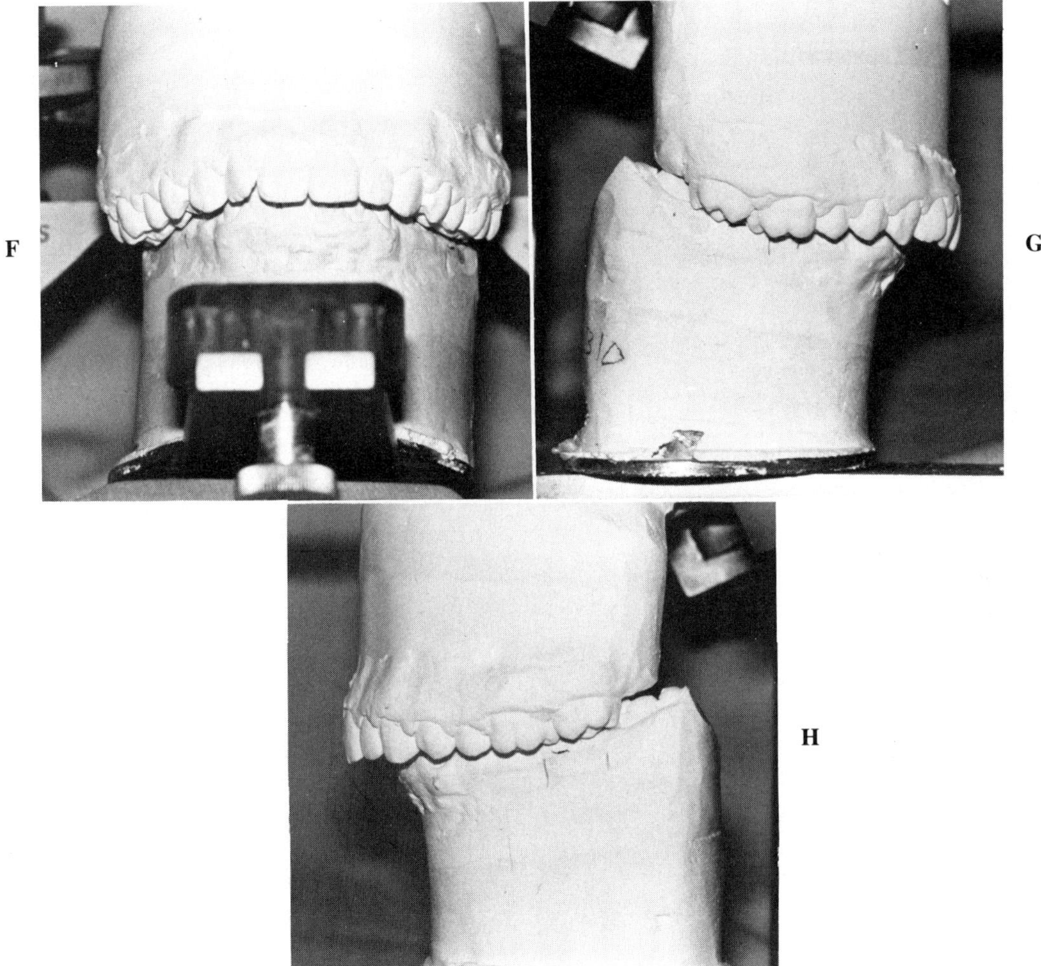

Fig. 3-12—cont'd.
F to **H,** Preoperative models.

Continued.

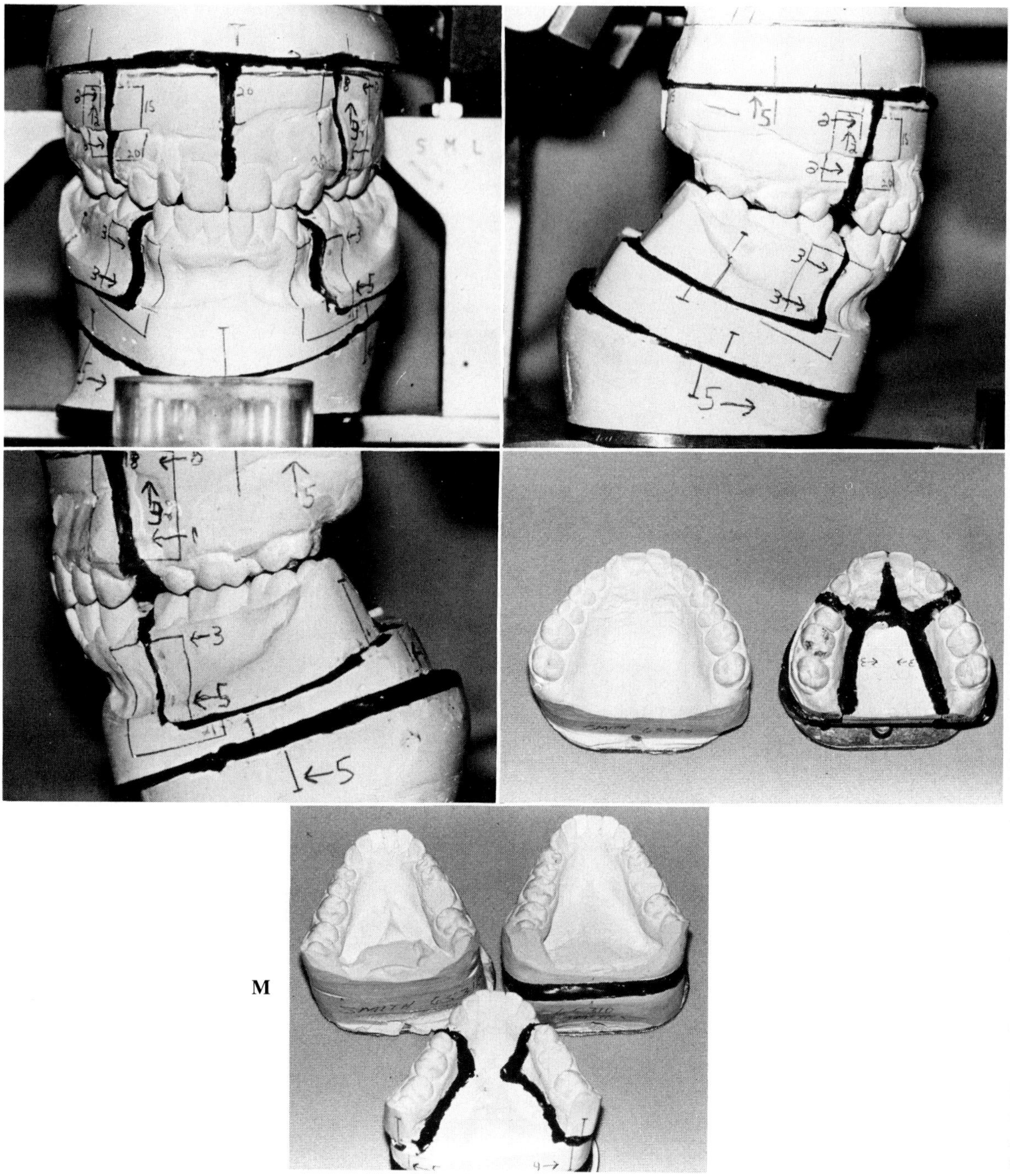

Fig. 3-12—cont'd.
I to **M,** Surgical models illustrating correction of the malocclusion, arch width discrepancy, and mandibular retrognathism via a four-segment total maxillary alveolar osteotomy, bilateral mandibular posterior subapical osteotomies, and sagittal osteotomies of the mandibular rami.

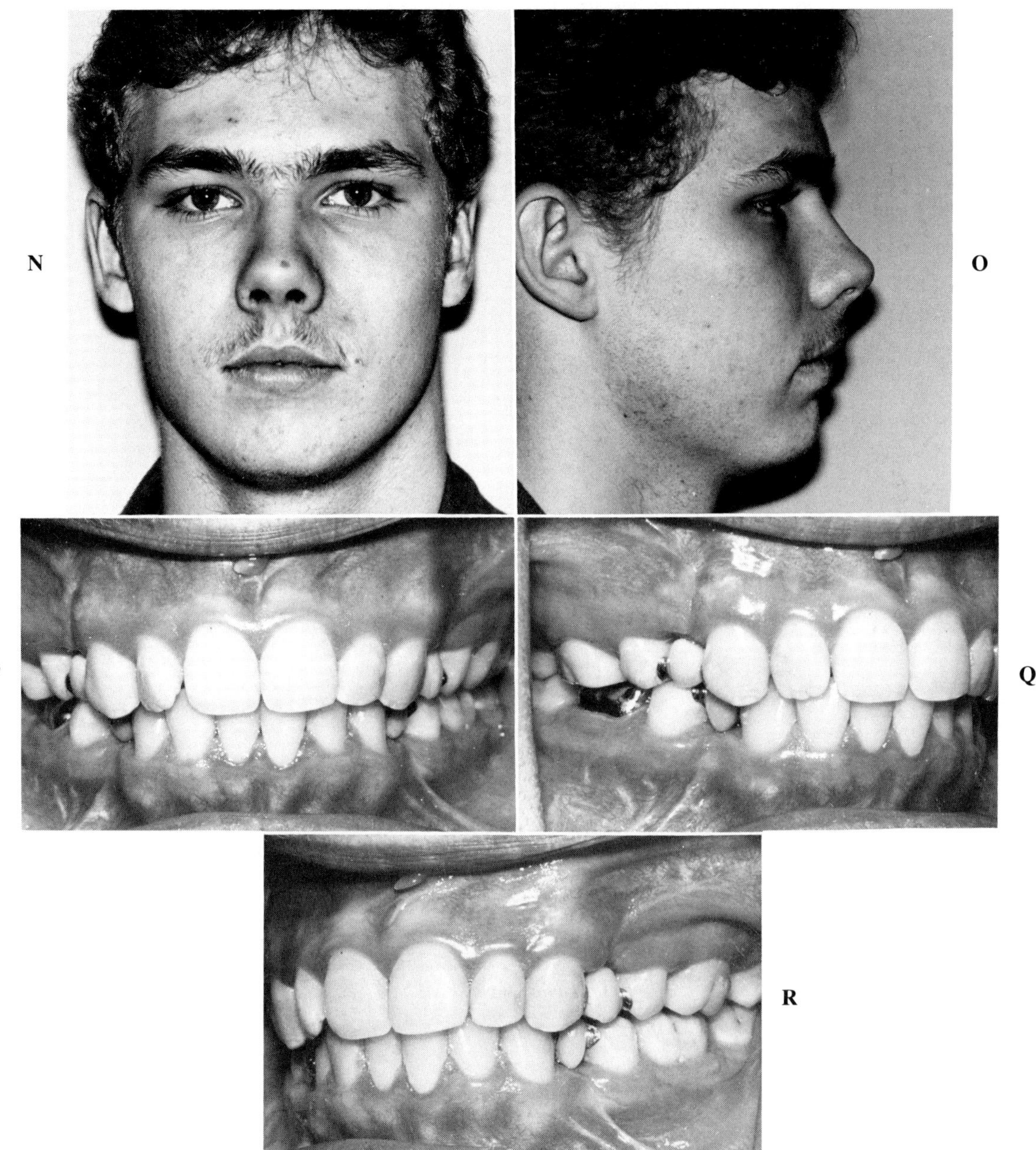

Continued.

Fig. 3-12—cont'd.
N to **R,** Postoperative views. The mandibular retrognathism has been corrected. After narrowing and recontouring of the maxillary dentoalveolus, posterior expansion of the mandibular dentoalveolus, and mandibular advancement. Fixed partial dentures are replacing the first premolars, removed during surgery.

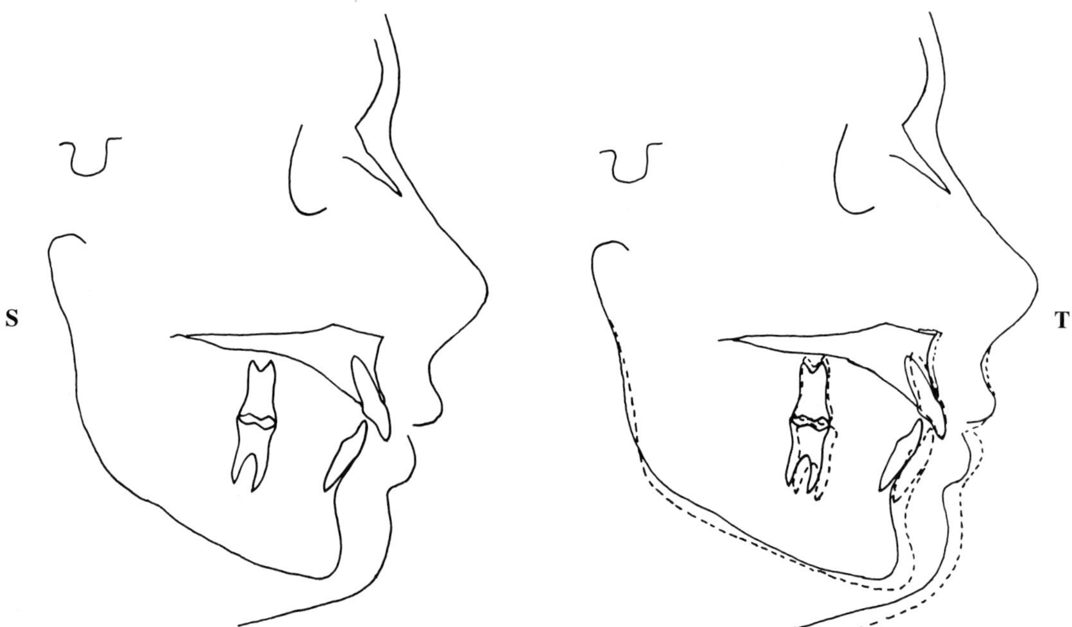

Fig. 3-12—cont'd.
Case 8. **S,** Preoperative cephalometric tracing. **T,** Composite preoperative and postoperative tracings after correction of the Class II malocclusion, arch width discrepancy, and mandibular retrognathism with total maxillary alveolar osteotomy, bilateral posterior mandibular subapical osteotomies, and sagittal osteotomies of the mandibular rami.

REFERENCES

1. Azaz, B., and Shteyer, A.: Modification of the muco-periosteal flap design in anterior maxillary osteotomies, Br. J. Oral Surg. **16**:253, 1977.
2. Bell, W.H.: Revascularization and bone healing after anterior maxillary osteotomy: a study using adult rhesus monkeys, J. Oral Surg. **27**:249, 1969.
3. Bell, W.H.: Correction of maxillary excess by anterior maxillary osteotomy, Oral Surg. **43**:323, 1977.
4. Bell, W.H., and Jacobs, J.D.: Surgical-orthodontic correction of maxillary retrusion by LeFort I osteotomy and Proplast, J. Maxfac. Surg. **8**:84, 1980.
5. Bell, W.H., and Levy, B.M.: Revascularization and bone healing after posterior maxillary osteotomy, J. Oral Surg. **29**:313, 1971.
6. Bell, W.H., and McBride, K.L.: Immediate surgical repositioning of anterior and posterior maxillary dento-osseous segments, J. Oral Surg. **34**:943, 1976.
7. Bell, W.H., and McBride, K.L.: Correction of the long face syndrome by LeFort I osteotomy, Oral Surg. **44**:493, 1977.
8. Bell, W.H., and Sinn, D.P.: Turbinectomy to facilitate superior movement of the maxilla by LeFort I osteotomy, J. Oral Surg. **37**:129, 1979.
9. Bell, W.H., et al.: Bone healing and revascularization after total maxillary osteotomy, J. Oral Surg. **33**:253, 1975.
10. Bresolin, D., et al.: Mouth breathing in allergic children: its relationship to dentofacial development, J. Dentofac. Orthop. **83**:334, 1983.
11. Cheever, D.: Displacement of the upper jaw, Med. Surg. Rep. Boston City Hosp., p. 156, 1870.
12. Cohn-Stock, G.: Die chirurgische immediatregulierung der Kiefer, Speziell die chirurgische Behandlung der prognathie, Vjschr Zahnheilkund. **37**:320, 1921.
13. Epker, B.N., Superior surgical repositioning of the maxilla: long-term results, J. Maxillofac. Surg. **9**:237, 1981.
14. Epker, B.N., and Wolford, L.M.: Middle-third facial osteotomies: their use in the correction of congenital dentofacial and craniofacial deformities, J. Oral Surg. **34**:324, 1976.
15. Epker, B.N., et al.: Indications for simultaneous mobilization of the maxilla and mandible for the correction of dentofacial deformities, Oral Surg. **54**:369, 1982.
16. Gross, B.D., and James, R.B.: The surgical sequence of combined total maxillary and mandibular osteotomies, J. Oral Surg. **36**:513, 1978.
17. Hall, H.D., and Roddy, S.C.: Treatment of maxillary alveolar hyperplasia by total maxillary alveolar osteotomy, J. Oral Surg. **33**:180, 1975.
18. Hall, H.D., and West, R.A.: Combined anterior and posterior maxillary osteotomy, J. Oral Surg. **34**:126, 1976.
19. Isaacson, R.J.: Maxillary growth aberrancy with special reference to maxillary hyperplasia, J. Oral Surg. **39**:898, 1981.
20. Kole, H.: Surgical operations on the alveolar ridge to correct occlusal abnormalities, Oral Surg. **12**:277, 1959.
21. Kole, H.: Results, experience, and problems in the operative treatment of anomalies with reverse overbite (mandibular protrusion), Oral Surg. **19**:427, 1965.
22. Kufner, J.: Experience with a modified procedure for correction of openbite. In Walker, R.V., editor: Transactions of the Third International Conference of Oral Surgery, London, 1970, E & S Livingstone, Ltd.
23. Mohnac, A.M.: Maxillary osteotomy for the correction of malpositioned fractures: report of case, J. Oral Surg. **25**:460, 1967.
24. Moloney, F., et al.: Surgical correction of vertical maxillary excess: a re-evaluation, J. Maxillofac. Surg. **10**:84, 1982.
25. Paul, J.K.: Correction of maxillary retrognathia: report of a case, J. Oral Surg. **27**:57, 1969.
26. Schendel, S.A., et al.: Superior repositioning of the maxilla: stability and soft tissue osseous relations, Am. J. Orthod. **70**:663, 1976.
27. Schuchardt, K.: Experiences with the surgical treatment of some deformities of the jaws, prognathia, micrognathia and openbite. In Wallace, A.B., editor: Transactions of the Second Congress of International Society of Plastic Surgeons, London, 1959, E & S Livingstone, Ltd.
28. Stoker, N.G., and Epker, B.N.: The posterior maxillary osteotomy: a retrospective study of treatment results, Int. J. Oral Surg. **3**:153, 1974.
29. Teuscher, U., and Sailer, H.F.: Stability of LeFort I osteotomy in Class III cases with retropositioned maxillae, J. Maxillofac. Surg. **10**:80, 1982.
30. Turvey, T.A.: Management of the nasal apparatus in maxillary surgery, J. Oral Surg. **38**:331, 1980.
31. Turvey, T.A.: Simultaneous mobilization of the maxilla and mandible: surgical technique and results, J. Oral Surg. **40**:96, 1982.
32. Wassmund, J.: Lehrbuch der praktischen Chirurgie des Mundes und der Kiefer, vol. 1, Leipzig, 1935, Hermann Meusser.
33. West, R.A., and Epker, B.N.: Posterior maxillary surgery: its place in the treatment of dentofacial deformities, J. Oral Surg. **30**:562, 1972.
34. West, R.A., and McNeill, R.W.: Maxillary alveolar hyperplasia, diagnosis and treatment planning, J. Maxillofac. Surg. **3**:239, 1975.
35. Westwood, R.M., and Tilson, H.B.: Complications associated with maxillary osteotomies, J. Oral Surg. **33**:104, 1975.
36. Wolford, L.M., and Epker, B.N.: The combined anterior and posterior maxillary ostectomy: a new technique, J. Oral Surg. **33**:842, 1975.
37. Wunderer, S.: Die prognathie Operation mittels frontal gestieltem Maxillafragment, Ost. Z. Stomatol. **59**:98, 1962.

CHAPTER 4

Considerations for genioplasty

Michael E. Lessin

The chin, lips, and nose have a long-acknowledged esthetic interrelationship and have been the basis of many attitudes toward favorable or unfavorable esthetic concepts and behavioral patterns. Although the background for surgical alteration of the bony chin is established in the European literature, and was introduced by Trauner and Obwegeser[25] to the American literature in 1957, it was not until Obwegeser's visits to America in the 1960s that a dramatic increase in intraoral surgery of the maxillomandibular complex was seen. Certainly, it has been during the last two decades that a larger body of cases has been statistically analyzed and newer techniques of genioplasty (horizontal osteotomy of the chin) have been presented.[2-5,11,12]

This chapter is written from the viewpoint of a clinician with teaching responsibilities. The cases selected and presented are from a narrow population spectrum, many without the benefit of conservative orthodontia because of financial or work requirements; others are without prolonged follow-up because of the dynamics of a transient population. Despite these limitations, surgery was still performed with reasonable expectations and generally satisfactory results. Whereas a combined orthodontic, oral, and maxillofacial surgical treatment plan may be desirable, we have recognized that not all patients are candidates for comprehensive orthodontia and that compromises not detrimental to the patient sometimes can be made.

INDICATIONS AND TREATMENT PLANNING

Although many patients are seen in our practice upon referral from their orthodontists, a large majority are seen on referral from their primary general dentist or physician. We hope that patients seen from the orthodontist are in the treatment planning stage so a viable coordinated treatment plan can be established and followed. Communication of goals and plans continues to be of utmost importance between participants.

Using the data-based problem-oriented evaluation and treatment system continues to be the most efficient way to define and treatment plan correction of chin abnormalities as well as other occlusofacial disharmonies. The data base has been well defined[8]; unfortunately many clinicians tend to ignore the efficient use of the statement of the problem in the patient's own words. What we may see as a relatively minor problem, for instance, a recessive chin, may have a greater position in a patient's mind and must be addressed. Elements of the psychosocial history may be important as well.

Separation of pure chin abnormalities is a minority in our practice, and generally appears in patients treated to a Class I occlusion orthodontically without the benefit of oral and maxillofacial surgery. The largest problems seen in pure chin abnormalities continue to be recessiveness or prominence, excessive or deficient height, asymmetry, and lip incompetence in association with recessiveness or excessive height. Unless it can be ascertained at the time of initial interview that the patient is not to be treated for occlusal disharmony as well, our data base includes those materials necessary for completeness.

After talking with the patient, we perform a complete intraoral and extraoral examination directing our attention to the frontal and profile views with the patient's head resting in the visual axis. The use of a *detail sheet* to note occlusal problems, midline hard and soft tissue shifts, and nasal, lip, and chin disharmonies is recommended. Visual inspection for lip competence and tooth exposure with lips in repose is a must, as is evaluation of the smile line and gingival exposure. Clinical use of the Holdaway line and zero meridian are useful in the evaluation of lips, nose and chin position as well.[14]

From this detailed examination a clinical impression of the deformity or deformities may be listed. If occlusal relationships are to be evaluated, study impressions are obtained and the casts mounted appropriately on suitable articulators.

Radiographs obtained for evaluation include a lateral head plate, a panographic film, and a true posteroanterior head plate for use in evaluating asymmetry problems if clinically apparent. Both hard tissue and soft tissue cephalometric analyses are performed, and also a PA cephalometric evaluation if asymmetries are being addressed.

The difference in racial standards does not appear in our analyses but must be considered during the evaluation of the cephalometric abnormalities. The soft tissue analysis of Legan and Burstone[15] contains a wealth of information regarding the nose, lips, chin and neck; and since we treat patients and not cephalometric standards, it may provide us with the greatest wealth of cephalometric information that can be coordinated with clinical findings and planning.

Additionally, the lateral head plate is also analyzed to gain information regarding thickness of the bony chin at the symphysis available for genioplasty. Extraoral and intraoral photographic evaluation is accomplished and is a must for permanent records.

A compilation of clinical, occlusal, and ra-diographic analyses leads to a final description of problems that, we hope, may be treated with surgery of the bony or soft tissue elements (that is, the lips and nose), either with or without coordinated orthodontic care. This chapter deals primarily with genioplasty; but in view of the fact that genioplasty may be only part of a detailed treatment plan of the maxillomandibular elements, a discussion of model surgery will be deferred except when genioplasty is part of the total mandibular procedures to be performed, accuracy of measurement of planned movements of the total mandible being extremely important to planning the genioplasty properly.

PREDICTIONS

Many analyses[3,4,18,22] have been performed to detail the concomitant soft tissue changes created by movement of the bony chin alone or with simultaneous movement of the mandible. That movement of the total mandible or chin affects the soft tissue chin and the lower and upper lips is undisputed and well summarized.[6,21] Soft tissue changes of the chin secondary to genioplasty associated with maxillary impaction have also been analyzed.[11]

Advancement genioplasty utilizing a minimal soft tissue dissection technique is extremely predictable, leading to a 75% soft tissue–hard tissue response at pogonion.[18,20] Reduction genioplasty alone, however, is not as predictable, results quoted ranging from 40% to 75%[4] whereas combined mandibular setback with advancement genioplasty appears to allow for a 1:1 soft tissue–hard tissue change, perhaps because of differences in soft tissue tension secondary to the mandibular repositioning.[3,22] Busquets and Sassouni[6] have also documented an approximate 44% change in position of the lower lip as pogonion is advanced. Gallagher et al.[11] demonstrate a 1 to 0.87 hard tissue to soft tissue change in advancement genioplasties performed concomitantly with large maxillary impactions and mandibular autorotations.

What this means to the clinician is that a fairly accurate way exists to predict soft tissue contours resulting from bony chin alteration with the use of overlays and cutouts[20] and indeed it is useful in planning and, in a limited fashion, as a patient education guide. The soft tissue analysis is extremely helpful in judging whether or not alterations produced may be beneficial to the patient in light of the effect upon the lower face–throat angle, lower vertical height-depth ratio, lower lip protrusion, and mentolabial sulcus.[15]

We do not dwell upon prediction tracings excessively, nor do we present them to the patient unless hard pressed to do so. The changes expected as a result of the planned surgical procedure are explained to the patient, in general terms, at the case presentation session. As Bell et al.[5] so appropriately state: "In the final analysis, irrespective of the cephalometric prediction study and soft tissue predictions, the final results must be esthetically pleasing to the patient and the clinician." Some patients may demand too much accuracy from the predictions, which may lead to patient displeasure and perhaps ultimately to litigation.

Some other clinical observations are pertinent to this discussion:

1. We believe that patients who are severely lacking in chin prominence can virtually never be overaugmented since the thickness of bone available for advancement at the symphysis prohibits overaugmentation, much less achievement of a desired profile in many cases. This problem may be addressed with the two-step genioplasty or a second procedure genioplasty.

2. Although reduction genioplasty is demonstrated repeatedly in the literature, we believe that despite the good bony reduction obtainable, a large number of patients have resultant contour excess of the submental area not accounted for in any prediction and may have on frontal view an unsatisfactory squaring of the mentum and associated soft tissue redundancy. Prevention or treatment of this unesthetic appearance has not been, in our minds, satisfactorily resolved.[24]

3. The question whether or not to perform associated genioplasty with mandibular advancement in pubescent growing males has arisen. Our experience confirms that in adolescent patients continued chin growth is often not significant in lacking patients, and we therefore generally choose to do the genioplasty if indicated.

SEQUENCING OF PROCEDURES

After treatment planning is complete, a presentation appointment with the patient and, as applicable, the parents of an unemancipated minor, the spouse, or other appropriate individuals is held. If combined care is planned, a joint clinician meeting may be desirable.

The surgery, hospitalization, functional and cosmetic expectations, and sequelae should be adequately discussed to ensure that all concerned parties are "operating on the same frequency" and not expecting too much or too little. It is interesting that, although great efforts are made to guarantee informed consent at our institution, questions or comments made by the patient or other concerned parties indicate continued need for reinforcement of plans, proposed outcome, and sequelae. Continued communication with the referring dentist or physician regarding treatment is again emphasized and pays multifold dividends.

In planning the sequence of procedures, necessary nasal or other soft tissue surgery (that is, lip reduction) is best performed after completion and healing of proposed maxillomandibular osteotomies. Infrequently lack of nasal airway competence may force septoplasty or adenoidectomy primarily.

Cases in which advancement genioplasty is to be performed concurrently with maxillomandibular osteotomy are generally those in which bilaterally symmetric ramal movements are planned. We prefer to do the genioplasty at the beginning of the case, when swelling is minimal and when horizontal osteotomy would not interfere with an occlusion and osteotomy stabilized and in intramaxillary fixation.

When asymmetric movements of the mandible are planned or when vertical augmentation or correction of transverse asymmetries is to be addressed, we prefer to do the genioplasty at a separate surgical session, anytime after 6 weeks postoperatively. The patient may then be mobilized and intubated more easily and the surgical planning will be enhanced after reevaluation, clinically and radiographically, as needed.

If mandibular anterior alveolar segmental osteotomy is to be performed in association with genioplasty and adequate bony height is not present (5 mm or more of bone between the horizontal osteotomy cut of the alveolar procedure and proposed genioplasty), then genioplasty is again deferred until at least 8 weeks after the mandibular anterior alveolar segmental osteotomy.

When insufficient bony height is available for two-step horizontal advancement and inadequate horizontal advancement is predicted or obtained, a second genioplasty may be planned 4 to 6 months after the initial procedure. The second procedure has allowed us to improve desired contour in several cases. Proper sequence planning and the use of additional surgical sessions if needed, per our criteria, have led to more satisfactory results.

SURGICAL TECHNIQUE

To perform genioplasty, our surgeons operate from the head of the table looking down on the surgical site. General anesthesia is administered via low-profile nasotracheal intubation, preferably utilizing a Bain nonrebreathing circuit. Relative hypotension is desirable. The surgical technique we use is that of minimal tissue dissection with resultant broad pedicle— as advocated by Epker and Wolford,[7] McBride and Bell,[17] and Bell and Gallagher[4]—with some differences in instrumentation.

Local anesthetic and vasoconstrictor is injected into the mandibular vestibule from first molar to first molar. If orthodontic wires are in place or if arch bars have been applied for maxillomandibular osteotomy, we have found it consistently easier to place the teeth in occlusion and apply minimal fixation prior to performing genioplasty.

The lip is extended and the incision is created from just above the mental foramen and bundle, which may be palpated, extending through the lower lip mucosa between the depth of the vestibule and the vermilion extending posteriorly to the opposite side (Fig. 4-1, *A*). The incision is then carried obliquely through mentalis muscle, care being taken to avoid the mental neurovascular bundles. Subperiosteal dissection is used superiorly to expose the apices of the teeth and to extend posteriorly in a horizontal manner, along the path of the proposed osteot-

omy, beneath the mental nerves (freeing them), to the inferior border of the mandible at the second premolar or first molar area. Minimal dissection is done inferiorly, leaving as much mentalis muscle and periosteum attached as possible. A modified Aufricht or piriform rim retractor with lip removed (Fig. 4-1, *B*) is inserted on a side, the acute bend allowing for better visualization of the inferior border and mental nerve (Fig. 4-1, *C*).

A no. 701 bur is placed in a Stryker rotating handpiece, and the midline is scribed vertically and lightly into the cortex. The proposed horizontal osteotomy is scribed into the cortex, to medullary bone, beginning at the inferior border, extending to the midline and carefully remaining 3 to 4 mm inferior to the mental foramen and root apices. Another modified Aufricht retractor is then placed on the opposite side and the continuation of the proposed osteotomy is again scribed lightly into the cortex in a similar fashion (Fig. 4-1, *C* and *D*). Attention is focused upon symmetry of the proposed cut by direct visualization and measurement as necessary. Once symmetry is confirmed, completion of scribing into medullary bone is assured.

We then prefer to use a reciprocating Stryker saw blade without a ribbed edge (Fig. 4-1, *E*). After it has been placed in the scribed surface at the inferior border of one side or the other, the Aufricht is removed. As the reciprocating blade is used at full speed, the handle of the reciprocator is lifted to ensure complete cutting at the inferior border. Fingers are placed extraorally in the submental area to help sense when the cut is completed in that area. The cut proceeds toward the midline, with care to protect the mental nerve as necessary. The fingers extraorally follow the saw blade toward the midline to ensure completeness of cut. To avoid ledges, care must be continually taken to cut at the same angle to bone. Once the midline is passed, the operator has two choices. The saw blade may be removed and reinserted on the uncut side and the osteotomy cut completed on the opposite side in a similar manner, or the clinician may continue in the same direction and by altering the position of the handle effectively cut from

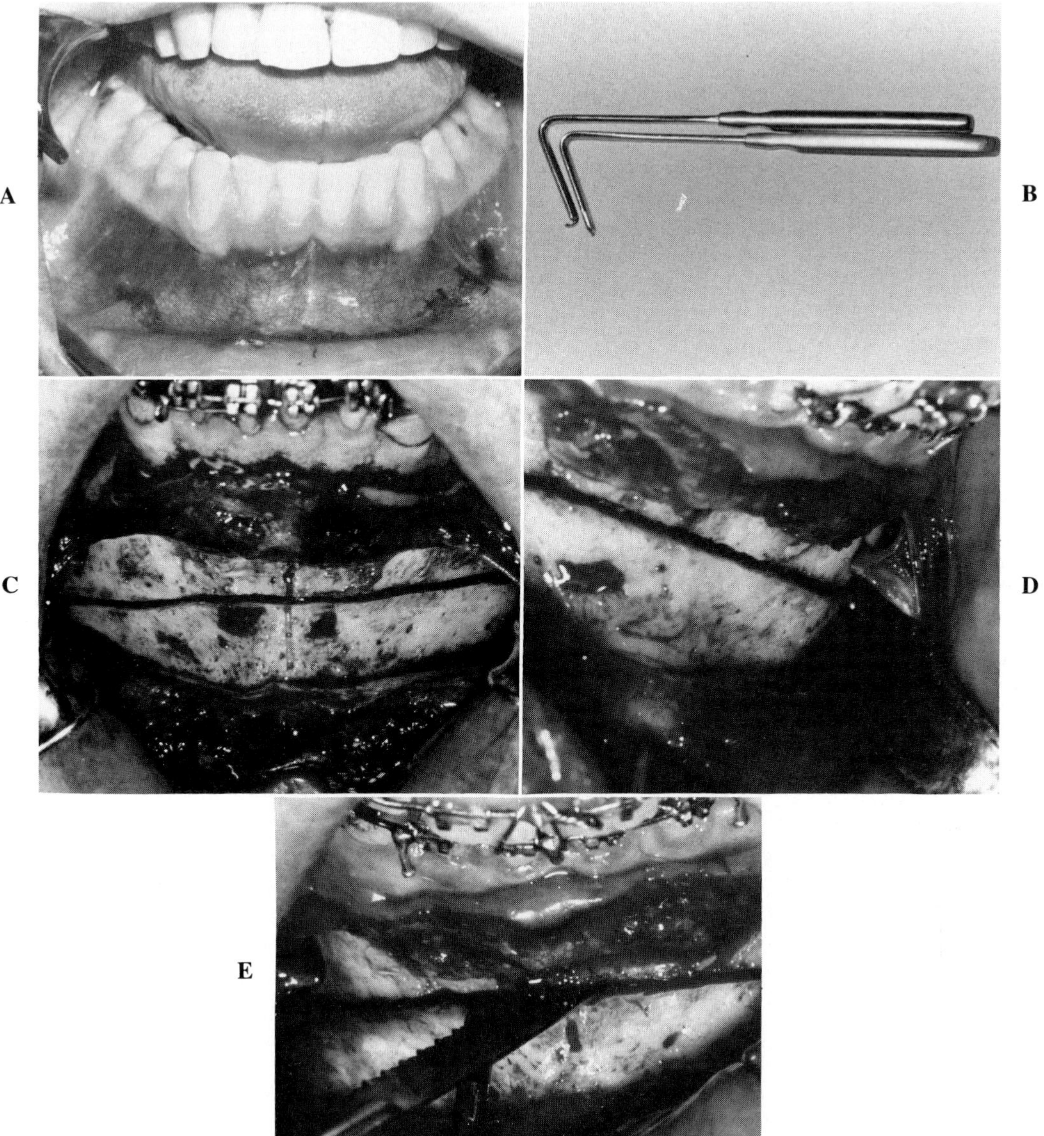

Fig. 4-1.
A, Incision outlined into the lip. **B,** Piriform rim retractor and modified version with the lip removed to create an Aufricht-type retractor. **C,** Proposed osteotomy outlined with a no. 701 bur. The midline has been scribed. **D,** Modified Aufricht retractors in place, enhancing vision. The proposed osteotomy lies well below the root apices and mental foramina. **E,** Use of a reciprocating saw to complete the osteotomy. The teeth are in light fixation, and the surgeon's fingers are positioned extraorally to palpate the blade as it penetrates the bone.

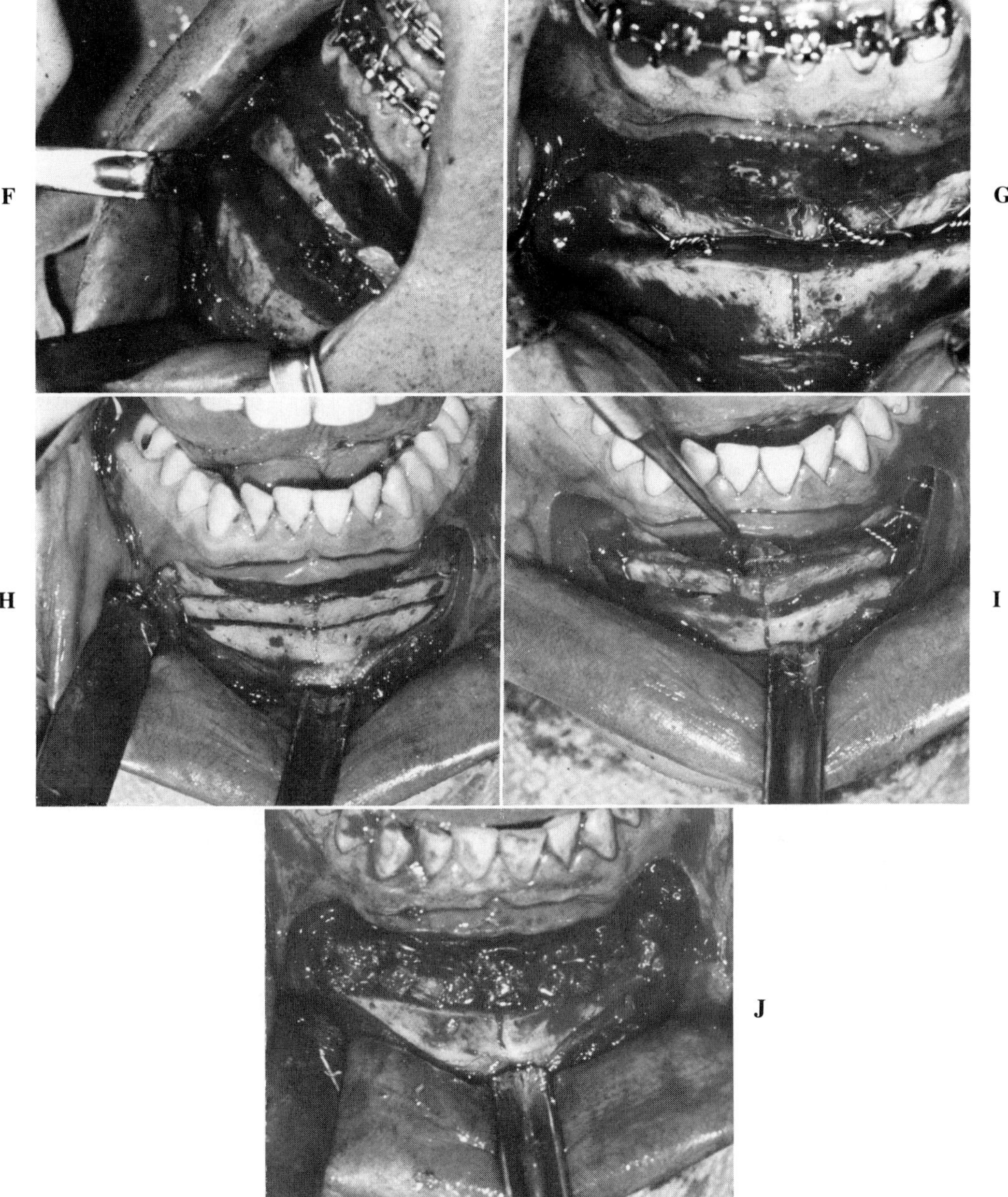

Fig. 4-1—cont'd.
F, Osteotomy completed. The distal (inferior) fragment is well pedicled. **G,** Distal (inferior) fragment advanced and wired appropriately through the labial cortex of the proximal (superior) bone and the lingual cortex of the distal (inferior) fragment. **H,** Two-step advancement genioplasty outlined. **I,** Two-step advancement completed and wired. The inferior or two-step cut was completed first, and then the superior cut. After placement of wires the superior step is advanced and tightened where desired and then the inferior (second) step is advanced and tightened. **J,** Cancellous bone graft placed to improve the contour along the horizontal steps of a two-step genioplasty.

the "inside out," using the scribed line for saw guidance; this has proved to be very effective. If the horizontal osteotomy has been thoroughly completed, the bony mentum will separate quite distinctly and remain pedicled to the mentalis muscle as well as the geniohyoid and digastric muscles and periosteum (Fig. 4-1, *F*).

It should be noted here that several modifications may be performed.

Modifying the direction in which the saw blade is held will allow for either shortening or lengthening of the chin as desired when advanced. If a wedge is to be removed for shortening or correction of vertical asymmetry, the wedge is scribed as desired. In completing the wedge ostectomy, the inferior cut is completed first to allow for stability in completion of the superior cut.

Midlines are adjusted and appropriate advancement or retrusion attempted. A tracheal hook and finger pressure have been useful for manipulating the free segment.

Three intraosseous holes are drilled through the labial cortex of the superior proximal stable bone, angled through medullary bone, one just off the midline and bilaterally in the canine-premolar region. If advancement is to be accomplished, holes are drilled in the free inferior distal segment to correspond with the superiorly placed holes, extending from medullary bone through lingual cortex. Intraosseous stainless steel wires are passed through corresponding holes in a circular or figure-8 fashion and tagged.

The modified Aufricht retractors are again placed and the tracheal hook and finger pressure used to position the inferior fragment as desired. Care is taken that the midline is in a desired position and that the lateral portions or wings of the inferior fragment project equally. Once satisfactory positioning is obtained, the lateral wires are twisted tight, followed by the midline wire (Fig. 4-1, *G*).

If posterior positioning of the inferior distal fragment is to be accomplished or pure shortening without advancement, all holes in the inferior fragment are also placed through labial cortex, exiting through medullary bone. In retrusion, prior to passing and twisting the wires, the lateral projections may be trimmed to pre-

vent irregular contour in the submental area.

Recently the use of Steinmann or Kirschner wires has been described[26,27] for fixation in large chin advancements, with or without associated bone grafting. We have not found them to be necessary thus far, even in large advancements.

Closure is performed in two layers; we prefer a polyglycolic acid suture for the deep closure and 4-0 chromic in a horizontal running mattress fashion for the mucosa. Polyglycolic acid suture in the oral environment takes considerably longer to absorb, generally creates a hygiene problem on the closure site, and may need to be removed. The deep closure never provides exact coaptation in advancement or vertical augmentations and generally ties muscle to periosteum, leaving gaps (though not appearing to be of consequence).

Two-step genioplasty for advancement may be performed if adequate bone is present to allow for at least a 4 to 5 mm superior step as well as an adequate inferior step. Certainly more soft tissue dissection is usually required, still attempting to maintain as much soft tissue attachment to the inferior portion as possible (Fig. 4-1, *H*). As in wedge ostectomy, the inferior (second step) is cut free first and then the superior step is accomplished. Holes are drilled as in one-stage genioplasties, allowing for advancement and fixation of each step, to a greater degree than if only one step is accomplished (Fig. 4-1, *I*). Periosteal scoring may be necessary to facilitate soft tissue closure.

For patients in whom two-step genioplasty is not feasible or whose extremely thin bone and retrusiveness do not allow adequate or desired advancement, a second genioplasty may be performed 4 to 6 months after the first. The incision and dissection through scar are more difficult, as expected, but the clinical appearance of the previously osteotomized bone is remarkable. Previously placed wires are usually partially covered with bone, and the horizontal table created by advancement is generally filled with new bone (Fig. 4-5, *I*). Some areas of bone scar may be seen. The old wires can most often be removed and the genioplasty continued as previously described.

In addition to allowing for a well-vascularized one-step or two-step genioplasty, the minimal dissection broad-pedicle technique allows division or wedge removal of the inferior (distal) fragment for widening or narrowing as desired while assuring adequate blood supply to maintain vitality of the smaller pedicles produced.[5,17]

After release of fixation, if applied, the oropharynx is suctioned free of debris and the throat pack removed. The sublingual area should then be inspected for excessive edema or hematoma. At completion a Microfoam tape* pressure dressing is applied over the chin for at least 24 hours to aid in the elimination of dead space and better soft tissue conformation. The minimal dissection broad-pedicle technique inherently decreases the amount of dead space available for hematoma formation. Longer-term use of the pressure dressing has not proved necessary.

Our technique calls for antibiotic administration at the initiation of the case (penicillin 2 million units preferably, if no allergy exists, with clindamycin 300 mg as a secondary drug in allergic individuals). Antibiotics continue to be administered at intervals, changing from IV to oral medication generally on the first postoperative day, and are continued 7 to 10 days. When oral drugs are administered, erythromycin is generally substituted for clindamycin. We realize that there would be some argument to stopping antibiotic administration immediately after surgery, but we continue to maintain that in the presence of hematoma, in an oral environment, with the concurrent administration of steroids, the continued antibiotic therapy is indicated. One hates to argue with success; and since we have had no infections in our intraoral genioplasty sites over the last 10 years, we are hesitant to change at this time. We do not consider this prophylactic but rather, in this environment, therapeutic.

Steroids are administered also at the initiation of treatment (dexamethasone 8 to 10 mg) and continued IV push every 6 hours. If an IV remains in place on the first postoperative day, IV steroids are continued (dexamethasone 8 mg

every 6 hours). However, if the IV is not in place after the morning dose, on postoperative day 1 the patient is administered methyl prednisolone acetate 80 mg IM on day 1 and 80 mg IM in one dose on day 2, even if then on an outpatient status. Some doctors may choose methyl prednisolone succinate as their primary IV steroid choice; either dexamethasone or methyl prednisolone appears satisfactory as long as high doses are administered.

Diet is progressed as tolerated to a dental soft consistency for patients not in fixation because of additional surgery. The pressure dressing is removed after 24 hours, and the patient returns gradually to an acceptable hygiene program and diet. Patients treated with genioplasty alone are generally released on the first postoperative day and followed closely as outpatients.

ALLOPLASTS

The use of alloplastic materials (Silastic) for augmentation of the chin has generally found favor with the plastic surgeon and otorhinolaryngologist and continues to be a mainstay in their approach to the contour-deficient chin.[24]

Robinson and Shuken[21] described bone resorption beneath 12 Silastic implants in a series of 14 implanted subperiosteally from extraoral and intraoral approaches. Bell[2] described an intraoral supraperiosteal pocket approach that also resulted in some degree of subimplant resorption in about half his cases.

For oral and maxillofacial surgeons the supraperiosteal Silastic implant has been succeeded by the intraoral horizontal osteotomy for advancement genioplasty. Contour appears more natural, and the difficulties from using any alloplastic materials (such as infection, migration, and pseudocapsule) have been eliminated.

The use of Proplast, a Teflon fluorocarbon polymer with vitreous carbon fibers, for chin augmentation implant has been described.[14,17] Biocompatibility and porosity, to allow tissue ingrowth, have indeed made Proplast a useful material for correction of contour defects or for bulking as necessary. However, those who advocate the implantation of large blocks of shaped Proplast through a subperiosteal intraoral approach offer no advantages, whether in operative time, results, or postsurgical prob-

<hr>

*Medical Products Division, 3M Co., Minneapolis.

lems, of this technique over the horizontal osteotomy for advancement genioplasty. We have not had the opportunity to implant an entire Proplast chin, nor have we encountered an indication that would make us choose this alternative. Smaller portions of Proplast to augment the lateral wings of an advancement genioplasty appear to be useful at times, and we have had successful experience with these.

We recently removed a large Proplast implant from the inferior border of the mandible in an infected patient. The implant had been placed at another institution and fixated as recommended 6 months previously and the patient treated with antibiotic solution. Pain and fluctuance had developed and the patient sought treatment. Culture and sensitivity tests revealed no bacterial growth from the aspirant, with WBCs too numerous to count. Upon removal of the implant from an extraoral approach, it was found to be totally mobile, with no tissue ingrowth and an apparent pseudocapsule present.

Although Proplast is a useful material to have at hand for use when indicated, we would encourage the oral and maxillofacial surgeon to continue to make the horizontal osteotomy of the chin the mainstay operation for correcting a contour-defective chin. The use of a hydroxyapatite implant along the horizontal cut to fill in resultant gaps or for lateral bulking has not yet been reported in genioplasty but would appear to merit investigation.

BONE GRAFTS AND GENIOPLASTY

Bone grafting in association with genioplasty procedures is generally necessary on only two occasions: to fill large gaps and for vertical augmentation.

When advancement genioplasty creates gaps with no bone-to-bone contact or with large steps along the horizontal table between the advanced inferior fragment and the labial cortex of the superior mandible, cancellous bone grafting may be useful (Fig. 4-1, *J*).

In the treatment of the short face syndrome, vertical augmentation genioplasty requires that a corticocancellous block be interpositioned to increase anterior mandibular facial height.[9,28] These patients have an extremely prominent chin, a deep labiomental fold, and generally a Class II malocclusion. Correction of the malocclusion does not as a rule improve the problem of the prominent chin and deep labiomental fold, and attempts at reducing the prominence of the chin with reduction genioplasty are moreover cosmetically unacceptable. For planning purposes bony vertical augmentation appears to show a 1:1 relationship with vertical soft tissue response and the expected 75% soft tissue response for any incorporated horizontal bony advancement as well.[26]

The use of autologous iliac crest, corticocancellous blocks, and autologous cancellous bone is well documented; and more recently the use of allogeneic, freeze-dried, lyophilized corticocancellous blocks and cancellous chips alone or as composite (autologous-allogeneic) grafts has been extremely well detailed.[1,8,10,16] That allogeneic bone is replaced by creeping substitution of host bone and that bone morphogenetic protein present in the allogeneic bone has an osteoinductive effect upon host cells seem to be a common conclusion of the research. Minimum antigenicity is of no apparent concern.[1]

Without a doubt, the genioplasty site, with its rich vascularity and ability to stabilize the components adequately and maintain soft tissue closure, is ideal.

Although we do not hesitate to harvest autologous iliac crest and cancellous marrow, during the last 4 years numerous genioplasties have been performed in which allogeneic cancellous bone or corticocancellous blocks were implanted either for the saving of time or because the patient did not want to have the iliac crest violated.

Allogeneic cancellous chips have been packed or onlayed when a sizable horizontal advancement resulted in large gaps, and a large step and allogeneic corticocancellous blocks and chips have been used for vertical chin augmentations. In one case an allogeneic rib portion was utilized with extremely satisfactory results (Fig. 4-7).

Although these cases have not been adequately analyzed statistically, all patients healed well without increase in sequelae and with clinically satisfactory and stable results.

Radiographically a change in densities occurs, indicating a replacement over time, with eventual total or near total replacement by host bone.

The technique for vertical augmentation differs little from the previously described technique. Special effort is made to ensure a properly placed incision, well into the lip to allow for excellent closure and to adequately release the mental neurovascular bundle to allow for stretching. The horizontal osteotomy of the chin is completed, and intraosseous holes are placed appropriately. The graft, having been properly reconstituted with saline previously, is shaped and contoured with rotary instruments to the desired proportions. In our cases a thickness of 4 to 5 mm has appeared desirable. Holes may be placed in the graft to allow for threading of the intraosseous wires, but generally this is not necessary except at the midline. The graft and inferior fragment are positioned as desired, with proper midline position, and the wires tightened. Allogeneic corticocancellous blocks or chips may be wedged or packed as necessary. Closure is accomplished in two layers. Periosteal scoring may be necessary to allow for adequate closure. The use of a pressure dressing to minimize hematoma formation and the administration of antibiotics intraoperatively and postoperatively are again emphasized. Steroids are also used as previously described.

MORBIDITY

Intraoperatively soft tissue injury, particularly from the reciprocating saw, is a possibility. Careful use of the instrument with adequate finger palpation generally limits the extent of this problem. Nonjudicious dissection or extreme retraction on the mental neurovascular bundle may lead to avulsion and its problems, which is certainly regrettable and usually avoidable.

Even with relative hypotensive anesthesia, the genioplasty remains an apparently bloody procedure, with blood loss dependent upon the individual circumstances. However, replacement with blood products has not been indicated. The apparent vascularity of the pedicled fragment should give good assurance of survival and demonstrates the wisdom of maintaining maximum soft tissue attachment.

Immediately postoperative morbidity includes sublingual edema and ecchymosis, which are minimized with good technique and the use of steroids. These have certainly not been a critical problem in any of our patients. Paresthesia or degrees thereof are evident for variable periods. If avulsion has not occurred intraoperatively, recovery to near normal or normal levels is to be expected over the course of time but certainly requires good preoperative and postoperative counseling.

Most commonly postoperative sequelae include incision dehiscence secondary to improper incision placement and excessive swelling or hematoma from nonuse or poor use of pressure bandages. Generally careful irrigation and hygiene techniques make this a short-lived problem since granulation and epithelialization proceed rapidly. Continued use of antibiotics during this period is advised.

In the case of grafts being exposed, loss of grafts or more often loss of portions of the graft are possible. Continued irrigation with 0.25% neomycin solution is indicated. We have had no exposure of grafts in this area. Attempts to reclose over an exposed graft are contraindicated and generally lead only to more exposure and loss.

Continued paresthesia or other nerve related disorder is possible, although in simple genioplasty alone without nerve avulsion near complete recovery of sensation within 3 months to 1 year appears to be the rule and residual neuropathy is not a problem for most patients. Even with avulsion of the mental neurovascular bundle, a certain degree of recovery is to be expected.

Hypertrophic scar is uncommon but can occur along the mucosal incision. Most commonly this results from excessive tissue bites taken while performing the running horizontal mattress suture closure. This may create a hygiene problem or altered lip appearance or function and may require revision after scar maturity occurs.

In association with hypertrophic scarring, a poorly placed incision as well may cause an abnormal pull on attached mucosa or gingiva, leading to gingival dehiscence in the incisor-canine area. Correction is easily obtained with free gingival grafting techniques.

It is interesting that although the incision for genioplasty is created through an area rich in minor salivary glands and ducts we have not witnessed resultant mucocele in any of our genioplasty patients; nor has sublingual gland disease been reported, although the glands may be seen to incur surgical insult.

STABILITY

The minimal dissection broad-pedicle technique has allowed for cosmetically more predictable, acceptable, and stable results. No observed regression has been reported for genioplasties. However, continued evaluation of the vertical augmentation genioplasty appears to be necessary, especially with allogeneic bone. Certainly, as with all genioplasties, a postoperative period of 2 to 4 months appears to improve the clinical appearance as remodeling at the leading edge and apposition at the cut inferior border and junction of the alveolar bone with the horizontal osteotomy occur.[18]

CASE PRESENTATIONS
CASE 1 (Fig. 4-2)

A 19-year-old boy was evaluated for a complaint of retrusive chin.

Problem list
Esthetics

Good facial contour and symmetry with marked facial convexity secondary to a prominent nose and moderately deficient chin

Hard tissue cephalometric analysis

Increased angle of convexity secondary to deficient chin, 16 degrees
Slight increase in angle of the mandibular incisiors to mandibular plane, 101 degrees

Soft tissue analysis

Increased angle of facial convexity
Increased lower face–throat angle
Increased nasolabial angle

Occlusal analysis

Class I molar and canine relationships
Minor anterior tooth rotations
Increased mandibular incisor to basal bone angulation

Treatment plan

No consideration of orthodontic treatment by the patient
Horizontal osteotomy of the chin to
Increase its prominence
Maintain vertical height

Follow-up

The minimal dissection broad-pedicled techniques for advancement genioplasty were utilized to gain maximum allowable advancement to 10 mm. A more harmonious nose-lip-chin balance was obtained as well as improved neck-throat contour. Normal healing without positional change has been evident.

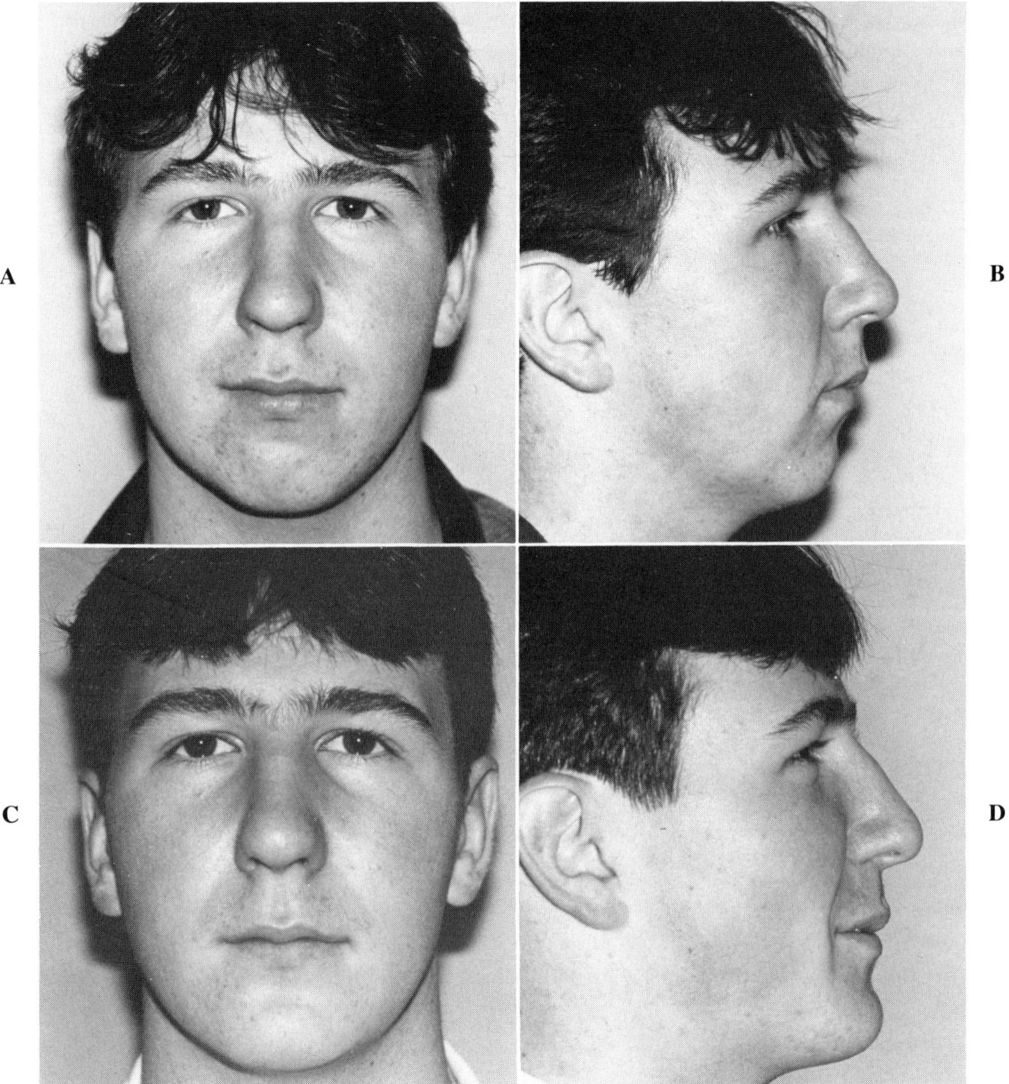

Continued.

Fig. 4-2.
Case 1. **A** and **B,** Preoperative facial appearance. **C** and **D,** Six-month postoperative appearance. An advancement genioplasty of 10 mm improved the nose-lip-chin relationship and neck-throat-chin contour.

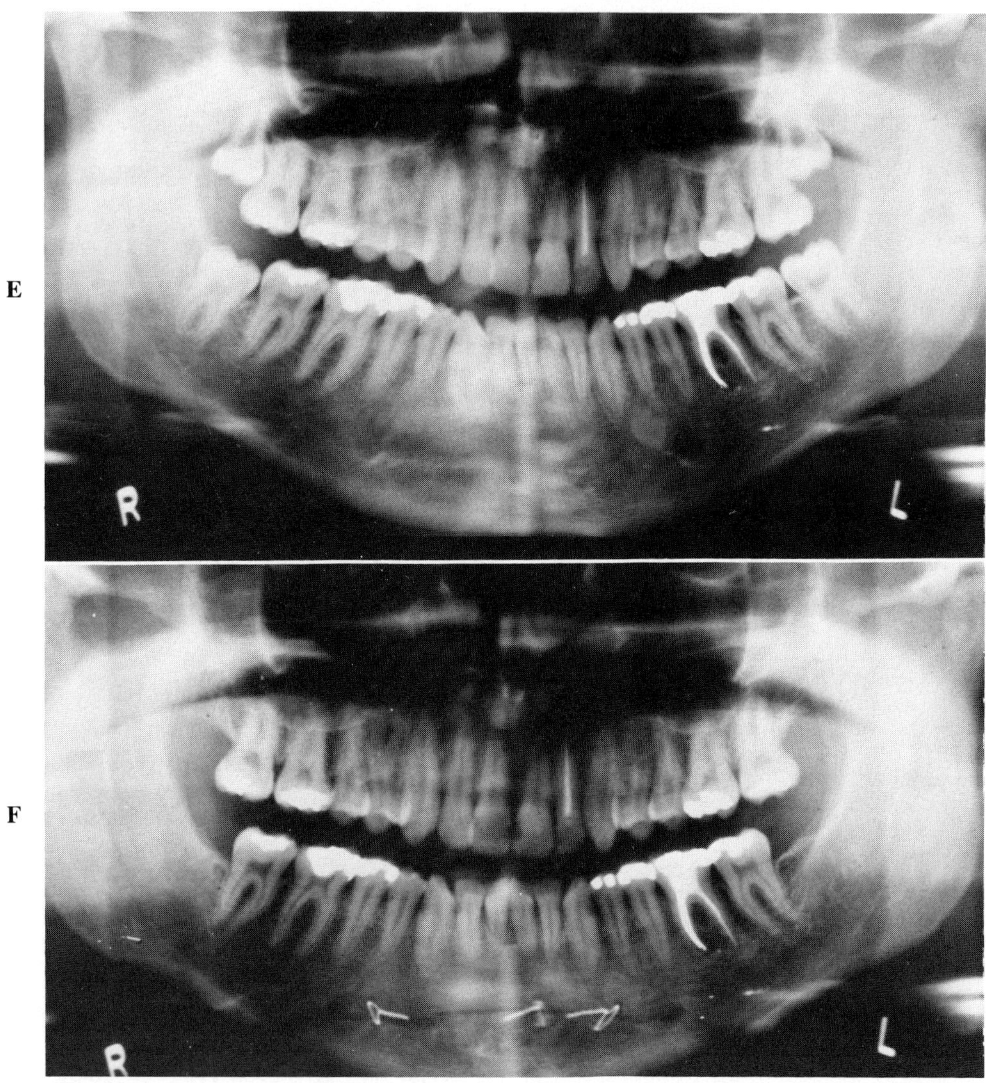

Fig. 4-2—cont'd.
E and **F**, Panolipse radiographs preoperative and postoperative of the advancement genioplasty.

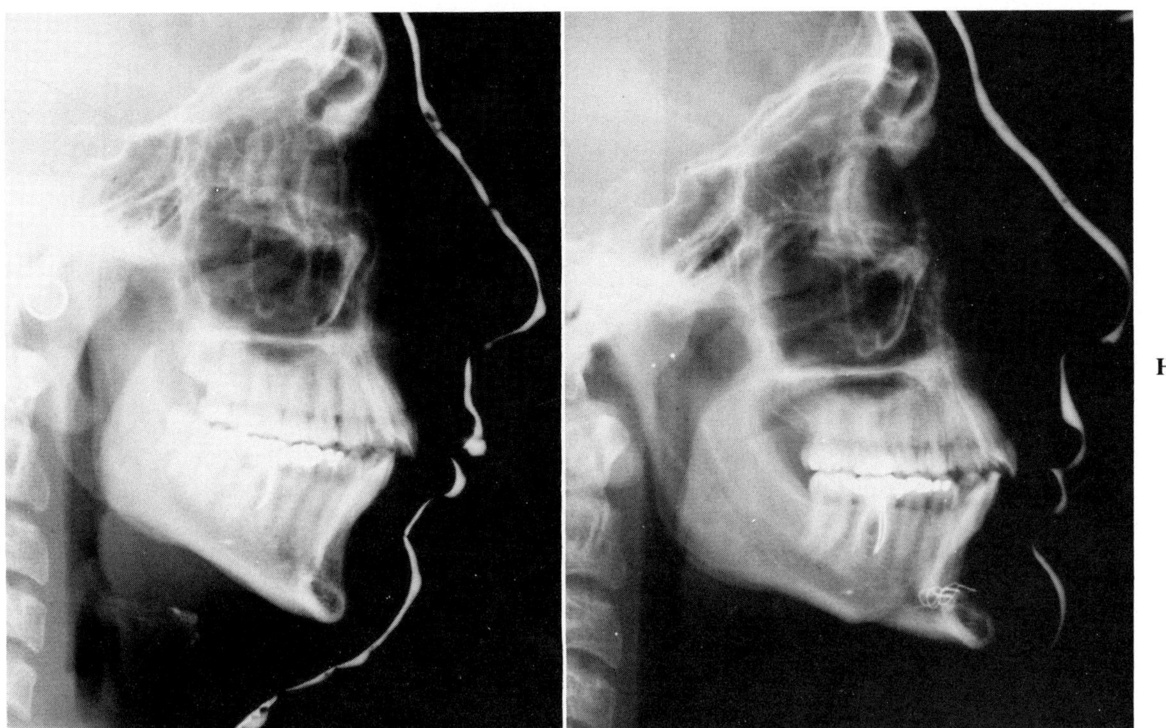

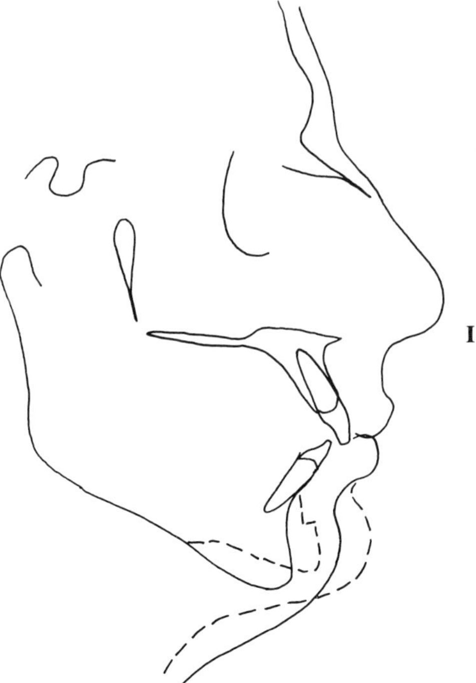

Fig. 4-2—cont'd.
G, Preoperative cephalogram. **H,** Six-month postoperative cephalogram. Bony apposition and recontouring of the genioplasty site. **I,** Composite cephalometric tracings. *Solid line,* Preoperative; *broken line,* postoperative.

CASE 2 (Fig. 4-3)

This case demonstrates the use of genioplasty to improve esthetics following orthodontics without surgical input. A 21-year-old woman who had previously undergone orthodontic therapy to conclusion was evaluated for complaints of undesirable facial profile and lack of chin prominence.

Problem list

Esthetics

Good facial contour and symmetry with moderate facial convexity, chin deficiency, and prominent nose

Hard tissue cephalometric analysis

Moderate mandibular retrusion (S-N-B, 72 degrees)
High mandibular plane angle (Go-Gn to S-N, 53 degrees)
High FMA (Go-Gn to FH, 44 degrees)
Short mandibular length (Go-Pog, 60 mm)
Increased angle of convexity (15 degrees)
Increased lower third facial height

Soft tissue analysis

High angle of facial convexity (30 degrees)
Deficient soft tissue pogonion position
Increased lower facial length
Increased nasolabial angle (124 degrees)
Deficient mentolabial sulcus (1 mm)

Occlusal analysis

Class I molar and canine relationship
Absent four first premolars
Adequate overjet and overbite

Treatment plan

Removal of the impacted upper right third molar
Two-step advancement genioplasty to
  Increase chin prominence
  Decrease chin height

Follow-up

The patient underwent two-step genioplasty to gain the maximum advancement of 10 mm. The superior first step segment was 5 mm in height; the inferior second step was 7 mm. Great improvement in nose-lip-chin balance was obtained as well as an improved soft tissue lower vertical height/depth ratio. Soft tissue chin contour was greatly improved. Long-term stability could not be evaluated because of patient transfer.

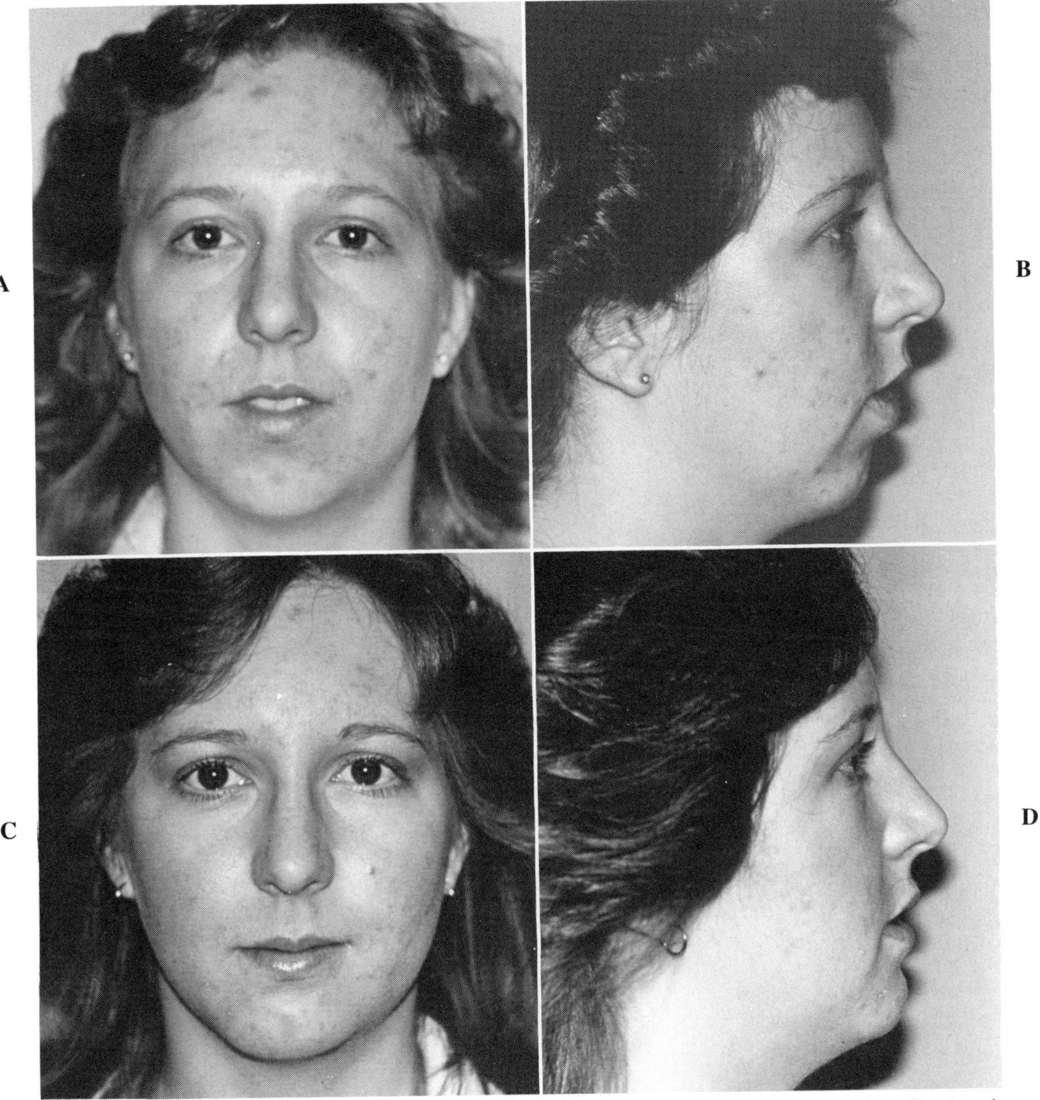

Continued.

Fig. 4-3.
Case 2. **A** and **B,** Preoperative appearance. **C** and **D,** Three month postoperative appearance. A two-step advancement genioplasty improved the facial contour. The patient was lost to follow-up because of her relocation.

E

F

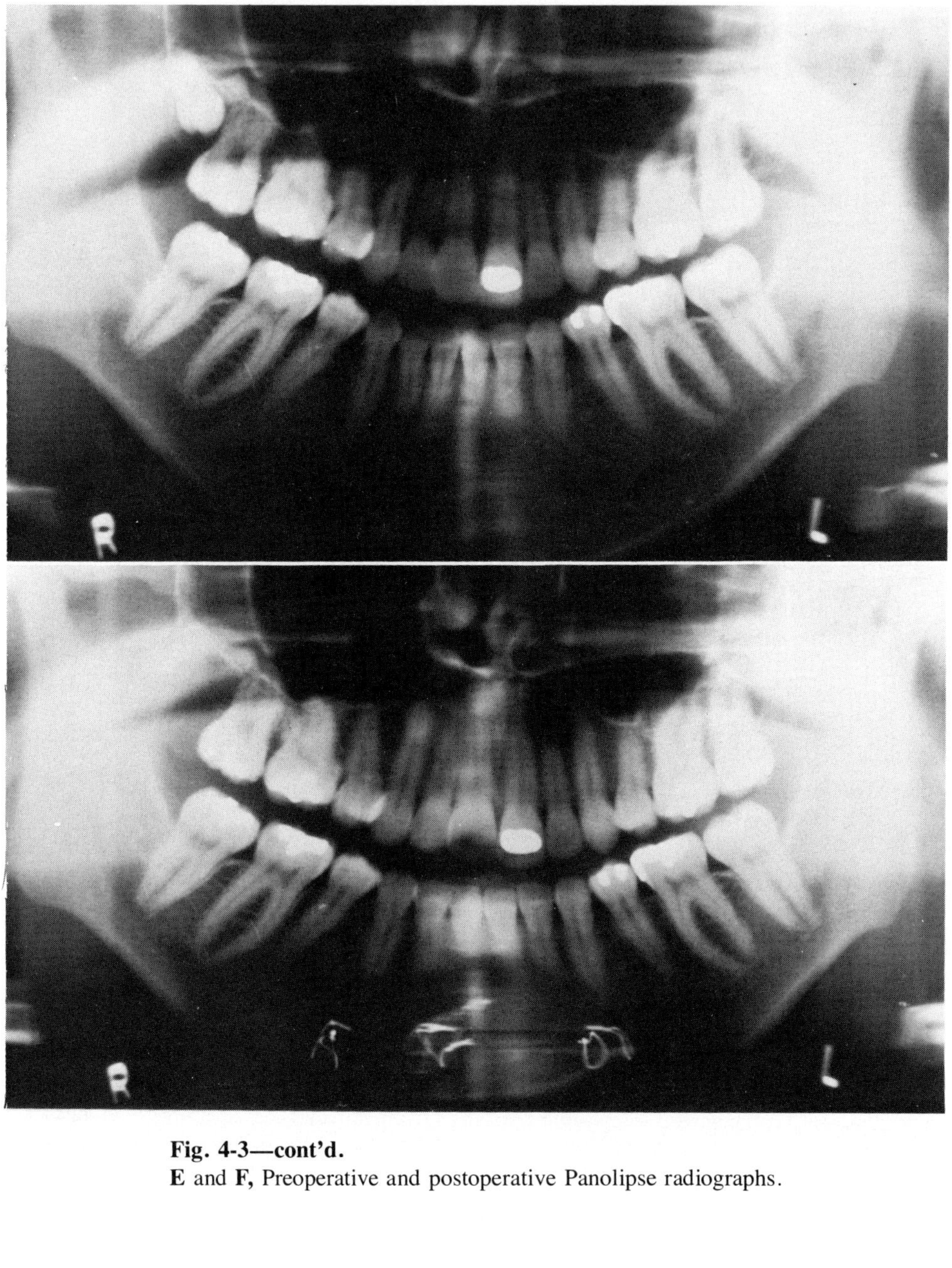

Fig. 4-3—cont'd.
E and **F,** Preoperative and postoperative Panolipse radiographs.

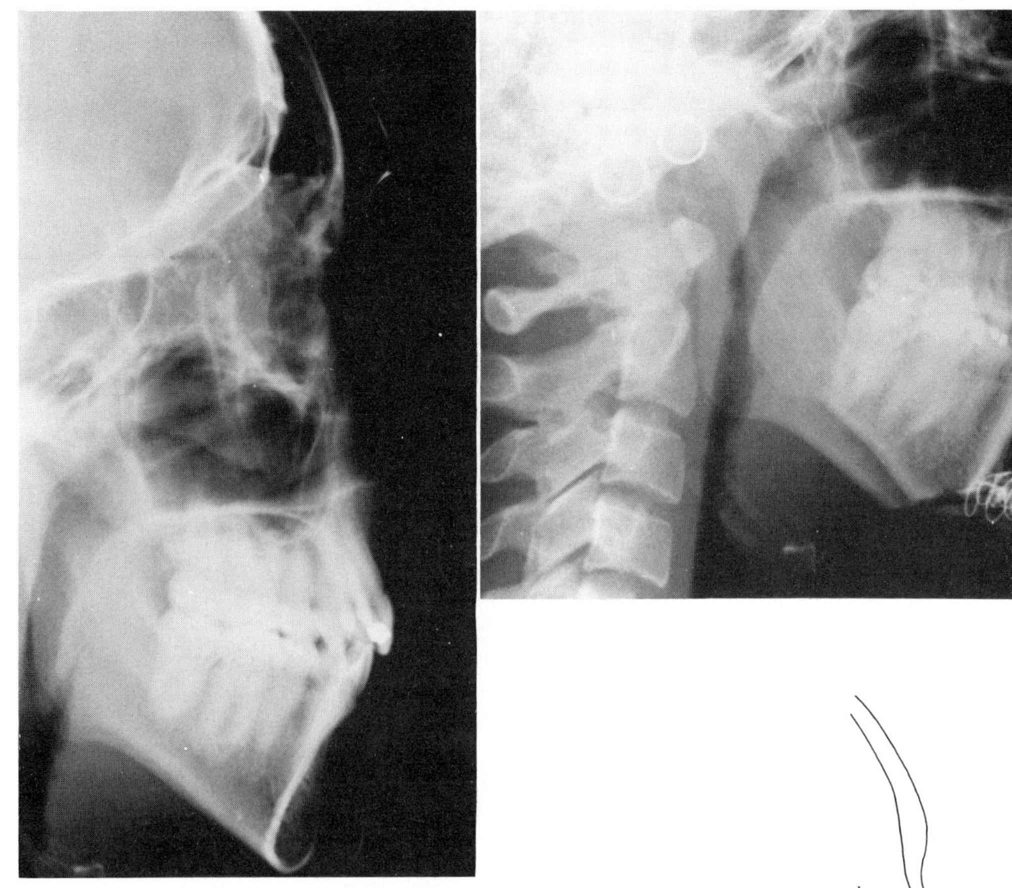

Fig. 4-3—cont'd.
G and **H,** Preoperative and postoperative cephalograms.
I, Composite cephalometric tracings. *Solid line,* Preoperative; *broken line,* postoperative.

CASE 3 (Fig. 4-4)

This case demonstrates a wedge ostectomy combined with advancement genioplasty to level the chin. A 34-year-old man, previously examined at another installation, referred himself for evaluation of his abnormal bite and facial asymmetry. He had received orthodontic care for several years as a teenager.

Problem list

Esthetics

Facial assymetry with increased right prominence
Deviation of chin to the left
Canted inferior border of the chin, right lower than left
Lower lip fullness

Hard tissue cephalometric analysis

Normal A-N-B (3 degrees)
Increased facial angle (N-Pog to FH, 90 degrees)
Increased mandibular plane angle (Go-Gn to S-N, 47 degrees)
FMA (Go-Gn to FH, 33 degrees)
Excessive mandibular length

Soft tissue analysis

Decreased angle of facial convexity (3 degrees)

Panograph

Long right condylar length

Occlusal analysis

Class III malocclusion
Shift of mandibular midline to the left
Left cross-bite
Slight cant to the right posterior maxillary occlusion
Good arch form and width
Compensated angulation of the mandibular anterior teeth
Edge-to-edge anterior occlusion

Treatment plan

Orthodontic care not feasible
Occlusion equilibration preoperatively
First procedure, mandibular setback via extraoral vertical subcondylar osteotomies and coronoidotomies to
Correct the Class III occlusion and mandibular prognathism within limits
Allow for asymmetric repositioning and shift
Second procedure, wedge ostectomy and advancement genioplasty to
Level the apparent inferior border discrepancy of the chin
Provide slight advancement after wedge removal

Follow-up

After mandibular setback procedures the patient was reevaluated for correction of chin asymmetry. Midline position was determined to be adequate. A 4 mm wedge ostectomy on the right, tapering to 0 on the left, was performed to level the chin as well as a 6 mm horizontal advancement of the distal fragment.

Improved occlusion, although imperfect, and improved facial asymmetry were accomplished and well received by the patient. Changes continue to be stable.

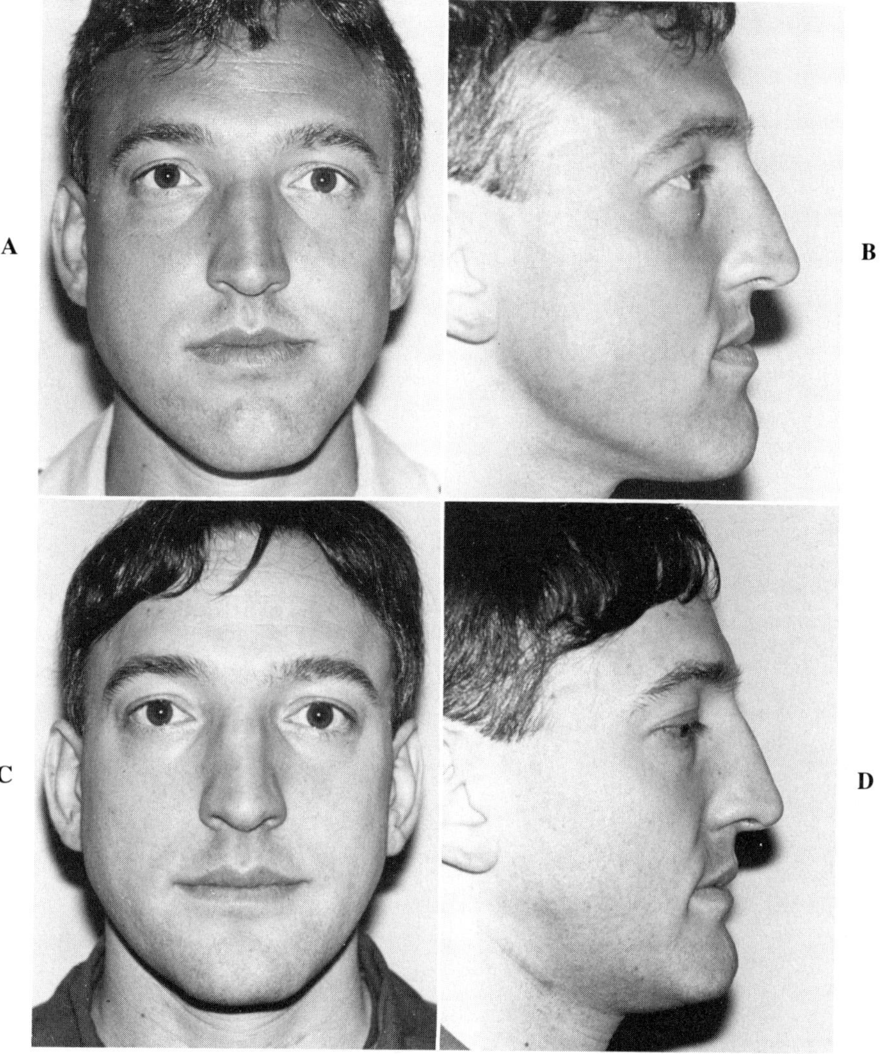

Fig. 4-4.
Case 3. **A** and **B,** Preoperative appearance. Notice that the right inferior border of the chin is lower than the left. **C** and **D,** Six months after a mandibular repositioning and wedge ostectomy–advancement genioplasty to level the chin and readjust its relative prominence.

E

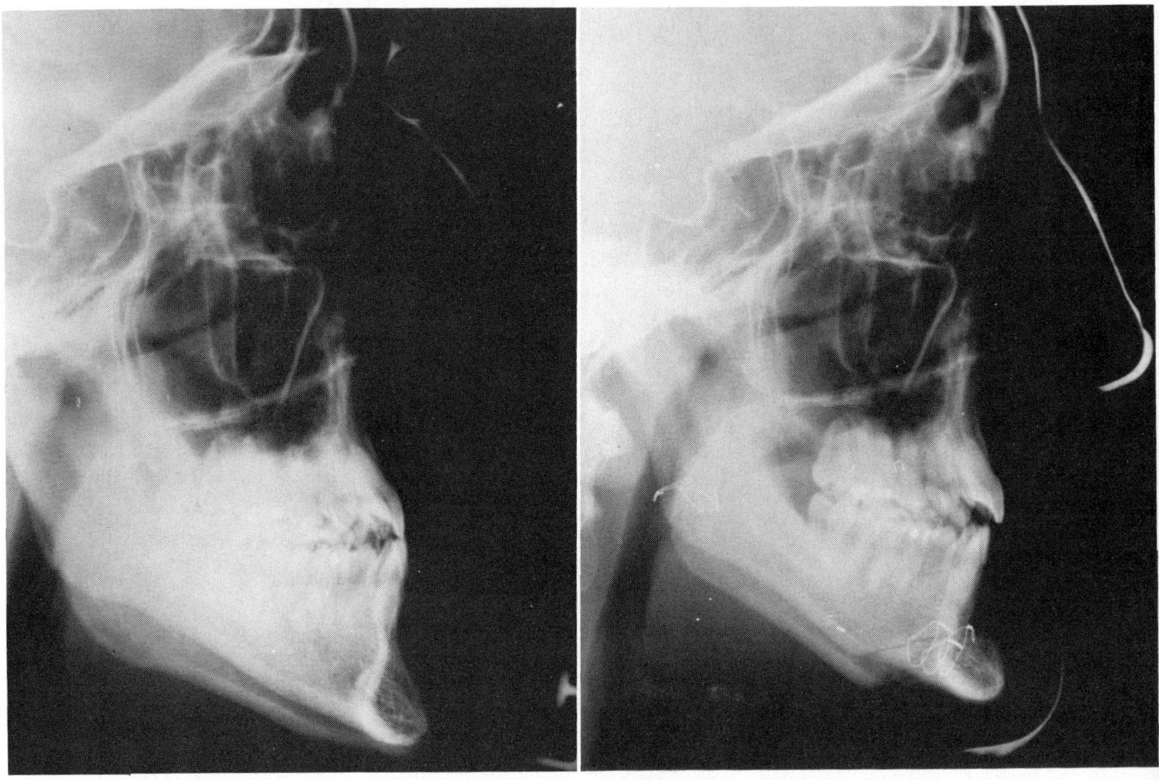

Fig. 4-4—cont'd.
E, Preoperative and, **F,** 6-month postoperative cephalograms. Excellent recontouring and bony apposition have been achieved along the horizontal leading edge of the genioplasty and at the inferior border cut.

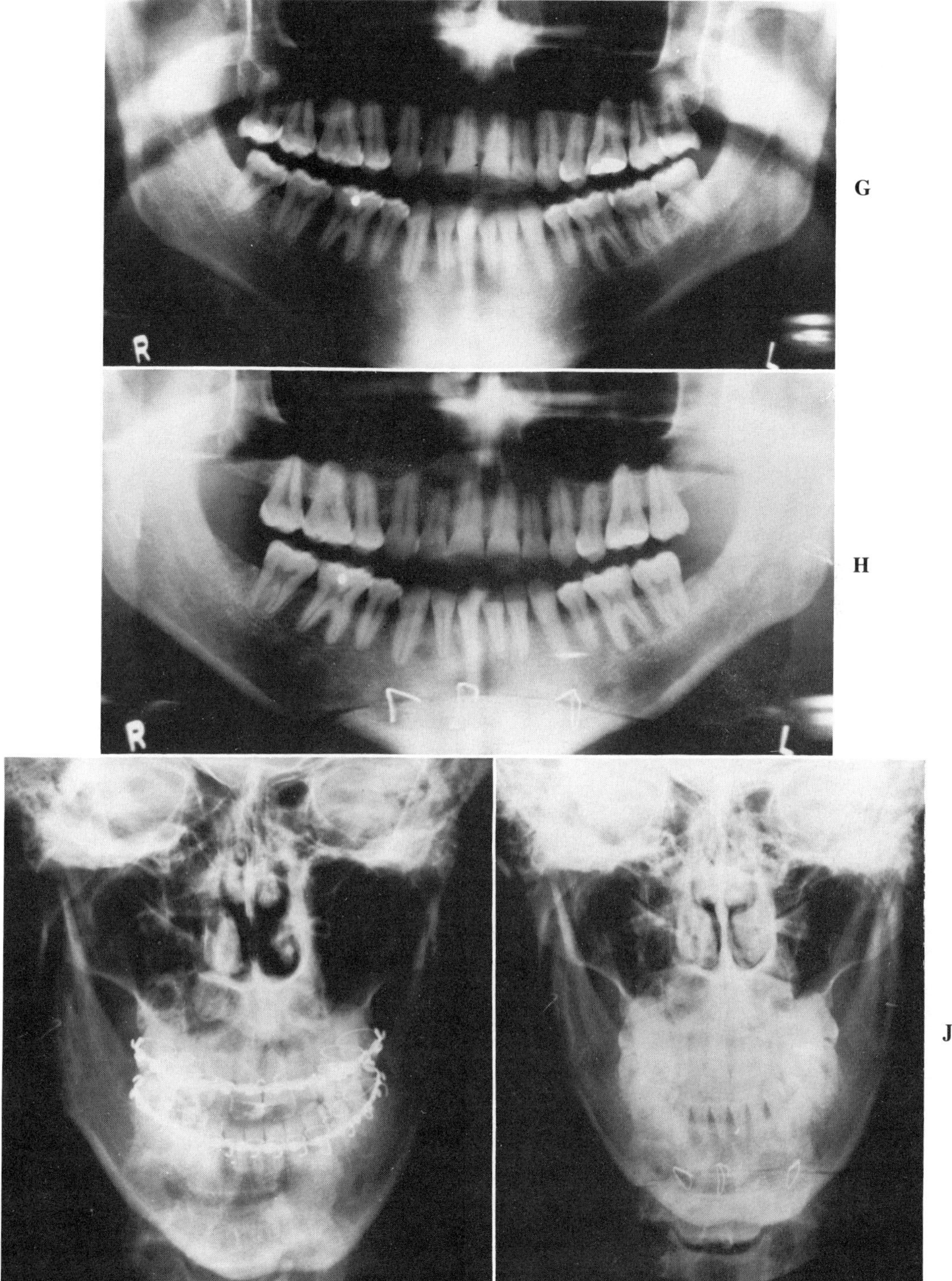

Fig. 4-4—cont'd.
G and **H,** Preoperative and postoperative Panolipse views. **I,** PA radiograph after ramus osteotomy. It is used to assess symmetry prior to the genioplasty. **J,** Final postoperative radiograph 6 months after the wedge ostectomy of 4 mm on the right tapering to 0 on the left and the advancement of the chin. Acceptable symmetry and levelness have been achieved.

CASE 4 (Fig. 4-5)

This case demonstrates the use of a second planned advancement genioplasty. A 24-year-old woman transferred her orthodontic care to the locale. Her new orthodontist referred her for surgical assistance in the correction of her malocclusion.

Problem list
Esthetics

Good facial symmetry; long thin face, prominent nasal dorsum, short upper lip, lip incompetence, excessive exposure of maxillary incisors in repose; also excessive facial convexity and chin deficiency

Hard tissue cephalometric analysis

S-N-A, 83 degrees; S-N-B, 74 degrees
High mandibular plane angle (Go-Gn to S-N, 45 degrees)
High FMA (Go-Gn to FH, 41 degrees)
Excessive lower third facial length

Soft tissue analysis

High-angle facial convexity (28 degrees)
Inadequate labiomental sulcus
Decreased vertical lip/chin ratio (Sn-Stm$_s$ to Stm$_i$-Me',* 1:2.5), consistent with the short upper lip

Occlusal analysis

Orthodontic appliances in place
Maxillary first premolars and mandibular second premolars previously extracted
Class II molar and canine relationship
Overjet 7 mm
Anterior open-bite tendency
Posterior maxillary arch width deficiency

Sn, Subspinale; *Stm$_s$,* stomion superius; *Stm$_i$* stomion inferius; *Me',* soft tissue menton.[15]

Treatment plan

Maxillary intrusion via total maxillary alveolar osteotomy with midline split to
Decrease the amount of incisor exposure in repose
Widen the maxillary arch
Decrease the relapse tendency to open-bite
Mandibular advancement to
Correct Class II malocclusion
Decrease lower facial height
Advancement genioplasty to decrease facial convexity
Rhinoplasty
Second advancement genioplasty
Postoperative orthodontic refinement, stabilization, and retention

Follow-up

Three months after total maxillary alveolar osteotomy (TMAO) and bilateral sagittal split osteotomy (BSSO) to obtain the planned occlusion, advancement genioplasty was performed. Extreme thinness of the bone allowed only a 4 mm advancement. A second advancement genioplasty was planned to improve contour. Orthodontic refinement continued; and although excessive notching and remodeling of the right mandibular proximal fragment was noted radiographically, cosmesis and occlusal result remained stable. The patient underwent rhinoplasty as planned. One year after the first genioplasty, a second one was performed, allowing another 4 mm horizontal advancement of the chin. Additional improvement in facial contour resulted. The patient completed orthodontic therapy and maintains a stable occlusal and cosmetic result and remains very pleased.

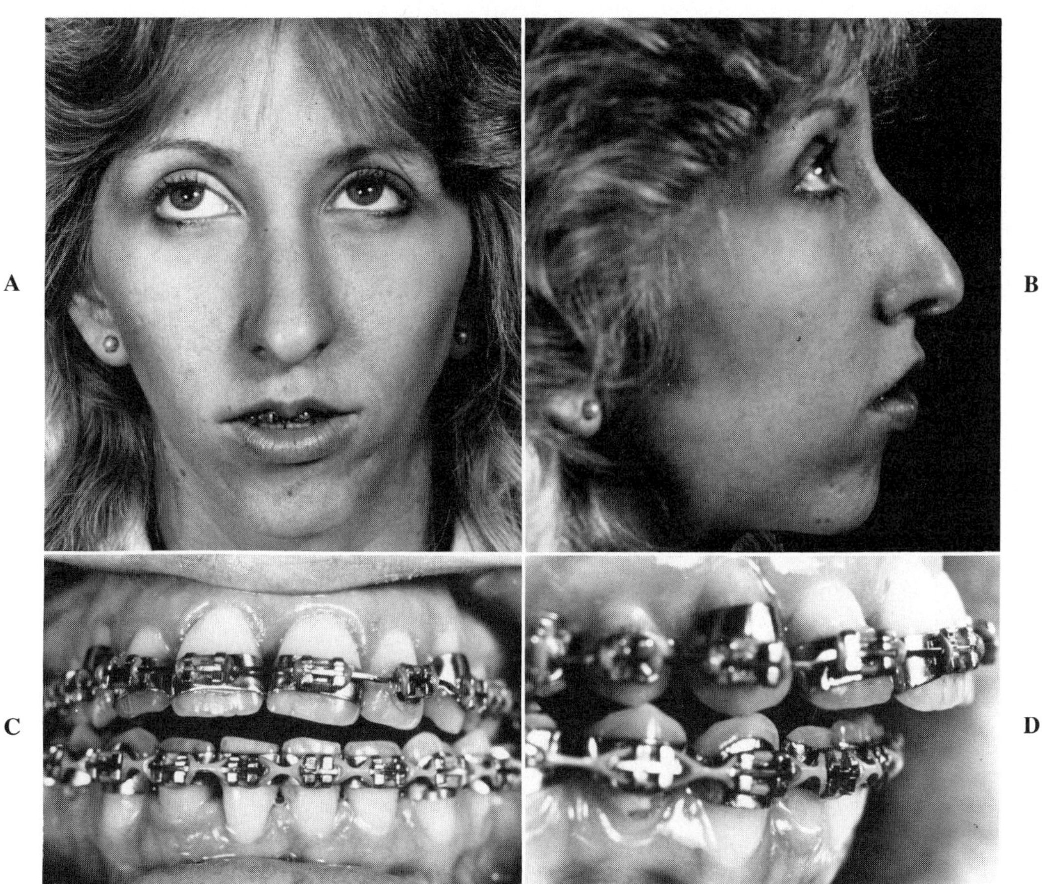

Fig. 4-5.

Case 4. **A** to **D,** Pretreatment facial appearance.

Continued.

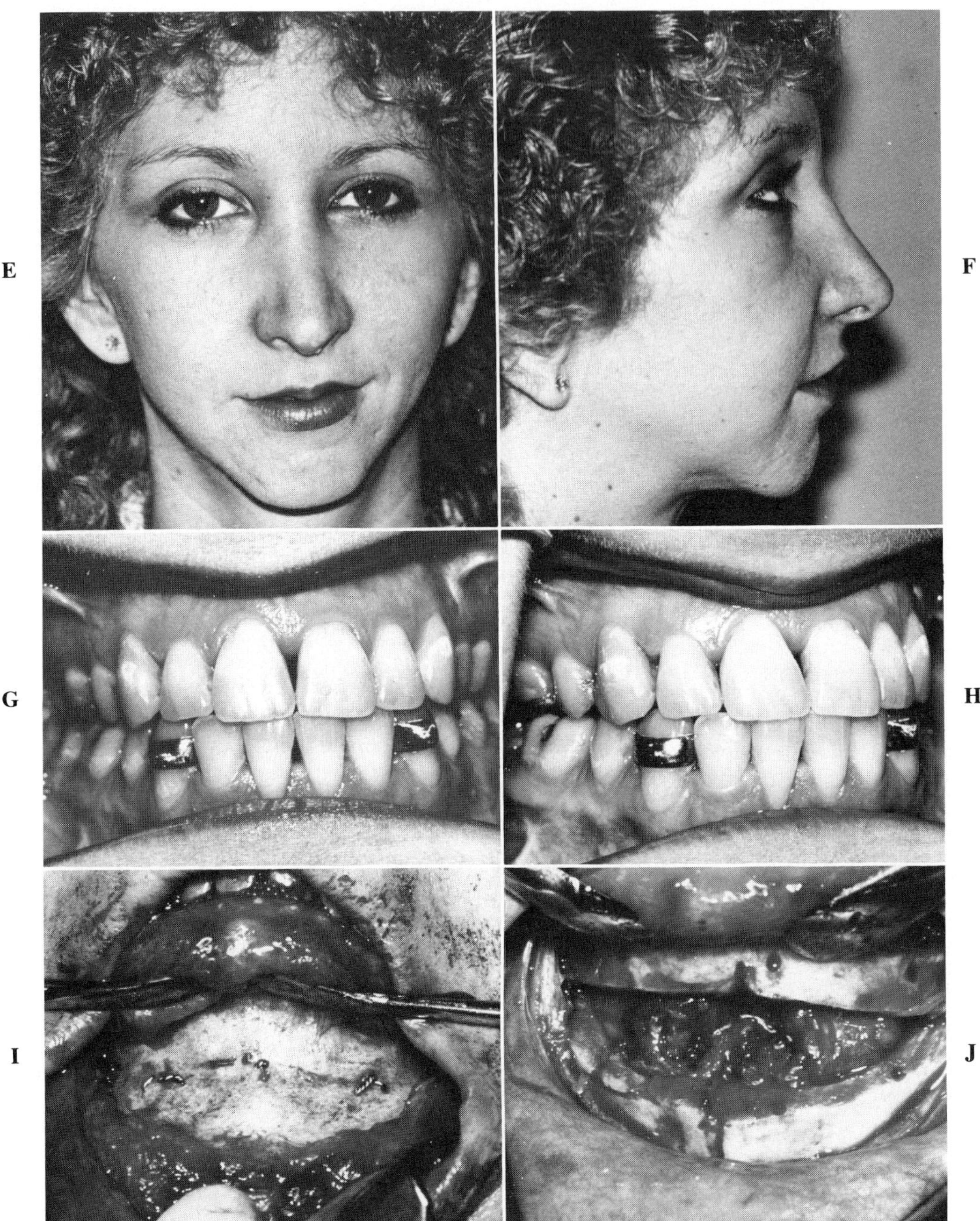

Fig. 4-5—cont'd.
E and **F,** Appearance 9 months after TMAO for maxillary intrusion and sagittal osteotomies to advance the mandible and 3 months after initial advancement genioplasty. Rhinoplasty has been accomplished as well. **G** and **H,** Posttreatment occlusal views. **I,** During the second advancement genioplasty, notice the excellent healing, recontouring, and apposition of bone along the initial genioplasty site. Intraosseous wires placed for the initial genioplasty are partially embedded in bone. **J,** Second horizontal osteotomy cut completed. Notice the thinness of bone, which allows a minimal advancement of 4 mm.

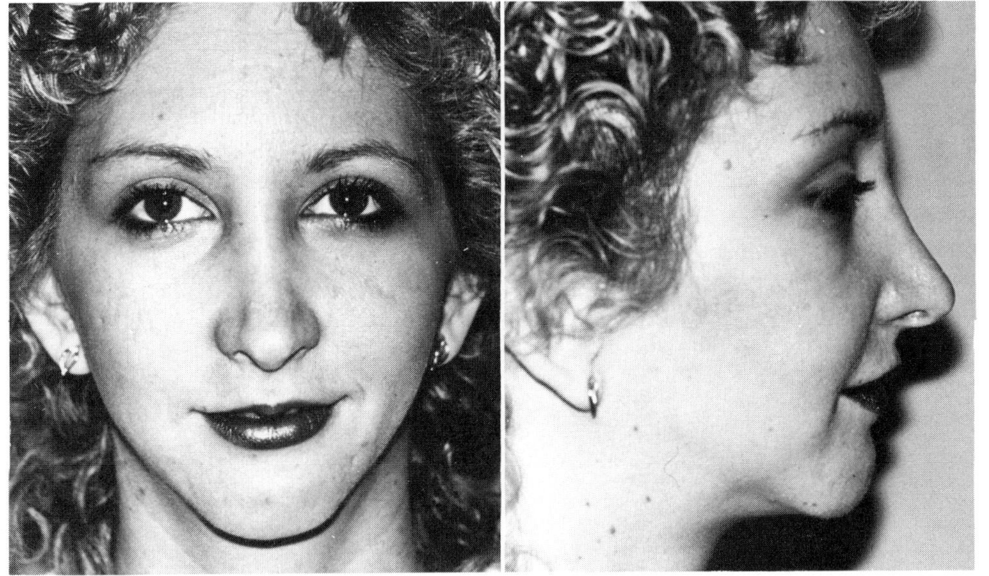

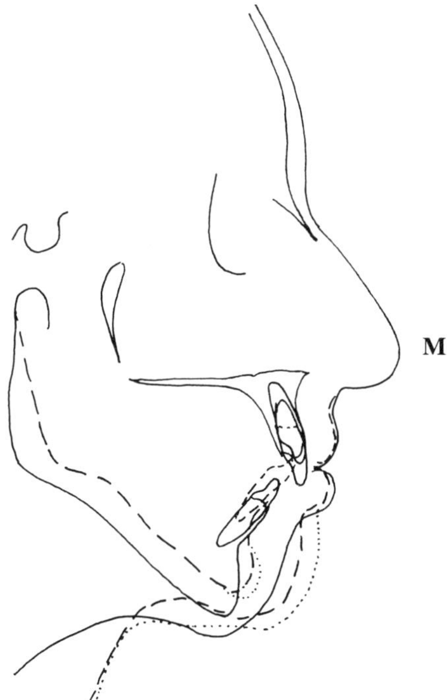

Fig. 4-5—cont'd.
K and **L,** Appearance 3 months after the second advancement genioplasty and 15 months after the original maxillary-mandibular osteotomies. **M,** Composite cephalometric tracings. *Solid line,* Preoperative; *broken lines,* postoperative TMAO, BSSO, and advancement genioplasty; *dotted line,* postoperative second genioplasty.

CASE 5 (Fig. 4-6)

This case demonstrates treatment of mandibular prognathism and relative lack of facial concavity. J.H., a 30-year-old black man was evaluated for a complaint of mandibular anterior tooth cross-bite.

Problem list

Esthetics

Good facial contour and symmetry with procumbent lower lip

Hard tissue cephalometric analysis

Bimaxillary protrusion (S-N-A, 91 degrees; S-N-B, 95 degrees) and relative mandibular prognathism
FMA (Go-Gn to FH, 32 degrees)
Increased mandibular length
Normal angle convexity (3 degrees)

Soft tissue analysis

Normal facial convexity
Relative maxillary and mandibular prognathism
Protrusive lower lip
Deficient labiomental sulcus

Occlusal analysis

Class III molar and canine relationship
Central incisor cross-bite
Dental crowding and linguoversion of the mandibular lateral incisors
Lingual position of the mandibular left first and second premolars

Surgical treatment

Orthodontics not considered by the patient
Staged osteotomy of the mandibular left premolars to correct linguoversion
Mandibular setback
Advancement genioplasty to return the chin to its relative preoperative prominence

Follow-up

Concurrent advancement genioplasty, although suggested to the patient, was deferred by him until after mandibular setback. Orthodontic treatment to correct individual tooth position was not possible. Four weeks prior to osteotomy the patient underwent lingual corticotomy mesially and distally to the first and second premolars under local anesthesia. A labial flap permitted completion of the osteotomy of teeth 20 and 21. Arch bars and mandibular lingual splint were placed, and bilateral extraoral vertical subcondylar osteotomies were performed to retrude the mandible 5 mm bilaterally. Intermaxillary fixation was kept in place for 6 weeks. It became obvious to the patient, as it had been to us during the treatment planning stage, that advancement genioplasty was necessary to improve facial convexity and undesirable submental and neck-throat contours. Three months after initial surgery, advancement genioplasty was performed to advance the chin 5 mm. Acceptable nose-lip-chin balance was obtained as originally planned along with better neck-throat contour. Soft tissue pogonion advanced 5 mm as compared to the pregenioplasty analysis. The occlusion remains stable and well maintained, and the patient is extremely happy with the results.

Text continued on p. 132.

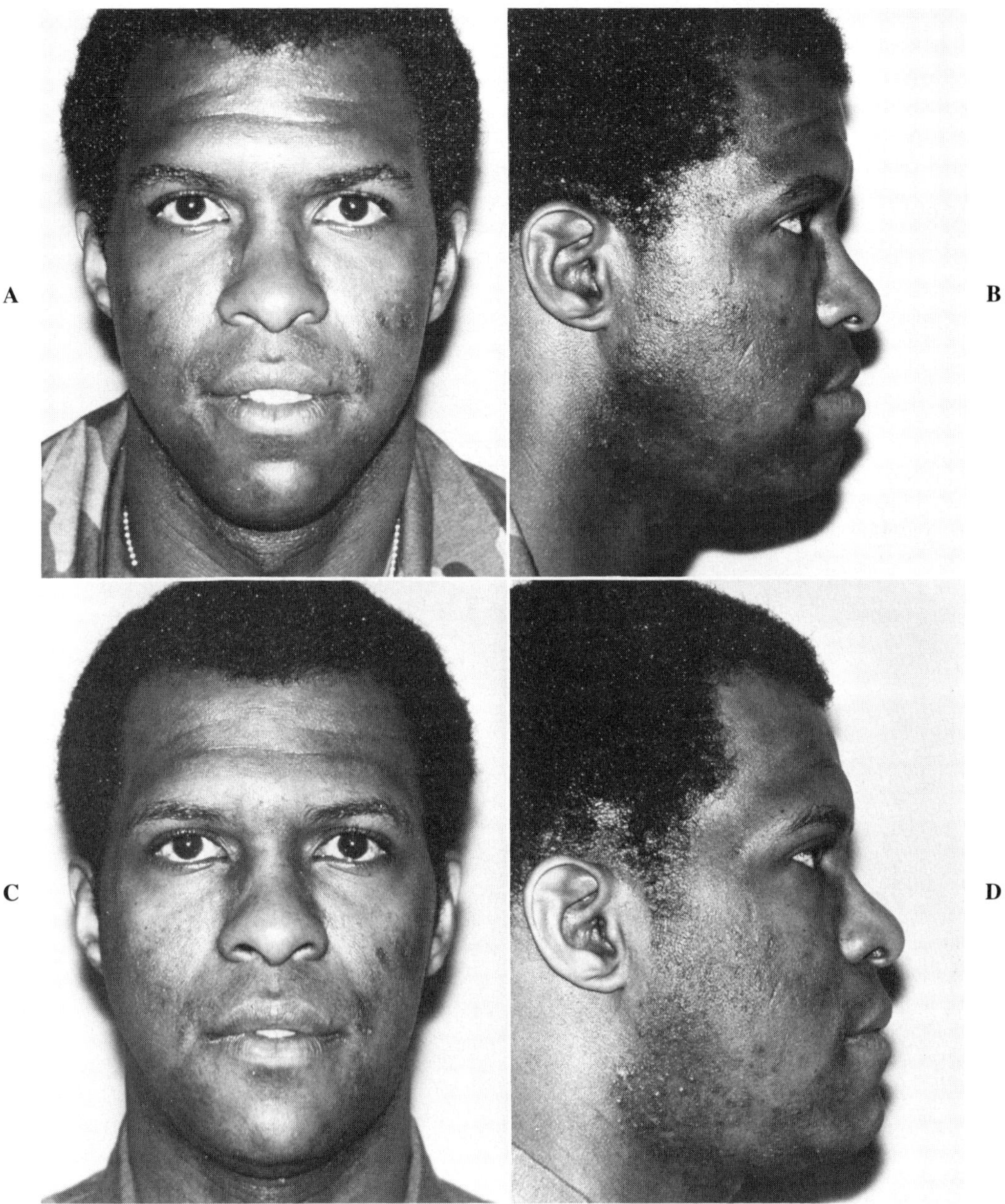

Fig. 4-6.
Case 5. **A** and **B,** Pretreatment facial appearance. **C** and **D,** Appearance 9 months after mandibular setback and 6 months after secondary advancement genioplasty.

Continued.

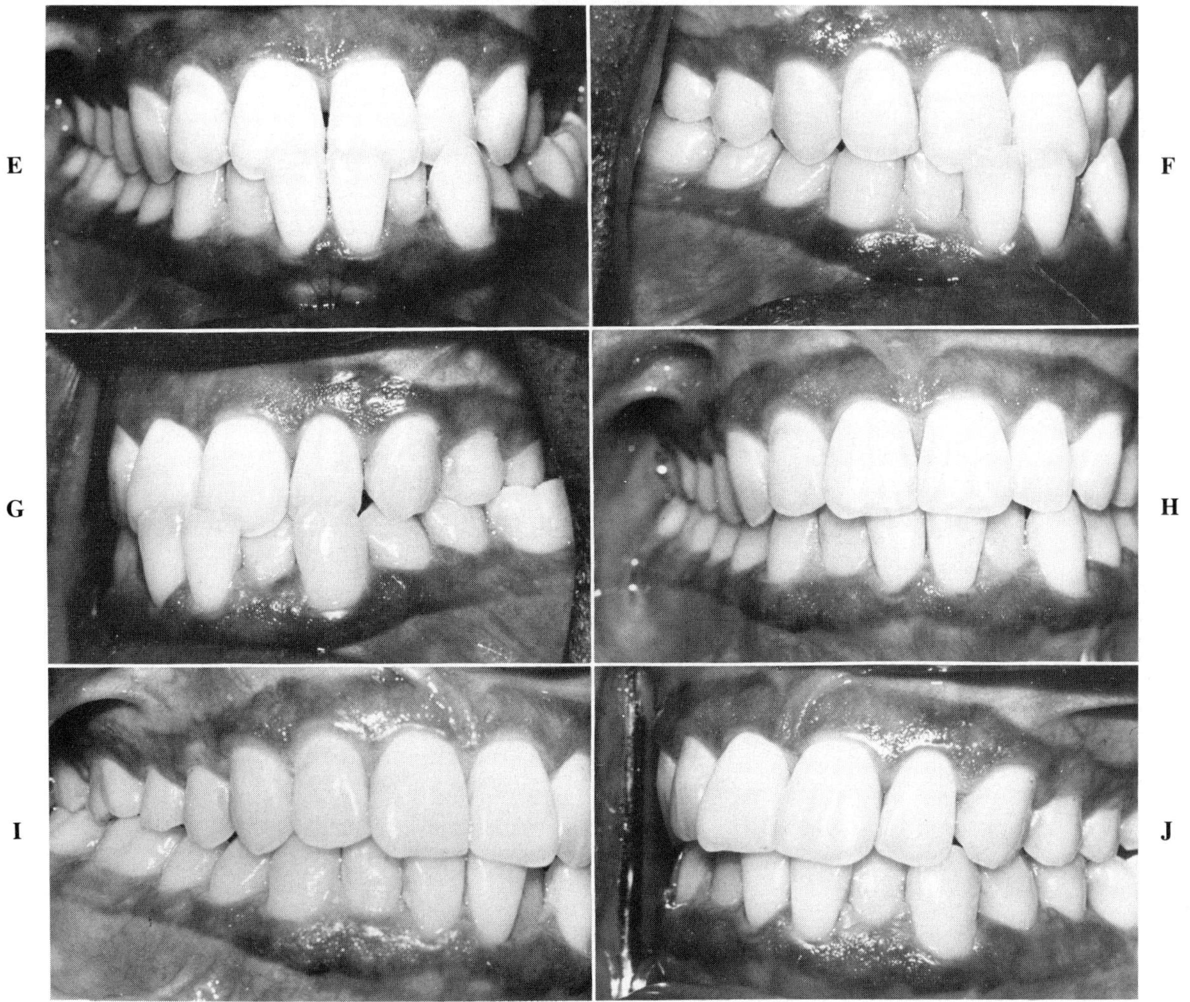

Fig. 4-6—cont'd.
E to **G,** Presurgical and, **H** to **J,** postsurgical occlusal views after mandibular repositioning and small segment osteotomy of the left mandibular premolars.

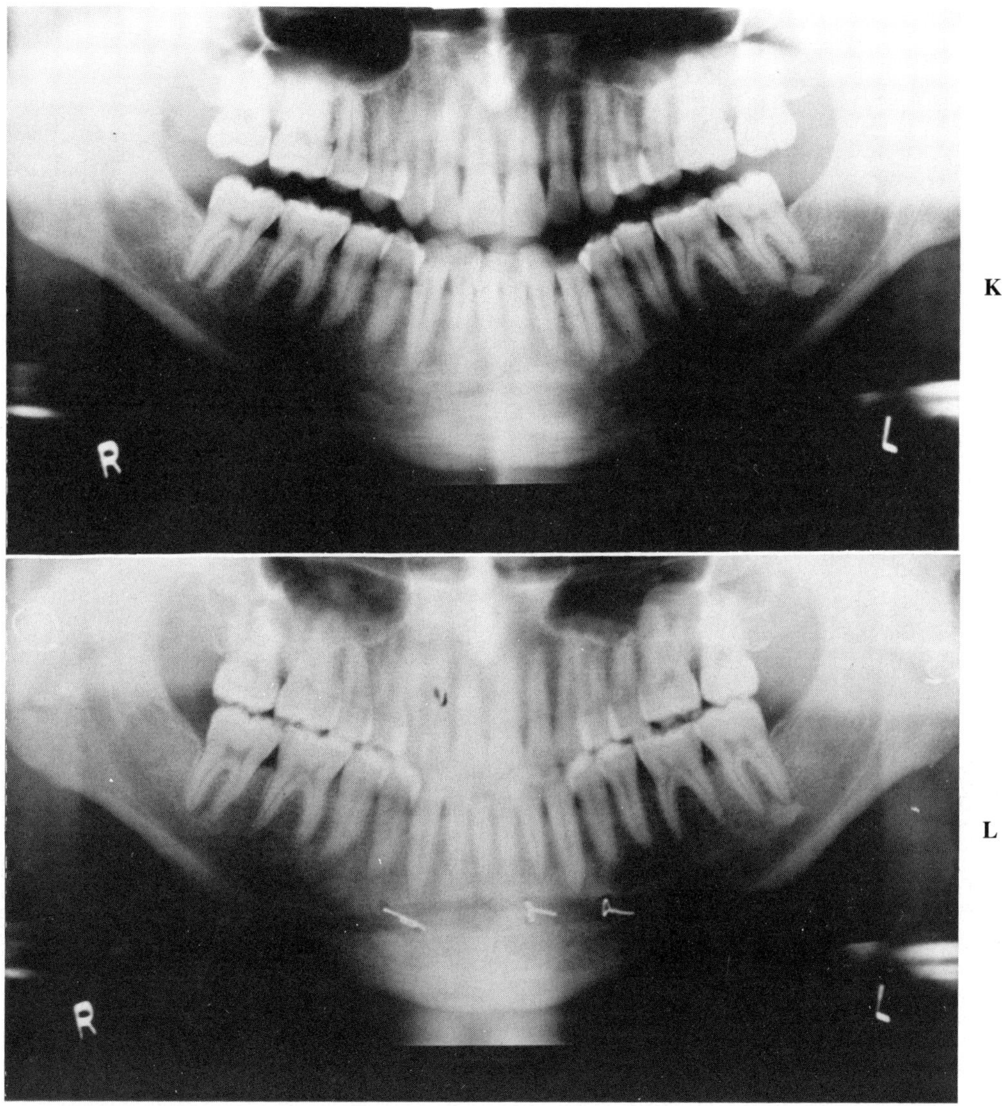

Continued.

Fig. 4-6—cont'd.
K, Preoperative and, **L,** postoperative Panolipse radiographs 6 months after ramus and small segment osteotomies and 3 months after advancement genioplasty.

M

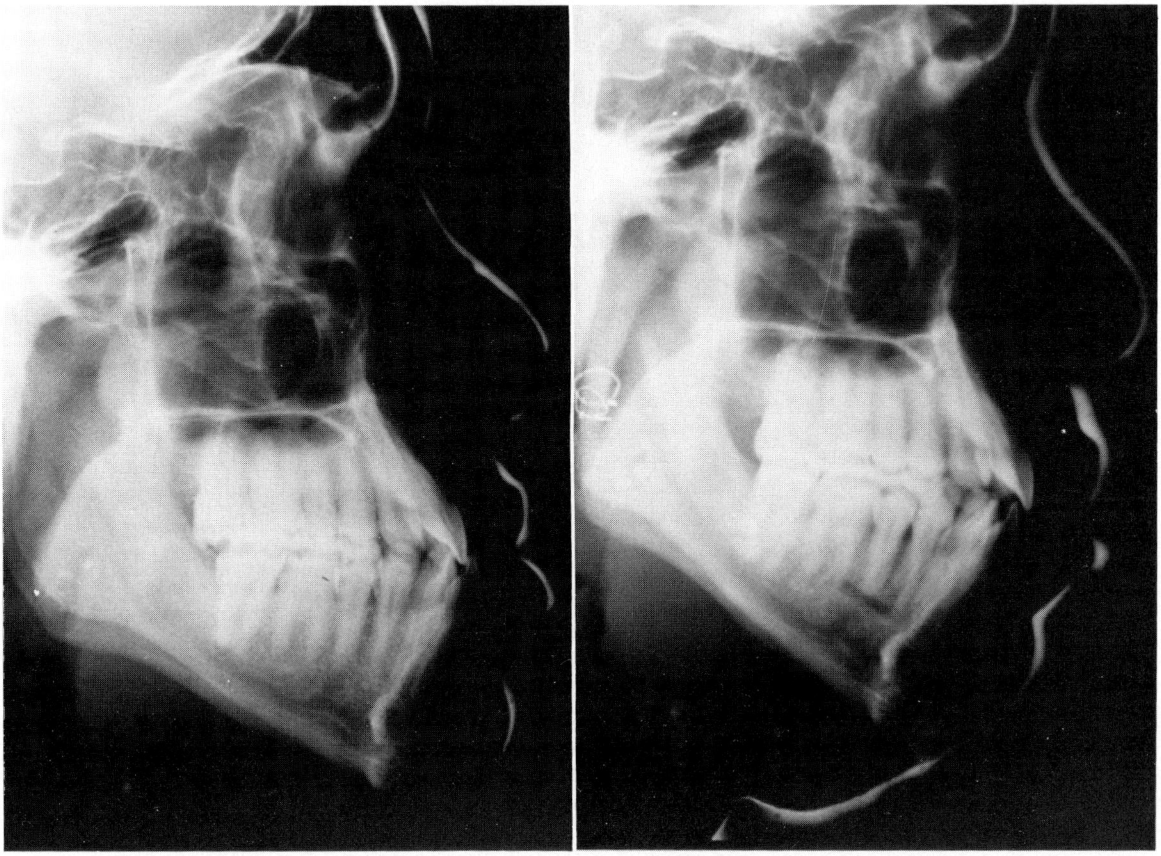

N

Fig. 4-6—cont'd.
M, Preoperative and, **N,** postoperative cephalograms after mandibular setback. Notice the poor lip-chin-neck soft tissue relationship.

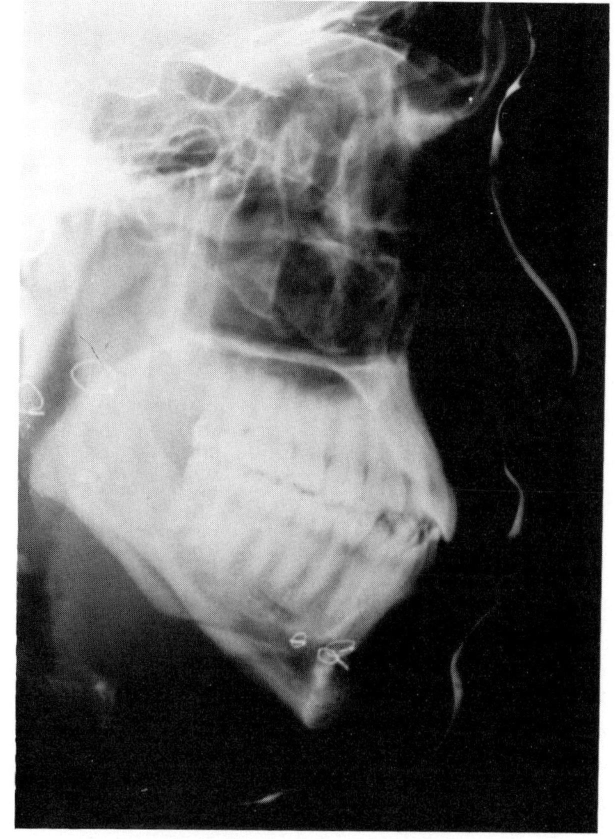 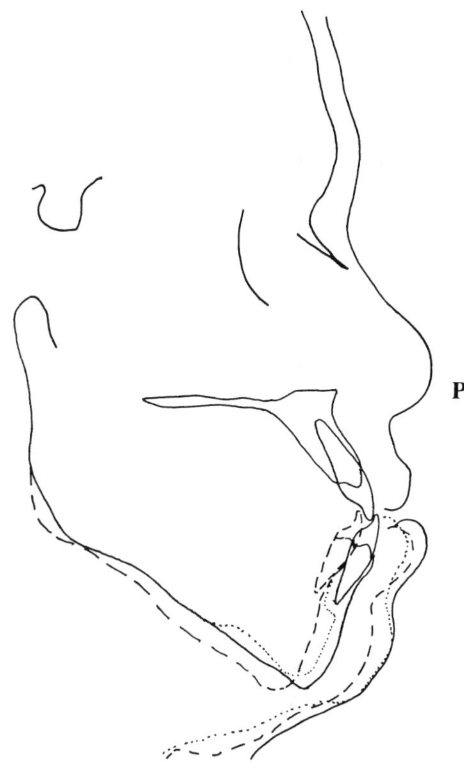

Fig. 4-6—cont'd.
O, Cephalogram 3 months after the advancement genioplasty. Improved lip-chin-neck soft tissue contour is evident. **P,** Composite cephalometric tracings. *Solid line,* Preoperative; *broken line,* postoperative EVSO; *dotted line,* postoperative advancement genioplasty.

CASE 6 (Fig. 4-7)

This case demonstrates the use of allogeneic bone in vertical augmentation genioplasties. A 14-year-old boy, presently undergoing orthodontic care, was referred for surgical evaluation of his malocclusion.

Problem list

Esthetics

Good facial contour and symmetry; short lower facial third; deep labiomental groove and everted lower lip

Hard tissue cephalometric analysis

S-N-A, 83 degrees; S-N-B, 75 degrees
Low mandibular plane angle (Go-Gn to S-N, 20 degrees)
Low FMA (Go-Gn to FH, 17 degrees)

Soft tissue analysis

High-angle facial convexity (30 degrees)
Short lower third vertical height ratio (1.5/1)
High lower face–to–throat angle (129 degrees)
Obtuse nasolabial angle (134 degrees)
Increased depth mentolabial sulcus (11 mm)

Occlusal analysis

Class II occlusion
Overjet 10 mm
Overbite 9 mm
Good arch form and width, orthodontically prepared

Treatment plan

Mandibular advancement to a Class I relationship
Vertical augmentation advancement genioplasty with interpositional allogeneic bone to
Increase the vertical chin height 6 mm at the midline and reduce the labiomental fold
Advance the chin 6 mm horizontally and improve the nose-lip-chin relationship
Finishing orthodontics and retention

Follow-up

The patient underwent concurrent genioplasty and sagittal split osteotomies. Allogeneic rib was available and contoured as the interpositional graft. One-year follow-up showed excellent stability of the obtained bony and soft tissue changes. The 2-year follow-up demonstrates excellent bony stability with almost complete replacement of the allogeneic bone by host bone. Minor soft tissue changes consistent with growth and maturation were found. The patient and parents remain satisfied with cosmesis and function. *Text continued on p. 140.*

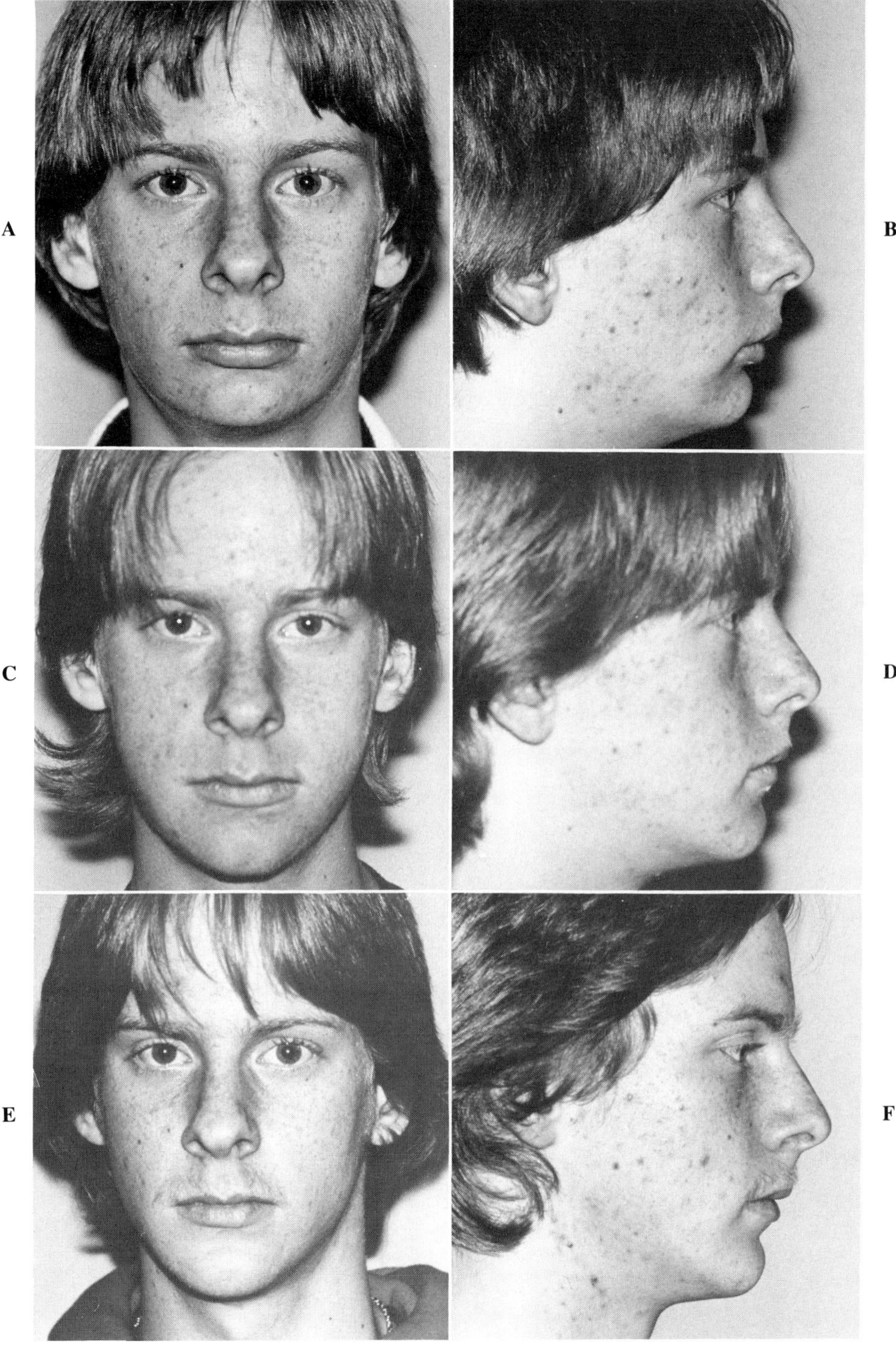

Continued.

Fig. 4-7.
Case 6. **A** and **B,** Preoperative facial appearance. **C** and **D,** One-year postoperative appearance after mandibular advancement and vertical augmentation-advancement genioplasty utilizing allogeneic rib. **E** and **F,** Two-year postoperative view. Further maturation and growth with good maintenance of vertical improvements.

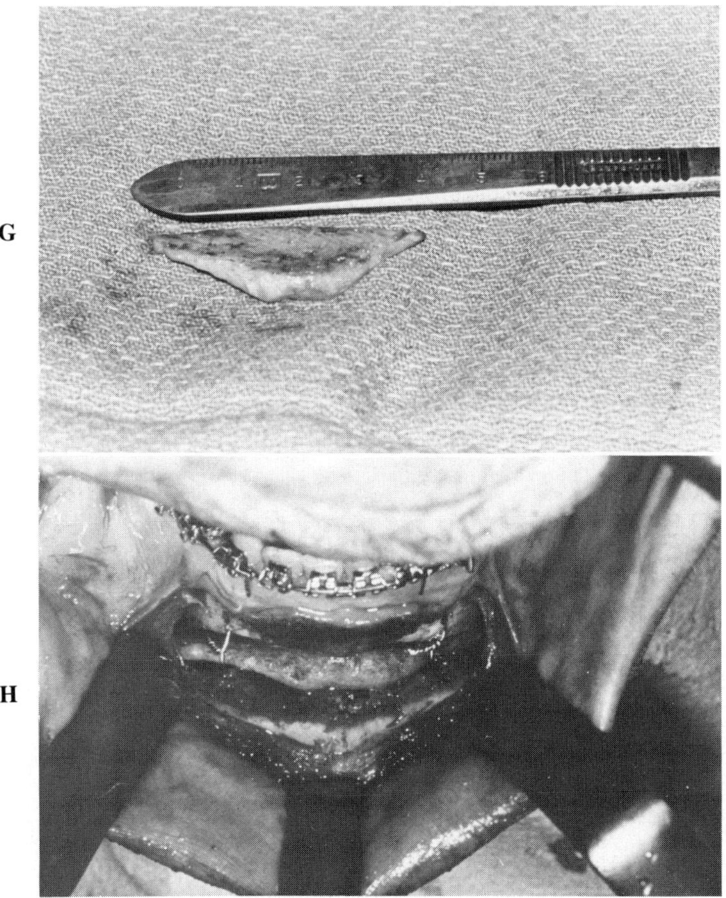

Fig. 4-7—cont'd.
G, Allogeneic rib shaped for vertical augmentation of 6 mm at the midline. **H,** Rib wired into place and the inferior fragment advanced.

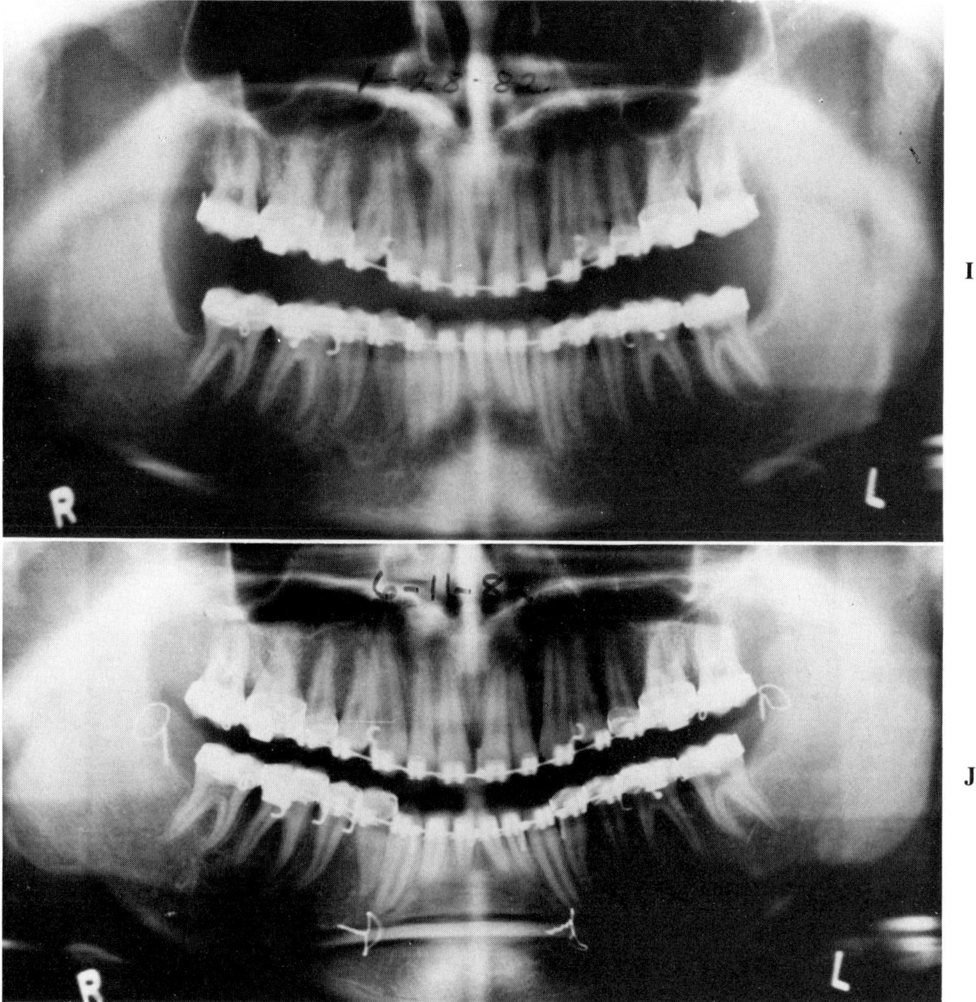

Continued.

Fig. 4-7—cont'd.
I and **J,** Panolipse radiographs, preoperative and 2 months postoperative.

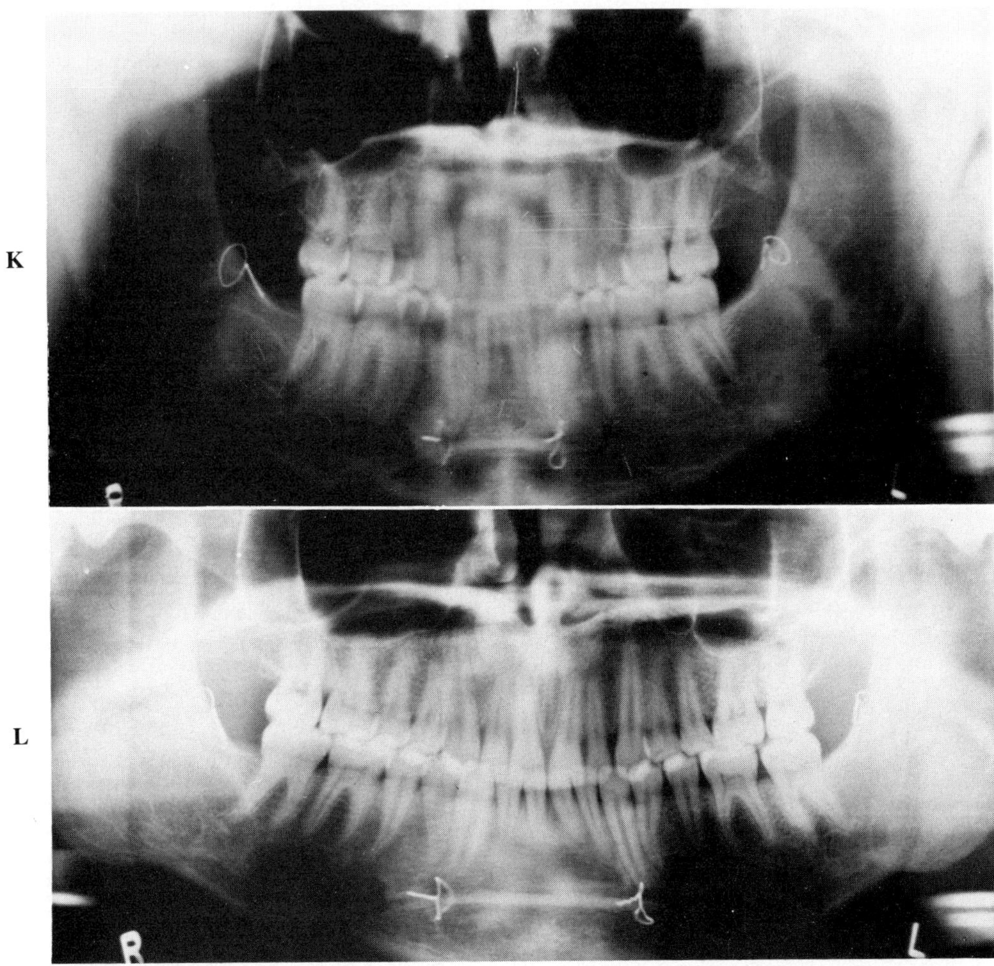

Fig. 4-7—cont'd.
K and **L,** Panolipse radiographs, 1 year postoperative (good consolidation of the genioplasty site) and 2 years postoperative (almost complete replacement of allogeneic bone with host bone).

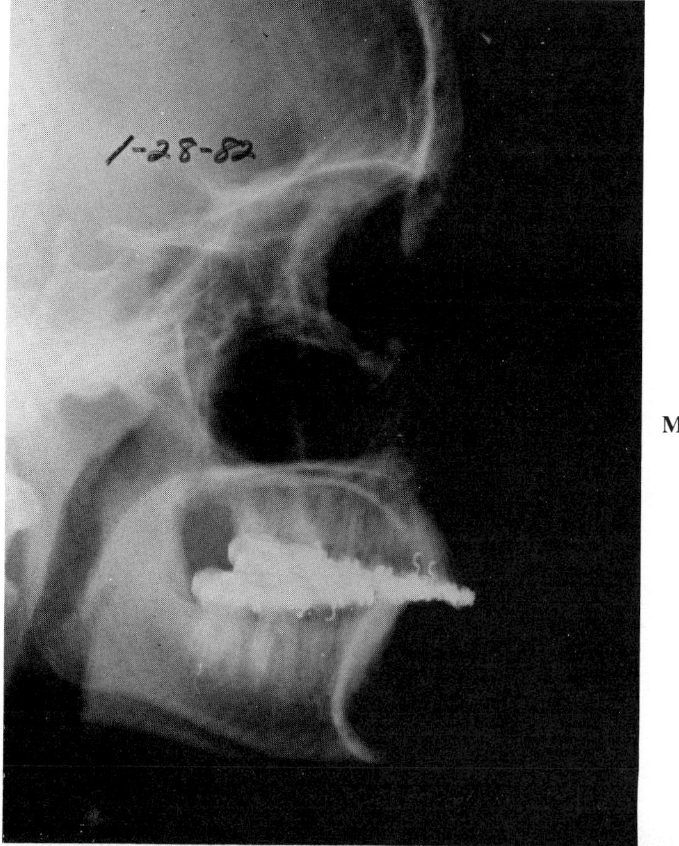

M

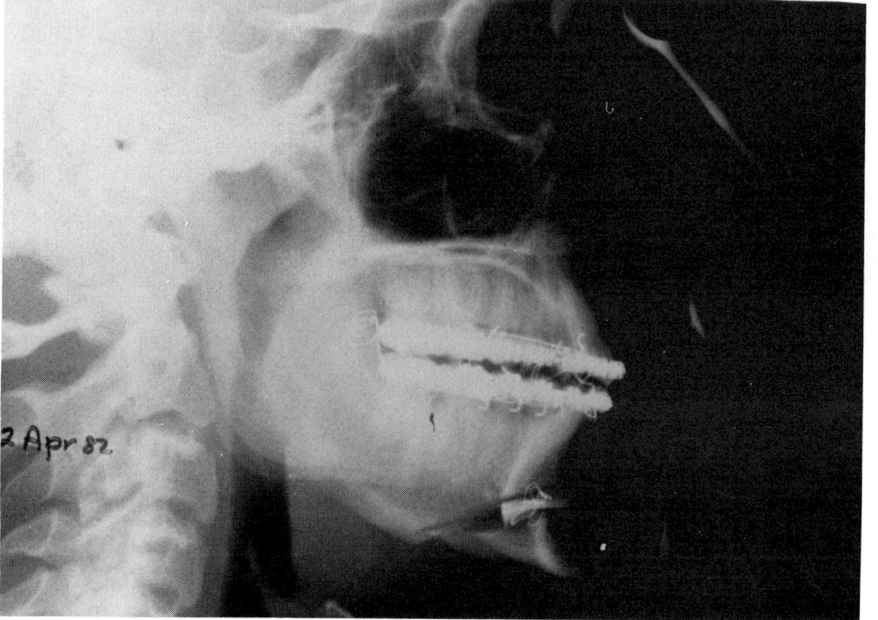

N

Fig. 4-7—cont'd.
Continued.
M and **N,** Cephalograms showing the preoperative and immediately postoperative conditions.

Fig. 4-7—cont'd.
O and **P,** Cephalograms showing the 1-year and 2-year postoperative conditions. Note the almost complete replacement of allogeneic bone with host bone at 2 years.

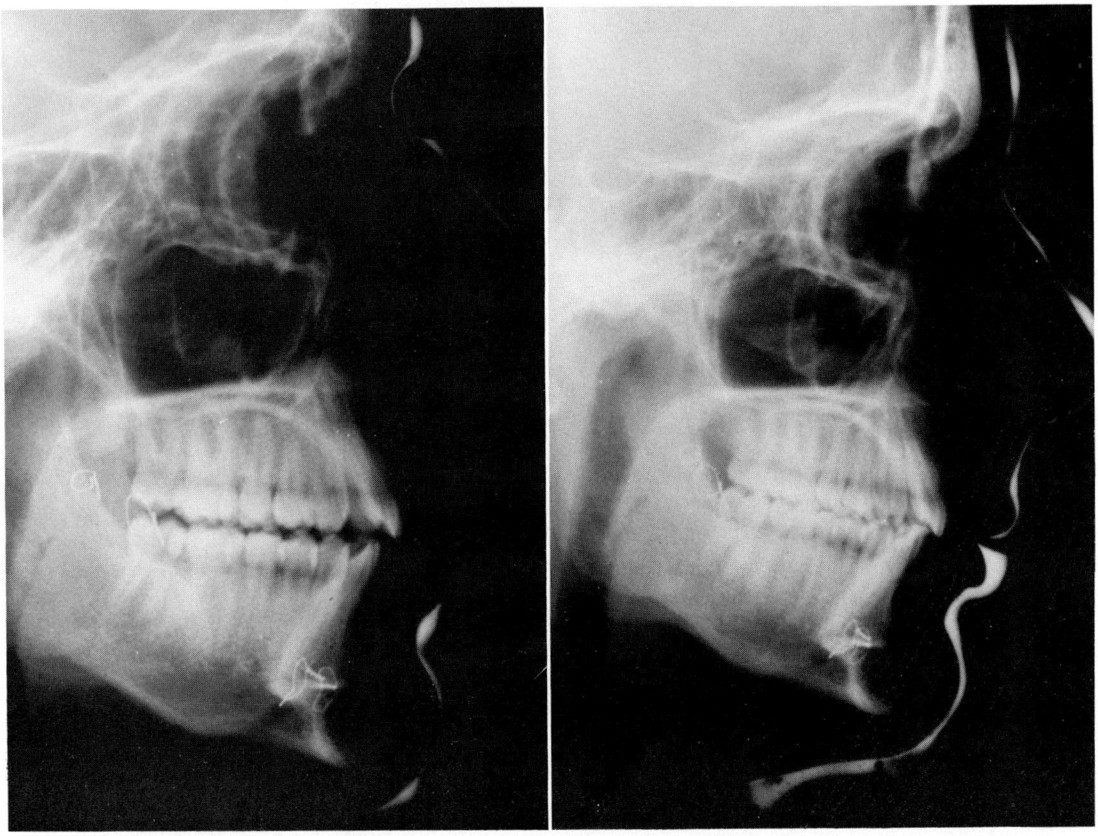

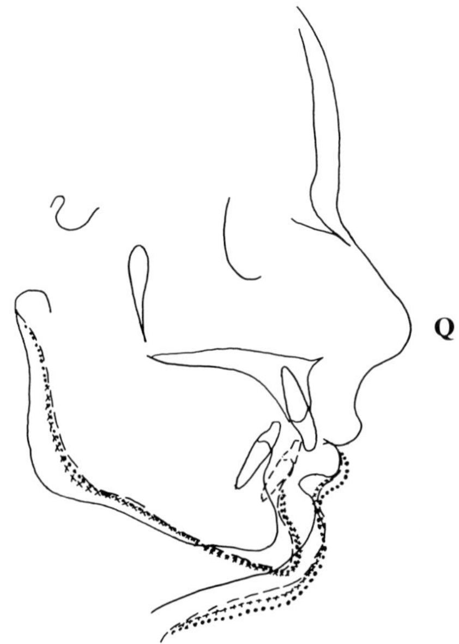

Fig. 4-7—cont'd.

Q, Composite cephalometric tracings. *Solid line,* Preoperative; *broken line,* immediately postoperative; *dotted line,* 1 year postoperative; **x** *line,* 2 years postoperative.

CASE 7 (Fig. 4-8)

A 15-year-old boy was evaluated for complaints of showing too much teeth and a lack of chin prominence.

Problem list

Esthetics

Good facial contour and symmetry with excessive exposure of the anterior maxillary teeth upon repose and excessive gingival exposure when smiling; poor lip competence with mentalis strain; excessive facial convexity.

Hard tissue cephalometric analysis

S-N-A, 81 degrees; S-N-B, 74 degrees
Increased FMA (Go-Gn to FH, 30 degrees)

Soft tissue analysis

Increased angle facial convexity (22 degrees)
Retrusion of soft tissue pogonion
Long steep lower facial third
Excessive incisor exposure

Occlusal analysis

Slight Class II occlusion
Good arch width and form
Minor tooth positional discrepancies and rotations
Overjet 5 mm
Overbite 5 mm

Treatment plan

Orthodontics was not possible
Maxillary impaction with total maxillary alveolar osteotomy to reposition the maxillary alveolus 7 mm anteriorly and 5 mm posteriorly
Mandibular autorotation
Horizontal advancement genioplasty to
Improve facial convexity deformity
Improve lip competence and decrease muscle strain

Follow-up

Procedures were performed concurrently; the genioplasty, done first, obtained 9 mm of advancement. Excellent positioning of the maxilla and autorotation of the mandible provided a stable occlusion. Planned incisor exposure was obtained. Genioplasty added to the excellent cosmesis, improving facial form and lip competence while eliminating mentalis strain. Three-year follow-up remains stable.

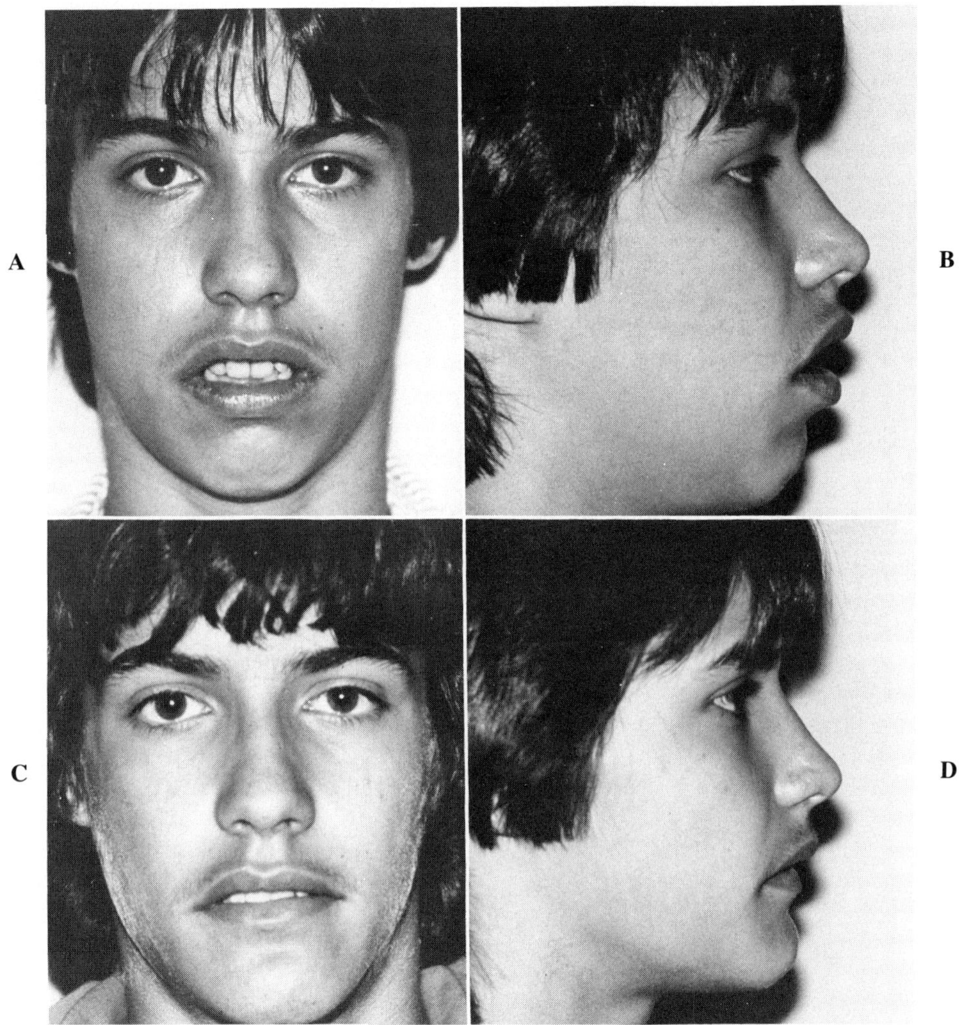

Continued.

Fig. 4-8.
Case 7. **A** and **B,** Presurgical facial appearance. **C** and **D,** Postsurgical appearance following maxillary intrusion by a total alveolar procedure and advancement genioplasty.

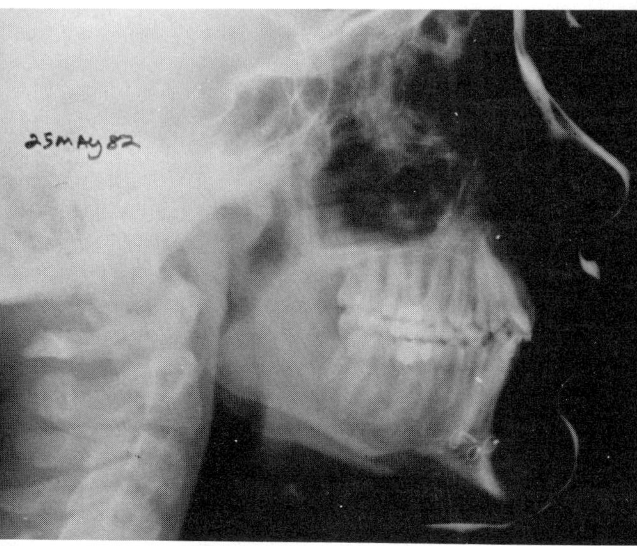

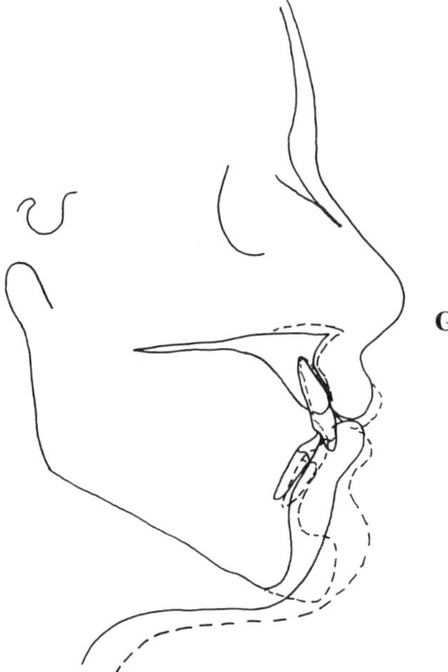

Fig. 4-8—cont'd.
E, Pretreatment and, **F,** 6-month posttreatment cephalograms. Consolidation, apposition, and recontouring at the genioplasty site are proceeding nicely. **G,** Composite cephalometric tracings. The repositioned maxillary alveolus, autorotated mandible, and advanced chin all have improved the facial contour. *Solid line,* Preoperative; *broken line,* postoperative.

CONCLUSION

Throughout the ages facial esthetics has been of concern. Surgical correction of the contour-deficient or excessive chin has undergone an evolution that now sees the implantation of substances generally inert and bioacceptable. Implantation has been surpassed, however, by innovative techniques of horizontal osteotomy of the chin, otherwise known as genioplasty. The development of the minimal–tissue detachment broad pedicle has created results that are generally more stable and cosmetically acceptable and beneficial than any prosthetic device could ever be. The treatment of multiple deformities of the chin now can be directly addressed with a stable biologically sound surgery that may be altered according to patient requirements and the art and science possessed by the surgeon.

The use of allogeneic bone grafting techniques in genioplasty appears to present a new source of available treatments for the protrusive chin found in anterior mandibular short face syndromes. It will be some time before all is known about this technique, but currently it appears stable with good predictability.

As with all aspects of oral and maxillofacial surgery, the clinician is challenged to make new and better use of what is a most versatile procedure.

REFERENCES

1. Bays, R.A.: Current concepts in bone grafting. In Irby, W.B., and Shelton, D.W., editors: Current advances in oral and maxillofacial surgery, vol. 4, St. Louis, 1983, The C.V. Mosby Co.
2. Bell, W.H.: Correction of the contour deficient chin, J. Oral Surg. **27:**110, 1969.
3. Bell, W.H.: Correction of mandibular prognathism by mandibular setback and advancement genioplasty, Int. J. Oral Surg. **10:**221, 1981.
4. Bell, W.H., and Gallagher, D.M.: The versatility of genioplasty using a broad pedicle, J. Oral Maxillofac. Surg. **41:**763, 1983.
5. Bell, W.H., et al.: Reduction genioplasty: surgical techniques and soft tissue changes, Oral Surg. **51:**471, 1981.
6. Busquets, C.J., and Sassouni, V.: Changes in the integumental profile of chin and lower lip after genioplasty, J. Oral Surg. **39:**499, 1981.
7. Epker, B.N., and Wolford, L.M.: Dentofacial deformities: surgical-orthodontic correction, St. Louis, 1980, The C.V. Mosby Co.
8. Fonseca, R.I., et al.: Revascularization and healing of onlay particulate allogeneic bone grafts in primates, J. Oral Maxillofac. Surg. **41:**153, 1983.
9. Freihofer, H.P.M.: Surgical treatment of the short face syndrome, J. Oral Surg. **39:**907, 1981.
10. Frost, D.E., et al.: Healing of interpositional allogeneic lyophilized bone grafts following total maxillary osteotomy, J. Oral Maxillofac. Surg. **40:**776, 1982.
11. Gallagher, D.M., et al.: Soft tissue change associated with advancement genioplasty performed concomitantly with superior repositioning of the maxilla, J. Oral Maxillofac. Surg. **42:**238, 1984.
12. Hinds, E.C., and Kent, J.N.: Genioplasty: the versatility of horizontal osteotomy, J. Oral Surg. **27:**690, 1969.
13. Hinds, E.C., and Kent, J.N.: Surgical treatment of developmental jaw deformities. Chap. 9, The Chin, St. Louis, 1972, The C.V. Mosby Co.
14. Kent, J.N., et al.: Proplast in dental facial reconstruction, Oral Surg. **39:**347, 1975.
15. Legan, H.L., and Burstone, C.J.: Soft tissue cephalometric analysis for orthognathic surgery, J. Oral Surg. **38:**744, 1980.
16. Marx, R.E., et al.: The use of freeze-dried allogeneic bone in oral and maxillofacial surgery, J. Oral Surg. **39:**264, 1981.
17. McBride, K.L., and Bell, W.H.: Chin surgery. In Bell, W.H., et al.: Surgical correction of dentofacial deformities, vol 2, Philadelphia, 1980, W.B. Saunders Co.
18. McDonnell, J.P., et al.: Advancement genioplasty: a retrospective cephalometric analysis of osseous and soft tissue changes, J. Oral Surg. **35:**640, 1977.
19. Profitt, W.R., et al.: Systematic description of dentofacial deformities: the data base. In Bell, W.H., et al.: Surgical correction of dentofacial deformities, vol 1, Philadelphia, 1980, W.B. Saunders Co.
20. Profitt, W.R., et al.: Treatment planning for dentofacial deformities. In Bell, W.H., et al.: Surgical correction of dentofacial deformities, vol. 1, Philadelphia, 1980, W.B. Saunders Co.
21. Robinson, M., and Shuken, R.: Bone resorption under plastic chin implants, J. Oral Surg. **27:**116, 1969.
22. Sheidman, G.B., et al.: Soft tissue changes with combined mandibular setback and advancement genioplasty, J. Oral Surg. **39:**505, 1981.
23. Shelton, D.W., and Schow, S.R.: Personal communication, 1982.
24. Toranto, I.R.: Mentoplasty: a new approach, Plast. Reconstr. Surg. **69:**875, 1982.
25. Trauner, R., and Obwegeser, H.: The surgical correction of mandibular prognathism and retrognathia with consideration of genioplasty, Oral Surg. **10:**677, 1957.
26. Trimble, L.D., and West, R.A.: Steinman pin stabilization after horizontal mandibular osteotomy, J. Oral Maxillofac. Surg. **40:**461, 1982.
27. Turvey, T.A., et al.: Kirschner wire stabilization of the horizontal osteotomy of the inferior border of the mandible, Oral Surg. **54:**513, 1982.
28. Wessberg, G.A., et al.: Interpositional genioplasty for the short face syndrome, J. Oral Surg. **38:**584, 1980.

CHAPTER 5

Orthognathic surgery—the practical use of functional principles

ROBERT A. BAYS

In the workup and surgical management of facial deformities, every effort should be made to accomplish goals based upon sound anatomic and physiologic principles. Stresses and strains present in the stomatognathic system may significantly alter the outcome of surgery. The challenge is to utilize these factors to advantage wherever possible rather than oppose them.

Comprehensive descriptions of orthognathic workups and treatment are available in many articles and texts. It is assumed that the reader has a fundamental background in this field so the rudimentary information need not be reiterated here.

The purpose of this chapter is to describe several techniques utilized in the management of orthognathic problems and, in so doing, to explain the rationale behind these techniques. Clinical research will be cited where appropriate. As with any discussion of surgical procedures, some of the recommendations are based solely on the clinical experience and bias of the author and should be regarded as such.

IMPORTANCE OF THE TEMPOROMANDIBULAR JOINT IN ORTHOGNATHIC SURGERY

Orthognathic surgery can be divided into operations that involve the maxilla (totally or in segments), only the mandible (totally or in segments), or any combination of these. All procedures, however, that involve movement of the entire maxilla or mandible must have some influence on the temporomandibular joints (TMJs). Segmental osteotomies may also influence the occlusion so that TMJ function is altered. Preliminary studies[23] have indicated that orthognathic surgery can undesirably affect TMJ function although little is actually understood of the influence of surgical changes on these joints.

Orthognathic surgery patients should be evaluated for TMJ signs and symptoms prior to treatment and at various intervals during treatment. This is not to say that the unaware patient should be unduly sensitized to the TMJs; but a thorough evaluation of masticatory muscle pain or associated headaches, TMJ tenderness, clicking, crepitus, locking, or limitation of opening is necessary before any surgical intervention that will alter the masticatory apparatus is contemplated.

There is value in this for several reasons: Obviously patients with definite TMJ and myofascial pain dysfunction (MPD) will be screened and treated, if possible, prior to orthognathic treatment (Fig. 5-15). Also they will be made aware of any problems so that no doubt exists, as treatment progresses, regarding what signs or symptoms are present at the onset of treatment. Finally, and perhaps most importantly, in a small but significant percentage of patients, centric relation (CR) or any stable reproducible position of the mandible cannot be achieved until the TMJ dysfunction is managed. Many Class II patients have postured their mandible forward for such a long time that their temporal and masseter muscles are extremely sensitive and they simply cannot achieve a comfortable occlusion. More important, chronic anterior positioning of the mandible will cause a shortening of the lateral pterygoid muscles, which may prevent seating of the condyles until the original muscle length can be reestablished. Preoperative splint treatment, physical therapy, or biofeedback may be valuable in allowing an accurate and reproducible CR to be found; but without a CR mounting the orthognathic treatment plan may be inappropriate. The importance of CR mounted models for workup, model surgery, and splint construction in specific instances will be discussed.

Almost every text or serious orthognathic treatise expounds upon the value of CR mounted models, at least for some cases.[7] Methods of attaining CR, however, are often not included. For the sake of this discussion CR may be described as the mandibular position in which the condyles are located upward and forward adjacent to the posterior slopes of the articular eminences with the intermediate zone of each articular disc so interposed that the posterior thick band is superior to the transverse ridge of the condyle. This position should be dictated by the muscles of mastication without the influence of tooth intercuspation. The muscles of mastication should be comfortable and free of significant myofascial pain to do this.[4,27,32]

It is realized that no "golden point" that is CR actually exists but that instead there is a range in which the condyles, discs, masticatory muscles, and ligamentous attachments are able to function in relaxed harmony. The size of this comfortable range varies from patient to patient. These are dynamic relationships and are not completely served by a static definition. Nevertheless, this functional range can be reasonably identified by a person with a dental degree and a modicum of interest. Furthermore, identification of CR has numerous benefits in all phases of orthognathic treatment.

Many persons without any symptoms at all have significant discrepancies between CR and centric occlusion (CO) or maximum intercuspation (MI). Why then should we be concerned?

First, patients who have had CR-CO discrepancies without symptoms have obviously adapted to them quite well. But if the occlusion is altered, which changes or "deprograms" proprioception during intermaxillary fixation, will this be tolerated? If a patient has been fortunate enough to adapt to the CR-CO discrepancy, should we hope that he will adapt to a new CR-CO difference? I believe that we should aspire to the most ideal CR-CO relationship within our grasp. It is extremely unfortunate when TMJ complaints arise in a patient after orthognathic treatment, especially if there was no problem prior to treatment. We should therefore plan treatment of all orthognathic surgery from CR (with seated condyles) and finish to CR. In this inexact science we will then have the most reproducible preoperative position from which to proceed and the postoperative position for finishing our orthodontic manipulations and achieving TMJ health.

In patients who are symptomatic attempts should not be made immediately to *conclusively* identify CR until the symptoms are brought under control.[4,27,32] Clinical experience has repeatedly shown that after splint treatment of MPD a small retrognathism may become larger (Fig. 5-1, *A* to *D*), a large open-bite may be revealed as the condyles seat during splint treatment (*E* to *H*), or a symmetric-appearing mandible may become asymmetric as the condyles seat (*I* to *L*). In the last situation, the reason the condyles do not fully seat in the glenoid fossae of such patients is that if either or both condyles have been functioning downward and forward the lateral pterygoid muscles shorten their functional length, preventing condylar seating. This situation can exist in the face of MPD of the temporal, medial pterygoid, and masseter muscles. Successful superior repositioning splint (CR splint) therapy will render these muscles comfortable gradually and will permit condylar seating as the lateral pterygoids increase their functional length. If mandibular ramal surgery is performed on a patient with MPD and unseated condyles, placement of the condyles by any means into the fossa will not be possible because of this shortened muscle state.

The number of cases in which these changes

Fig. 5-1.
Three cases illustrating the differences observed between CR occlusion obtained in the presence of MPD and that found after successful superior repositioning splint therapy. In each case the true CR occlusion was unattainable until the muscle dysfunction had been eliminated. Retrognathism, **A** and **B,** before and, **C** and **D,** after treatment.

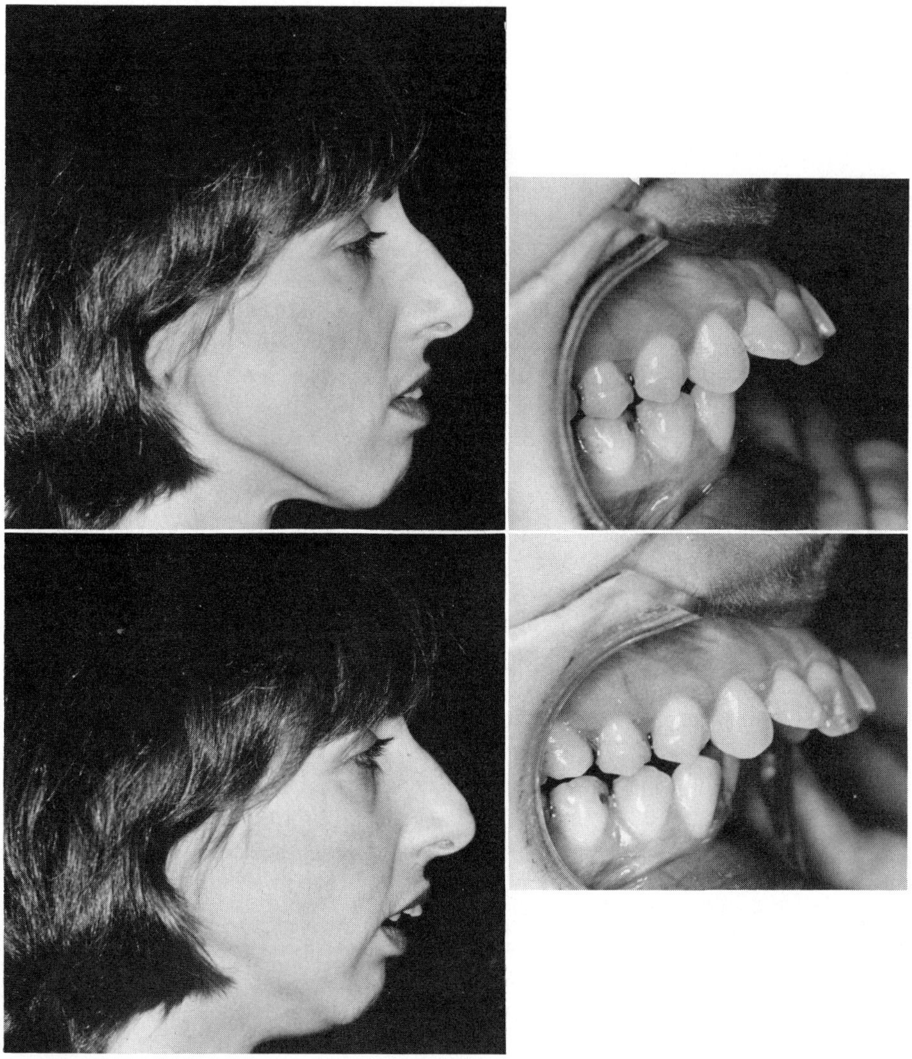

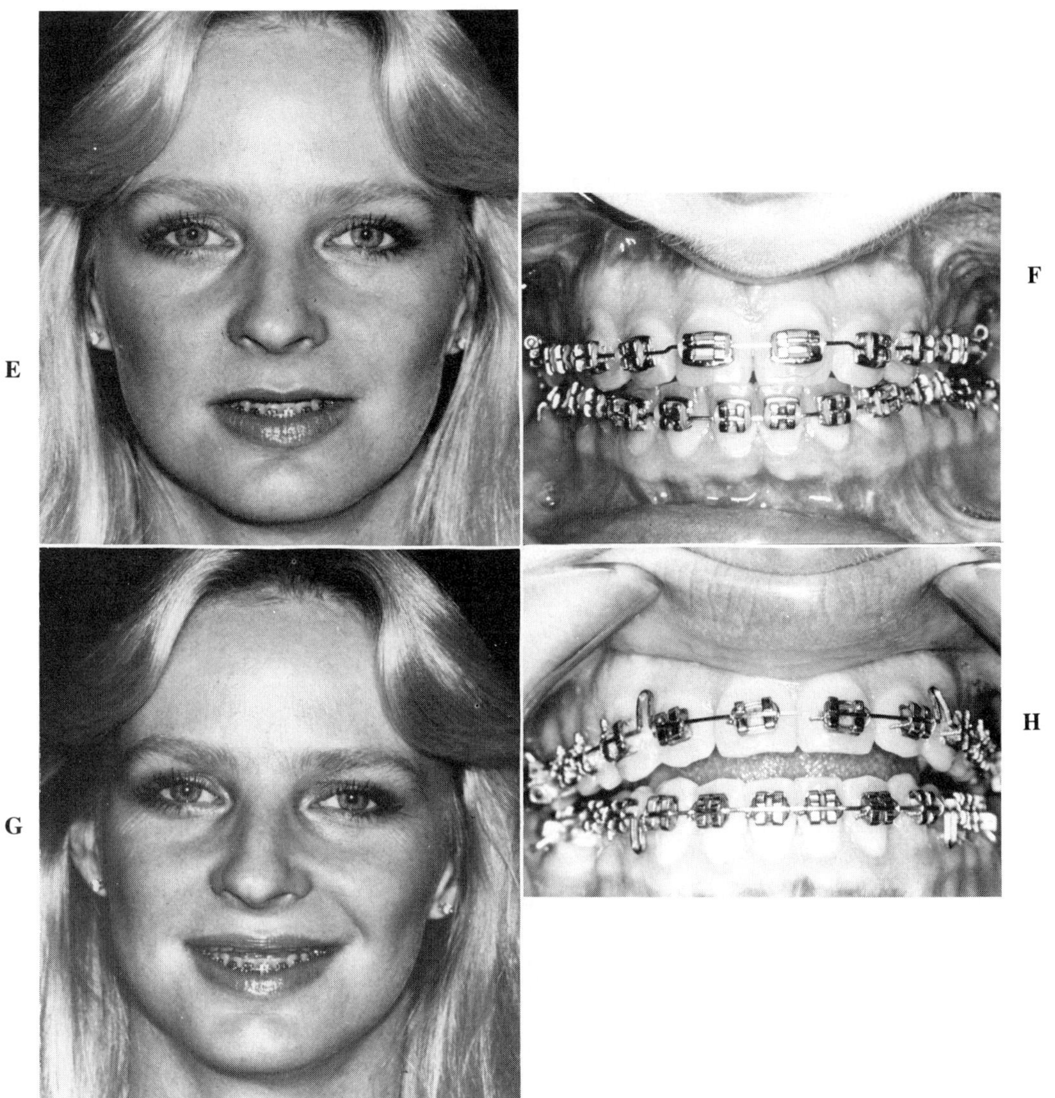

Continued.

Fig. 5-1—cont'd.
Open-bite, **E** and **F,** before and, **G** and **H,** after treatment.

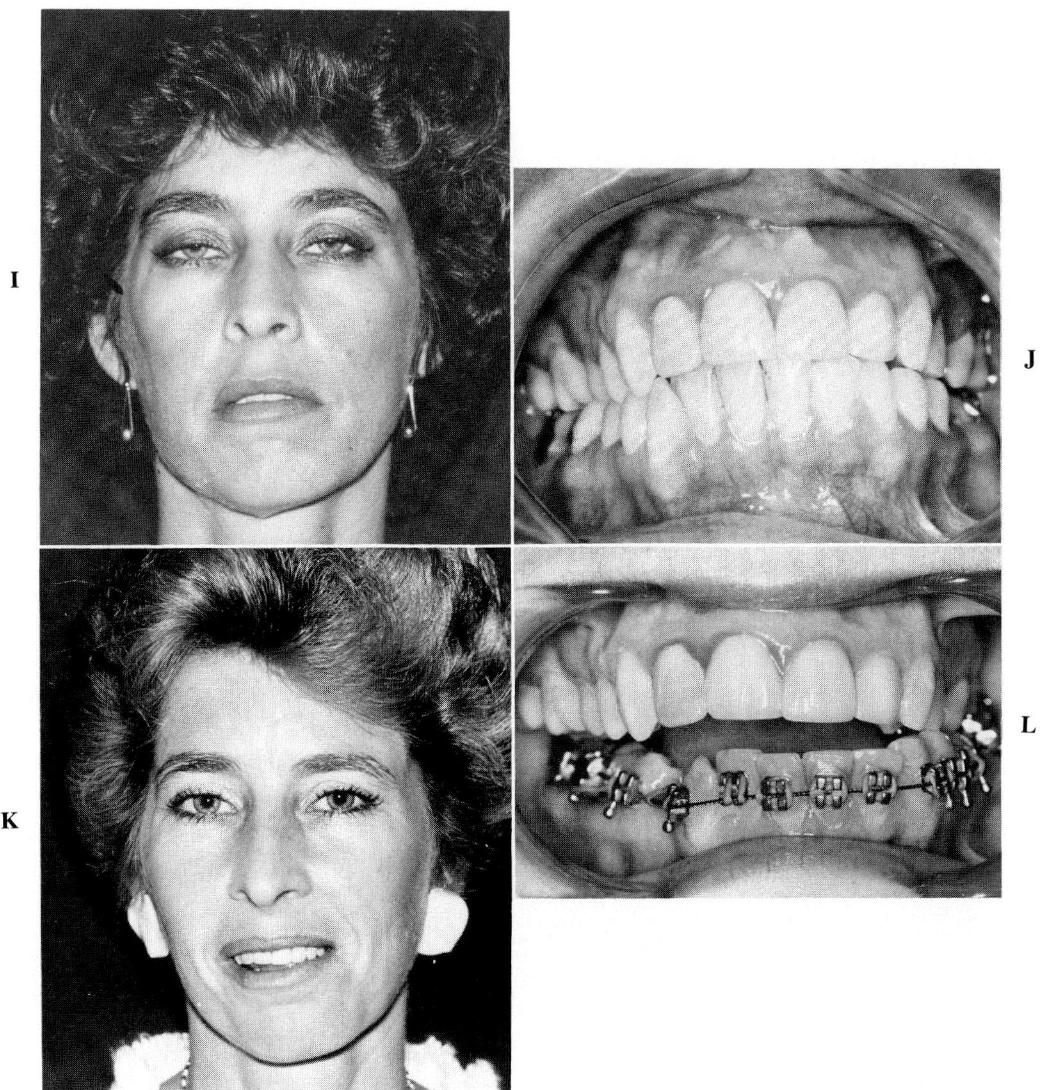

Fig. 5-1—cont'd.
Mandibular asymmetry, **I** and **J,** before and, **K** and **L,** after treatment.

occur under the influence of TMJ splints is not insignificant. Therefore, if masticatory pain and/or TMJ complaints are present prior to treatment, splint therapy to alleviate them is also crucial in diagnosing the CR position of the mandible. Even if the patient's presenting complaints do not include myofascial or TMJ dysfunction, it is the responsibility of the treating clinician to detect and eliminate such problems prior to orthognathic treatment. Once the patient has been taken to a comfortable seated condylar position that is repeatable, the orthognathic surgeon can rest assured that it is both stable and reproducible. If the deformity can be corrected while leaving the TMJ at this comfortable functioning position, a stable and comfortable result will be attained. Unfortunately, the situation in which MPD or TMJ dysfunction has not been identified preoperatively often occurs in patients in whom TMJ complaints develop postoperatively. There is thus no time in orthognathic surgery when an in-depth accurate knowledge of the patient's true deformity, including the state of TMJ health, is not absolutely necessary or at least helpful.

In patients with TMJ-related findings that are incidental at the time of orthognathic evaluation, correction of the malocclusion may eliminate these signs and symptoms. However, the determination of CR may be difficult or impossible without initial splint therapy. Additionally, a splint acts as a diagnostic aid to determine whether a correction of the malocclusion will alter the TMJ problem. In mild cases incidental TMJ problems may be noted and observed rather than treated during preoperative orthodontic therapy and then reassessed prior to surgery, but a comfortable CR mounting is still necessary before final surgical diagnosis and treatment planning.

WHY MOUNTED MODELS?

Most orthognathic surgeons have recognized the need for CR mounted models on a semiadjustable articulator for the majority of orthognathic procedures. Although there is some disagreement as to the necessity for this in all types of orthognathic surgery, the following outline presents the rationale for the use of mounted models in *all* orthognathic surgical cases:

1. Mandibular surgery
   a. To determine the magnitude and nature of the mandibular movement
   b. To determine the planned postoperative occlusion (can goals be accomplished?)
   c. To permit easier functioning into an interocclusal wafer postoperatively
   d. To reveal more open-bite than clinically apparent (requiring maxillary surgery)
   e. To help predict the size of the osteotomy defects (condyles may be difficult to seat intraoperatively, which may not be readily apparent unless model surgery is available)
2. Maxillary surgery
   a. To determine the arc of rotation of the mandible
   b. To reveal anteroposterior (AP) changes at the upper incisors
   c. To determine the planned postoperative occlusion
   d. To permit easier functioning into an interocclusal wafer postoperatively
   e. To reveal asymmetric movements, transverse or vertical, which would necessitate mandibular surgery to level the occlusal plane or match the midline
3. Bimaxillary surgery
   a. To permit accurate positioning of the maxilla
   b. All the benefits of maxillary surgery alone
   c. All the benefits of mandibular surgery alone
4. Segmental surgery that does not reposition either total arch
   a. To determine the planned postoperative occlusion
   b. To permit easier functioning into an interocclusal wafer postoperatively

Mandibular surgery
MAGNITUDE AND NATURE OF MOVEMENT

CR mounted models on a semiadjustable articulator are valuable for assessing the magnitude and nature of mandibular movement in all planes of space. The models can be marked to reveal the size and shape of the lateral defect in a sagittal split advancement or the lateral segment of bone to be removed in a sagittal split setback.

Fig. 5-2 demonstrates the clockwise or counterclockwise rotations that may occur and also reveals the nature of asymmetric changes. A mark on the buccal surfaces of the molars to measure horizontal changes will not show the size or shape of the change to be expected at the lateral osteotomy site. This knowledge can be crucial if the planned advancement or setback is difficult to achieve at the time of surgery. Just pushing the condyles as far posteriorly as possible during surgery will not always result in an acceptable condylar position, especially if the condyles have been chronically functioning out of the fossae. An inferoanterior condylar position (condylar sag) at the end of surgery is the single most significant factor in relapse after mandibular surgery.[24] If the case is accurately planned and the osteotomy site is as predicted, the condylar segment position will be very close to ideal. Although such accuracy and double check are not always necessary, they sometimes are and one cannot predict in which cases they will or will not be. Furthermore, the modern concept of condylar position in CR as just defined would dictate against pushing the condyle superoposteriorly as far as possible at the time of surgery since this could contribute to disc dislocation and impingement on the retrodiscal tissue. Accurate preoperative planning with mounted models on a semiadjustable articulator will permit surgical positioning of the proximal segment where it was planned rather than guessing. Inferior border wiring (Fig. 5-6) of the sagittal split allows the muscles of mastication to seat the condyles upward and forward, with the planned advancement between proximal and distal segments maintained by the inferior border wire and intermaxillary fixation. This is an example of allowing the forces acting on the mandible to work favorably.

Planned Postoperative Occlusion

No attempt will be made to discuss thoroughly the theories of occlusion. However, the goal of almost all orthognathic surgery is to achieve the best occlusion possible. Much electromyographic evidence supports the concept that disocclusion of the posterior teeth in lateral or protrusive excursions is desirable.[1,4,27] The only way to evaluate the planned postoperative occlusion is to have mounted models on a semiadjustable articulator. After the mandibular model has been repositioned, the occlusion can be checked. Lateral check bites are not necessary since minor alterations can be made in the postoperative orthodontic treatment phase.

Easier Postoperative Functioning

If one plans to leave the interocclusal wafer in place after release of intermaxillary fixation, it should be constructed from the articulator-mounted models to ensure a clear path of closure.

Revealing Open-Bite Tendency

Occasionally the very process of obtaining a CR will reveal more of an open-bite tendency than was previously recognized. A small open-bite may be closed by mandibular advancement in certain cases, but experience has shown that in many retrognathic patients as the condyles are fully seated by the muscles of mastication a significant anterior open-bite develops because of pivoting around the second molars. This open-bite tendency is not obvious from the centric occlusion position (Fig. 5-1, *E* to *H*). If no attempt is made to seat the condyles for mounted models or for diagnostic purposes, it is altogether possible that the surgeon may miss the open-bite tendency in his workup. In such cases maxillary surgery to close the open-bite may be indicated.

Obviously, early recognition of an open-bite tendency is desirable. However, in some cases the bite may be very slightly open prior to orthodontic treatment but open more as the result of preoperative orthodontic preparation. Only mounted models at the time of preoperative workup will reveal the amount of counterclockwise rotation to be expected. It is then up to the surgeon to decide how much of this rotation is permissible before maxillary surgery is considered.

Predicting Osteotomy Defect

A clear knowledge of the size and shape of the defect at the lateral vertical cut in a sagittal split advancement osteotomy has one additional

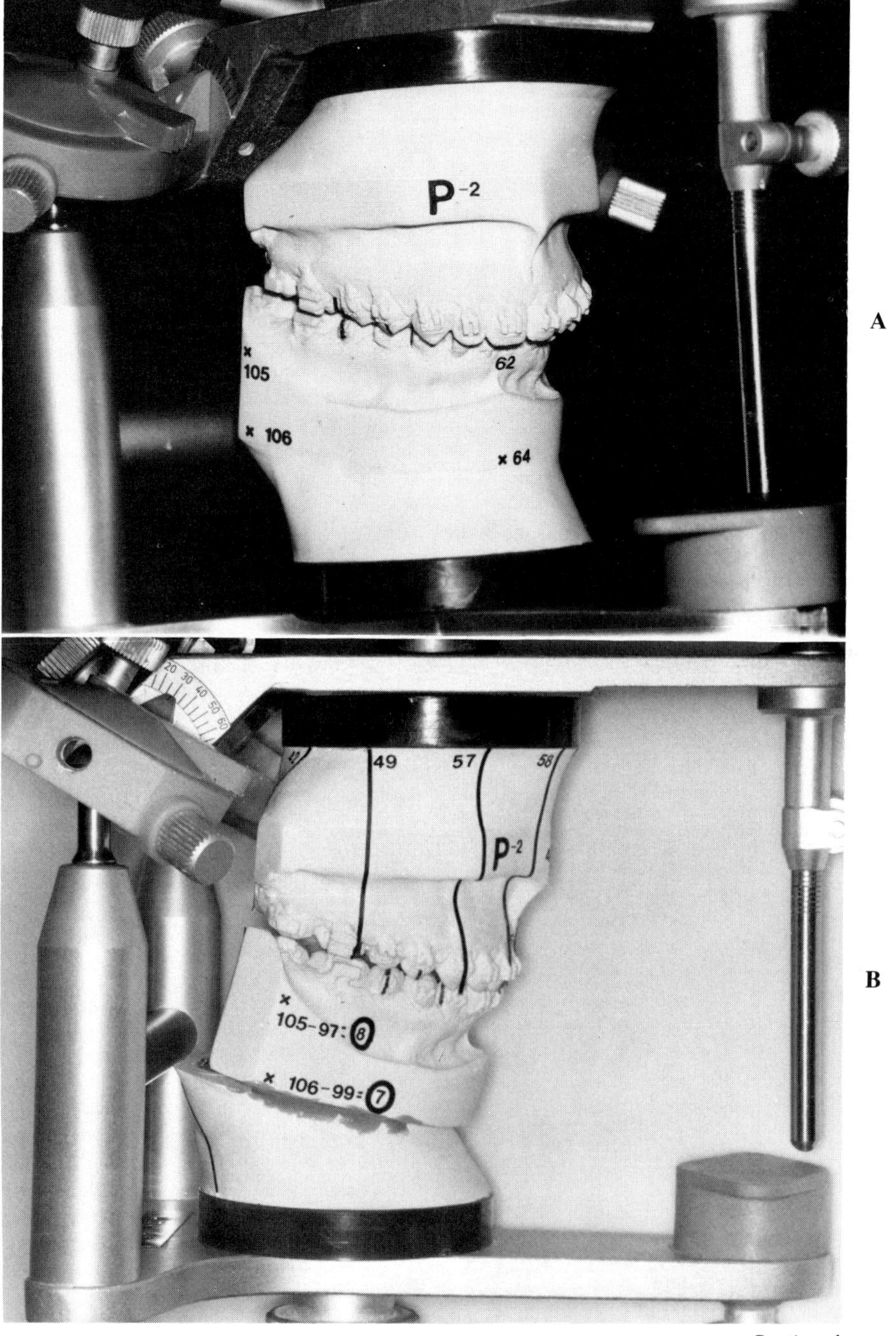

Continued.

Fig. 5-2.

Mounted models for mandibular surgery marked in such a way that the lateral vertical osteotomy site (Dal Pont) can be measured before and after the surgical moves. All measurements are made from the xs to the closest side of the pin. The position of the pin is marked on the maxillary model. Note: In bimaxillary cases the pin position for measurement must be marked after the maxillary model has been positioned so the autorotation will not be measured. **A,** Preoperative markings. **B,** Mandible repositioned forward. Note that the pin is lifted off the table. Therefore plaster must be removed between the base and the mandibular model until the pin can be returned to the table at the original setting.

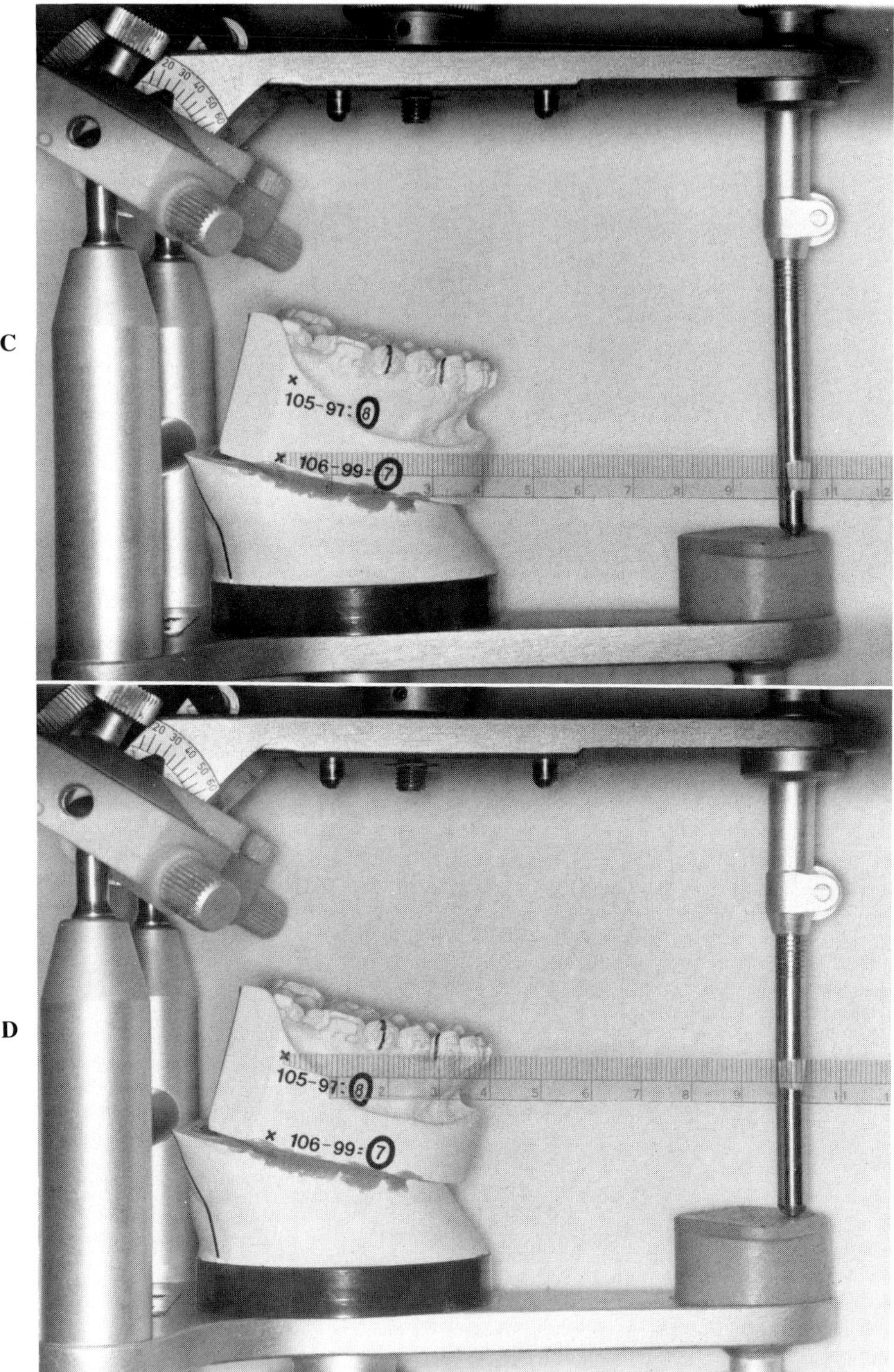

Fig. 5-2—cont'd.
C and D, Measurement of the inferior and superior aspects of the Dal Pont osteotomy.

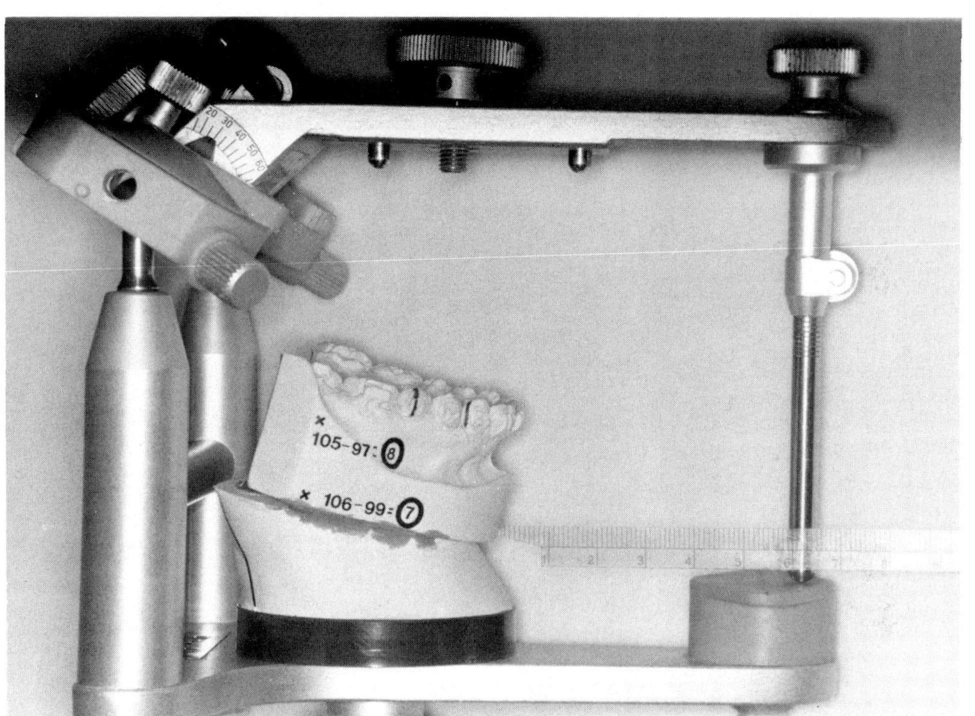

E

Fig. 5-2—cont'd.
E, Measurement of pogonion to be used for prediction tracing purposes.

use. On rare occasions, cases are seen in which it is impossible to achieve the planned opening at the vertical osteotomy sites even after conscientious mobilization, manipulation, and paralyzation of the patient. In such an instance the patient is in intermaxillary fixation, and so we know that the distal fragment has been moved to the desired occlusion. However, if the anticipated opening at the vertical osteotomy site cannot be achieved, it must be assumed that the patient's condyle cannot be fully seated under general anesthesia. This situation would go completely unrecognized if the model surgery had not made one aware of the amount of advancement to be expected at the vertical osteotomy site. In such rare cases the surgeon must be aware that condylar positioning is not appropriate and must develop strategies to overcome this.

In these cases when it is impossible to even approximately achieve the predicted degree of change between proximal and distal segments, an overcorrection of the occlusion may be considered to overcome the condylar sag that will be present. In such a case, if the condyle is blindly pushed up and back, condylar sag will result and relapse will be seen when the intermaxillary fixation is released. Although cases in which great difficulties are encountered in achieving something close to the planned condylar position are uncommon, they do occur and it is unwise to risk not knowing whether the condyle of the proximal segment is seated or not.

The reason for the inability to seat a condyle during surgery is unclear. It may be due to the TMJ disc position in the abscence of muscle tone. It was shown by McMillan[20] that total condylar seating during general anesthesia is difficult and falls slightly short of ideal. In the phenomenon presently being described (which has been observed only rarely) the condyle was several millimeters shy of a seated position. Again, detecting that the desired advancement between proximal and distal segments had not been achieved was possible only because mounted models had been made and measurements accurately taken. Otherwise the reason for ''relapse'' would not have been understood. If this problem is appreciated at the time of surgery, overcorrection of the occlusion to the point where the vertical defect of the sagittal osteotomy is the size planned preoperatively seems warranted. This may require alteration of the splint at the time of surgery to an end-to-end or Class III relationship of the teeth (that is, overcorrection). The important point is that if the models are carefully made and mounted the defect in the vertical osteotomy site should be as planned.

Maxillary surgery
Determining Arc of Rotation

Because the mandible is not mobilized, maxillary position is determined first by the intercuspation of the teeth and second by the arc of rotation around the mandibular condyles. The amount of pure AP change achieved by a given vertical alteration in maxillary position varies and is dependent on the length of the lever arm from the condyle to the anterior maxilla and the gonial angle. It is known that if the gonial angle is large (Fig. 5-3, *A*) the arc of rotation will have more of an anterior component whereas in small-angle cases rotation around the mandibular condyle moves the maxilla more vertically (Fig. 5-3, *B*). The obvious value of mounted models for this purpose is generally accepted.

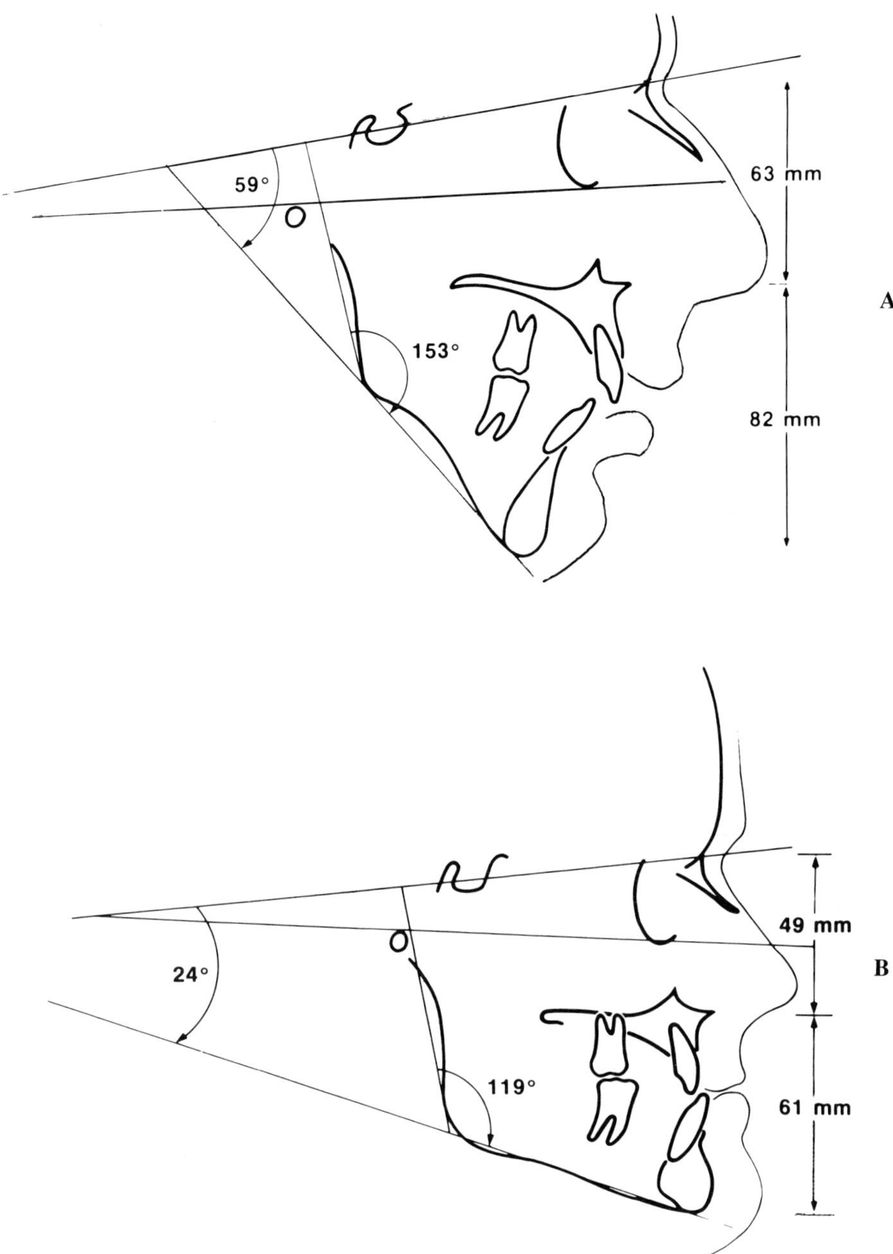

Fig. 5-3.
Facial types: **A,** dolichocephalic or high angle and, **B,** brachycephalic or low angle.

AP Changes at Upper Incisors

The anterior and posterior maxillae are rarely repositioned an equal amount. If the posterior maxilla is moved superiorly more than the anterior, the incisors will be torqued posteriorly even though the anterior nasal spine is moved forward (Fig. 5-4). This can increase the nasolabial angle. An awareness of this is not always possible solely from the cephalometric prediction tracings because no intercuspation is possible with radiographs. Properly marked mounted models will reveal the exact anteroposterior postoperative position of the incisors (Fig. 5-10). This is crucial to the prediction of the final facial profile.

Postoperative Occlusion

As with all of the other procedures described, the planned postoperative occlusion can be evaluated for interferences and other discrepancies.

Easier Postoperative Functioning

Mounted models will allow function into the surgical occlusal wafer with greater ease. This is more important in maxillary surgery, especially if the jaws are not wired together, because the stable maxilla can be made mobile by a traumatic occlusion or prematurity in the splint. In most cases, if the mandible is not surgically mobilized, the maxilla need not be wired into intermaxillary fixation. This is, in fact, desirable because the occlusion can be checked postoperatively with the patient awake and able to move the mandible with the muscles of mastication. Intermaxillary fixation after maxillary surgery may disguise a displaced condyle until release of the fixation, at which time it is too late to adjust the maxillary position without additional surgery and general anesthesia.

A foolproof method for performing maxillary surgery without mandibular surgery is to construct an accurate occlusal wafer and use the orthodontic archwires and wafer to stabilize the maxilla with suspension wires or use the stable pins (described later). After the maxilla is fixed to the cranial base, intermaxillary fixation is released on the operating room table and the patient is "functioned" into the splint to check the accuracy of the maxillary position. The day

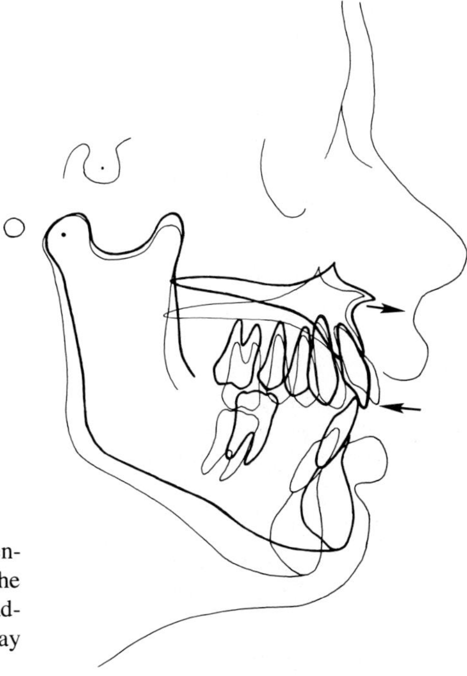

Fig. 5-4.
Clockwise rotation of the maxilla for closure of openbite. This results in posterior repositioning of the maxillary central incisors even though ANS is advanced. Lack of awareness of this phenomenon may lead to a loss of upper lip support.

after surgery the occlusion is again checked in the clinic or in a treatment room with good light, suction, and assistance. In rare cases the maxillary position may not be acceptable. If so, loosening of the suspension wires or pins and repositioning the maxilla are quite feasible. These usually can be accomplished without any problems; however, a sedative may be added to the IV to relax the patient, which surely is preferable to intermaxillary fixation on the operating table resulting in an unseated condyle that is not detected until release of fixation. Intermaxillary fixation can be instituted the day after surgery if it is deemed necessary for immobilization of the maxilla; but if the occlusion is stable, this is rarely necessary.

REVEALING ASYMMETRIC MOVEMENT

On occasion, when the maxillary model is repositioned into an ideal occlusion, the intercuspation will require asymmetric repositioning of the maxilla. This may mean that the maxillary midline will be drawn to one side of the facial midline or that the occlusal plane will be canted. If this is the case, mandibular surgery must at least be considered. Only reexamination of the patient and consultation with all involved can determine whether mandibular surgery is appropriate in these cases.

Bimaxillary surgery
ACCURATE MAXILLARY POSITIONING

Traditionally the maxilla is positioned using the intact mandible, and in such cases the intermediate wafer is made from the mounted models. A useful way to employ the mounted models is to perform both maxillary and mandibular surgery on the models and construct the final splint (Fig. 5-5, *A*). The mandibular model is repositioned to the original mounting *(B)* (or a second uncut mounted mandibular model is used) for construction of an intermediate wafer between the mandibular model and the final wafer, which is on the maxillary arch *(C)*. In this way the final wafer can be wired to the teeth at the time of maxillary positioning and left there.

This works best in superior repositionings of the maxilla and in some advancements, but it opens the bite excessively when the maxilla is inferiorly repositioned. Therefore in maxillary inferior repositioning it is best to make a separate intermediate wafer as thin as possible.

ALL BENEFITS OF MAXILLARY SURGERY

The exactness of maxillary position need not be as precise regarding the occlusion when mandibular surgery is performed simultaneously, but the esthetic result may suffer if positioning is not close to the predicted.

ALL BENEFITS OF MANDIBULAR SURGERY

Once the maxilla has been repositioned, the mandible and mandibular condyles must still be accurately fixed into position.

Segmental surgery that does not reposition either arch
PLANNED POSTOPERATIVE OCCLUSION

The determination of the planned occlusion postoperatively is as important in these cases as in the others, especially if the surgery is to be done in preparation for prosthetic reconstruction.

EASIER POSTOPERATIVE FUNCTIONING

The ability to function into the occlusal wafer postoperatively can be facilitated as described with the other types of surgery.

MANDIBULAR SURGERY— TECHNICAL CONSIDERATIONS

Proximal segment positioning is the single most important issue in mandibular surgery. Studies have revealed that failure to seat the condyle in the glenoid fossa at the time of surgery is probably more responsible for relapse during and at the release of intermaxillary fixation than any other single factor.[18,24] As stated earlier, attempts to drive the condyles upward and backward are ill-conceived in light of our understanding of TMJ function.

As awareness of TMJ function has increased within our profession and the public in general, greater demands have been made for accurate surgical positioning in orthognathic surgery. This is not only due to TMJ considerations but also for the sake of accuracy and precision. Surgery is and will always remain an art form de-

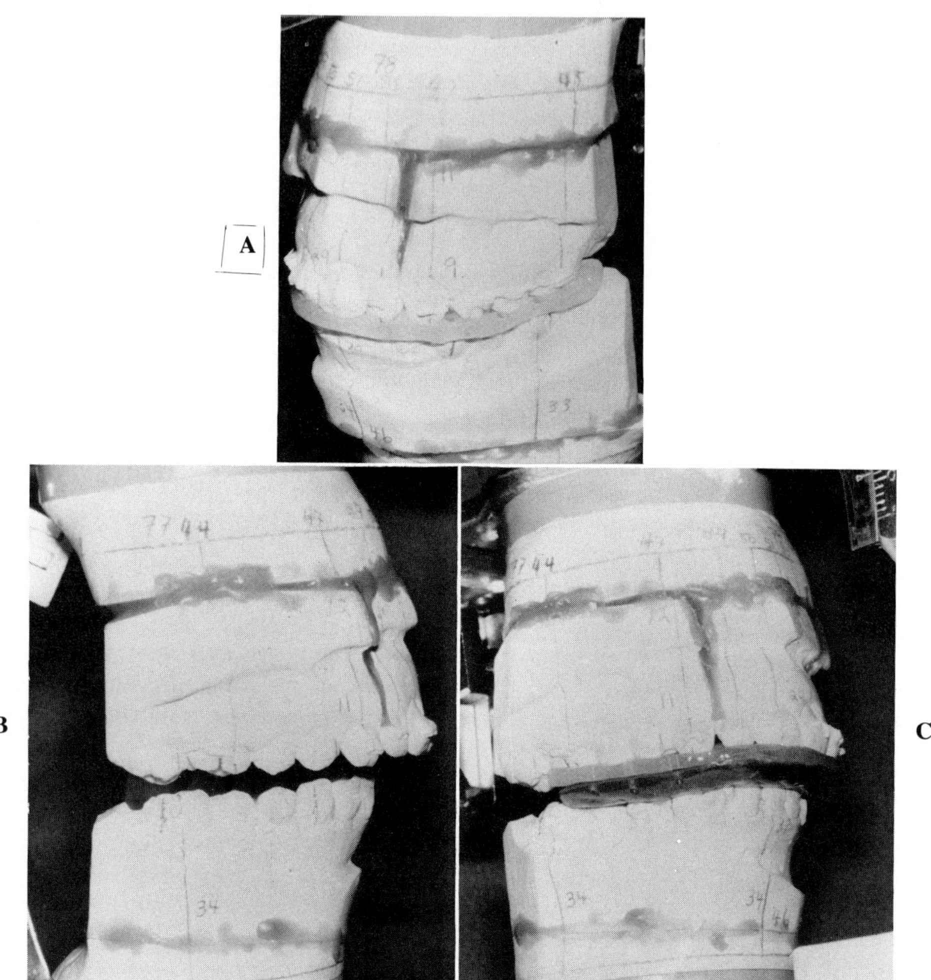

Fig. 5-5.
Surgical wafer construction in bimaxillary surgery. **A,** Maxillary and mandibular models positioned with the final surgical wafer in place. **B,** Mandibular model returned to the original position (or a second uncut mandibular model can be used). Note that the pin setting also has been returned to the original vertical so the maxillary positioning will be easier at surgery. **C,** Intermediate wafer constructed between the mandibular model and the final surgical wafer.

pendent upon individual skills and judgment; however, most of us need all the tangible help we can get to achieve the desired results.

Of the intraoral mandibular ramal osteotomies currently available, the sagittal split technique as described by Trauner and Obwegeser[29] and modified by Dal Pont[9] and Hunsuck[15] offers the most control of the proximal fragment. It is my procedure of choice for most mandibular advancements, retrusions, and asymmetric rotations, although for extreme moves other procedures may be substituted. Because of the individual variations surrounding these extreme cases, no attempt will be made to set guidelines as to how many millimeters a mandible or maxilla can be moved by means of a specific technique. This implies a simplistic solution. However, many factors dictate the choice of procedures, not the least of which are the experience, skill, and preference of the operator.

The following description of proximal segment management will adequately serve for most mandibular repositionings. The method uses the muscles of mastication to direct the condylar segment upward and forward against the posterior slope of the eminence. If the proximal and distal segments are repositioned accurately, the muscles attached to the proximal segment will seat the condyle naturally. This is based upon the assumption that the proximal segment is not rigidly fixed to the distal segment, which would make rotation of the proximal segment impossible.

Inferior border wiring is recommended for several reasons:

Most important, it puts the pivotal point around which the proximal segment will rotate as far from the muscle pull as possible (Fig. 5-6, *A*). Therefore the vector established by the combined forces of the muscles of mastication is a broad arc directed upward and forward. If the changes seen between fragments at the vertical osteotomy site on the lateral buccal cortex are correct, then the inferior border wire will permit the physiologic seating of the condyles by the muscles.

Another benefit is that less anterosuperior (counterclockwise) rotation of the proxi-

mal segment is permitted.[26] Therefore the gonial angle is preserved and the proper articular surface of the condyle faces the glenoid fossa rather than rotating anterosuperiorly.

Also less condylar sag is seen, which apparently decreases relapse over the long term.[26] This method represents the best attempt to leave the proximal segment where it was preoperatively and where the muscles have positioned it.

Success of inferior border wiring is dependent upon (1) CR mounted models on a semiadjustable articulator, (2) model surgery marked so the size and shape of the vertical osteotomy defect on the lateral border of the mandible are known, and (3) a surgical splitting procedure that facilitates positioning and wiring.

1. CR mounted models have been discussed. A helpful technical hint is to trim the mandibular model so the height of the bone approximates the height of the mandibular body at the second molar region. Then the base is lubricated slightly so it can be tapped free of the mounting without having to saw the model free.

2. Model surgery is performed by marking the models as illustrated in Fig. 5-2 at points corresponding to pogonion, the lower incisors, the external oblique ridges bilaterally (which correspond to the top of the vertical osteotomy), and the inferior borders bilaterally. Measurements are made from these points out to the pin of the articulator. Pin position is noted and marked on the model for future reference. The model is tapped free of the base, repositioned into the desired occlusion, and fixed to the base. With the same measurements, new points can be placed bilaterally on the lateral aspects of the model and the expected surgical defect can be recreated. Also measurements are made from pogonion and the lower incisors for assistance with the prediction tracings. The original pin position should be used. If the movement of the model lifts the pin off the table, the maxillary model should be removed for the purpose of measuring.

3. The splitting procedure is not greatly different from such procedures described elsewhere. There are a few differences, however,

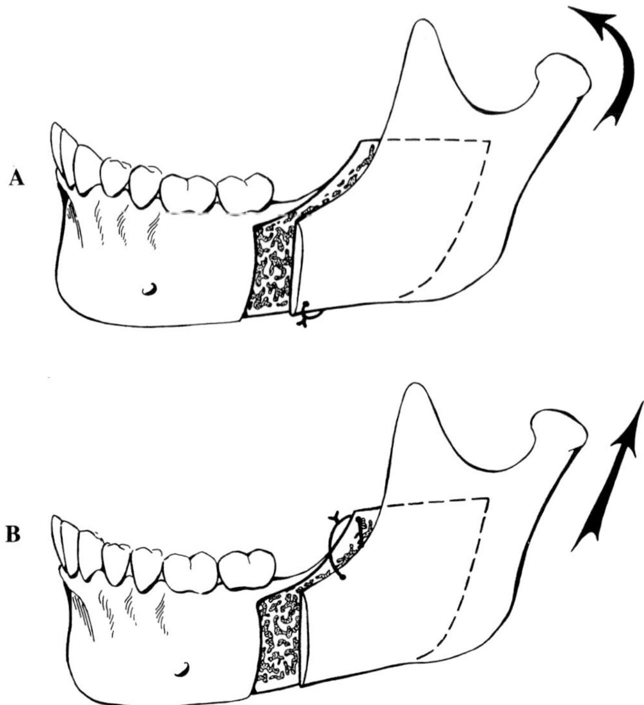

Fig. 5-6.
Biomechanical advantage gained by inferior border wiring of sagittal split osteotomies. **A,** Inferior border wiring permits the muscles of mastication to seat the condyles upward and forward against the posterior slopes of the eminences. This provides a pivot point at the farthest possible distance from each condyle. Wire placement is dictated by the measurements made on the model. Thus any defect on the lateral aspect is predicted by the model surgery. **B,** Superior border wiring drives the condyles upward and backward, which may dislocate a disc or permit superoanterior rotation of the proximal segment.

that are important to success. One of the most important is preservation of the bone below the inferior alveolar neurovascular canal so that inferior border wiring is possible. Also, the Hunsuck split[15] should not occur too close to the inferior alveolar canal on the medial aspect of the ramus because it may involve the canal or lead to placement of the neurovascular bundle in the wrong fragment. Either of these will involve some altered neurosensory changes postoperatively. The technique described next is designed to fulfill these goals while achieving a controlled cutting of the mandible rather than an uncontrolled split.

Surgical technique

The sagittal split osteotomy is performed essentially according to the methods of Trauner and Obwegeser,[29] Dal Pont,[9] and Hunsuck[15] (Fig. 5-7). The following modifications are used to facilitate a clean split with a nerve in the distal segment and ample bone on both segments at the inferior border. The significance of the latter point will become evident as we discuss the inferior border wiring technique.

1. The mucoperiosteal incision is made from the level of concavity of the anterior border of the ramus along the external oblique ridge to the second molar region. The incision must be lateral enough to be sutured with the patient in intermaxillary fixation. Only enough periosteum is elevated to perform the osteotomies. The periosteum is elevated from the anterior border of the ramus up to a level approximately even with the sigmoid notch. The curved Kocher* self-retaining retractor is placed on the

____
*Walter Lorenz Co., Jacksonville, Florida.

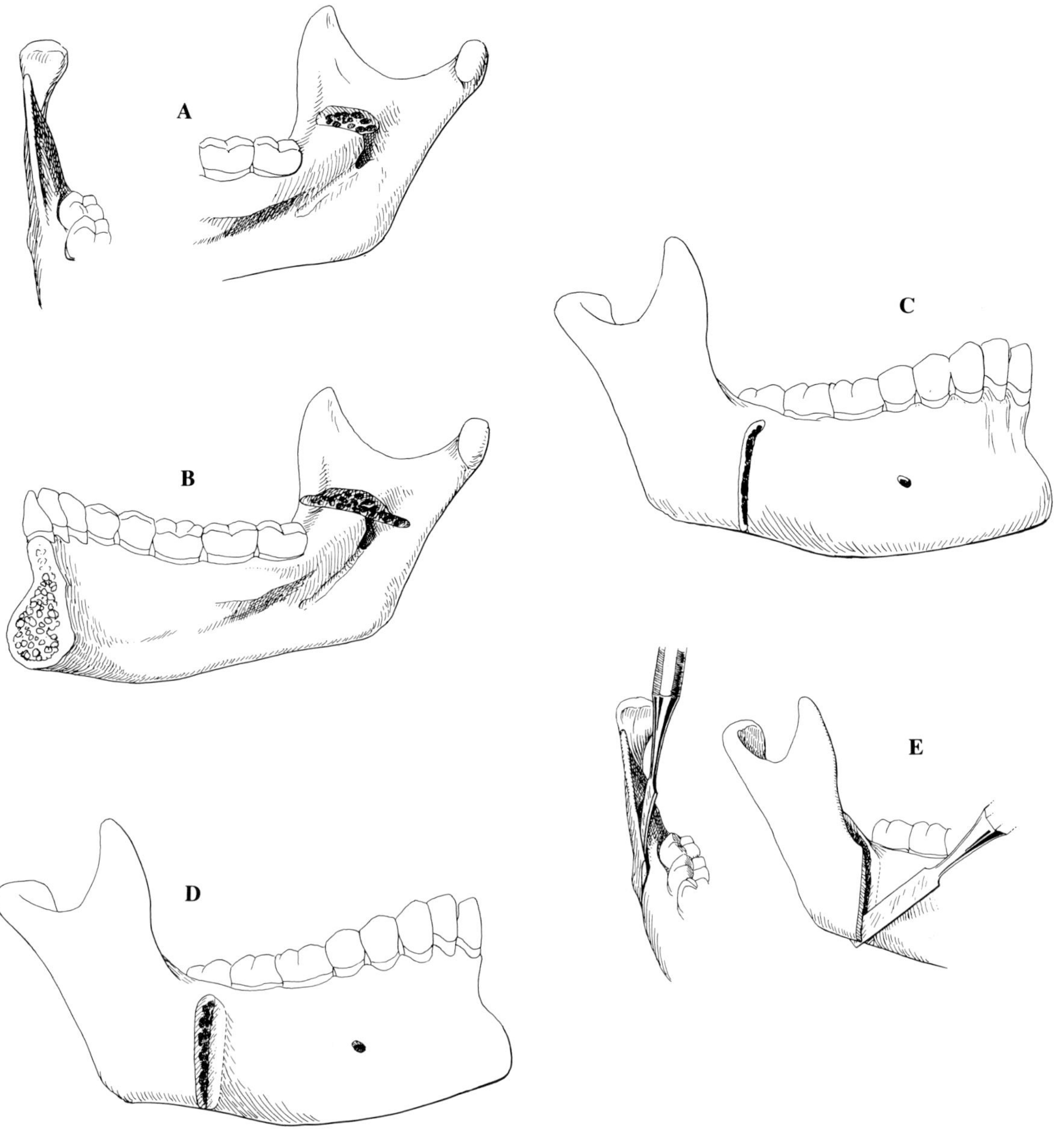

Continued.

Fig. 5-7.
Sagittal splitting osteotomy technique that facilitates inferior border wiring, muscular positioning of the proximal segments, and protection of the inferior alveolar neurovascular bundles. **A,** Generous removal of the internal oblique ridge facilitates visualization of the medial ramus. **B,** Medial ramal horizontal osteotomy. Carried well posterior to the mandibular foramen, into the widened posterior border but not through it. **C,** Lateral vertical (Dal Pont) osteotomy. Penetration to bleeding bone and exactly halfway through the inferior border. **D,** Anterior lip of this osteotomy. Generously removed with a large bur to permit positioning of the chisel. **E** *(right),* Cement spatula chisel placed at the inferior border with soft tissue protection underneath by the ramus retractor. This permits exact splitting of the inferior border. *(left),* Wide connecting cut made as lateral as possible. This permits placement of the chisel under the lateral cortex without endangering the neurovascular bundles.

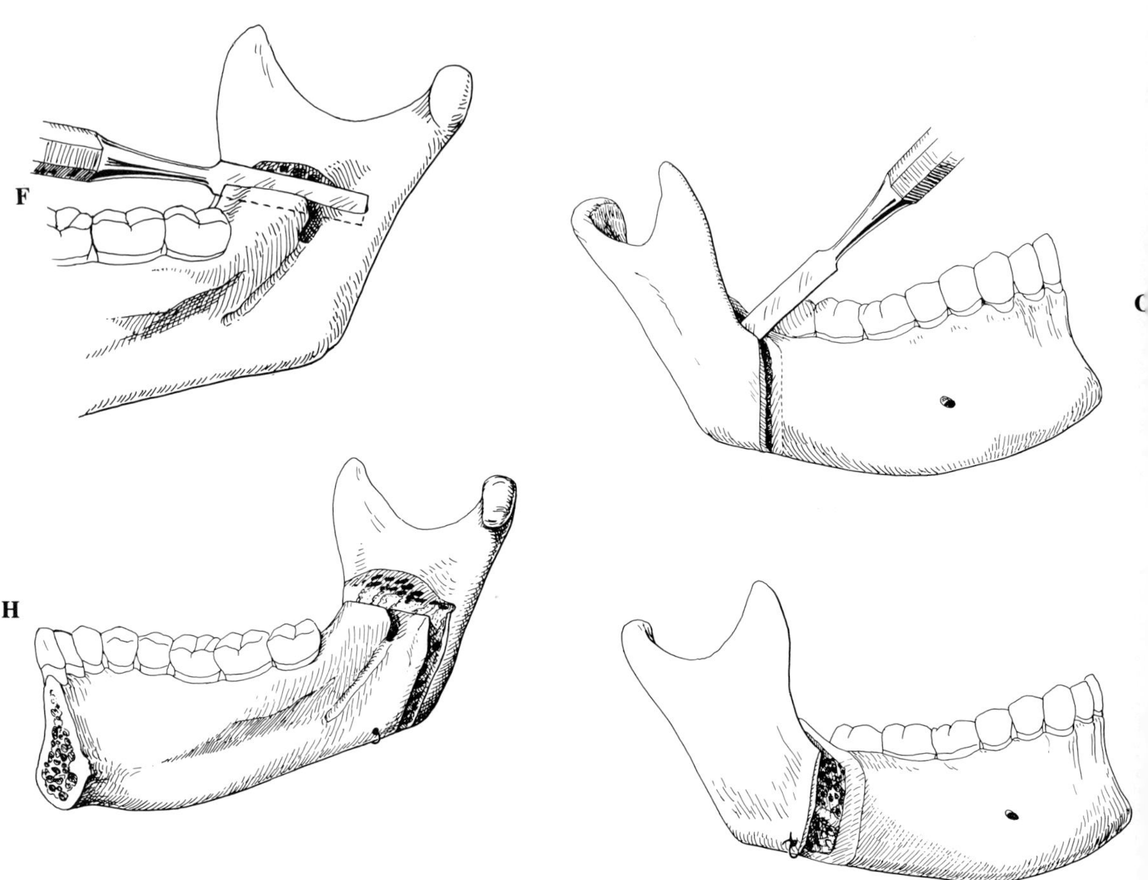

Fig. 5-7—cont'd.

F, Chisel driven posterior to the mandibular foramen. This ensures splitting of the horizontal medial ramus osteotomy to its full extent. Extreme lateral direction is necessary so the chisel will just "skin" under the lateral cortex of bone. **G,** Completion of the osteotomy. A sharp cement spatula chisel moves from the Dal Pont osteotomy to the horizontal osteotomy and back at increasingly greater depths. Its extreme lateral orientation protects the neurovascular bundles. Cutting rather than breaking avoids undesirable splits. If chisel orientation is always toward the lateral plate, total cutting of the mandible can be achieved without damage to the inferior alveolar neurovascular bundles. Nearly perfect splitting will occur in almost every case, with the neurovascular bundles appropriately and safely remaining in the distal fragment. **H,** Medial aspect of the ramus after successful advancement of the mandible and inferior border wiring. **I,** Lateral aspect after successful splitting and advancement with inferior border wiring. Note: The wires are placed in such a way as to create a defect consistent with what is expected from the model surgery.

anterior border of the ramus. Medially two periosteal elevators are used to work posteriorly along the ramus above the greatest concavity of the anterior border of the ramus until the sigmoid notch is located with a Woodson* elevator. The subperiosteal dissection proceeds posteriorly and inferiorly until the depression above the mandibular foramen is felt. The sigmoid notch location helps in this orientation.

Often the internal oblique ridge is so full that it obstructs visibility of the medial aspect of the ramus (Fig. 5-7, *A*). A groove is made in this ridge at the anticipated level of the horizontal osteotomy to facilitate access for the subperiosteal dissection and subsequent horizontal cut (Fig. 5-7, *B*). A large egg-shaped bur works well for making this groove, which should be placed prior to completion of the subperiosteal dissection if one cannot see all the medial ramus to be osteotomized.

2. Usually a Hargis* retractor is used for medial retraction. However, it is not hooked around the posterior border but is placed so the projection at its end contacts the subcondylar widening of the ramus. This holds the retractor blade away from the bone, which safely improves access. A slight torque of the blade will permit placement of a suction tip alongside.

When visualization is achieved with or without the groove in the internal oblique ridge, the horizontal osteotomy is made with a Lindemann* bur using a back-and-forth motion. Special care must be taken on the patient's right side because if the bur "grabs and runs" on that side it will be carried down into the neurovascular bundle. The horizontal cut extends posteriorly into the neck of the condyle, where it begins to widen (Fig. 5-7, *B*). It has been recommended that this cut stop at the depression above the mandibular foramen. However, this may cause a split through the foramen along the canal, resulting in nerve injury, so it should not be done. Instead, the horizontal medial ramal osteotomy should be extended almost to the posterior border but not through it (Fig. 5-7, *B*).

A frequent error is to make this cut too shallow, especially at the posterior aspect, so the

splitting occurs along the neurovascular canal. It is helpful, especially in very thin rami, to tap a cement spatula chisel posteriorly in this cut to a point posterior to the mandibular foramen. Then, if the chisel is directed against the lateral plate, there will be no problem in completing the cut posterior to the mandibular foramen without injuring the nerve. This maneuver helps ensure a clean split posterior to the lingula (Fig. 5-7, *F*).

3. The vertical (Dal Pont) osteotomy (Fig. 5-7, *C*) is made next; but contrary to other descriptions, it should not be carried more than halfway around the inferior border. Instead, it should continue just halfway. If the Lindemann bur is used on a convex lateral cortex, care must be taken to avoid penetrating more than just the cortex at the height of the contour lest damage to the nerve result. At the same time, however, failure to penetrate the cortical bone completely may cause an unfavorable split.

The lateral aspect of the ramus is fairly flat whereas the lateral aspect of the mandibular body is more convex. The junction of these two planes is a good place for the vertical osteotomy. After this has been completed to (but not into) bleeding bone, a large egg-shaped bur is used to flatten the anterior lip of the osteotomy from superior to inferior (Fig. 5-7, *D*). This will permit access for a narrow cement spatula chisel to be tapped down under the lateral cortical plate through the inferior border (Fig. 5-7, *E*). If this is not done, the anterior lip of the osteotomy will cause the chisel to twist, with a sharp edge directed medially toward the neurovascular bundle.

4. A Steiger* or fissure bur is used to join the horizontal and vertical cuts so the connecting osteotomy is very lateral. One should be able to chisel straight down under the buccal plate of bone (Fig. 5-7, *E*). This cut can hardly be too lateral as long as the mandibular marrow space is entered. There is no advantage to making this cut narrow; in fact, a wide cut is needed to allow the chisel access.

5. The inferior border split should be made exactly through the middle of the inferior bor-

---

der so there is sufficient bone on both fragments to permit wiring. To facilitate this, a cement spatula chisel is placed at the superior side of the inferior border and malleted through proximal to the bur cut (Fig. 5-7, *E*). This starts a split exactly at the inferior border. The same chisel is used at all points along the osteotomy incisions where one wants the split to occur— that is, the junction of the inner surface of the buccal plate with the cancellous bone (Fig. 5-7, *E*). Care should be taken at the height of the mandibular contour because the neurovascular bundle may be just under the cortical plate. If one is not careful, a narrow vertical cut may torque the chisel edge into the canal. This is the reason for removing the lip of bone anterior to the vertical cut (Fig. 5-7, *D*). The horizontal cut is started by malleting a cement spatula chisel until it is posterior to the mandibular foramen. This will ensure that the split does not occur through the foramen and canal (Fig. 5-7, *F*).

6. After the chisel has been used as described, a broader cement spatula chisel is directed laterally against the buccal cortex. One should work from vertical to horizontal along the connecting cut, being careful not to cut too deep (Fig. 5-7, *G*). The most common beginner's mistake is not directing the chisel laterally enough for fear of penetrating the buccal cortex. This endangers the neurovascular bundle. The chisel will not penetrate the buccal cortex but will "skin" along just inside it, leaving the neurovascular canal intact in the distal fragment (Fig. 5-7, *E* to *G*).

7. If the neurovascular bundle is retained in the proximal segment or becomes lacerated, the splitting cuts have been made improperly (probably with insufficient lateral direction of the osteotome). *The lateral direction of the chisel must be exaggerated.* With strict adherence to this technique, one should expect a near-perfect split almost every time. However, it does not guarantee that there will be no paresthesia, especially in patients over 35 years of age. Nevertheless, I have found that postoperative neuropathies with this technique are less frequent than reported in the literature and are rarely ever permanent.

8. After the segments have been separated, the curved stripper is placed between them and the distal fragment is stripped of medial pterygoid attachment. Great care must be taken at the posterosuperior aspect of the distal segment, for the neurovascular bundle may be damaged with the stripper as it enters the foramen.

9. The knowledge gleaned from the model surgery is utilized in this step. The objective is to make the vertical defect on the lateral border look just like the results of model surgery in both anteroposterior width and shape (Fig. 5-7, *H* and *I*). If this is done and the mounting was correct, the proximal segment will be in the right anteroposterior position and close to the proper superior position. Wiring at the inferior border will then allow the muscles of mastication to seat the condyle on the posterior slope of the eminence, which will correct any inferior sag of the condyle.

10. The patient should *not* be in intermaxillary fixation during placing of the inferior border holes and passing of the wires. A hole is drilled in the most inferoanterior corner of the proximal fragment. It is necessary to hold the patient in occlusion while the hole position is determined for the distal segment. The positioning of the hole in the distal segment is determined by adding 2 or 3 mm to the amount that the lateral osteotomy is expected to open. This will compensate for the position of the hole in the proximal fragment and for wire laxity. An instrument of known width (such as a Lambotte* osteotome) is used as a measuring device. The hole is made obliquely in a medioinferior direction so it emerges at the most inferior aspect of the medial cortex.

A 28- or 26-gauge wire is used, because larger ones are not malleable enough. The proximal fragment should not be distracted any more than is necessary to cut the holes and pass the wires.

Passage of the wire through the proximal segment is not difficult since the segment can be rotated; however, passage through the distal segment may be more problematic. If the surgical assistant holds the mandible by the chin and anterior teeth, pulling it forward and to the opposite side, the distal segment hole will be more

---

*Walter Lorenz Co., Jacksonville, Florida.

accessible. After the hole is placed, a classical Obwegeser* retractor is positioned so its cupped end is just under the hole and a wire is directed inferiorly through the hole until it hits the cup of the retractor. The retractor can be moved laterally as this occurs, which deflects the wire back toward the operator so it can be retrieved. The two ends of the wire are clamped or lightly twisted but are not tightened yet.

11. The throat pack is removed, and the patient placed in final intermaxillary fixation. The inferior border wires are tightened by using a ligature director (Woodson instrument with notches cut in the ends) to help hold the wire perpendicular to the bone and the proximal fragment in position. The left inferior border wires should be twisted counterclockwise to maintain the appropriate position between the two fragments.

When the final position duplicates closely what was expected from the model surgery, the postoperative condylar position is invariably excellent. This has been the case clinically as well as radiographically. Conversely, if the proximal segment is not in the position predicted by the model surgery, the postoperative position will usually show some deviation from the preoperative position. This may or may not be clinically evident depending upon the magnitude of the discrepancy.

12. The wire twist should not be placed at the inferior border because the patient may palpate it some months after surgery. Rather it should be positioned in the lateral wire hole of the proximal segment.

13. Eighth-inch Hemovac drains are inserted bilaterally through puncture wounds in the vestibule anterior to the mandibular canines. The wounds are then closed in the usual manner.

Positioning the maxilla

Various descriptions of maxillary positioning during surgery have implied that this is achieved either by preoperative measurements or by the arc of rotation around the temporomandibular joint. Actually both systems must be used to achieve accurate maxillary position-

---

*Walter Lorenz Co., Jacksonville, Florida.

ing during surgery of the maxilla alone or as the first stage of a bimaxillary procedure. Model surgery, cephalometric tracings, and prediction tracings are important; but in the final analysis the maxillary position must be determined intraoperatively using the mandibular arc of rotation. Although studies[18,20] suggest that perfect positioning may be impossible to obtain on the operating table under general anesthesia, the arc of rotation nevertheless remains the best system available. The following paragraphs describe how the oral and maxillofacial surgeon can achieve a maxillary position that satisfies the goals of acceptable function and esthetics.

The value of cephalometric tracings, workup, and prediction tracings has been overrated. As scientists and surgeons we have been trained to think in terms of numbers, statistics, and analyses. Although these are valuable in the workup of patients with dentofacial deformities, we must be aware that no system has been developed that accurately analyzes, predicts, and delivers the precise three-dimensional accuracy and precision needed for the correction of such deformities. The practice of orthognathic surgery, therefore, is an art as well as a science.

Of all the tools available, model surgery is perhaps the most valuable in preparing for the orthognathic correction of dentofacial deformities. It has been undersold as a mechanism for achieving a suitable occlusal relationship, which, of course, is important, but the information gleaned from it also has far-reaching implications in the esthetics as well as function of the stomatognathic system. A key to success is to avoid becoming burdened by the numbers regarding deviation from the norm (mean cephalometric values obtained from computer-based cephalometric analyses). Rather this information should be used, along with one's knowledge of the function of the masticatory apparatus, to arrive at a logical and sensible treatment plan for the functional and esthetic correction of a particular deformity. It can thus be concluded that the approach to a patient's deformity is not consistent with a single formula solution. Careful model surgery, cephalometrics, prediction tracings, and exhaustive analysis of physical characteristics will lead to a satisfactory treatment plan for orthognathic surgery.

If we assume that the foregoing has been accomplished, positioning the maxilla at the time of orthognathic surgery becomes perhaps the most crucial issue in the overall functional and esthetic result. This is true because maxillary movement is rarely unidimensional or bidimensional but tends to be three dimensional. From an esthetic point of view the crucial factors are the *vertical, transverse,* and *anteroposterior* positions of the central incisors relative to the lip, nose, and facial contour. The workup of the patient with the mandible in the seated condylar position is crucial; otherwise, the predicted position of the maxilla may be significantly different from the final position in either the anteroposterior or the transverse dimension. Vertical positioning of the maxilla can also be altered if a seated condylar position is not used. However, vertical positioning is more likely to be influenced by the presence or absence of solid bony contacts and the loss of orientation by tilting, tipping, or torquing motions of the maxilla. For example, in a superior repositioning of the maxilla, if the posterior maxilla moves more superiorly than the anterior aspect, the entire maxilla (that is, the center of gravity) will move upward while the anterior nasal spine may tilt somewhat forward and the incisors may tilt somewhat posteriorly (Fig. 5-4). If this fact is not appreciated by the surgeon, an inappropriate loss of upper lip support at the upper incisor level may be achieved inadvertently. Accurate three-dimensional model surgery will prevent such miscalculations. The ensuing description is designed to show how to position the maxilla at the time of orthognathic surgery in all *three* planes of space using the tools of model surgery, cephalometric predictions, and seated condylar position.

VERTICAL POSITIONING

The decision as to vertical changes needed in a tooth-lip relationship is a complex one. Unfortunately, formulas used to determine the necessary changes may not be applicable in many situations.[5] No mathematical formula exists for determining the proposed vertical maxillary position. Generally, if the maxilla is too short or too posteriorly displaced, it is un-

usual to overcorrect in an inferior or anterior position; however, if the maxilla is too long or too prominent, it is perilously easy to overcorrect posteriorly or superiorly, to the detriment of esthetics and function.

It is therefore recommended that in the inferior or anterior movements of the maxilla an attempt be made to move the maxilla into at least the normal range cephalometrically. The possibility that it will be moved too far forward or too far inferiorly is remote. The more common problem, overcorrection, is encountered in cases of vertical maxillary excess with or without maxillary protrusion. In these cases a number of factors must be considered. Generally, the rule-of-thumb to be followed is that *undercorrection* is far better than overcorrection. There is no scientific evidence that lip competence has any meaning in the function of the stomatognathic system. Is it necessary for the lips to be in contact at all times except during function? From an esthetic point of view, it is clear that lip competence is not desirable. One need only look at Western society's obvious conception of beauty to realize that visibility of the teeth during smiling and functional activities as well as at rest is considered a desirable feature. From a functional point of view, lip competence would seem to be important only if excessive drying of the teeth, gingiva, or mucosa occurs to the detriment of the health of these structures. It appears that 2 to 5 mm of visible tooth exposure during rest does not adversely affect the health or function of the teeth, gingiva, or mucosa but does significantly contribute to improved esthetics of the face. Therefore it is recommended that 2 to 5 mm of tooth should remain visible at rest in patients after orthognathic surgery with a preoperative diagnosis of vertical maxillary excess or maxillary protrusion (Fig. 5-8).

To decide upon the amount of vertical or posterior repositioning of the maxilla to be achieved in these cases, one should look at the patient at rest, during smiling, and when speaking. An assessment should be made of the amount of mucosa that shows above the mucogingival junction and the visibility of the root eminences or any other unesthetic intraoral structures. A superior or posterior repositioning of the

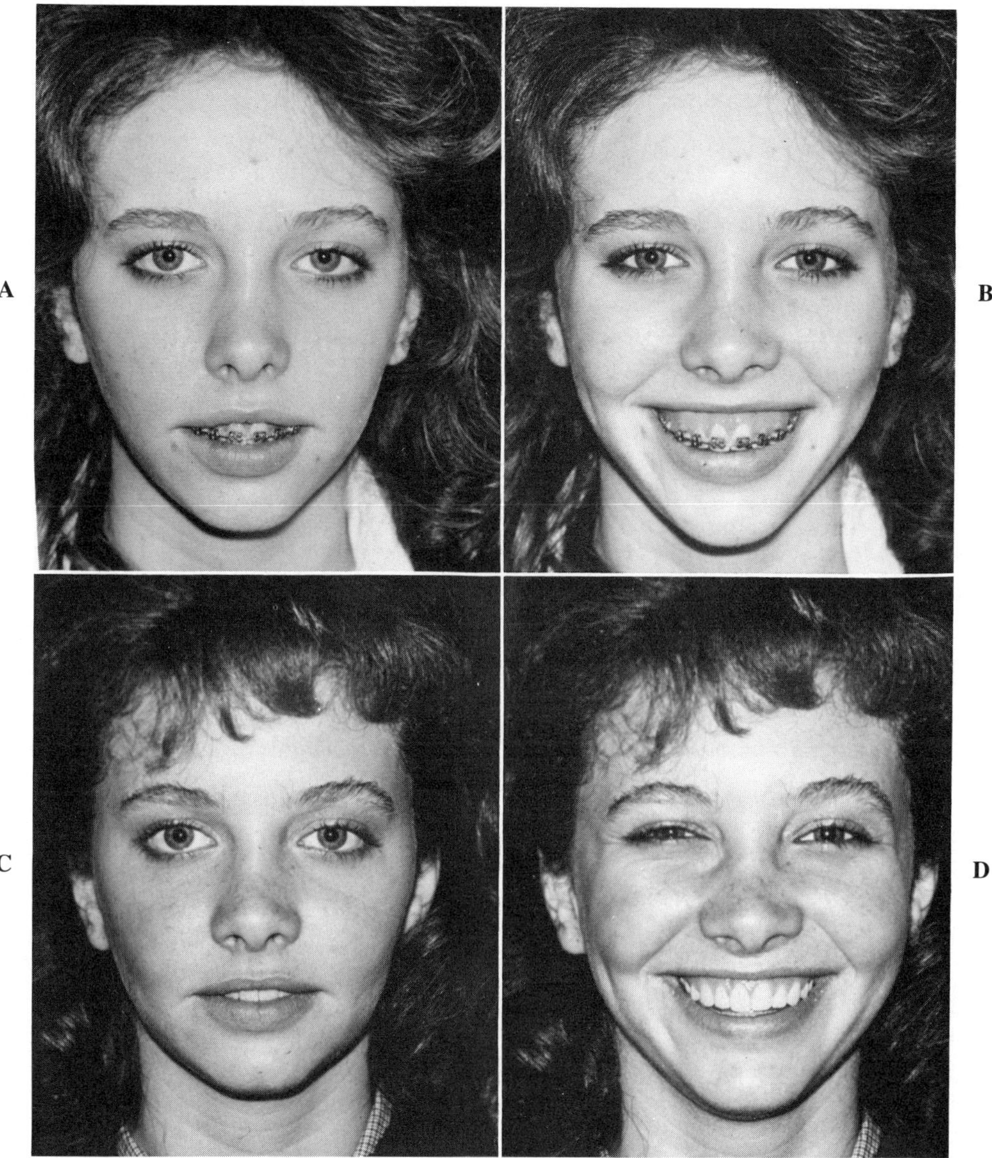

Fig. 5-8.
Appropriate superior repositioning of the maxilla for esthetics. **A** and **B,** Preoperative evaluation. Only the amount of unesthetic tissue showing is measured, and superior repositioning is planned on this basis. **C** and **D,** Postoperative result. The maxilla has not been excessively elevated. "Lip competence" was not achieved, nor would it have been desirable.

maxilla should then be determined on the basis of covering these unsightly intraoral structures and nothing more. It is recommended that in this calculation the amount of shortening of the upper lip not be considered. However, later in this discussion it will be shown how measures can be taken to minimize shortening of the upper lip so this shortening does not have to be considered as a major factor in the long-term esthetics of the face.

There are several extenuating circumstances that may alter the aforementioned observations. Patients who have inflamed anterior maxillary gingiva secondary to crown and bridge work or periodontal disease may require greater repositioning of the maxilla than the average patient to camouflauge this unsightly appearance (Fig. 5-9, *A*). Conversely, patients with very short maxillary clinical crowns who expose an excessive amount of maxillary teeth, gingiva, and root eminences during function must not be repositioned as far superiorly as others (Fig. 5-9, *B*). In these cases it is impossible to eliminate the exposure of maxillary gingiva and root eminences during smiling and still leave the patient with an acceptable amount of maxillary tooth showing at rest. The admonition is to err on the side of conservatism rather than to overcorrect.

Any discussion of the vertical position of the maxilla should emphasize that when the maxilla has been positioned superiorly postoperative instability has resulted in additional superior movement.[13,16] Therefore, if one moves the maxilla superiorly to the exact desired position, postoperative instability may contribute to an additional superior repositioning (another argument in favor of conservatism in superior repositioning of the maxilla).

In summary, the decision on the amount of vertical repositioning needed in the presence of vertical maxillary excess is a subjective one on the part of the surgeon and the patient. It is based on an evaluation of the lip-tooth relationship during rest, smiling, and speech. When all the evaluations have been made, the surgeon must determine and perform the *minimal* amount of movement superiorly to achieve the goal of esthetics, disregarding any potential shortening of the lip that may occur.

Anteroposterior Positioning

AP positioning of the maxilla has more numerical guidelines than does vertical positioning. The final decision, however, must be based on the clinical evaluation of the patient. The factors to be considered are (1) the nasolabial angle, (2) the labiomental fold, (3) the facial

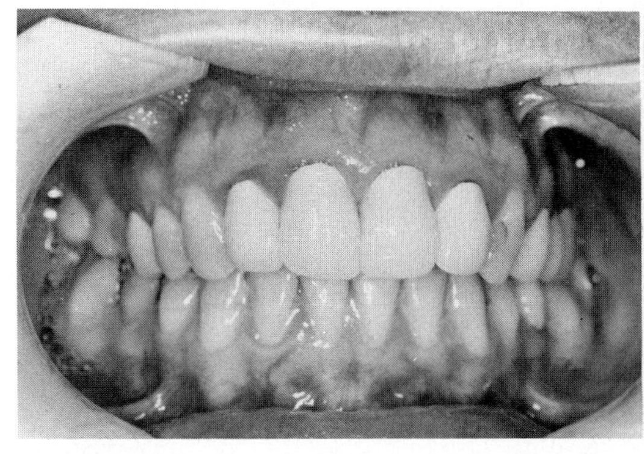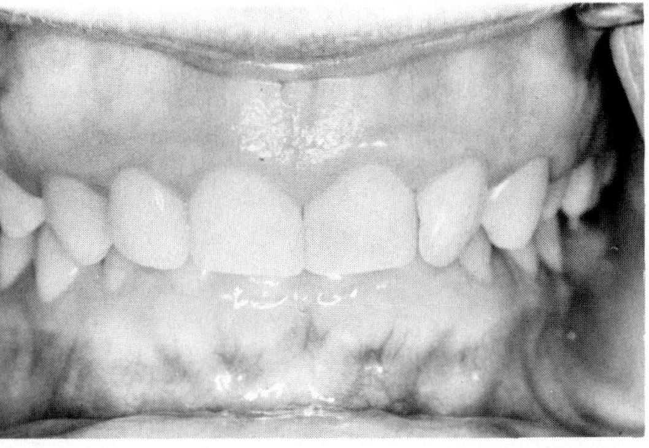

Fig. 5-9.
A, Unsightly gingiva secondary to anterior crown irritation. This may require slightly greater superior positioning. Crown length can be increased if necessary to compensate. **B,** Small clinical crowns. Gingival appearance during smiling cannot be totally eliminated lest the teeth not show at rest, which would create an unpleasant appearance.

convexity, (4) the overall nasal prominence, and (5) the upper lip–tooth relationship. Many cephalometric analyses address the proper relationship of the maxilla and the maxillary incisors to the overall craniofacial balance. However, the numbers that they record are often not relevant to the specific esthetic demands of a particular patient. Again, we must return to the axiom that if there is a question the maxilla must not be positioned too far superiorly or posteriorly resulting in an unesthetic loss of lip support. Perhaps the most common error is to perform one-jaw maxillary surgery in a situation when superior repositioning of the maxilla will not quite couple the upper incisors with the mandibular anterior teeth after autorotation of the mandible. Therefore the temptation is to move the maxilla either more superiorly than is desirable or superiorly and posteriorly to couple the anterior teeth. The result is a maxilla too superior or too posterosuperior for the esthetics of the upper lip, nasolabial angle, or overall facial convexity. If after maxillary surgery the maxilla does not occupy the predicted position, it is invariably too superior, too posterior, or both relative to the planned position. Therefore, when autorotation of the mandible does not quite meet with anterior occlusal coupling, bimaxillary surgery is almost always indicated.

It is obvious from this discussion that the anteroposterior positioning of the maxilla is primarily an esthetic decision. This implies not that function of the TMJ and the occlusion should be ignored but simply that esthetics should not be compromised in a vertical or anteroposterior direction to avoid bimaxillary surgery. Maxillary surgery in cases of mandibular retrognathism with the maxilla repositioned posteriorly has the same effect as the orthodontic four-premolar extraction in mandibular retrognathism: loss of upper lip support, retrogenia, and an unesthetic facial convexity.

TRANSVERSE POSITIONING

Transverse mediolateral positioning of the maxilla can be dictated only by the harmony achieved with the upper lip, the nose, and the overall symmetry of the face (Fig. 5-10). During the model surgery it is essential that the facial midline be represented so any deviation

from the midline of the mounted model can be noted. The most important midline is the one between the maxillary dentition and the upper lip. The dental midlines between maxillary and mandibular teeth are important but not crucial so long as the skeletal midlines are matching. A common pitfall in maxillary surgery, especially when mandibular surgery is not performed, is that the occlusion dictates a slight deviation of the maxilla to one side. If the magnitude of this deviation is less than 1.5 mm, it may not be crucial; but anything greater than 1.5 mm is immediately obvious from an esthetic point of view. The realization during model surgery that the maxilla must be deviated more than 1 to 1.5 mm from the midline may require a consideration of mandibular surgery also. For this reason mounted models are important, not only for vertical and anteroposterior relationships but also for transverse ones. Illustrations that will guide the clinician in the model surgery and cephalometric workup so the midlines can be maintained and evaluated are presented in Fig. 5-10.

It is obvious from this discussion that the vertical, anteroposterior and transverse orientations of the maxilla in the incisor area are determined by esthetic considerations. However, this observation must not be misconstrued as implying that the functional aspects of the TMJ and the mandible have been disregarded. In fact, once these three dimensions are established for the anterior maxilla the posterior maxillary position is determined by the functioning of the mandible and the masticatory apparatus. Therefore the model surgery and prediction tracings should be performed with the vertical, anteroposterior, and transverse relationships of the anterior teeth in mind. The remainder of the maxilla is positioned by the autorotation of the mandible from the seated condylar position on mounted models. When the position of the maxilla has been determined by these esthetic considerations and the models articulated in the most desirable position, it is possible to determine whether the mandibular arc of rotation has caused the maxilla to deviate from the planned position in the vertical, anteroposterior, or transverse direction. If we assume that the maxilla can be maintained in an

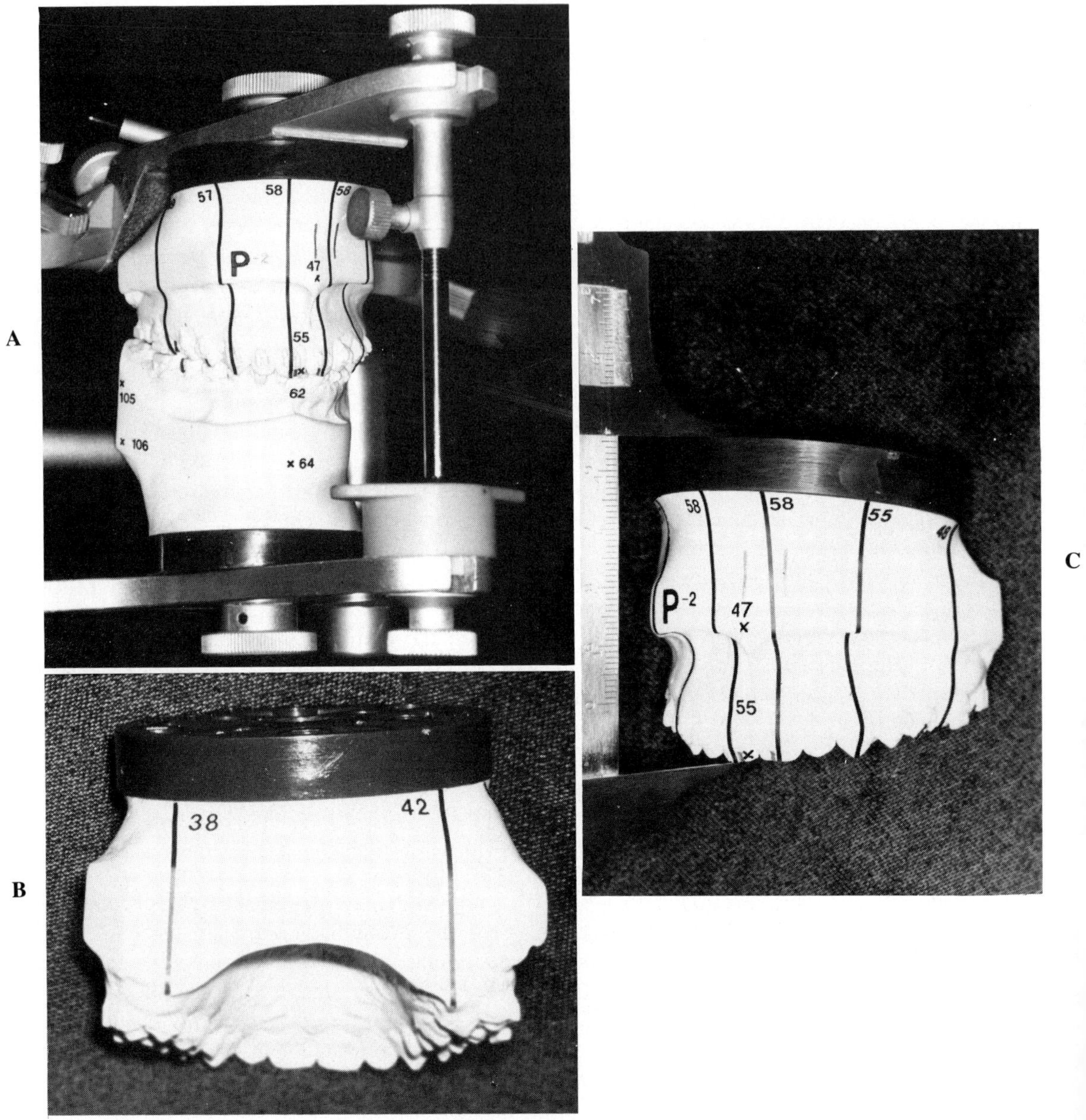

Fig. 5-10.
Mounted models for maxillary surgery marked so all three planes of space can be evaluated both before and after model surgery. For the *vertical* dimension measurements are made at four points on each side of the maxillary cast—central incisors, canines, first molars, and posterior aspect of the casts. A Boley gauge is used to measure from the top of the mounting ring to the incisal edges of the teeth. It is held perpendicular to the mounting ring surface (Frankfort horizontal). For the antero-posterior dimension (**A** to **C**) the anterior nasal spine and incisal edge of the maxillary central incisor are measured horizontally to the pin of the articulator. Pin position is marked on the model, and all AP measurements are made with the pin in this position. For the transverse dimension (**D**) the articulator is held so the operator is looking at the models directly from the front using one eye only. Marks are placed on the base of the mounting so they are just visible on each side of the pin and extend from the base down onto the maxillary model. Two marks are made (**E**) on the incisor teeth also so each can be seen on either side of the pin. **A** shows the mounted models with *vertical* lines placed, *anteroposterior* xs at ANS and the central incisor, and *transverse* markings on the maxillary base and superior aspect of the model as well as on the incisors bilaterally. **B** shows the posterior markings for *vertical* measurements on the maxillary model. **C** shows measurement of the *vertical* with a Boley gauge.

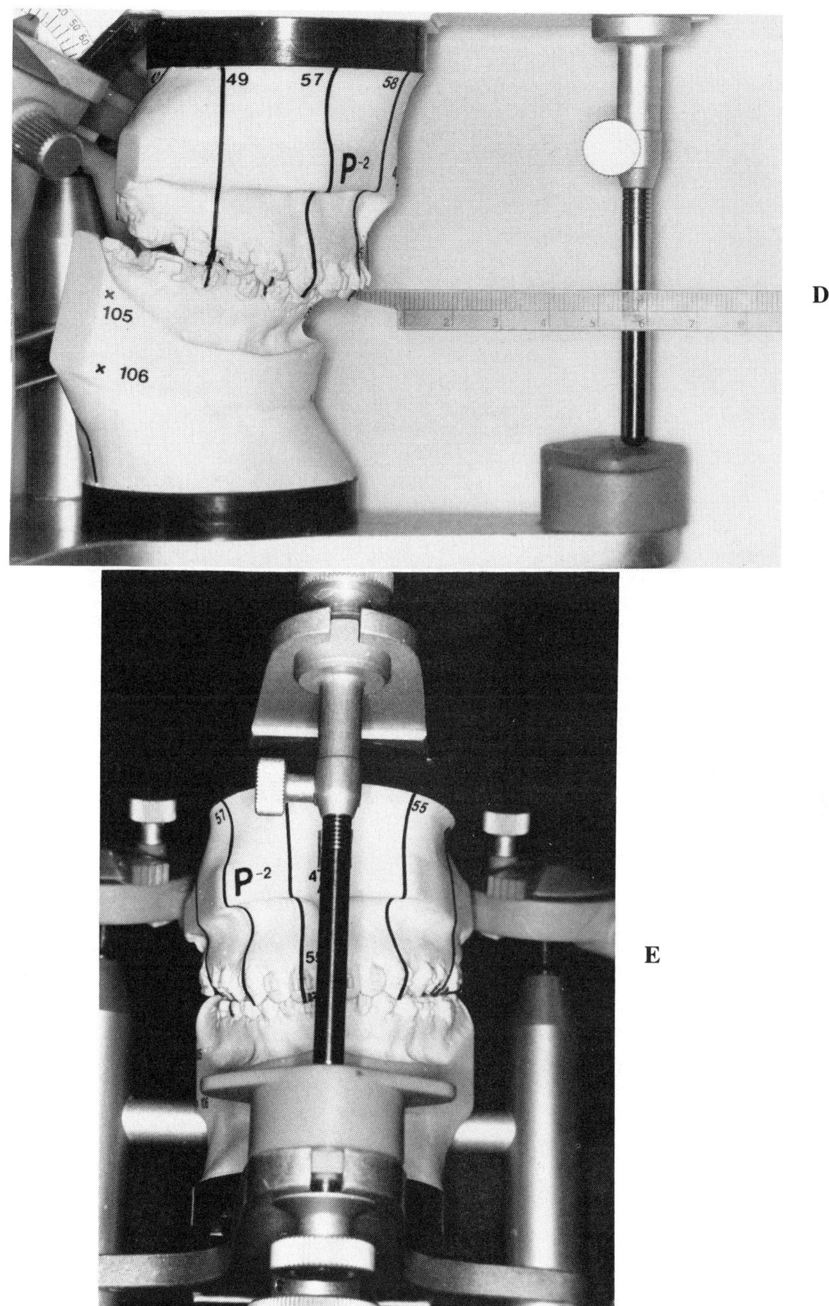

Continued.

Fig. 5-10—cont'd.

D, Measurement of the *anteroposterior* from the maxillary incisor to the recorded pin position. **E,** Markings made to be just visible on each side of the pins for *transverse* measurements.

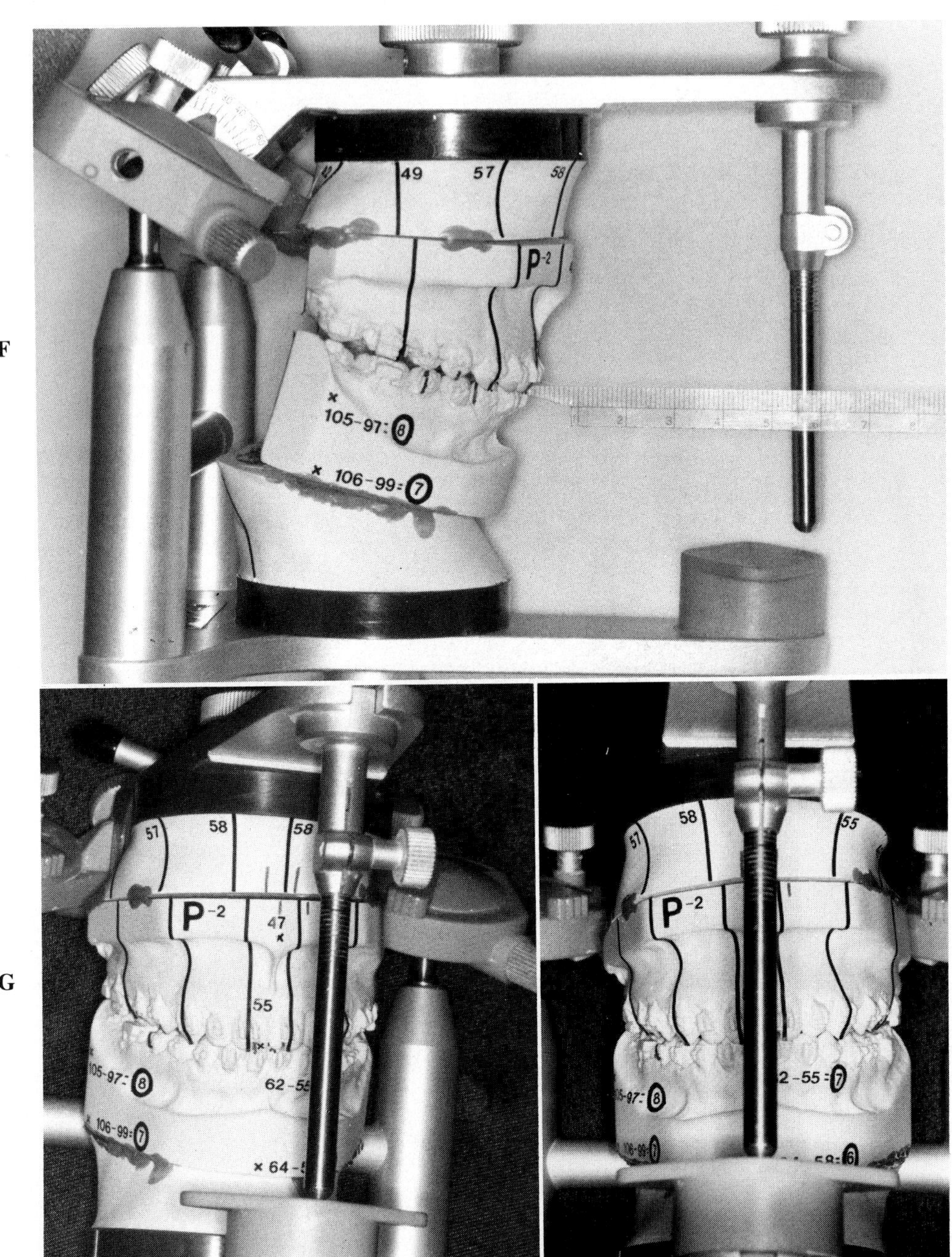

Fig. 5-10—cont'd.

F, Following model surgery, *anteroposterior* measurements are repeated. Note: Although the superior aspect of the maxillary cast (ANS) may have been advanced, the maxillary incisors may actually have been posteriorly displaced. (See Fig. 5-4.) Vertical lines on the model are not sufficient for evaluating this phenomenon. Measurement, as illustrated, is the best method for determining the anteroposterior position of the maxillary incisors. **G,** Oblique view of a maxillary model that has been tilted some to level the occlusal plane. Note that the *transverse* markings on the base and top of the model are no longer aligned. **H,** By aligning the markings on the base with those on the incisor teeth, however, the maxillary incisors can be returned to the original midline.

ideal position anteriorly following the arc of rotation of the mandible and that the posterior occlusion can be maintained in an ideal position, then maxillary surgery alone is indicated.

MODEL SURGERY

The models are marked according to Fig. 5-10 so the vertical, anteroposterior, and transverse evaluations can be made. The maxilla is then repositioned according to the esthetic guidelines just outlined. Measurements are made in all planes of space to ensure proper positioning. The mandible is autorotated into occlusion; and if the maxilla is not moved off an acceptable position, then maxillary surgery alone can be performed.

MAXILLARY SURGERY— TECHNICAL CONSIDERATIONS

Details of specific maxillary movements are described elsewhere in this chapter. However, a number of factors common to all maxillary movements can be discussed here. Once the maxilla has been mobilized from the cranial base and wired into intermaxillary fixation via a preformed occlusal wafer, the important part of maxillary surgery begins.

At this point in the surgery the surgeon must be concerned primarily with condylar position. The physiologic position of the condyles is a superoanterior orientation relative to the glenoid fossae against the posterior slopes of the articular eminences. The surgeon must position the condyles of the maxillary-mandibular complex in an upward and forward direction prior to autorotation (Fig. 5-11, *F*). The importance of this stage of the surgery cannot be overestimated. Since the most likely points of bony interference are in the areas of the pterygoid plates and the maxillary tuberosities, it is quite possible to rotate the maxilla-mandible inappropriately around the TMJs due to the lack of awareness of a premature pivot point in these posterior bony areas (Fig. 5-11, *C*). The sur-

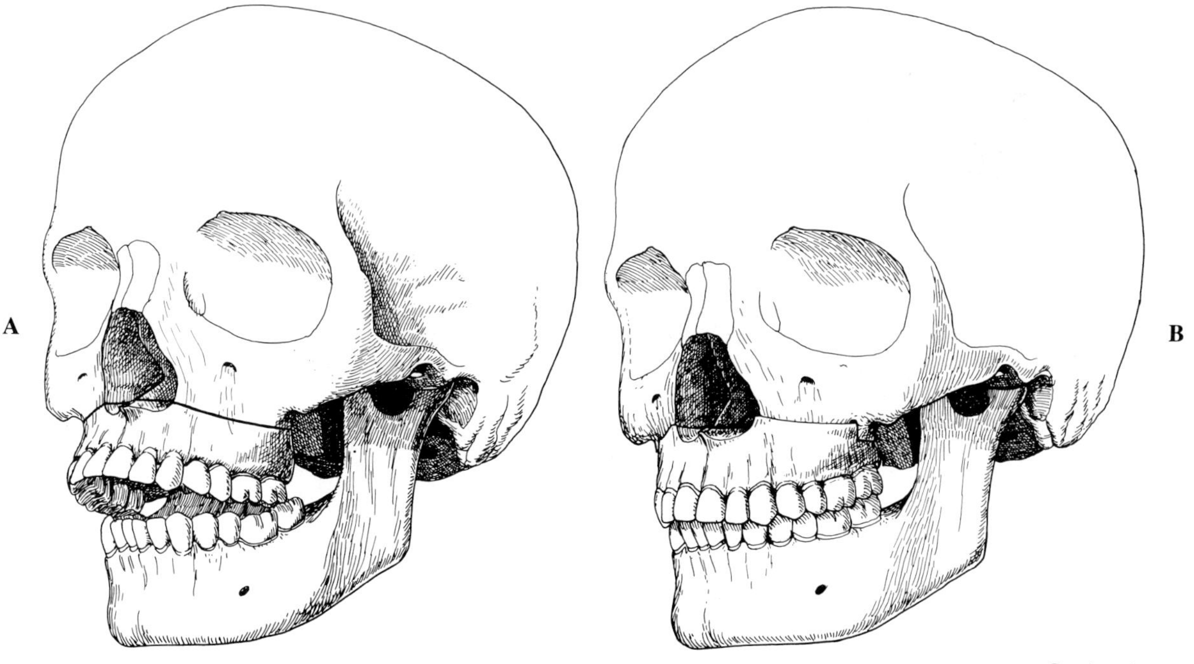

Fig. 5-11.

Continued.

Intraoperative maxillary repositioning. **A,** Preoperative skeletal open-bite. **B,** Desired postoperative interbony relationship using the technique as described in the text.

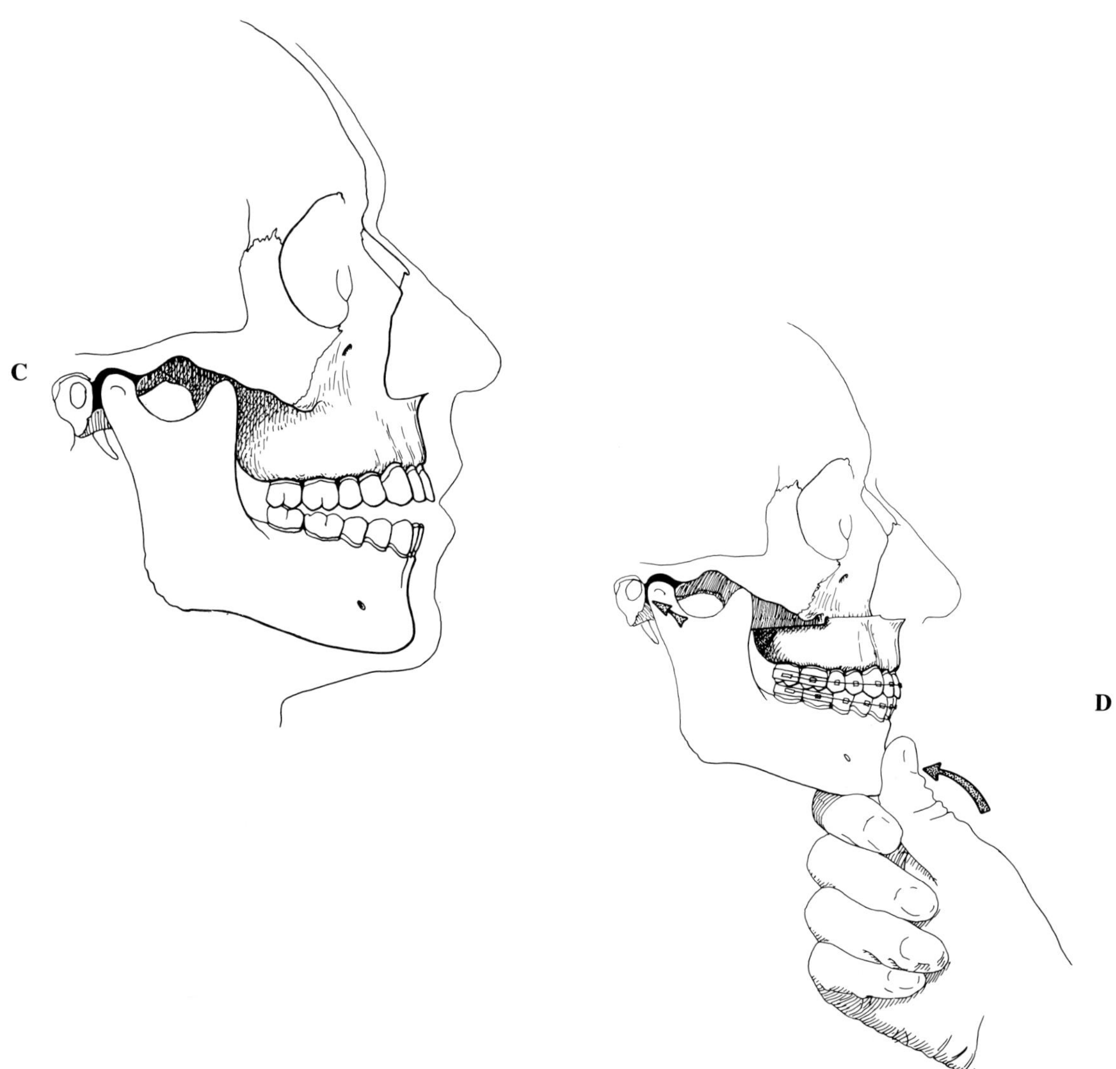

Fig. 5-11—cont'd.
C, Open-bite with the condyle seated. **D,** Incorrect positioning of the maxilla at surgery: using the mandible in intermaxillary fixation. Anterior bony contact may be achieved by pivoting the condyle downward and posteriorly (as illustrated here). Therefore insufficient bone is removed posteriorly to facilitate closure of the open-bite. If the patient is wired into intermaxillary fixation, the open-bite will not be recognized until fixation is released.

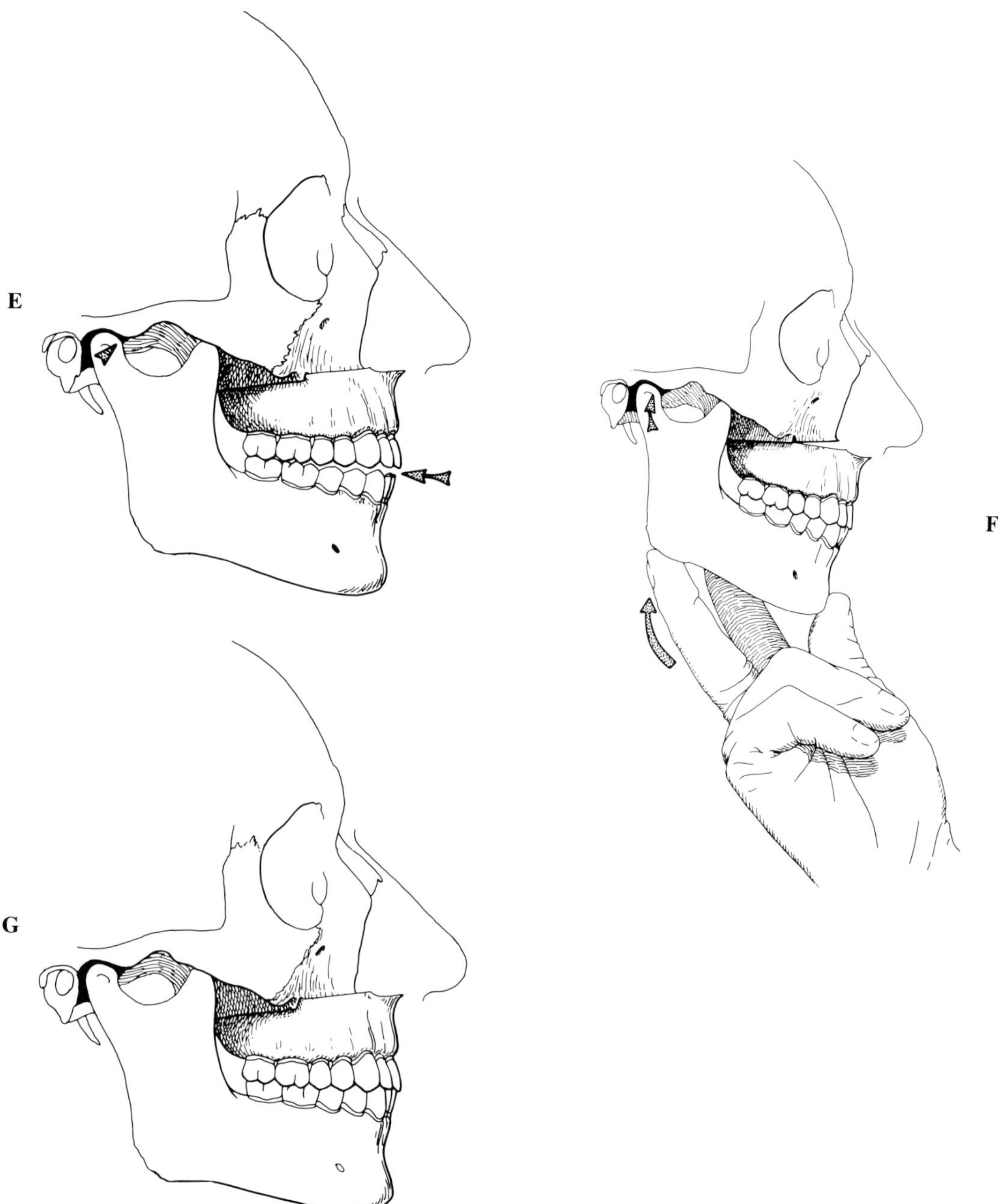

Fig. 5-11—cont'd.
E, Postoperative open-bite if the technique just illustrated is used for maxillary positioning. **F,** Proper positioning of the condyles during surgery by autorotating the maxilla and mandible wired together permits recognition of posterior bony contact. Note that the direction of finger pressure is upward and forward. **G,** Removal of bone only at the point of contact permits enhanced bony contact **(B)** and avoids excessive bone removal.

geon must be fastidious in attempting to position the joints appropriately and then must rotate the entire complex around the arc of rotation of the TMJs until the first contact of bone occurs, either at the piriform rims or at the zygomatic processes.

Next, the anteroposterior, vertical, and transverse positions of the maxilla must be evaluated. Any concern about these prior to elimination of the posterior pivot points is premature and may result in distraction of the mandibular condyles from the fossae and a postoperative open-bite. Once these posterior pivot points have been removed, a similar obligation exists to rotate the entire complex around the TMJs until the appropriate vertical relationship is achieved (Fig. 5-11, *G*). The anteroposterior and transverse relationships have already been dictated by the fact that the maxilla and mandible are wired together. For this reason preoperative model surgery and planning are important. Once the desired vertical relationship has been achieved, the maxilla should be fixed in position by whatever means is deemed appropriate. Methods of fixation, including stable pin fixation, are discussed in other parts of this chapter (facing page). When the maxilla is finally in a stable position, the intermaxillary wiring is removed and the mandible is manipulated as has already been described so the condyles will be seated superoanteriorly against the posterior slopes of the eminences. The mandible is autorotated into occlusion so the position of the maxilla can be checked. If it autorotates precisely into the desired occlusion (as determined by an interocclusal wafer or a tooth-to-tooth contact), then the maxilla can be considered to be in an appropriate position also. However, since the studies[20] have indicated that the mandibular condyles cannot always be perfectly seated under a general anesthetic, the maxilla may not be in the precise position desired at this time—which is the primary reason why intermaxillary fixation after maxillary surgery is not desirable.

It is far preferable to leave the patient out of intermaxillary fixation until the day following surgery and then to reevaluate the occlusion. If the occlusion on the day after surgery is acceptable, then no further treatment is necessary and the patient can be left to function on a liquid diet. However, if it is not acceptable, this is the most opportunistic time to alter maxillary position. Were the maxilla to be wired into intermaxillary fixation on the operating table with the condyles drawn slightly out of the glenoid fossae, this would not be apparent until the release of intermaxillary fixation (Fig. 5-11, *D* and *E*). Evaluation of the occlusion on the first postoperative day gives the surgeon an opportunity to determine whether slight malpositioning of the maxilla has occurred and to make minor corrections. It does not condone sloppy surgical technique or careless positioning of the maxilla, however, but merely indicates that accurate positioning of the mandibular condyles under a general anesthetic is not always possible. Therefore, since the maxilla is positioned with the mandible as a guide, conceivably the maxilla will not be perfectly in position on the operating table. The surgeon must permit alterations in the fixation system to take place postoperatively or else risk an inappropriate maxillary position.

Corrections that can be made the day after surgery are small ones but may be very significant in the final occlusion. A hospital dental clinic or treatment room with suction and adequate lighting is recommended for the postoperative evaluation. If corrections are to be made, sedation can be added to the IV as necessary. In experienced hands such corrections are only rarely necessary, but occasionally they are and in these cases poor results can be avoided.

Summary

The desired *transverse* and *anteroposterior* positions of the maxilla are determined from the model surgery and cephalometric prediction tracings. The maxillary position in these two planes is set by the occlusal wafer and IMF on the operating table. If the condyles are seated as effectively as possible when the maxilla is positioned, the transverse and anteroposterior positions of the maxilla should be as planned at model surgery. Measurements made intraoperatively are valuable only in verifying these positions.

The desired *vertical* position of the maxilla is determined mainly by the physical examination of the patient. It is calculated and fixed on the operating table by measuring from holes placed bilaterally in the piriform rims at the level of the inferior turbinates. These holes are used for suspension wires or pin placement and should be created with this in mind. Prior to surgical mobilization of the maxilla, a measurement is made from each hole to the bracket on the maxillary canine bilaterally. These values are recorded for future use. Since there is no accurate method for measuring the vertical position of the incisors, the canine measurements must be used. This is feasible if the model surgery has positioned the incisors in the desired vertical position and the vertical changes at the canines have been measured. As the maxilla is being positioned with the mandibular condyles seated, these measurements from the holes to the maxillary canine brackets can be made until desired vertical positioning is achieved.

Maxillary stabilization and fixation

In the previous section a method for the workup, planning, and positioning of the maxilla in orthognathic surgery was described. These descriptions generally are applicable to almost any movement of the maxilla. In this section specific problems of fixation and stabilization will be considered. A system for stable pin fixation of the maxilla[2,3] has proved to be extremely useful in numerous types of maxillary repositioning. A brief review of this system is presented.

The system[3] consists of 0.045-inch stainless steel orthodontic wire fashioned preoperatively on a skull and pins that are bent as illustrated in Fig. 5-12, *A*. Stainless steel bone screws (2.7 mm) from the mandibular bone plating system or the finger plate system are utilized for fixation of the pins. In these kits a 2 mm drill and tap are also provided.

1. Bilateral obliquely directed holes are placed in the piriform rims so they will penetrate the attachment of the inferior turbinate in the lateral walls of the nose (Fig. 5-12, *B*). These can be drilled prior to movement of the maxilla and used for measurement marks, and they give maximum bony support to the screws holding the anterior pins.
2. Holes also are placed in the zygomatic region and directed posteriorly so they

penetrate the infratemporal sides of the zygoma.

3. After the holes have been drilled and tapped and it is clear that they can be used, the pins are held in position and the final adaptations made with the three-prong orthodontic pliers.
4. The pins are attached to the bone by the bone screws, and final adjustments of contour or length are made. The end of each pin that contacts the orthognathic archwire is scored somewhat with a bur to improve its attachment to the acrylic.
5. With the maxilla held in the desired postoperative position, cold-cure acrylic is flowed onto the interface between pin and orthodontic archwire, care being taken that the orthodontic bracket on each side of the pins is incorporated into the acrylic and that a certain amount of acrylic runs into the interproximal space. Care must also be taken that the acrylic does not directly contact the gingiva.
6. When the acrylic has hardened, intermaxillary fixation is removed and the occlusion tested.

Minor discrepancies in the occlusion can be adjusted by bending the pins; however, more significant changes require removal of the acrylic, repositioning of the maxilla, and reapplication of the acrylic. Once it has been determined that the maxilla is fixed in the desired position, any finishing procedures such as bone grafting can be accomplished and the wound closed. The wounds are closed around the pins. Care must be exercised that the tissue is not gathered posterior to the pin since this will tether the lip. Therefore, to avoid an undesirable position, one should always suture anterior to the pin first.

Maxillary superior repositioning

In the past it was customary to determine the amount of bone that had to be removed so the maxilla could be appropriately repositioned superiorly. Unfortunately, the wedge shape of the maxilla (with the superior aspect wider than the dentoalveolar area) often left large gaps between the bony interfaces as the maxilla was moved superiorly. Shifting, tilting, or advancing the maxilla could also reduce bone-to-bone

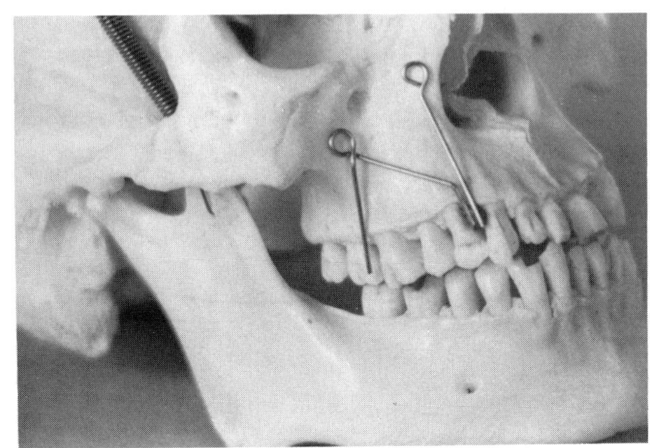

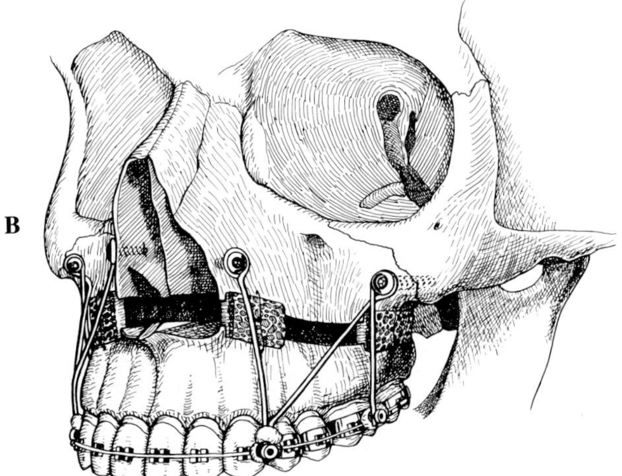

Fig. 5-12.
Stable maxillary pin fixation system. **A,** Pins fabricated from 0.045 round orthodontic wire. The skull is used for estimating length and position. **B,** Pins placed with inferior repositioning of the maxilla and interposed bone graft. The anterior screws are diagonally directed so the attachment of the inferior turbinate to the piriform rim on the inner side can be utilized for additional bony support. Posterior screws are positioned in a directly anteroposterior direction so they will engage the thicker part of the zygomatic buttress.
From Bays, R.: J. Oral Maxillofac. Surg. **43:**60, 1985.

contact. The method described next avoids this needless removal of bone and provides a far more secure interface between the maxilla and the cranial base. Nevertheless, its success is dependent upon two factors: accurate model surgery and the selection of the proper procedure (total down-fracture osteotomy).

Accurate model surgery is essential so the changes in the area of the piriform rim and zygomatic buttress will be known and will result in an ideal maxillary incisor position. Unfortunately, it is nearly impossible to measure the maxillary incisor position on the operating table. The maxillary canine and maxillary first molar positions, however, can be measured for comparison with the patient. At the beginning of maxillary surgery, holes are made in the maxilla for suspension wires or pin fixation bilaterally in the zygomatic buttresses and bilaterally in the piriform rims at the level of the attachment of the inferior turbinates. These will approximate the measurements made on the models at the maxillary first molars and maxillary canines. A caliper can then be used to measure from the bottom of each hole to the bracket on the canine and the buccal tube on the first molar. These measurements are recorded for later use in determining the vertical position of the maxilla. The anterior, posterior, and transverse positioning of the maxilla is almost completely dependent upon the arc of rotation of the mandible.

The total down-fracture maxillary osteotomy, regardless of segmentalization or amount of vertical change to be made, is the procedure of choice because access is gained for the appropriate removal of bony interferences that would prevent proper positioning of the maxilla. Studies[12,30] have indicated that, if the surgery is performed properly, nasal airway impingement is not significant after maxillary down-fracture and superior repositioning. Admittedly there is added bone-to-bone contact with the total alveolar osteotomy, but this may contribute to difficulties in positioning the maxilla properly with the arc of rotation of the mandible (especially if only the maxilla is repositioned). For the down-fracture technique described here, no bone is removed during the maxillary osteotomy per se. A LeFort I down-fracture is performed and the appropriate amount of bone removed from the nasal septum and septal crest of the maxilla, medial walls of the sinuses, and area around the descending palatine neurovascular bundles.

Management of descending palatine vessels

Guidelines for the management of the descending palatine neurovascular bundles have not been clearly established. On the one hand, it is obvious that if the descending palatine arteries and veins can be preserved and remain patent the blood supply to the maxilla should be better than if these vessels are sacrificed. On the other, the questions of how much stretching, torquing, or crimping of these vessels can be tolerated without a loss of patency are unanswered. The blood flow studies and revascularization studies comparing LeFort I maxillary osteotomies with and without sacrifice of these vessels have not disclosed what actually constitutes a significant distance. Some studies[7] indicate that the blood supply to the maxilla is adequate following sacrifice of the descending palatine arteries and veins. Others[10,22] suggest that a high percentage of the blood to the maxilla comes through these vessels. If these vessels are severed and ligated, however, it is still not known what percentage of the blood is transferred by collateral circulation to the maxilla through soft palate anastomoses.

Most of the blood to the maxilla comes through the posterior superior alveolar arteries and the greater palatine arteries.[21,22] By necessity, the posterior superior alveolar arteries are sectioned during the surgical procedure. The most often quoted evaluation of maxillary blood flow following LeFort I osteotomy[22] uses the microsphere technique, but it does not answer the questions posed because the descending palatine arteries were inadvertently severed during the procedure. The evaluation of maxillary blood flow then was conducted by comparing maxillary procedures in which the arteries were intact versus those in which the arteries were severed but not ligated. Careful evaluation of the data indicates that blood flow to the maxilla in cases in which the arteries were severed was less than when the arteries were left intact. However, blood flow above the osteotomy site in the severed group was also dramatically decreased whereas that to the areas above the osteotomy site in the intact group either decreased only slightly or actually increased. In addition, the blood flow to the soft palate was decreased significantly (47%) in the severed group but increased significantly (85%) in the intact group. These two facts would seem to indicate that the blood flow to not only the maxillary pedicle but also the soft palate and the tissues above the osteotomy site is compromised by severing the descending palatine arteries. The probable explanation for this is that with bleeding unligated arteries no pressure head can be developed for the collateral circulation through the soft palate whereas with the descending palatine arteries ligated collateral circulation from the soft palate can develop a pressure head. (Also the maxillae were returned to their original position rather than moved into a new position.)

Most clinicians have observed that in the one-, two-, and three-piece maxillary osteotomies the descending palatine arteries and veins are not necessary for adequate perfusion of the maxilla. In the four-piece osteotomy, however, with the anterior segment divided in the midline, an anterior pedicle of soft tissue should remain. Whether preservation of the descending palatine arteries and veins minimizes or lessens the need for this anterior pedicle is not known.

If there were no liability in preserving the descending palatine arteries and veins, one might ask why not do it? Recently 15 cases of severe postoperative bleeding after LeFort I maxillary osteotomy were reported.[19] In nearly half of these cases the descending palatine arteries were directly implicated as the bleeding source and in several others the bleeding came from nearby areas. It was not stated whether the descending palatine arteries were ligated at the time of surgery; but from the case reports it would seem that they were later ligated as a secondary procedure to stop the bleeding. Therefore, in view of the fact that they may not be necessary for perfusion of the maxilla and probably will not remain patent anyway, preserving the vessels may constitute a liability because of their vulnerability to laceration intraoperatively and postoperatively. It seems unlikely that properly clipped or ligated arteries which have been allowed to retract in their canals after ligation will lead to secondary hemorrhage. For these reasons I recommend, in most cases, the routine ligation and division of the descending palatine arteries and veins.

After the maxilla is mobilized completely, it is wired to the mandible with the interocclusal wafer in position and the maxilla and mandible are moved through the arc of rotation as already described for seating the maxilla in maxillary surgery (Fig. 5-11). The areas of bone contact can now be seen as the maxilla is positioned superiorly. Just enough bone is removed at the contact points to permit the superior repositioning planned on the surgical models and the tracings. Bone is removed until the maxilla around the arc of rotation of the mandible is seated superiorly to the desired level. In many cases this will result in the formation of slots or grooves in the zygomatic buttress wall or elsewhere along the maxillary wall (Fig. 5-11, *B*). Until the desired vertical dimension is achieved, one must be careful that the grooves do not inhibit the free arc of rotation of the maxilla and mandible together. This technique is particularly valuable when the maxilla is being shifted laterally or torqued in a transverse direction and also in cases of advancement or setback of the maxilla. The bony walls often do not match well; if a section of bone is removed prior to maxillary repositioning, much of it may be unnecessarily sacrificed.

The process of seating the maxilla around the arc of rotation of the mandible and removing bone only where contact exists can be likened to equilibrating the occlusion. If the condyles have been held upward and forward against the posterior slopes of the eminences while the maxilla and mandible were being rotated to the desired maxillary vertical position, it is assumed that the vertical, anteroposterior, and transverse positions of the maxilla will conform to the plan of the presurgical models. The maxilla then can be fixed into position with whatever system is deemed appropriate and the intermaxillary fixation removed.

The mandible is rotated into and out of occlusion with the maxilla, with the condyles seated to ensure that the maxilla is in the desired position and that the mandible does not seat into the splint prematurely. If bimaxillary surgery is being performed and there are small discrepancies in the occlusion, one may choose to proceed with the mandibular surgery so long as the maxilla is stable. If maxillary surgery alone is being performed, however, the maxilla must be stabilized in a position that will accommodate repeated mandibular rotation.

Maxillary inferior repositioning

Inferior repositioning of the maxilla offers a special challenge in orthognathic surgery because a discontinuity is created between the maxilla and the cranial base and there is a great relapse tendency.[8,11,14] Various mechanisms have been advocated for stabilization and fixation of the maxilla after inferior repositioning. In addition to conventional mechanisms of suspension wires, interosseous wires, bone plates, and bone grafting, adjunctive measures have been advocated—such as Steinmann pins[33] and Wessberg pins.[31] I have reported[2,3] on a technique for pin stabilization of the maxilla that has proved to be extremely stable, adjustable, and tissue compatible.

The following description for stabilization of the inferiorly repositioned maxilla does not require bone grafting from a distant site if the rigid pin fixation system is used. The system employs a series of slanted osteotomies in the maxilla that are preplanned so the maxilla will slide down the inclined plane of the cuts, maintaining bone contact as it is repositioned inferiorly. It may seem as though this would anteriorly reposition the maxilla. However, depending upon the inclination of the anterior versus the posterior osteotomies, this is not necessarily so.

Fig. 5-13 diagrammatically shows how the desired repositioning of the maxilla can be predicted using a cephalogram with the mandible in a seated condylar position. The anterior osteotomies in the piriform rim are angled so the maxilla will slide downward along them. Slanted osteotomies in the area of the zygomatic arch are placed at either steeper or shallower angles depending upon whether a forward, downward-forward, or downward repositioning of the maxillary anterior teeth is desirable. The maxillary archwire can be used as a horizontal plane from which to measure the angles of the various osteotomies.

The workup procedure is as follows: A routine cephalometric tracing is made with the entire maxilla and the maxillary teeth traced to include the piriform rim of the nose and an outline of the zygomatic buttresses. A template is made of the maxilla, including all the aforenamed structures. The maxillary template is moved into the desired postoperative position and taped securely. Lines can then be drawn from the template back to the original tracing to indicate the path that the maxilla has followed into its new position. These lines are placed at the piriform rims and the zygomatic buttresses approximately where the surgical osteotomies will be made. The angles formed between the osteotomy lines and the maxillary archwires are used at the time of surgery for orientation of the osteotomies. The osteotomy cuts at the time of surgery are made as illustrated (Fig. 5-13) by angling the reciprocating saw in a superior direction toward the infraorbital nerve. The exact angulation can be measured by using a piece of radiographic film that has been cut out and sterilized to indicate the angulation between the maxillary archwire and the osteotomy cut. The angle on the film should be slightly steeper than the planned angle so a small amount of bone can be removed to permit the proper positioning of the maxilla. The angled cuts through the zygomatic buttresses are somewhat more difficult to position. The landmarks, however, essentially involve the roots of the maxillary molars and the infratemporal surface of the zygomatic arch. The cut is angled so there will be solid bone on both the superior and the inferior aspects of the osteotomy. As with other maxillary osteotomies, following these bilaterally the rest of the lateral maxillary wall can be cut with saw, burs, or chisels. The maxilla is down-fractured and any areas of loose bone or interferences are removed. The descending palatine neurovascular bundles can be inspected and managed as stated earlier.

The maxilla is then wired into intermaxillary fixation with the interocclusal wafer interposed, and the maxilla-mandible is moved through the arc of rotation of the mandible. Care must be

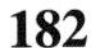

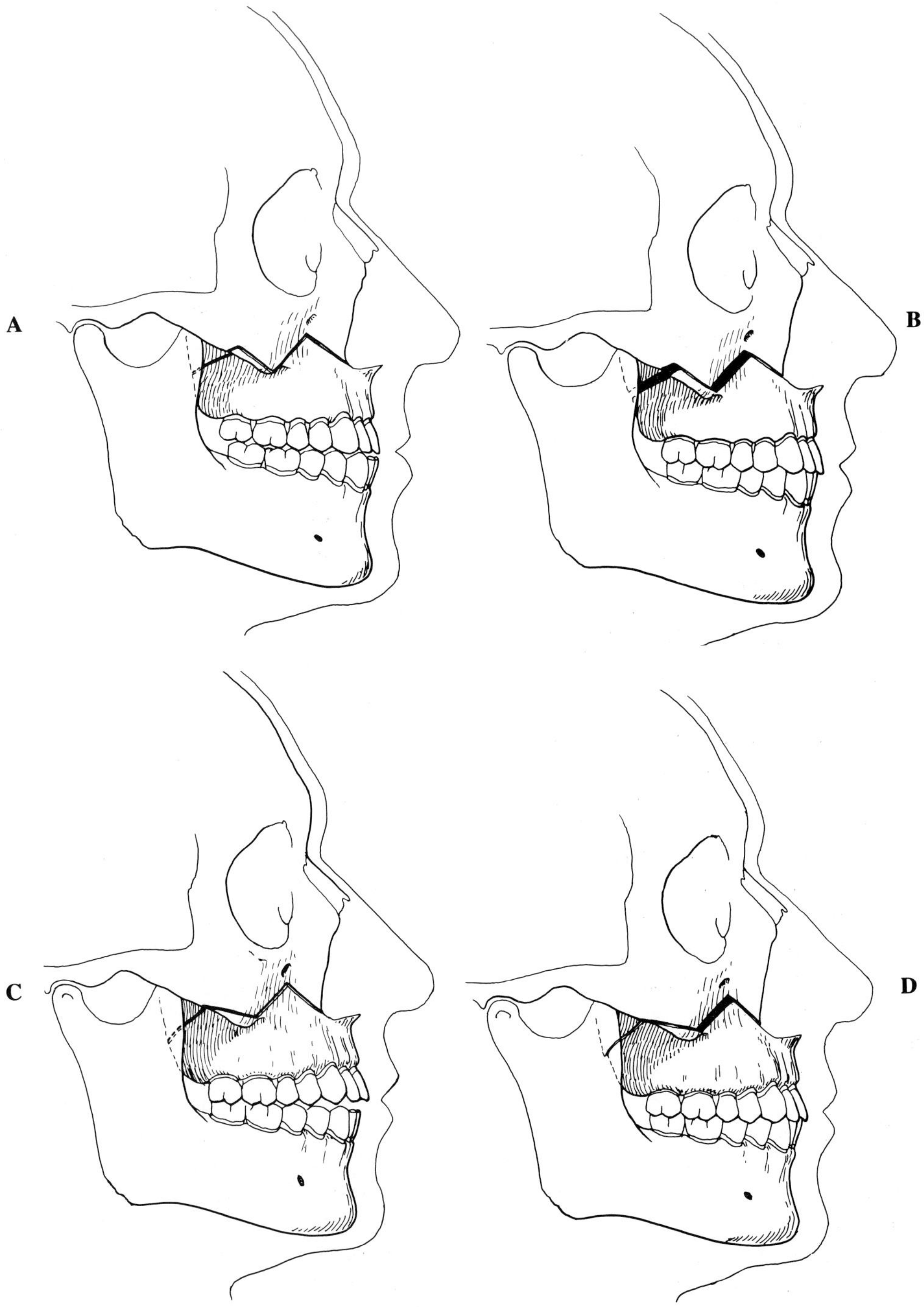

Fig. 5-13.
For legend see opposite page.

Fig. 5-13.
Inferior repositioning of the maxilla achieved with Z-osteotomies, which require little or no bone grafting if a stable pin system is used. The maxillary anterior teeth can be positioned inferiorly with *no* anterior movement, *some* anterior movement, or *considerable* anterior movement depending on the inclination of the osteotomies. **A** and **B,** Osteotomies in the piriform rims and zygomatic buttresses are parallel so the maxilla can be repositioned *inferoanteriorly* a prescribed amount. The angle of the cut is based on the prediction tracing, with the maxillary archwire as a reference line. Note that bony contact is maintained at the piriform rims and zygomatic buttresses bilaterally. **C** and **D,** If a pure *inferior* repositioning of the maxillary central incisors is desired, the anterior osteotomies must be much steeper than the posterior ones on each side. Even though ANS will be advanced somewhat, the maxillary incisors will be moved inferiorly **(D).**

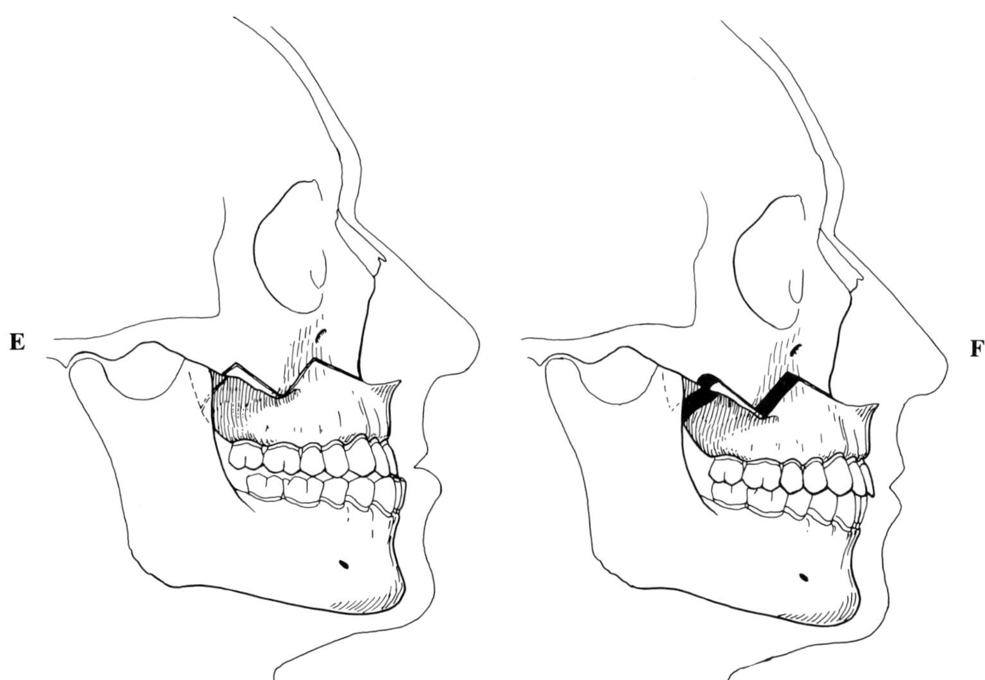

Fig. 5-13—cont'd.
E and **F,** If *anterior* and *inferior* repositioning in which the anterior exceeds the inferior repositioning is necessary, the posterior osteotomy **(E)** is steeper than the anterior. The maxilla is advanced and repositioned only slightly inferiorly **(F).**

taken that the condyles are seated until bone contact is made (Fig. 5-11). Measurement of vertical changes is performed as described previously by measuring from wire or pinholes to the archwire. Equilibration of bone contacts is performed until the desired vertical position of the maxilla is achieved and bone contact exists in the four critical areas: the piriform rims and the zygomatic buttresses bilaterally. The maxillary pin fixation system just described (Fig. 5-14) is applied. Following stabilization of the maxillary pin fixation system an evaluation of the osteotomy is made to determine whether additional bone contact (in other words, bone grafting) is necessary. I have found this to be rarely necessary. If, however, small blocks of bone should be necessary, they can generally be harvested from the zygomatic buttresses above the osteotomy cuts or from the genial or lateral aspect of the mandible through an intraoral approach. Maxillary inferior repositionings of up to 8 mm have been performed with excellent stability by this technique with no bone grafting whatsoever.[2] Perhaps the greatest drawback to the procedure is that if the maxilla must be inferiorly repositioned without any anterior movement a slight lingual torquing of the maxillary incisors will result and the anterior nasal spine will be somewhat advanced. This should be taken into consideration in the treatment plan by evaluation of the template tracings. Usually the incisor position is not altered more than 3 or 4 degrees. ANS removal or recontouring can be performed when necessary at the time of surgery.

Soft tissue management of maxillary surgery

When the LeFort I down-fracture technique is used, the maxilla becomes a pedicle with its blood supply based on the palatal soft tissues. The blood supply therefore comes to the anterior maxilla via the greater palatine arteries below the level of the greater palatine foramina. This is also true if the descending palatine arteries have been ligated above because of the anastomoses with the blood supply of the soft palate. The attached gingiva receives its blood primarily from the alveolar bone, as does the adjacent free mucosa.[21,22] The anterior maxillary gingiva and adjacent mucosa represent the tip of the pedicle; thus allowing a wide cuff of free mucosa attached to the anterior maxilla has no particular advantage in terms of maxillary blood supply unless an intact anterior pedicle is maintained from superior to inferior. We can therefore safely make our mucoperiosteal incision in the anterior region rather close to the mucogingival junction for the sake of esthetics without fear of compromising the blood supply to the maxilla so long as the posterior mucosal incision leaves a wider base. The incision I advocate is a mucoperiosteal one that is high in the vestibule posteriorly at the zygomatic buttress and dips low to within 3 or 4 mm of the

Fig. 5-14.
Maxilla inferiorly repositioned by Z-osteotomy cuts and the maxillary stable pin fixation system. No bone grafting is necessary if the pin system is left intact for 12 weeks. Inferior movements of up to 8 mm with no more than 2 mm relapse have been accomplished when this system is used.

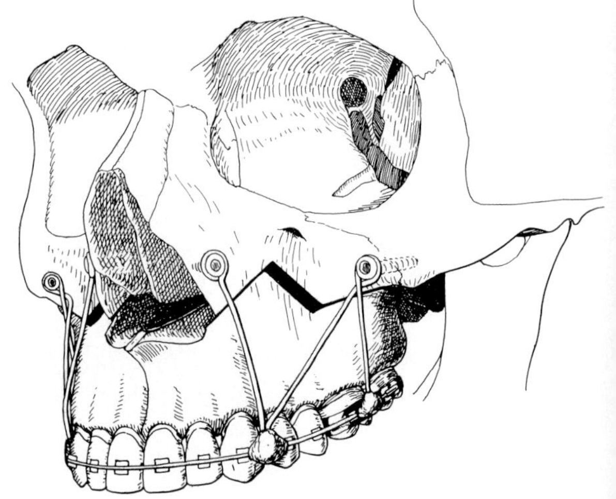

mucogingival junction from canine to canine. It eliminates some disruption of the muscles of facial expression attached to the upper lip. The subperiosteal dissection superiorly to the level of the infraorbital foramen and along the lateral rim of the nose will disrupt several muscles—the nasalis, levator labii superioris alaque nasi, levator labii superioris, and levator anguli oris. The origins and insertions of other facial muscles should not be involved directly.

Periosteal closure is achieved at the area of the canine, and this (at least in part) restores the length to the levator labii superioris. The levator labii superioris alaque nasi and nasalis can be closed in the midline underneath the anterior nasal spine with periosteal sutures especially if widening of the alar bases is undesirable. This constitutes the anatomic restoration of these muscles. A long-lasting absorbable material, such as polyglycolic acid, is used for these sutures. The mucosa is closed with small bites so that no inversion or shortening of the upper lip will occur. Regarding the V-Y closure,[25] it has been noticed that in the early postoperative stages an increased pillow of vermilion is created in the midline just below the philtrum at the expense of the vermilion of the corners of the mouth and lateral aspect of the lip. Although this may be "robbing Peter to pay Paul," it may very well prevent the flattened appearance and lack of contour of the upper lip characteristic of some maxillary cases. The long-term effects, if any, of this closure are yet to be determined. The aforedescribed incision and suturing method is advocated for one-piece, two-piece, and three-piece maxillary osteotomies. When the anterior maxilla will be divided in the midline, as in the case of the four-piece maxillary osteotomy, I prefer to avoid an incision from canine to canine, which leaves a pedicle of mucosa in the anterior region. A vertical incision between the central incisors is used for access to the nasal septum.

SURGICALLY ASSISTED RAPID PALATAL EXPANSION

Difficulties in expanding the maxilla orthopedically in patients who are beyond the age of 14 to 16 years are well known.[28] It is apparent that the lateral maxillary walls are perhaps most responsible for the difficulties in maintaining a widening of the maxilla.[17] There may have been a reluctance on the part of orthodontists to embrace surgically assisted rapid palatal expansion because of the necessity of admitting the patient to hospital and administering a general anesthetic.

The following description presents a technique that I have used routinely for expansion of the maxilla on an outpatient basis with intravenous sedation and local anesthesia. A Hyrax palatal expansion device is cemented into place preoperatively and routine preoperative instructions for intravenous sedation are given. The patient is also instructed to bring the expansion key at the time of surgery. Surgery is performed in the outpatient office utilizing the intravenous sedation technique of choice. Intravenous diazepam and fentanyl have been used successfully. Local anesthesia includes infiltration bilaterally in the mucobuccal fold of the maxilla, infraorbital nerve blocks, posterior superior alveolar nerve blocks, nasopalatine nerve blocks, and greater palatine nerve blocks. After successful anesthesia of the labial mucosa in the anterior region, infiltration anesthesia is achieved around the base of the nose, along the anterior nasal spine, and in the area of the lateral piriform rims. This may be supplemented intraoperatively as one dissects if the patient begins to experience some sensation. It has proved helpful to inject local anesthetic into the most superior aspect of the nasopalatine canal to achieve localized obtundation in the area of the nasal septum anteriorly. Mucoperiosteal incisions are made bilaterally from the zygomatic buttresses to the edges of the piriform rims. Subperiosteal dissection exposes the lateral maxilla from the pterygomaxillary junction anteriorly to the piriform rims. If no incision is made from canine to canine, the major support of the alar bases and anterior aspect of the upper lip will not be altered. A bone cut is made in the lateral maxillary wall from the zygomatic buttress to the piriform rim. Posterior to the buttress the cut is made above the roots of the molars and dips down to the lowest aspect of the pterygomaxillary junction. This procedure is feasible on an outpatient basis because no attempt is made to separate the maxilla from the pterygoid plates and no entry is made into the pterygomaxillary junction. Therefore the maxillary osteotomy passes posteriorly to the roots of the last molar and dips down toward the junction of the tuberosity and the pterygoid plates without contacting the plates.

In the anterior region the piriform rim cut is taken only posteriorly along the lateral nasal wall about 1 cm or less, just enough to ensure that the most solid bone in the piriform has been sectioned. After this is done bilaterally a chisel fashioned from a thin cement spatula is placed in the interdental papilla between the central incisors and malleted through until it can be palpated under the palatal mucosa. No soft tissue incision is necessary in this area, since the chisel will make an incision. The midline sectioning progresses superiorly step by step, one chisel width at a time, until the chisel can be felt parallel to the palate. At this time the jackscrew of the Hyrax appliance is turned until some separation of the central incisors is observed. To mobilize the hemimaxillae, periosteal elevators or large-handled osteotomes are used at the zygomatic buttresses and piriform rims and in the midline. The Hyrax appliance is continuously cranked as this mobilization process occurs until the operator is confident that there is a 1.5 to 2 mm opening between the central incisors and that the appearance of the osteotomy sites bilaterally indicates a symmetric widening of the maxilla and mobility of the hemimaxillae. Then the wounds are irrigated copiously and closed. Along with the intravenous sedation most patients receive intravenous steroids.

The postoperative course involves tapering steroid doses, systemic decongestants, and topical nasal spray as needed. Antibiotics are usually used. Patients are instructed not to turn the jackscrew for 3 to 5 days and then to turn it a quarter-turn every other day. They are then scheduled to see the orthodontist within the first 7 to 10 days after surgery, at which time the amount of additional expansion needed is determined. Expansion can proceed as much as one quarter-turn per day until a desirable amount is attained. No period of retention has been necessary following this procedure, and no separation of the nasal septum from the septal crest of the maxilla is required. Furthermore, there has not been any clinically apparent deviation of the septum upon intranasal examination following expansion. Thus there is no reason why the nasal septum should be any more deviated after this type of expansion than after routine orthopedic maxillary expansion. Undoubtedly some minor deviation to the base of the septum exists that is not clinically apparent, but the elimination of the need to separate the nasal septum from the septal crest of the maxilla and the pterygoid plates adds to the feasibility of this procedure on an outpatient basis. Another key to the prevention of complications is the elimination of posterior cutting on the lateral wall of the nose posterior to the piriform rim. Troublesome nasal bleeding may be encountered if the osteotomy is carried too far posteriorly in this region. The most likely area for postoperative bleeding is the anterior superior alveolar artery as it is sectioned at the piriform rim. Hemostasis must be achieved in this area prior to closure.

SEQUENCING OF TEMPOROMANDIBULAR JOINT AND ORTHOGNATHIC TREATMENT

Since many patients who exhibit dentofacial deformities also experience TMJ dysfunction, combined treatment of their dentofacial deformity and TMJ problems must often be coordinated. However, it must be stressed that no rigid plan can be outlined for the management of a specific patient because of the multiplicity of factors that contribute to these problems.

Combined treatment may be required in patients with:

1. Orthognathic deformities (without original TMJ complaints)
2. Myofascial pain dysfunction
3. Internal derangement of the TMJ
4. Combinations of the above

Fig. 5-15 displays several flow diagrams, which should be used *only* as general guidelines for patients with TMJ problems and dentofacial deformities.

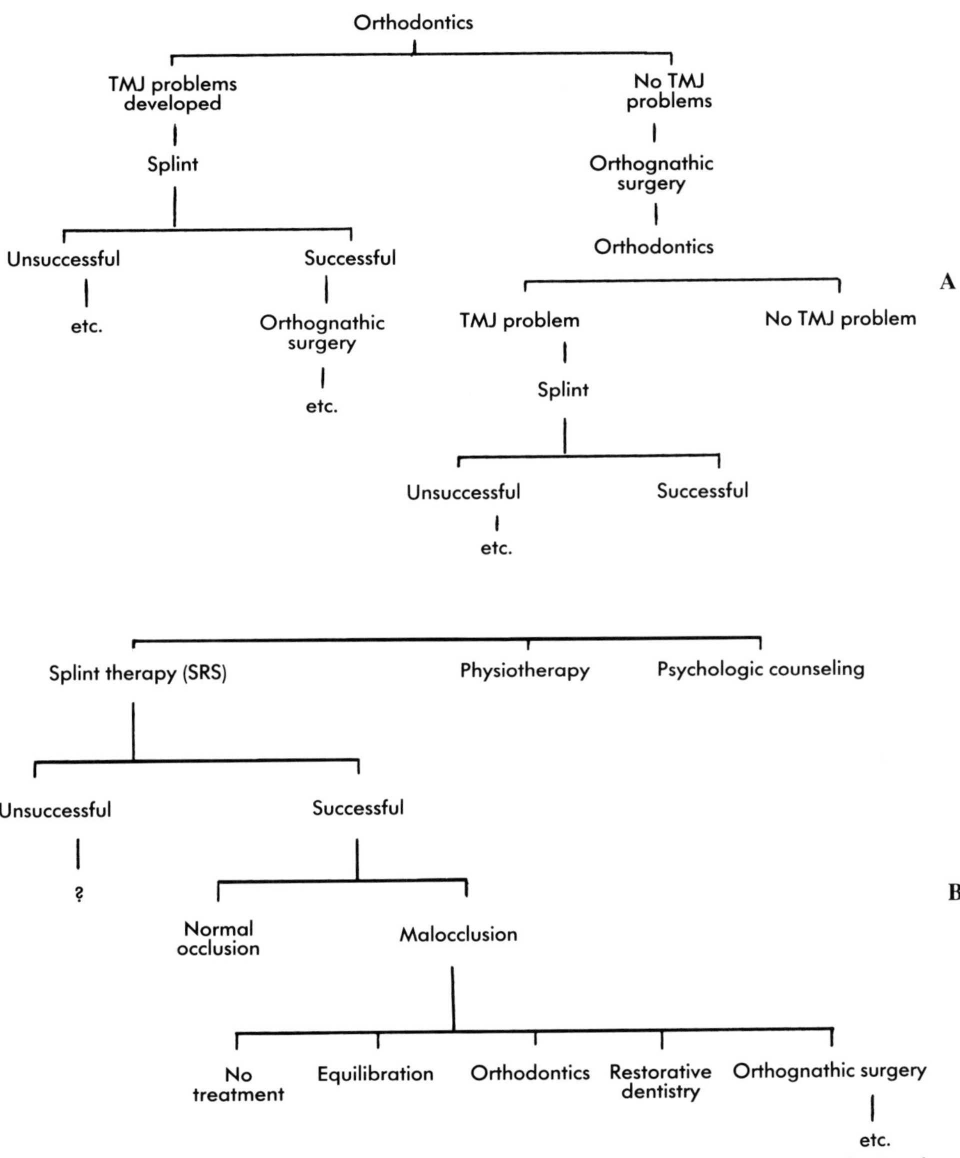

Fig. 5-15.
Flow diagrams as general guidelines for patients with TMJ problems and dentofacial deformity. **A,** Orthognathic deformity and no TMJ problem. **B,** Myofascial pain dysfunction (MPD).

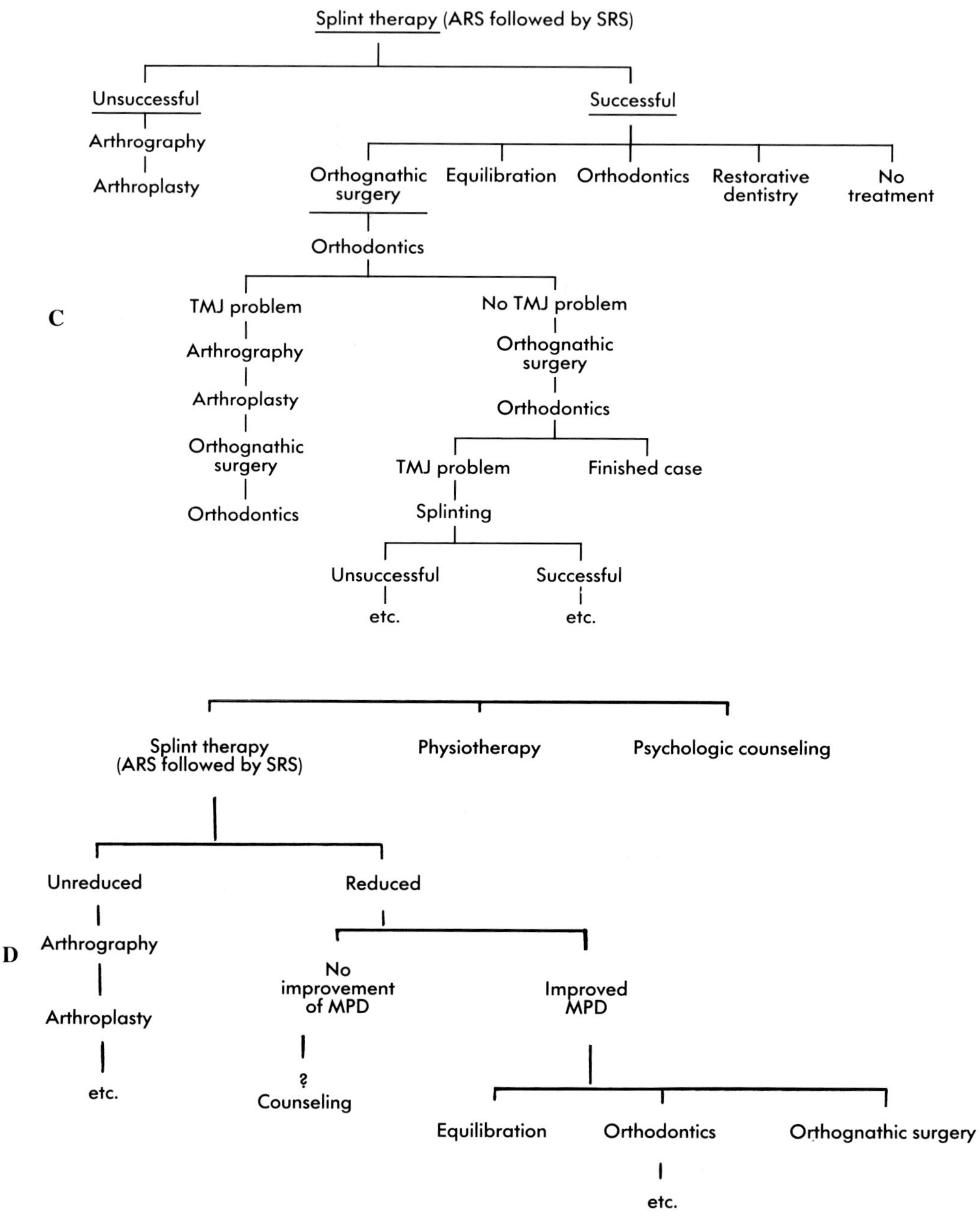

C

D

Fig. 5-15—cont'd.
C, TMJ disc dislocation. **D,** Combinations of MPD with TMJ dislocation.

In the patient with *orthognathic deformities* in whom TMJ problems develop during treatment (Fig. 5-15, *A*) it may be necessary during the preoperative phase of orthodontics to institute splint therapy—which, if successful, will permit continuation of orthognathic treatment, etc. However, if splint therapy is not successful, a reevaluation must be made and consideration given to arthrograms and TMJ surgery. Usually these problems can be managed with splint therapy until the time for orthognathic surgery.

Another possibility is the development of TMJ problems after orthognathic surgery, during the finishing phase of orthodontics. If the problem is of significant magnitude splint therapy should be attempted. Intermittent TMJ popping, clicking, or discomfort is not infrequent with postoperative orthodontics, especially under the influence of interarch elastics. Therefore practitioners should be cautious about becoming too aggressive until the completion of orthodontic treatment. In every case adequate splint therapy managed by a clinician experienced in the area of gnathology should be attempted prior to any consideration for TMJ surgery.

For the patient who presents with *myofascial pain dysfunction* (MPD) (Fig. 5-15, *B*) a flow diagram illustrates that treatment should be as conservative as possible—by splints, physical therapy, or biofeedback—and prior to any orthognathic workup or treatment. Success in management of MPD is relative. However, no attempt should be made to begin such workup on a patient with significant pain from the muscles of mastication. The cooperation and management of a physical therapist and clinical psychologist are also recommended. If conservative treatment is unsuccessful, it is questionable whether any orthognathic treatment should progress. If the patient can be managed successfully by conservative means, the degree of the malocclusion following completion of splint therapy will dictate the amount of treatment necessary to correct the malocclusion. The malocclusion is assessed while the condyles are in the position allowed by the splint. Treatment options may range from none at all to equilibration, orthodontics, restorative dentistry, or orthognathic surgery. These patients should be cautioned about and carefully instructed in the multifactorial nature of myofascial pain so intermittent mild episodes of discomfort are not interpreted as failure but rather something to be expected and managed in the early stages.

The third group of patients are those with *TMJ dislocation* or internal derangement of the disc (Fig. 5-15, *C*). Again, it is imperative that these patients be treated conservatively, usually with splints prior to any irreversible therapy (such as orthodontics or surgery). Splint therapy involves an anterior repositioning splint to recapture the disc and to reestablish the disc-condyle relationship. After this has been achieved, the patient is given a superior repositioning (CR) splint, which will allow the physiologic seating of the condyles by the muscles of mastication. Then the occlusion and jaw position can be evaluated for additional workup.

If the splint treatment is not successful, a surgical solution to the dislocated disc must then be approached. In such patients the ideal sequence is to proceed with orthognathic treatment and to reserve intracapsular surgery for the final stages. However, it has been my experience that most patients with significant discomfort or limitation of function from internal disc derangement will not permit additional orthodontic or surgical management of their malocclusion until the TMJ pain and dysfunction have been alleviated. In addition, since the patient's seated condylar position cannot be attained while the disc is dislocated, the degree and magnitude of the dentofacial deformity are difficult if not impossible to assess. If splint treatment is successful or if arthroplasty is necessary and is successful, the seated condylar position is attained by means of a superior repositioning splint. The degree of malocclusion is evaluated next so a treatment plan can be made. This could range from no treatment at all to equilibration, restorative dentistry, or orthodontics, to orthognathic surgery.

It is still possible that the internal derangement patient who has been successfully managed with splints earlier will have recurrent problems as preoperative and postoperative orthodontics occur throughout the orthognathic treatment. If intracapsular problems return, a reevaluation must be made as to whether orthodontic or orthognathic treatment should continue or a splint approach to the intracapsular problem be undertaken. Many patients have minor clicking and popping as well as discomfort in the postoperative phase of finishing orthodontics. Therefore not everyone in whom intermittent TMJ popping or clicking develops during postoperative orthodontics will need aggressive splint treatment.

Treatment for patients having a *combination of myofascial pain and disc dislocation* is often exceedingly difficult (Fig. 5-15, *D*). The approach recommended here is to use an anterior repositioning splint to recapture the disc and follow this by a superior repositioning splint to seat the condyles with the disc in place. If such a regimen is not possible, disc surgery may be necessary. It is extremely important in these cases that the patient be informed as to the difference between internal disc dislocation and myofascial pain. This will help eliminate confusion as to the purpose for disc surgery. If the disc can be repositioned with the anterior repositioning splint or with surgery, then a superior repositioning splint is used until the myofascial pain component of the problem is under control. Next a treatment plan can be made for the correction of whatever malocclusion and dentofacial deformity are observed. If no improvement can be made in the myofascial pain, the patient must be reevaluated before any irreversible treatment is instituted. As with all patients who have myofascial pain, physical therapy and psychology play an important role.

ACKNOWLEDGMENTS

I wish to express my sincere thanks to Beth Barber and Karin Paulin for their dedicated efforts in the preparation of this manuscript and management of the cases reported.

REFERENCES

1. Ahlgren, J.: The silent period in the EMG of the jaw muscles during mastication and its relationship to tooth contact, Acta Odontol. Scand. **27:**219, 1969.
2. Bays, R.: Stable, adjustable fixation system for maxillary osteotomies. Presented at the Southeastern Society of Oral and Maxillofacial Surgeons meeting, Orlando, Fla., 1984.
3. Bays, R.: Rigid stabilization system for maxillary osteotomies, J. Oral Maxillofac. Surg. **43:**60, 1985.
4. Beemsterboer, P., et al.: The effect of the bite plane on the electromyograph silent period duration, J. Oral Rehabil. **3:**349, 1976.
5. Bell, W.H., and Proffit, W.R.: Maxillary excess. In Bell, W., et al.: Surgical correction of dentofacial deformities, p. 272, Philadelphia, 1980, W.B. Saunders Co.
6. Bell, W.H., and Scheideman, G.: Correction of vertical maxillary deficiency: stability and soft tissue changes, J. Oral Surg. **39:**666, 1981.
7. Bell, W.H., et al.: Bone healing and revascularization after total maxillary osteotomy, J. Oral Surg. **33:**253, 1975.
8. Bell, W.H., et al.: Surgical correction of dentofacial deformities, p. 172, Philadelphia, 1980, W.B. Saunders Co.
9. Dal Pont, G.: Retromolar osteotomy for the correction of prognathism, J. Oral Surg. **19:**42, 1961.
10. Deeb, M., et al.: Evaluation of local blood flow after total maxillary osteotomy, J. Oral Surg. **39:**249, 1981.
11. Epker, B., et al.: Surgical-orthodontic correction of maxillary deficiency, Oral Surg. **46:**171, 1978.
12. Graham, C., et al.: The effect on nasal airway resistance of superior repositioning of the maxilla, J. Dent. Res. **56:**B63 (special issue), Abstract 45, 1977.
13. Harle, F.: LeFort I osteotomy (using miniplates) for correction of the long face, Int. J. Oral Surg. **9:**427, 1980.
14. Hedemark, A., and Freihofer, H.: The behavior of the maxilla in vertical movements after LeFort I osteotomy, J. Maxillofac. Surg. **6:**244, 1978.
15. Hunsuck, E.: A modified intraoral sagittal splitting technic for correction of mandibular prognathism, J. Oral Surg. **26:**249, 1968.
16. Kaminishi, R., et al.: Improved maxillary stability with modified LeFort I technique, J. Oral Maxillofac. Surg. **4:**203, 1983.
17. Kennedy, J., et al.: Osteotomy as an adjunct to rapid maxillary expansion, Am. J. Orthod. **70:**123, 1976.
18. Kundert, M., and Hadjianghelou, O.: Condylar displacement after sagittal splitting of the mandibular rami, J. Maxillofac. Surg. **8:**278, 1980.
19. Lanigan, D., and West, R.: Management of postoperative hemorrhage following LeFort I maxillary osteotomy. J. Oral Maxillofac. Surg. **42:**367, 1984.
20. McMillan, L.: Border movements of the human mandible. J. Prosthet. Dent. **27:**524, 1972.
21. Meyer, M., and Cavanaugh, G.: Blood flow changes after orthognathic surgery: maxillary and mandibular subapical ostectomy, J. Oral Surg. **34:**495, 1976.
22. Nelson, R., et al.: Quantitation of blood flow after LeFort I osteotomy, J. Oral Surg. **35:**10, 1977.
23. O'Ryan, F., and Epker, B.: Surgical orthodontics and the temporomandibular joint: Part II mandibular advancement via modified sagittal split ramus osteotomies, Am. J. Orthod. **83:**418, 1983.
24. Schendel, S., and Epker, B.: Results after mandibular advancement surgery: an analysis of 87 cases, J. Oral Surg. **38:**265, 1980.

25. Schendel, S., and Williamson, L.: Muscle reorientation following superior repositioning of the maxilla, J. Oral Maxillofac. Surg. **41:**235, 1983.
26. Singer, R., and Bays, R.: Comparison between superior and inferior border wiring techniques in sagittal split ramus osteotomy, J. Oral Maxillofac. Surg. **43:** 444, 1985.
27. Solberg, W., et al.: Nocturnal electromyographic evaluation of bruxism patients undergoing short-term splint therapy, J. Oral Rehabil. **21:**215, 1975.
28. Timms, D.: Rapid maxillary expansion, Chicago, 1981, Quintessence Publishing Co.
29. Trauner, R., and Obwegeser, H.: The surgical correction of mandibular prognathism and retrognathia, with consideration of genioplasty. I and II, Oral Surg. **10:** 677, 787, 1957.
30. Turvey, T., et al.: Alterations in nasal airway resistance following superior repositioning of the maxilla, Am. J. Orthod. **85:**109, 1984.
31. Wessberg, G., and Epker, B.: Intraoral skeletal fixation appliance, J. Oral Maxillofac. Surg. **40:**827, 1982.
32. Williamson, E., et al.: The effect of bite plane use on terminal hinge axis location, Angle Orthod. **47:**25, 1977.
33. Wolford, L., and Hilliard, F.: The surgical orthodontic correction of vertical dentofacial deformities, J. Oral Surg. **39:**883, 1981.

Preprosthetic oral and maxillofacial surgery: a rational approach for systematic evaluation and treatment planning

BRUCE N. EPKER
JAMES B. GETZ, JR.

Preprosthetic surgery has, by and large, lacked the specificity of evaluation and treatment planning commonly employed in the field of orthodontic-surgical correction of dentofacial deformities. This is due in part to two major problems: (1) the fact that surgeons have developed and learned selected surgical techniques to correct certain specific prosthetic problems, such as inadequate vestibular depth, and have utilized these too often, *regardless of the specific nature of the individual patient's existing prosthetic problems,* and (2) the fact that practitioners performing prosthetic dentistry have been reluctant to inform their patients of the potential benefits that can be derived from surgery or have failed to inform them of legitimate treatment options.

Compounding the first problem has been the fact that the oral and maxillofacial surgeon often makes the primary decision regarding what is, or are, the most relevant prosthetic problems in a given case instead of allowing the reconstructive dentist or prosthodontist who will be responsible for the prosthetic phase of treatment to do this. The result has been the common practice that various surgeons espouse "their favorite technique" regardless of the specific nature of the prosthetic problems as determined by the general dentist.

More appropriately, a surgical-prosthetic decision-making process should be predicated upon the questions: "What are the individual patient's specific prosthetic problems?" and "Can real prosthetic benefits be achieved for the patient as the result of surgery?" Most generally this means that any patient who would be able to *function significantly better* because of surgery, with an improvment in facial esthetics, is such a candidate. It also means that the dentist responsible for the prosthetic phase of treatment should actively participate in making the decision as to what specific prosthetic problems most deserve improvement.

The reasons for the second problem may be ignorance, economics, or some other situation. To make such decisions more objectively and quantitatively, it is necessary that a systematic patient evaluation be performed that will result in a definition of the *specific nature and severity of the actual prosthetic problems.* This approach will enable both the surgeon and the reconstructive dentist to identify which specific problems warrant consideration for surgical correction.

In this chapter we present a method for the systematic evaluation of the patient that will result in a quantitative index for diagnosing and treatment planning the surgical-prosthetic case, and we discuss sequentially the technique for systematic patient evaluation, the essentials of treatment planning, and some specific illustrations of this approach with case reports.

SYSTEMATIC PATIENT EVALUATION

The systematic patient evaluation consists of five interrelated categories that together form a clear picture of the specific nature and severity of existing problems in a surgical-prosthetic patient: (1) the previous prosthetic history, (2) a facial esthetic evaluation, (3) a cephalometric evaluation, (4) a dental model evaluation, and (5) an evaluation of the temporomandibular joints.

Previous prosthetic history

The primary importance of the previous prosthetic history in the overall evaluation is to determine the likelihood that the patient will be satisfied and will exhibit improved function, according to expressed need, as the result of any integrated surgical-prosthetic treatment. In this regard there are perhaps two general types of potential surgical-prosthetic patients: those who have been edentulous for many years, having had relatively few new dentures constructed during this time, and who, despite *significantly compromised anatomic relations,* can tolerate and function surprisingly well; and those who have had an unusually large number of new dentures constructed, often during a relatively short time, and who, despite only *moderately compromised anatomic* relations, are unable to tolerate and function satisfactorily. The first type of patient generally expects realistic improvement from treatment, not a miracle, and thus is usually an excellent candidate for integrated surgical-prosthetic treatment. Conversely, the second type, especially when the denture history exists in concert with unrealistic expectations, either esthetic or functional, is often a poor candidate and it is wise not to undertake surgical-prosthetic treatment unless its benefits have been realistically presented to and accepted by the patient. These and related essen-tial elements of the prosthetic history are useful in making certain definitive decisions. (See Form A.)

Facial esthetic evaluation

The first portion of the facial esthetic evaluation is used to help the clinician determine what, if any, changes in facial appearance the patient desires or anticipates from treatment. These expressed wishes are recorded along with the esthetic findings. (See Form B.)

We prefer to do the esthetic evaluation directly from the patient, who may be either standing or seated comfortably. All that is required is a millimeter ruler. It is important that the examination be done in a systematic manner. We place the major emphasis on front face because that is how individuals most often view themselves and are viewed by others. Although the actual details of the esthetic facial evaluation are recorded directly from the patient, facial photographs are essential to document these details.

The recommended essential facial photographs are front face in repose, front face smiling, and right profile in repose. In specific cases additional photographs may be desired.

The esthetic evaluation is recorded, and (it is emphasized) *only the abnormal findings* need be recorded. These findings will subsequently be useful in the treatment planning phase and will serve as a primary means for making the basic decision as to what surgical procedure would benefit the patient most.

FRONTAL ANALYSIS

Symmetry, balance, and *morphology* are the three major elements in the production of good frontal facial esthetics. Certainly no face is perfectly symmetric, yet the absence of any obvious asymmetry is necessary for good frontal esthetics. Facial balance is construed to mean that the upper, middle, and lower facial thirds are of nearly equal length. Although various morphologic configurations of faces exist, it is perhaps most important that the facial thirds be of the same basic morphologic configuration.

Upper third of face—hairline to eyebrows. The upper third of the face is the least important since it is easily disguised by hairstyle. Never-

Text continued on p. 198.

Form A. Previous prosthetic history

Length of time edentulous

   Maxilla

      Partially   __________________________ yr

      Totally   __________________________ yr

   Mandible

      Partially   __________________________ yr

      Totally   __________________________ yr

Sets of new dentures constructed during this time

   Maxilla

      Partial   __________________________ yr

      Full   __________________________ yr

   Mandible

      Partial   __________________________ yr

      Full   __________________________ yr

Last set of dentures constructed ____

Times dentures have been relined in last 2 years ____________________________________

General satisfaction with existing denture function _________________________________

Foods unable to eat ____

____

General satisfaction with existing denture appearance _____________________________

____

Esthetic improvement desired from treatment ______________________________________

____

Favorable or unfavorable prosthetic experiences among patient's family, relatives, or close

friends ____

____

Form B. Facial esthetic evaluation

Esthetic changes desired ____

____

Frontal esthetics

General facial characteristics

  Symmetry ____

    Balance (length)

      Upper third _______________________

      Middle third _______________________

      Lower third _______________________

  Morphology ____

Upper third of face (hairline to eyebrows)

  General shape and symmetry ____

Middle third of face (eyebrows to subnasale)

  Eyes and orbits

    Canthal symmetry (inner-outer) ____

    Ptosis ____

    Ectropion ____

    Entropion ____

  Nose

    Dorsum ____

    Tip ____

    Alar base (34 + mm) ____

  Cheeks

    Symmetry and projection of malar eminences ____

    Infraorbital rims ____

    Paranasal areas ____

  Ears

    Level and symmetry ____

    Deformities ____

Continued.

Form B. Facial esthetic evaluation—cont'd

Lower third of face (subnasale to menton)

  Balance

    Subnasale-stomion to stomion-menton (1:2) ______________________________

    Subnasale-vermilion to vermilion-menton (1:1) ______________________________

    Ratio upper to lower vermilion (1:1, 1/4) ______________________________

    Interlabial distance (0 to 3 mm) ______________________________

  Anterior teeth (prosthetic or natural)

    Uppers

      Exposure (mm):   Repose ______________   Smiling ______________

      Symmetry ______________________________

    Lowers

      Exposure (mm):   Repose ______________   Smiling ______________

      Symmetry ______________________________

    Midlines ______________________

      Dental ______________________

      Facial ______________________

  Chin

    Symmetry

      Left ______________________

      Right ______________________

    Shape ______________________

  Mandibular angles

    Symmetry ______________________

    Deficiency ______________________

    Hyperplasticity ______________________

Form B. Facial esthetic evaluation—cont'd

Profile esthetics

Upper third of face

Forehead ___________________________

Middle third of face

Nose

Prominence: Excessive ______________ Deficient ______________

Dorsum: Convex ______________ Concave ______________

Supratip break: Present ______________ Absent ______________

Nasolabial angle (90° to 110°) ______________________

Columella: Angled upward ______________ Angled downward ______________

Cheeks (malar eminences)

Convex ______________ Flat ______________ Concave ______________

Infraorbital rim projection ($\pm$ 2 mm) ______________________

Paranasal areas

Convex ______________ Flat ______________ Concave ______________

Tip-subnasale to subnasale-alar base (2:1) ______________________

Lower third of face

Lips

Upper (relative to subnasale perpendicular): Protrusive ________ Retrusive ________

Lower (relative to upper lip):   Protrusive ________ Retrusive ________

Labiomental fold: Deficient ________ Excessive ________

Chin projection: Retrusive ________ Protrusive ________

Neck-chin angle: Deficient ________ Excessive ________

Neck-chin length: Deficient ________ Excessive ________

theless, its general shape and symmetry should be noted and any abnormalities recorded. Except in craniofacial syndrome–related conditions, abnormalities in this area are rare.

Middle third of face—eyebrows to subnasale. We systematically evaluate the *eyes,* the *nose,* the *cheeks,* and the *ears* in the following order:

Eye evaluation begins with noting the vertical symmetry of the inner and outer canthi. Generally a true horizontal line will bisect these, and this is the most meaningful method of evaluating true oculoorbital symmetry. Next, notations are made of any abnormalities in the eyelid areas.

The nose is studied for form and symmetry, and any deformities in the alar base that could be prosthetically or surgically enhanced or worsened as a result of treatment are recorded.

Cheek evaluation consists of sequential assessment of the malar eminences, infraorbital rims, and paranasal areas for symmetry and normal projection. Care must be taken in these observations not to be misled by optical illusions created by the lower jaw or the nose being abnormally large or small. Palpation of the underlying structure is a useful technique in helping to evaluate these areas.

The ears are observed, and any asymmetry in their level (vertical location) or gross abnormalities are noted.

Lower third of face—subnasale to menton. When good esthetics exist, the normal vertical length of the lower third of the face is approximately equal to that of the middle third. In addition, the ratio of the vertical distance from subnasale to upper lip stomion and that from upper lip stomion to soft tissue menton is about 1:2. The ratio of the vertical distance from subnasale to the vermilion cutaneous margin of the lower lip to soft tissue menton is about 1:1. Disparities in these relations define the precise nature of existing lower-third-of-face imbalances. These measurements *must* be made with the facial musculature at rest and, in edentulous patients, the mandible in rest position.

The lips are extremely important to the overall esthetics of the face. They must be critically evaluated so that after prosthetic placement proper upper and lower lip support can be achieved. Any asymmetry must be recorded and notation made of whether it is an intrinsic lip deformity (as in many cleft patients), a facial nerve dysfunction, or an underlying dentoskeletal asymmetry, so it can be dealt with surgically or possibly compensated prosthetically.

The relations of the existing anterior teeth (whether natural or prosthetic) are important. After prosthetic placement the upper teeth in repose are normally exposed 0 to 3 mm beneath the upper lip with the lower teeth seldom showing. Generally there is less exposure in males than in females. Also, in repose, the lower lip usually manifests about 25% more vermilion than the upper lip does and an interlabial separation of 0 to 3 mm exists.

It must be remembered that during animation, symmetry is the single most important factor in producing an esthetic smile. Thus proper prosthetic lip support for symmetry of the upper lip both at rest and during movement must be achieved. It is also imperative that the dental midlines be essentially coincident with one another and with the *facial midline.*

The chin is evaluated first for symmetry in both right-to-left and vertical relationships. Morphology or shape is compared with that of the rest of the face. Often the chin is more pointed than the rest of the face.

Finally, the mandibular angles are assessed with regard to both their symmetry and fullness and whether they are deficient, normal, or excessive. This completes the frontal facial esthetics evaluation.

PROFILE ANALYSIS

Profile analysis is likewise done in a systematic manner.

Upper third of face. The forehead should normally slope from superior to inferior, with an accentuation or projection of the supraorbital rims.

Middle third of face. The middle-third-of-face analysis consists of a sequential examination of the *nose,* the *cheeks and orbital rims,* and the *paranasal areas.*

The configuration of the nose (nasal dorsum and tip) is evaluated, the dorsum being normally somewhat concave with a supratip break. The nasolabial angle is assessed next and is normally between 90 and 110 degrees. It is often defined as the angle between imaginary lines tangent to the columella and the upper lip. When it is abnormal, care must be used to distinguish the angulation. For this reason we prefer to use also the relation of the upper lip to subnasale perpendicular as a guide in determining protrusion or retrusion of the upper lip and dentition. (See Form C.)

The cheeks and orbital rims are evaluated in profile relative to the globes. The infra-orbital rims generally project 0 to 2 mm ahead of the most anterior projection of the globes, and the lateral orbital rims lie 8 to 12 mm behind this projection.

The paranasal areas, like the cheeks, are generally somewhat convex. The ratio of the linear distance, in the horizontal plane, from the nasal tip to subnasale to the alar base is normally 2:1. Values approaching 1:1 are suggestive of a lack of support for the alar base and indicate a maxillary or true middle third facial deficiency. It is important when viewing the paranasal areas not to be influenced by an abnormal chin projection, which may produce an optical illusion or may actually influence the soft tissue drape in this area. The patient with mandibular prognathism will

---

Form C. Cephalometric evaluation

Soft tissue relationships

	Normal	Patients
Vertical		
Go-Sn : Sn-Me	1:1	__________
Upper lip length (Sn-St)	20 ± 2	__________
Sn-St : St-Me	1:2	__________
Sn-Llv : Llv-Me	1:0.9	__________
Interlabial distance	0 to 3 mm	
Horizontal		
Subnasale perpendicular to		
Upper lip	0 mm	__________
Lower lip	−2 mm	__________
Chin	−4 mm	__________
Skeletal relationships		
Facial axis angle	90° ± 3°	__________
Facial depth	89° ± 3°	__________
Mandibular plane angle	24° ± 3°	__________
Maxillary depth	90° ± 3°	__________
Maxillary length : mandibular length	1:1.3	__________
Interarch distance	20 ± 5 mm	__________

appear to be paranasally concave whereas the one with a mandibular deficiency will appear convex.

Lower third of face. Observations in the lower third of the face sequentially include the *lips,* the *labiomental folds,* the *chin projection,* and the *neck-chin areas.*

Normally, in repose, the upper lip projects slightly anterior to the lower lip. Protrusion or retrusion of each lip is independently noted as it relates to the underlying prosthetic dental support.

A discernable labiomental fold gives definition to the face whereas lack of one, or an excessively deep one, detracts from this pleasant definition.

After assessment of the chin prominence with the mandible in rest position, the neck-chin area is evaluated. Normally this area exhibits an obtuse angle (135 degrees) and the distance from pogonion to the neck-chin angle is about 50 mm.

These relations give definition to the chin, whereas excessive obtuseness of the neck-chin angle detracts from chin definition.

Cephalometric evaluation

The cephalometric evaluation is performed in the specific manner presented so as to provide meaningful information concerning several important factors: (1) Are the vertical soft tissue relationships compatible with those recorded clinically or expressed as concerns of the patient? (2) Are the anteroposterior soft tissue relationships compatible with those recorded clinically or expressed as concerns of the patient? (3) Are the anteroposterior jaw and ridge relationships within normal limits so that a functional and esthetically acceptable prosthesis can be constructed? (4) Is the vertical interarch ridge distance adequate for the construction of a functional and esthetically acceptable prosthesis?

It is essential that the cephalometric radiographs of fully edentulous individuals be taken in mandibular rest position with the lips totally relaxed. Otherwise, the true skeletal relations may be distorted because of the usual forward and upward rotation of the mandible that occurs with increased ridge resorption.

Fig. 6-1 is a cephalometric tracing of a person in centric occlusion with existing dentures in place and the mandible in rest position. The actual values listed are those recommended for soft tissue and skeletal relationships. Normal values are given on the cephalometric evaluation form. It is beyond the scope of this chapter to discuss in detail each of the values listed, and the interested reader is referred to appropriate references at the end of the chapter. However, of primary importance is the fact that the nature of the existing skeletal and esthetic problems is significantly different on these two radiographs. Indeed, on one (Fig. 6-1, *A*) the primary problems appear to be anteroposterior in nature whereas on the other *(B)* they are primarily vertical or related to existing ridge heights.

Dental model evaluation

To be properly evaluated, dental models are related to one another in the proper vertical relationship—not arbitrarily or in an "overclosed" relationship. The articulated dental models are sequentially evaluated for (1) transverse ridge abnormalities, (2) size of the maxillary and mandibular ridges, (3) labiobuccal vestibular adequacy of the maxilla and mandible, (4) palatal depth and adequacy of the floor of the mouth, and (5) bony irregularities such as undercuts or knife-edge ridges. Abnormalities of the soft tissues are recorded, as determined from the clinical, radiographic, and dental model analysis. (See Form D.)

Notice the numerical values of 1 through 5 adjacent to the various anatomic relations listed on Form D. Values of *1* and *2* indicate that there is not a problem with the specific anatomic relationship which would preclude the construction of an optimally functional prosthesis. A *3* indicates that, although a functional prosthesis might be constructed, preprosthetic surgery would result in improved function and esthetics. The notations *4* and *5* are made when it is determined that, to achieve the desired functional and esthetic requirements of the specific patient, surgical improvement of the relationship is necessary.

It is obvious that there will be some interexaminer variation in this quantitative approach. However, two aspects are important:

Preoperative CO
101°
100°
87 mm
120 mm
68 mm
A
25°
17
21
18°
38
55
34
11°
141°
Preoperative CR
93°
95°
87 mm
120 mm
68 mm
B
32°
20
30
23°
62
42
32°
32
4°
145°

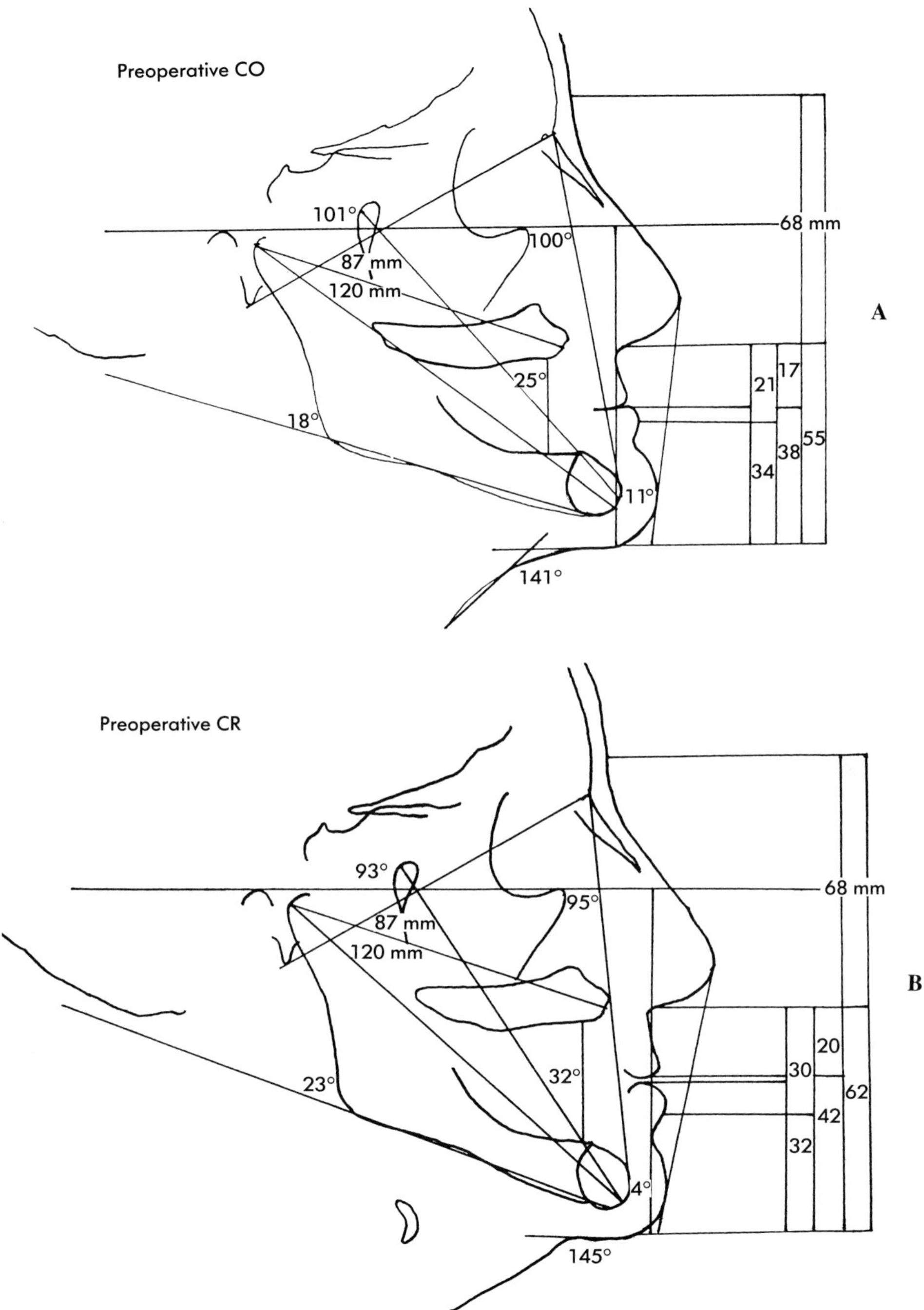

Fig. 6-1, A and **B.**

First, it has become apparent in our experience that this evaluation is quite reproducible from examiner to examiner. Second, the ultimate decision as to whether a given relationship is a 2 or a 4 is made by the dentist who will be constructing the denture for the patient and not by the oral and maxillofacial surgeon.

Temporomandibular joint evaluation

It is important diagnostically and prognostically in the evaluation of problems that might occur during treatment, or that *appear to result from* treatment, to evaluate the TMJs *prior to* the institution of treatment. A simple examination can be done in three parts: (1) evaluation of mandibular movements, (2) examination of TMJ symptoms, and (3) examination of TMJ signs. If significant abnormalities are disclosed in any of these, it is important that the joints be further evaluated and an *accurate diagnosis made* prior to the institution of treatment of any existing prosthetic problem. The following comments are intended to aid the clinician in making the initial examination and in determining whether a more detailed examination is necessary. (See Form E.)

Mandibular Movements

The evaluation of mandibular movements is appropriately recorded on the form.

Temporomandibular Joint Symptoms

In the evaluation of TMJ movements maximal interincisal, protrusive, and excursive movements are recorded. The edentulous person with prosthetic appliances will have a normal interincisal opening of about 50 mm as well as protrusive and excursive movements of approximately 6 mm. In the edentulous state, ridge relationships are measured and appropriate consideration given for the variable interincisal value resulting from the absence of teeth. If *deviations* of the mandible greater than 2 to 4 mm occur during opening, they are noted and

---

Form D. Dental model evaluation

Transverse jaw disharmonies

Buccal cross-bite	1	2	3	4	5
Lingual cross-bite	1	2	3	4	5

Maxillary ridge disharmonies

Size of ridge	1	2	3	4	5
Labiobuccal vestibule	1	2	3	4	5
Palatal depth	1	2	3	4	5
Bony irregularities	1	2	3	4	5
Soft tissue abnormality	1	2	3	4	5

Mandibular ridge disharmonies

Size of ridge	1	2	3	4	5
Labiobuccal vestibule	1	2	3	4	5
Floor of mouth	1	2	3	4	5
Bony irregularities	1	2	3	4	5
Soft tissue abnormality	1	2	3	4	5

Form E. Temporomandibular joint evaluation

Mandibular movements

    Maximum opening (50 mm) _______________________

      Deviation

          Left ____________________ mm   Right ________________ mm

      Protrusive (6 mm) ____________________

      Excursive (6 mm) ____________________

          Left ____________________   Right ____________________

TMJ symptoms (pain)

    Rest

        Left

        Right

    Movement

        Left

        Right

    Loading

        Left

        Right

TMJ signs (noise)

    Popping

        Left

            Less than 10 mm

            10 to 20 mm

            Greater than 20 mm

        Right

            Less than 10 mm

            10 to 20 mm

            Greater than 20 mm

        Functional or anatomic

    Crepitation

        Left

        Right

recorded. If opening is reduced or deviations exist, it is important to determine whether they are due to true *TMJ abnormalities* or to masticatory muscle problems. This can often be simply accomplished by asking the patient to touch the specific areas of soreness or tightness that prevent normal execution of these movements. **Far too often masticatory muscle pain or spasm is called TMJ dysfunction.** If muscle dysfunction exists, it can be eliminated via standard approaches and the patient reevaluated after the influences of muscle dysfunction upon jaw movement have been eliminated.

Symptoms can be explicity referred to *TMJ joint pain*. They are manifested as pain specifically localized in the preauricular and external auditory canal areas as determined by palpation. *When true TMJ pain exists, it is almost always accentuated by movement and loading of the joint.* This latter phenomenon can be achieved by having the patient bite hard on two tongue blades sequentially placed in each canine area and incisally. Biting in the left canine area will load the *right* joint and thus accentuate pain in that joint. Biting hard on the incisors will load *both* joints. When true joint pain exists and is increased with loading, laminagrams of the joints are generally indicated.

TEMPOROMANDIBULAR JOINT SIGNS

A large percent of the total population (40% to 80%) who are without symptoms have popping or clicking of their TMJs. The clinical significance of this in the absence of symptoms is not agreed upon. However, it is important to note that most patients who have popping exhibit an associated *premature protrusive movement* of the condyles as the pop occurs. The question is whether this noise is secondary to an underlying neuromuscular dysfunction (often habitual) or due to a true anatomic internal derangement. When a pop occurs early (at 20 mm of opening) and is not associated with locking, it is often functional. This question can be answered by having the patient undergo 2 to 4 weeks of jaw physiotherapy. Normal jaw movements are demonstrated and the patient is then informed that exercise must be performed four times a day in front of a mirror for 10 minutes each time to eliminate the premature protrusive movement; that is, the mandible must be opened and closed without deviations. *When this regimen is followed, the majority of patients (75% to 80%) readily eliminate the deviation, popping, and any associated symptoms.* These patients have a *functional pop* and do *not* generally require other methods of treatment. Patients who are not cured by this regimen may have a *true anatomic internal derangement* and be candidates for a more detailed evaluation such as a CT scan or arthrogram to establish the definitive diagnosis. The individual with an opening or closing lock, either with or without joint noise, generally has a true anatomic derangement and will likely require surgical correction.

Crepitation is uncommon in asymptomatic joints and may be an early sign of true degenerative joint disease. When it exists, it is best to obtain laminagrams of the joints for a better evaluation of the possible presence of early degenerative joint disease.

When, predicated upon the findings in this examination, a possible or probable organic TMJ disorder exists (such as significant hypomobility, severe deviation upon opening, locking, and pain localized to the joint), further detailed TMJ studies are indicated. It is beyond the scope of this text to detail the sequence of these additional evaluations. However, it is fundamentally important that the clinician *not* confuse myofascial pain dysfunction syndrome with a true TMJ problem.

At this point in the evaluation all factors relevant to making definitive surgical prosthetic decisions are sequentially listed and quantified so a reasonable treatment plan can be developed that will address the *specific* factors which preclude construction of an optimally functional and esthetic prosthesis. (This is accomplished on Form F.)

The use of this system of evaluation and treatment planning is important in that it dictates the specific nature and severity of any existing prosthetic problems but not the specific manner in which a problem is to be corrected. In other words, when the mandibular labial vestibule is rated 4, the surgeon treating the individual must decide upon the preferred method of improving it, whether by an Edlan flap, split-thickness skin graft, dermal graft, or palatal graft. However, conversely, it does identify the specific problems that warrant surgical correction and thus eliminates the tendency for all patients to be treated by a given surgeon's "favorite technique" regardless of the patient's specific problems.

ESSENTIALS OF TREATMENT PLANNING

Upon completion of the systematic patient evaluation and quantitation of the specific problems, two decisions must be made: (1) What is the priority of problems requiring surgical correction? (2) What specific methods will be utilized to correct them?

The first decision is easily made directly from the quantitative evaluation of the various anatomic prosthetic relations. Thus the reason for the system. The problem with the greatest value (provided it is greater than 3) is of highest priority and so on. Problems with values of 3 must be decided upon individually. Those with values of less than 3 are of no significant concern regarding possible surgical treatment.

The second decision, what specific surgical method will be utilized to correct the existing problems, is less readily made. This is due in large part to the lack of scientific information on the preference of one method versus another that is utilized to treat basically the same problem. Thus this phase of decision making will vary considerably among surgeons—which, however, does not detract from the important fact that if this system of diagnosis and treatment planning is utilized the proper problems will be treated, even though they are treated via different accepted surgical techniques. Finally, it is emphasized that the surgical methods selected to improve any prosthetic problems must also effect improvement in any abnormal existing esthetic relations. In this regard the correction of, for example, a Class III ridge relation must be done in either the maxilla or the mandible as dictated by esthetics and not arbitrarily.

Form F. Quantitative guide for surgical-prosthetic patients

Previous prosthetic history

Favorable ____

Unfavorable ____

None _____✓____

Esthetic facial evaluation

Frontal objectives _____*Increase fullness of lips*_____________

Profile objectives _____*Increase fullness of lips*_____________

Cephalometric evaluation
Anteroposterior jaw (ridge) disharmonies

Class III	1	(2)	3	4	5
Class II	1	2	3	4	5

Vertical jaw disharmonies

Excessive interarch distances	1	2	3	4	5
Insufficient interarch distances	1	2	3	4	5

Dental model evaluation
Transverse jaw disharmonies

Buccal cross-bite	1	2	3	4	(5)
Lingual cross-bite	1	2	3	4	5

Maxillary ridge disharmonies

Size of ridge	1	2	3	(4)	5
Labiobuccal vestibule	(1)	2	3	4	5
Palatal depth	1	(2)	3	4	5
Bony irregularities	1	2	3	4	5
Soft tissue disorders	1	2	3	4	5

Mandibular ridge disharmonies

Size of ridge	1	2	3	4	5
Labiobuccal vestibule	1	2	3	4	5
Floor of mouth	1	2	3	4	5
Bony irregularities	1	2	(3)	4	5
Soft tissue disorders	1	2	3	4	5

TMJ evaluation

Abnormal movements _____None_________________________________

____

Symptoms _________None_________________________________

____

Signs _________None_________________________________

____

Probable diagnosis ____

____

CASE REPORTS

The ensuing case presentations illustrate results obtained with systematic evaluation and quantitative assessment of the surgical-prosthetic patient.

CASE 1 (Fig. 6-2)

A and **B,** Mandibular rest position. **C** and **D,** The narrow maxilla. **E,** Note the transverse discrepancy between maxilla and mandible.

Treatment plan

Expansion of the narrow maxilla with autogenous cancellous bone. Secondary maxillary vestibuloplasty. Maxillary and mandibular full denture construction.

F, Surgical widening of the maxilla with autogenous cancellous bone. *left,* Pretreatment and, *right,* posttreatment dental models. **G,** *upper,* Maxilla after and, *lower,* maxilla before surgery. **H,** Maxilla before surgical expansion. **I,** Maxilla after surgical expansion and secondary epithelialization vestibuloplasty.

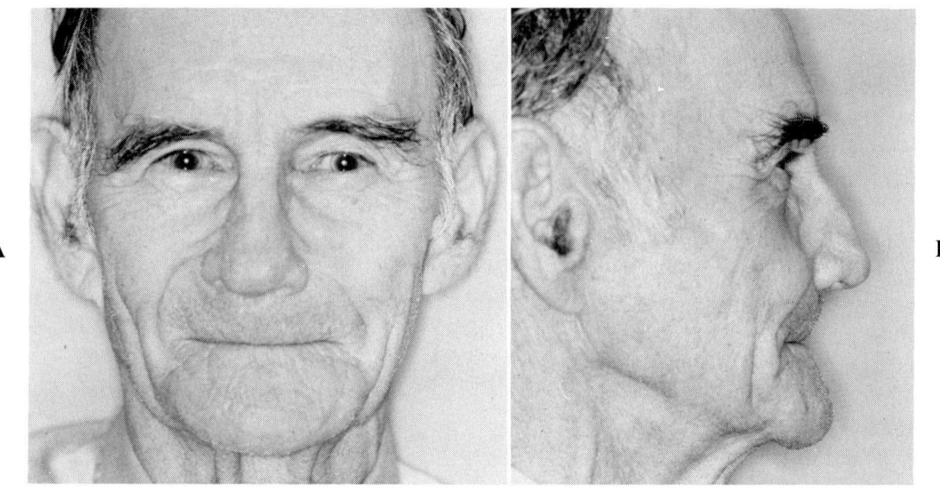

Fig. 6-2, A and **B.**

Continued.

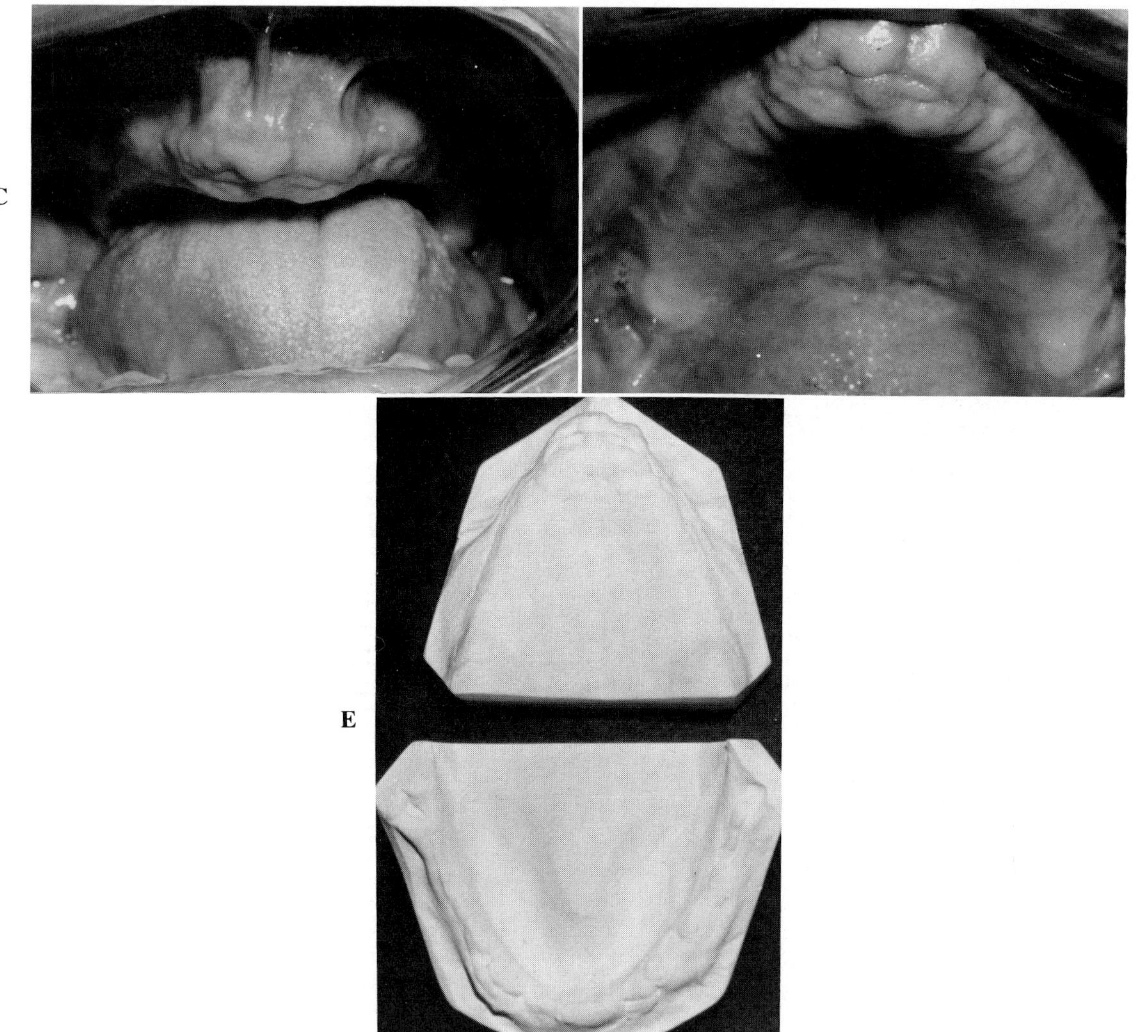

Fig. 6-2, cont'd. C, D, and **E.**

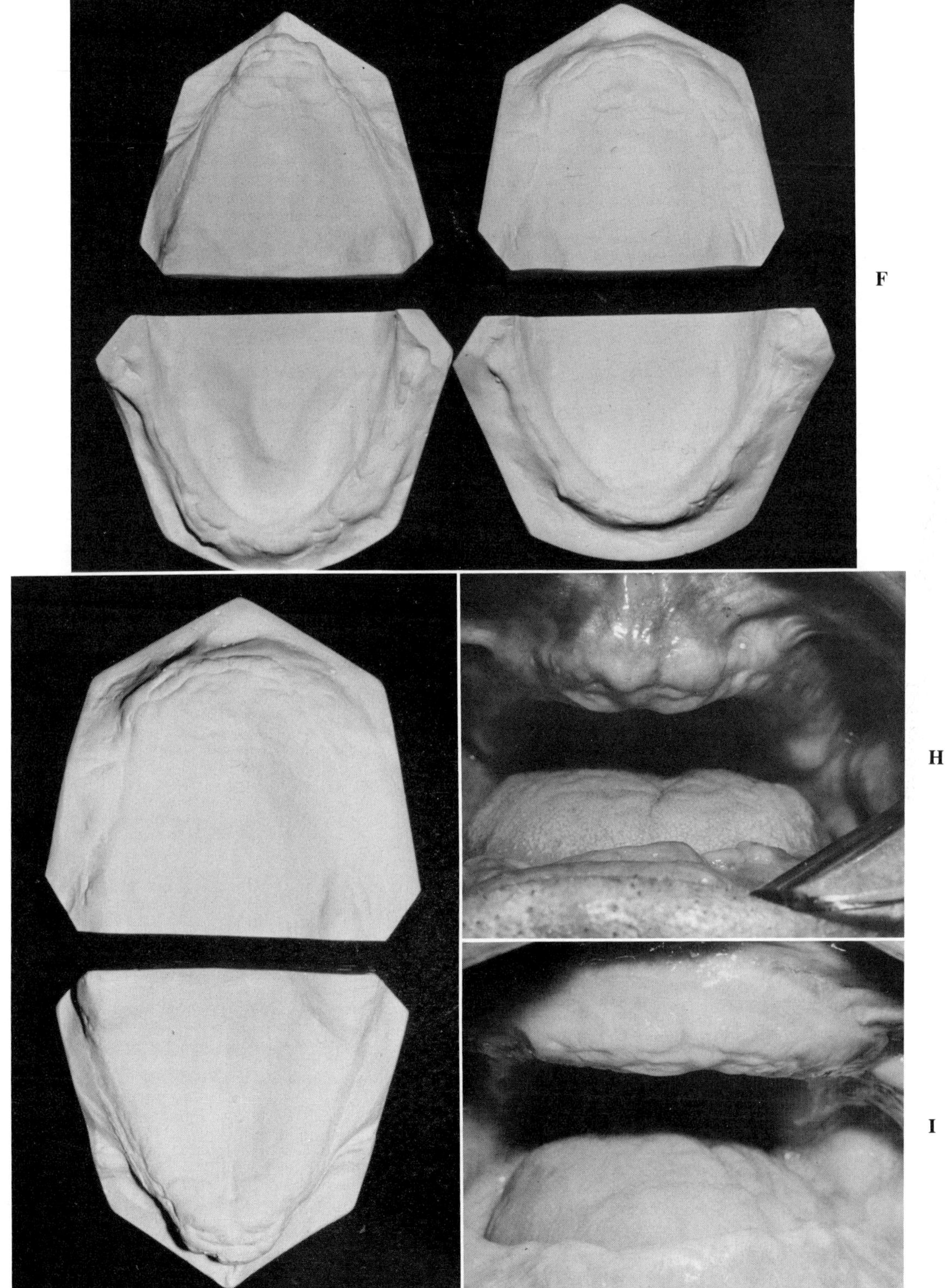

Fig. 6-2, cont'd. F to I.

Form F. Quantitative guide for surgical-prosthetic patients

Previous prosthetic history

Favorable ✓

Unfavorable

None

Esthetic facial evaluation

Frontal objectives *Increase fullness upper lip*
Wider alar bases

Profile objectives *Decrease prominence nose*
Decrease relative prominence chin

Cephalometric evaluation

Anteroposterior jaw (ridge) disharmonies

Class III	1	2	3	4	(5)
Class II	1	2	3	4	5

Vertical jaw disharmonies

Excessive interarch distances	1	2	3	4	5
Insufficient interarch distances	1	2	3	4	5

Dental model evaluation

Transverse jaw disharmonies

Buccal cross-bite	1	2	3	(4)	5
Lingual cross-bite	1	2	3	4	5

Maxillary ridge disharmonies

Size of ridge	1	2	3	4	5
Labiobuccal vestibule	1	2	3	4	5
Palatal depth	1	2	(3)	4	5
Bony irregularities	1	2	3	4	5
Soft tissue disorders	1	2	3	4	5

Mandibular ridge disharmonies

Size of ridge	1	2	3	4	5
Labiobuccal vestibule	1	2	(3)	4	5
Floor of mouth	1	2	3	4	5
Bony irregularities	1	2	3	4	5
Soft tissue disorders	1	2	3	4	5

TMJ evaluation

Abnormal movements *None*

Symptoms *None*

Signs *Occasional on right with wide opening (> 40 mm)*

Probable diagnosis *Asymptomatic pop — right TMJ beyond normal range of mandibular movement*

CASE 2 (Fig. 6-3)

A and **B,** Mandibular rest position. **C,** Pretreatment cephalometric analysis. **D,** Pretreatment dental models.

Treatment plan

High LeFort I maxillary advancement with autogenous bone grafting and maxillary and mandibular full denture construction.

E and **F,** After LeFort I maxillary advancement. **G,** Composite pre- and postsurgical cephalometric tracings. **H,** Posttreatment models. **I,** Posttreatment dentures. **J** to **M,** Ten-year posttreatment records.

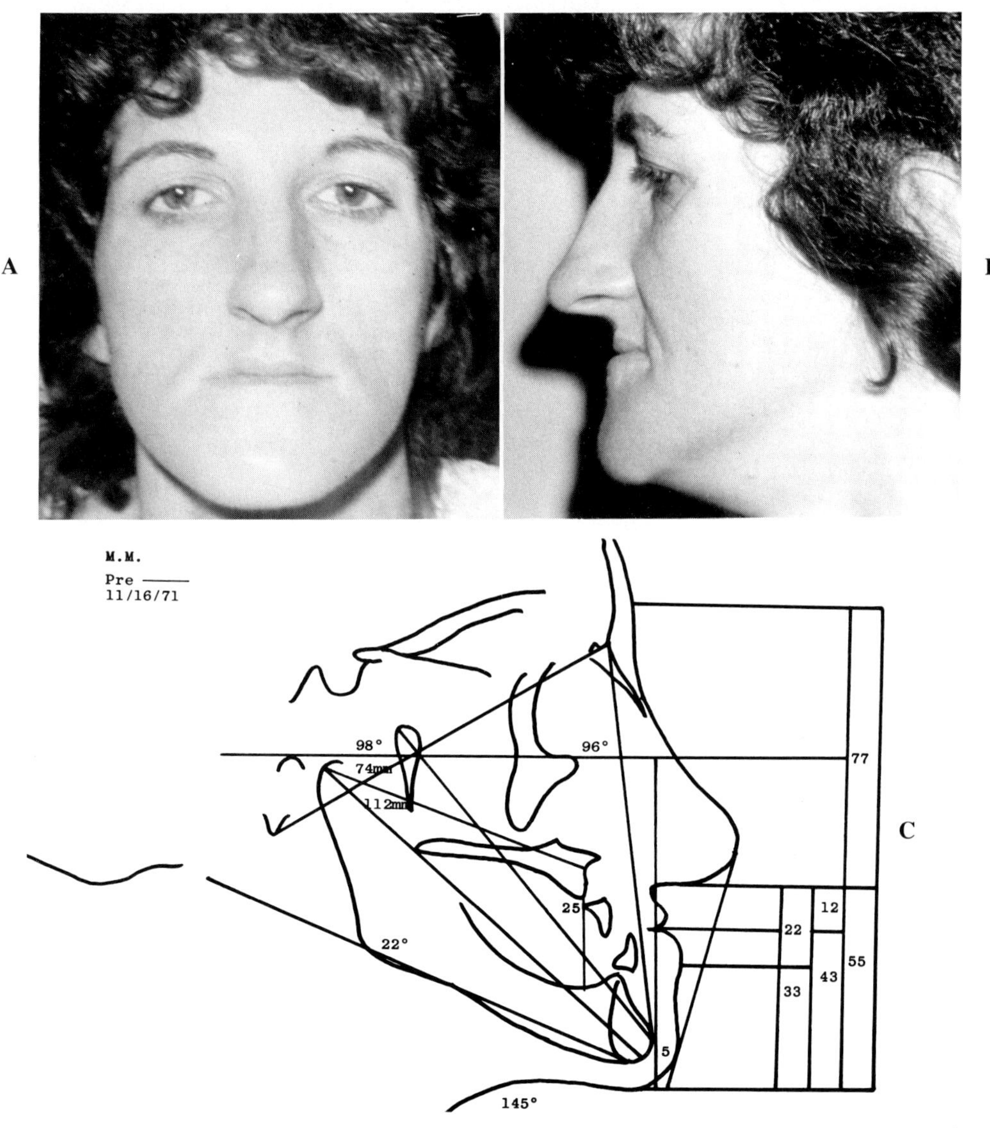

Fig. 6-3, A, B, and **C.**

Continued.

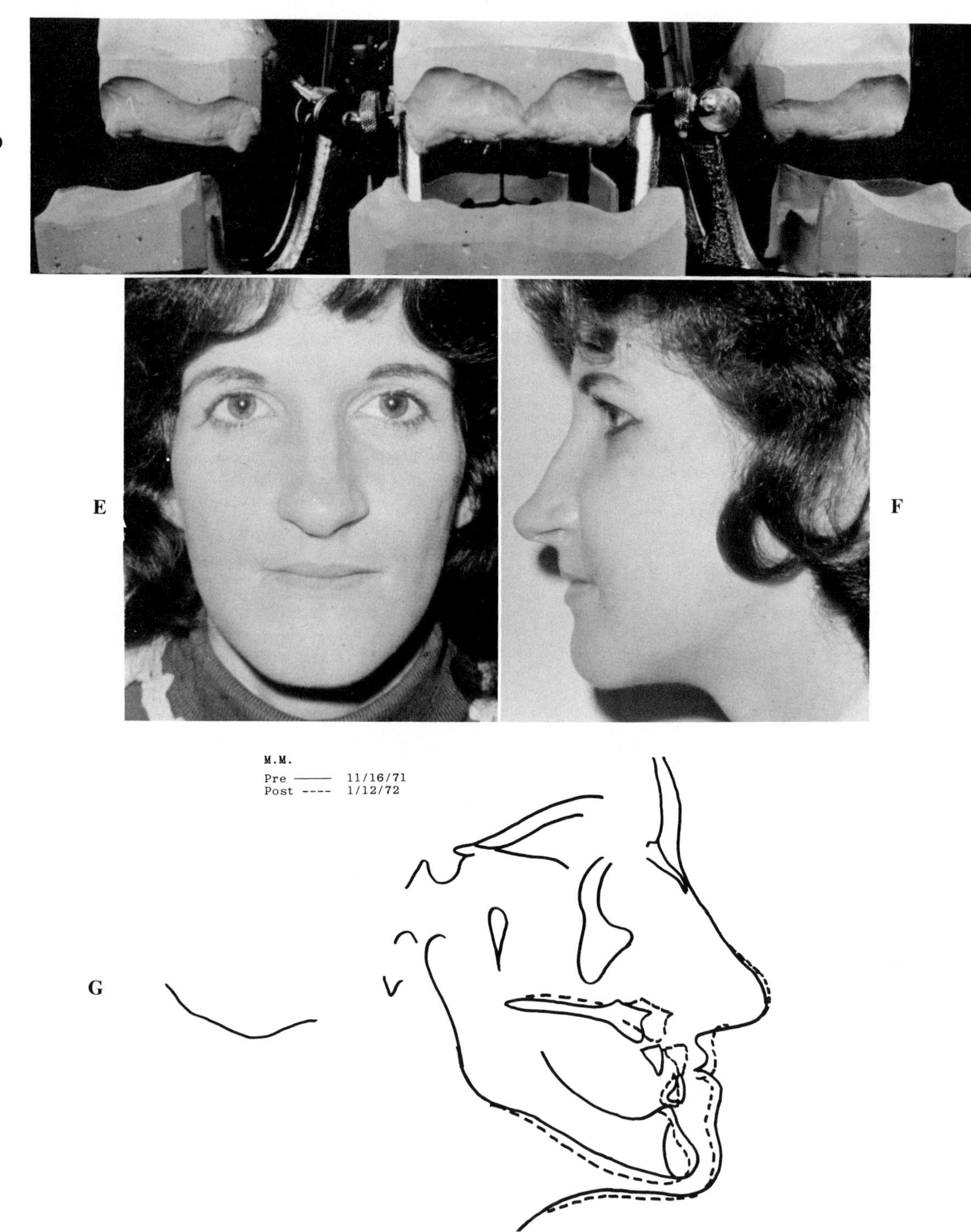

Fig. 6-3, cont'd. D to G.

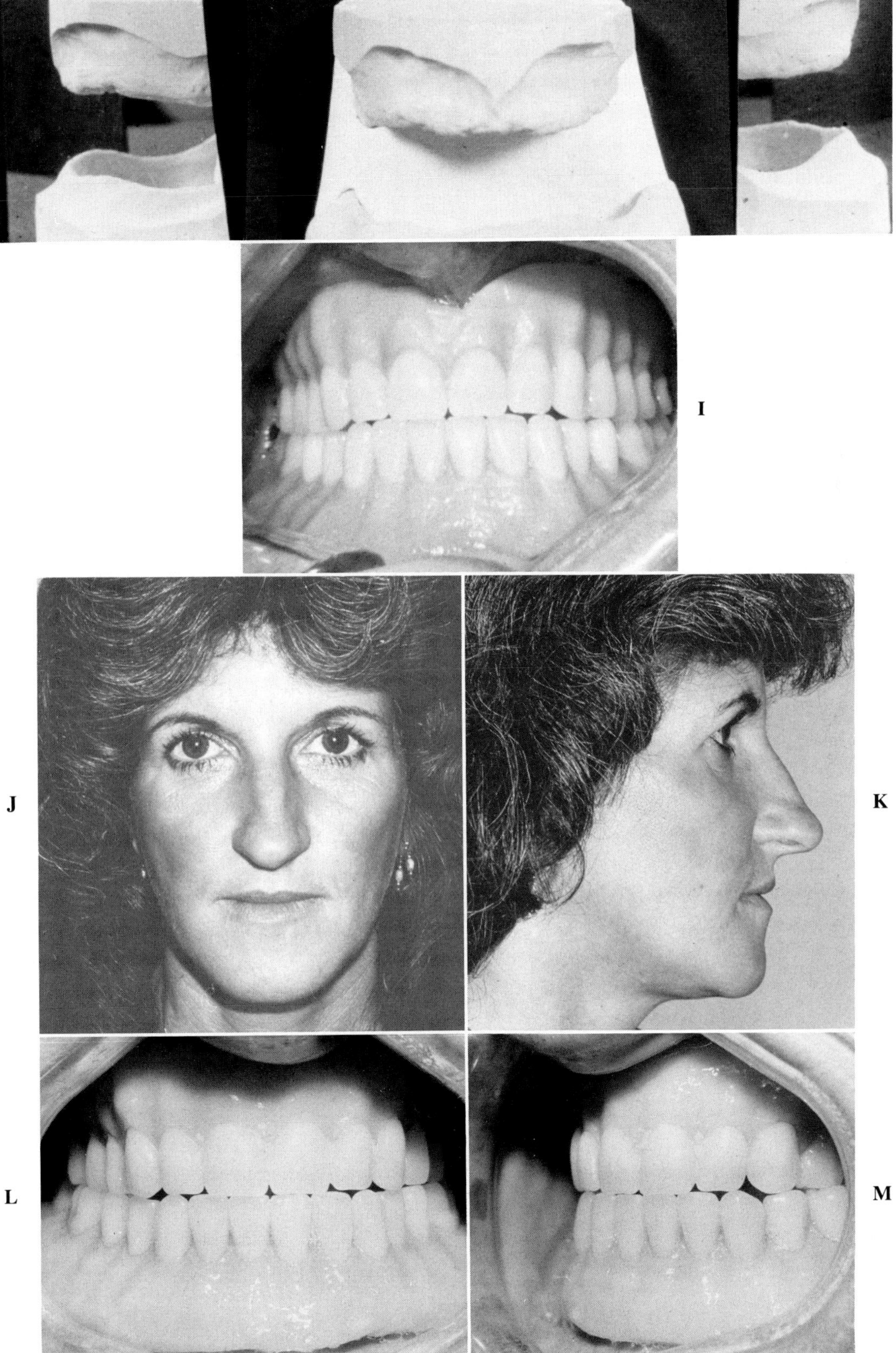

Fig. 6-3, cont'd. H to M.

Form F. Quantitative guide for surgical-prosthetic patients

Previous prosthetic history

Favorable ______ ✓ ____________________

Unfavorable ____________________

None ____________________

Esthetic facial evaluation

Frontal objectives ___ *None* ____________________

Profile objectives *Decrease prominence chin*
Increase fullness upper lip

Cephalometric evaluation

Anteroposterior jaw (ridge) disharmonies

| Class III | 1 2 3 4 ⑤ |
| Class II | 1 2 3 4 5 |

Vertical jaw disharmonies

| Excessive interarch distances | 1 2 3 ④ 5 |
| Insufficient interarch distances | 1 2 3 4 5 |

Dental model evaluation

Transverse jaw disharmonies

| Buccal cross-bite | 1 2 3 ④ 5 |
| Lingual cross-bite | 1 2 3 4 5 |

Maxillary ridge disharmonies

Size of ridge	1 2 3 4 5
Labiobuccal vestibule	1 2 3 4 5
Palatal depth	1 2 3 4 5
Bony irregularities	1 2 3 4 5
Soft tissue disorders	1 2 3 4 5

Mandibular ridge disharmonies

Size of ridge	1 2 3 4 5
Labiobuccal vestibule	1 2 3 4 5
Floor of mouth	1 2 3 4 5
Bony irregularities	1 2 3 4 5
Soft tissue disorders	1 2 3 4 5

TMJ evaluation

Abnormal movements ___ *None* ____________________

Symptoms ___ *None* ____________________

Signs ___ *None* ____________________

Probable diagnosis ____________________
____

CASE 3 (Fig. 6-4)

A and **B,** Pretreatment views. **C** and **D,** Pretreatment cephalometric tracings in centric occlusion (overclosed) and mandibular rest position. **E** and **F,** Pretreatment models mounted in proper vertical relationship.

Treatment plan

Inferoanterior repositioning of the maxilla with simultaneous expansion and interpositional autogenous bone grafting. Construction of new partial denture prostheses.

G and **H,** Model surgery to reposition the maxilla inferoanteriorly and expand it. **I** and **J,** Surgical splint construction. **K** and **L,** Posttreatment views. **M** and **N,** Pre- and postoperative and, **O** and **P,** pre- and postoperative occlusions.

Text continued on p. 221.

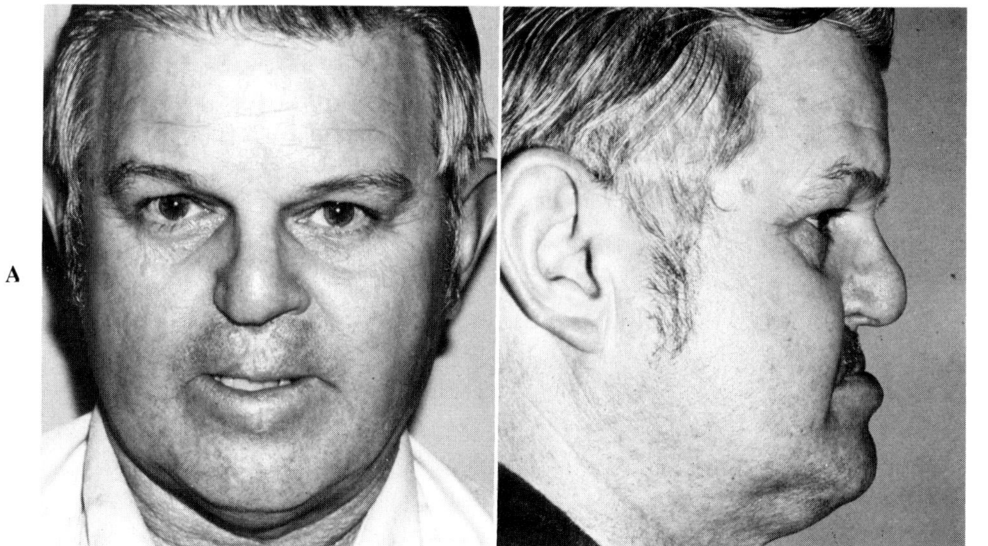

Fig. 6-4, A and B.

Continued.

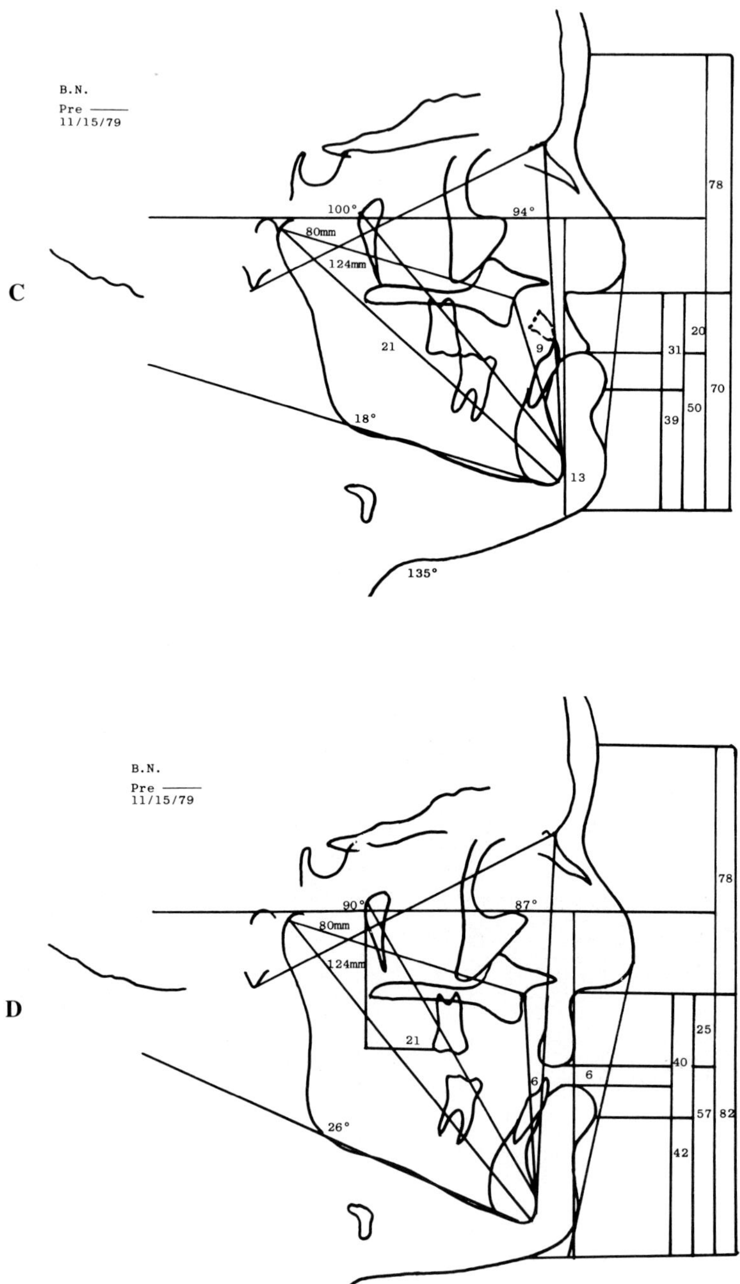

Fig. 6-4, cont'd. C and **D.**

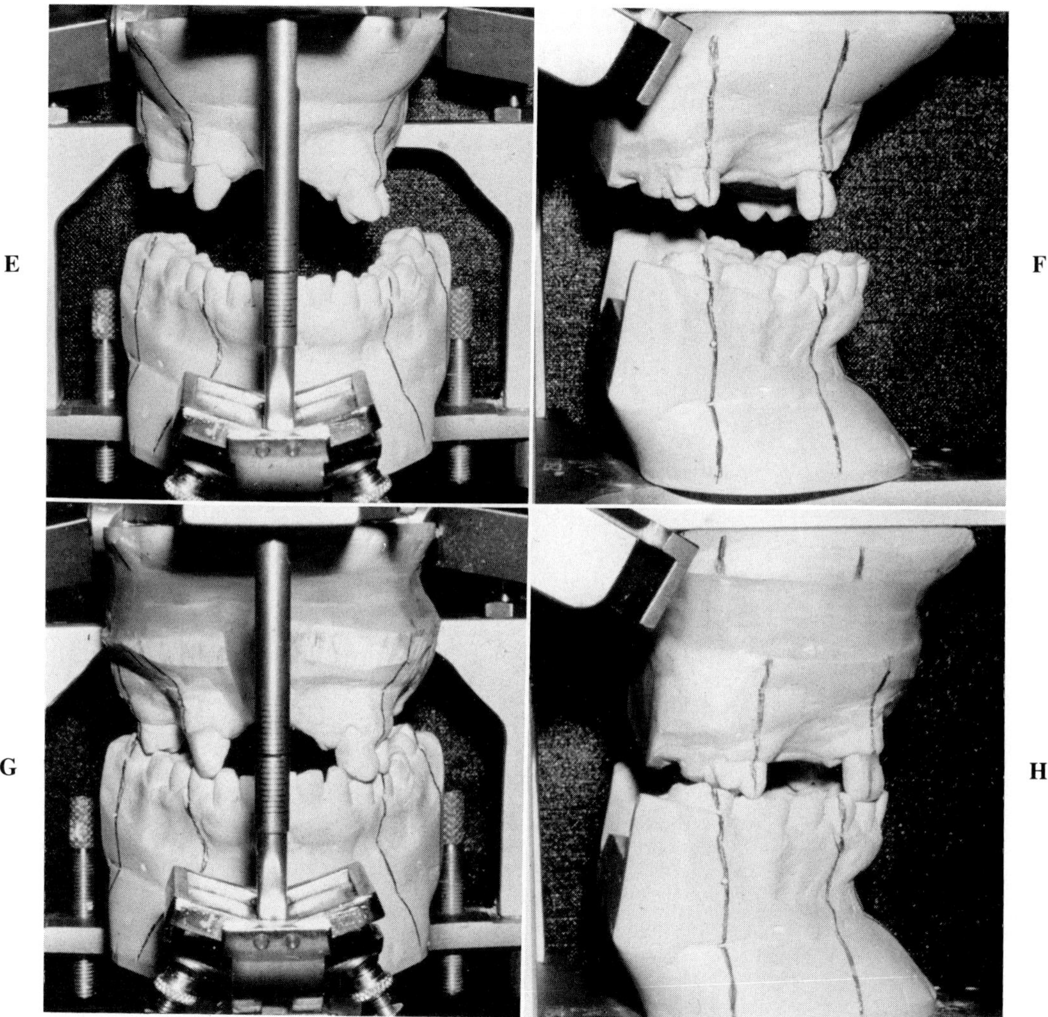

Fig. 6-4, cont'd. E to H.

Continued.

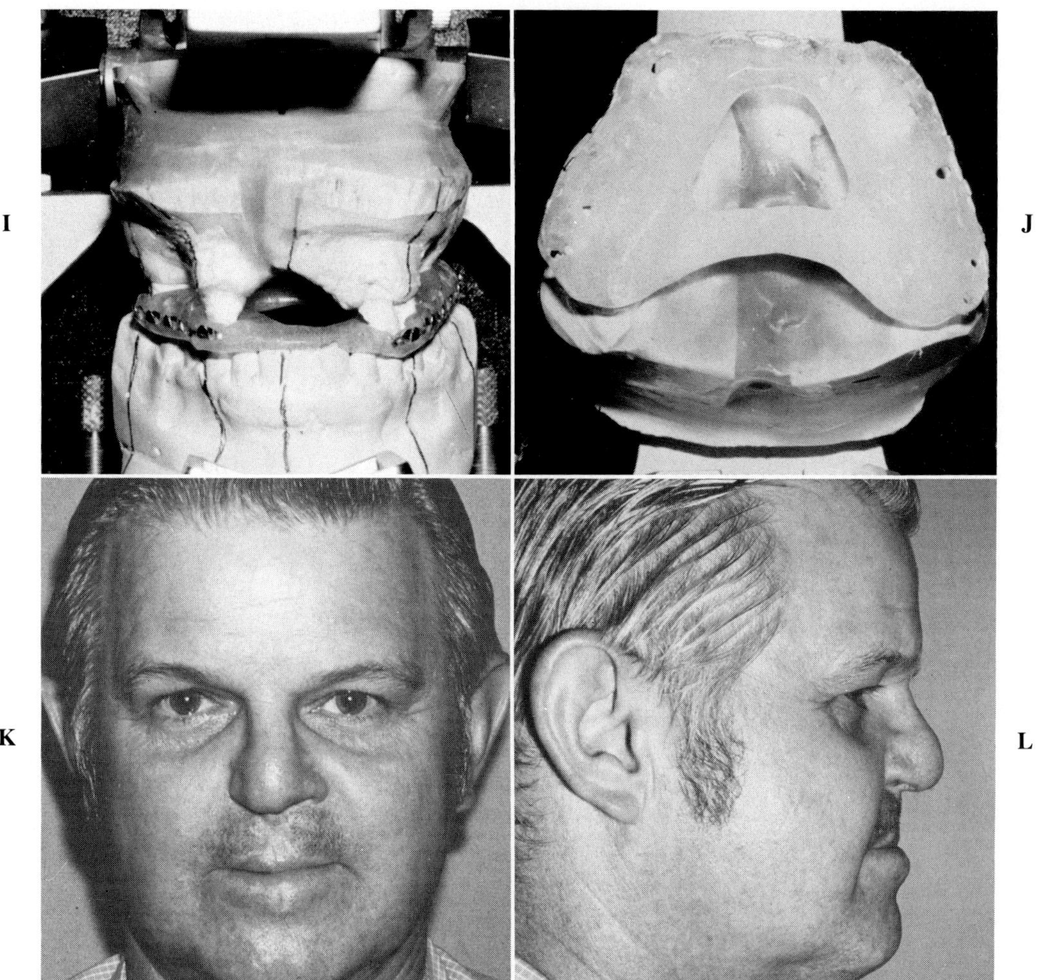

Fig. 6-4, cont'd. I to L.

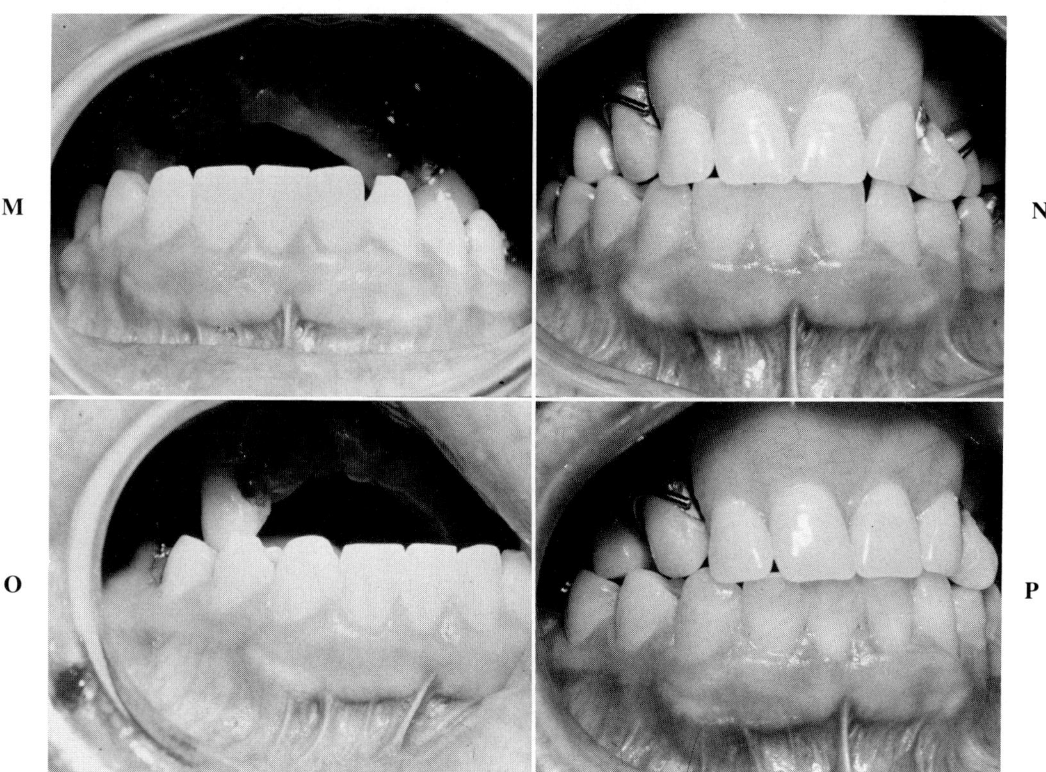

Fig. 6-4, cont'd. M to **P.**

Form F. Quantitative guide for surgical-prosthetic patients

Previous prosthetic history

Favorable ____

Unfavorable ___ ✓ (Esthetically) _______________________

None ____

Esthetic facial evaluation

Frontal objectives ___ Decrease exposure and
prominence of upper teeth

Profile objectives ___ Decrease lip prominence

Cephalometric evaluation

Anteroposterior jaw (ridge) disharmonies

Class III	1	2	3	(4)	5
Class II	1	2	3	4	5

Vertical jaw disharmonies

Excessive interarch distances	1	2	3	4	5
Insufficient interarch distances	1	2	3	(4)	5

Dental model evaluation

Transverse jaw disharmonies

Buccal cross-bite	1	2	3	4	(5)
Lingual cross-bite	1	2	3	4	5

Maxillary ridge disharmonies

Size of ridge	1	2	3	4	5
Labiobuccal vestibule	1	2	3	4	5
Palatal depth	1	2	3	4	5
Bony irregularities	1	2	3	4	5
Soft tissue disorders	1	2	3	4	5

Mandibular ridge disharmonies

Size of ridge	1	2	3	4	5
Labiobuccal vestibule	1	2	3	4	5
Floor of mouth	1	2	3	4	5
Bony irregularities	1	2	3	4	5
Soft tissue disorders	1	2	3	4	5

TMJ evaluation

Abnormal movements ___ None _______________________

Symptoms ___ None ________________________________

Signs ___ None __________________________________

Probable diagnosis ________________________________

CASE 4 (Fig. 6-5)

A and **B,** Pretreatment facial views. **C,** Pretreatment cephalometric tracing. **D** to **F,** Pretreatment occlusion.

Treatment plan

Segmental superior repositioning of the maxilla and anterior mandibular subapical ostectomy. Construction of new partial denture prostheses.

G to **I,** Model surgery. **J** and **K,** Posttreatment facial views **L,** Composite pre- and posttreatment cephalometric tracings. **M** and **N,** Pre- and posttreatment occlusion.

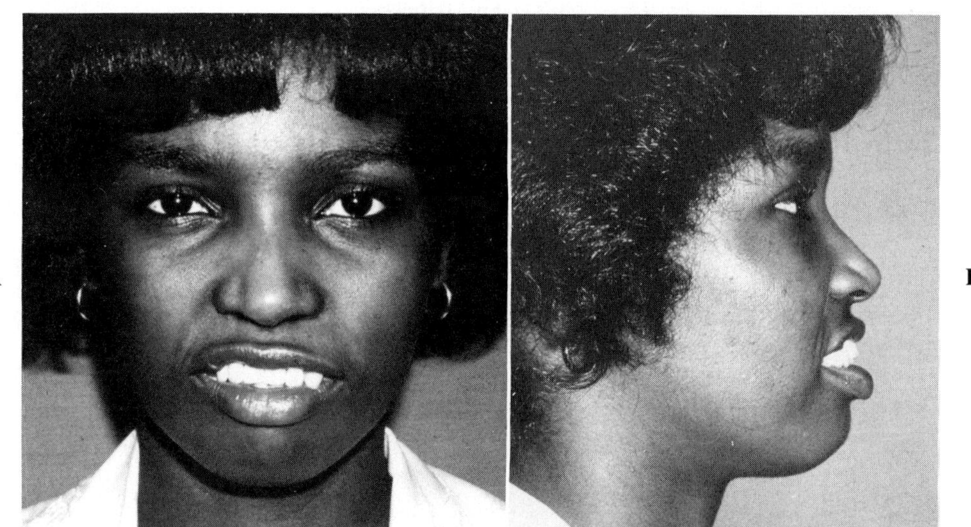

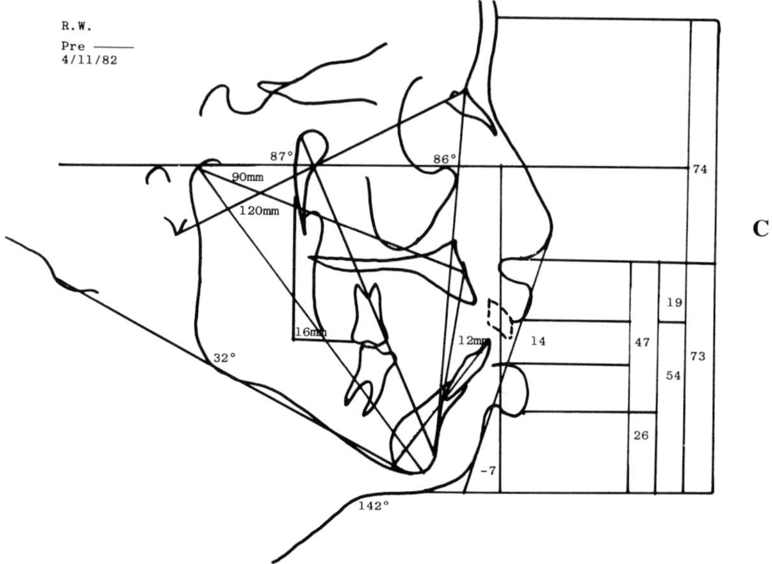

Fig. 6-5, A, B, and **C.**

Continued.

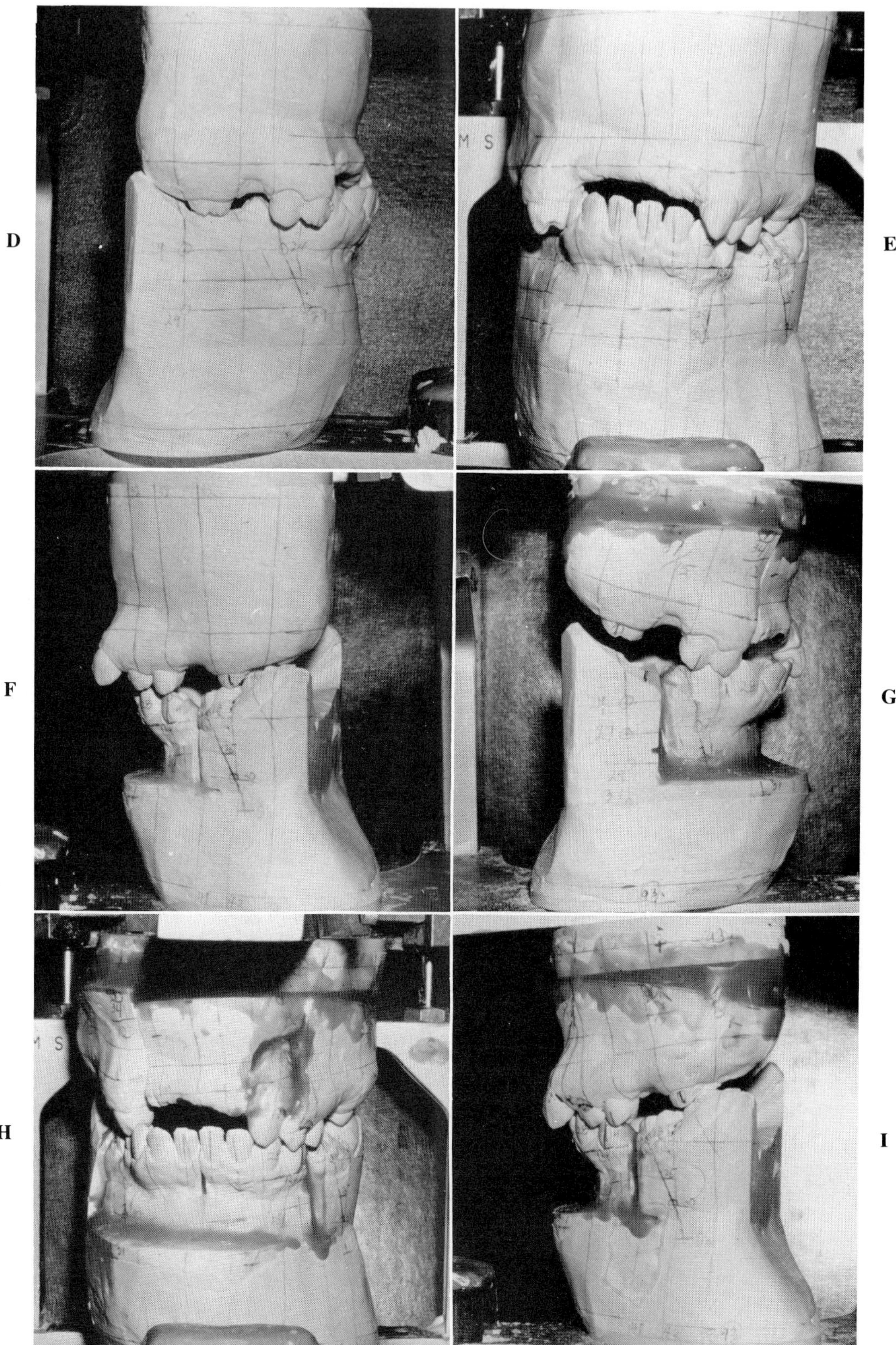

Fig. 6-5, cont'd. D to **I.**

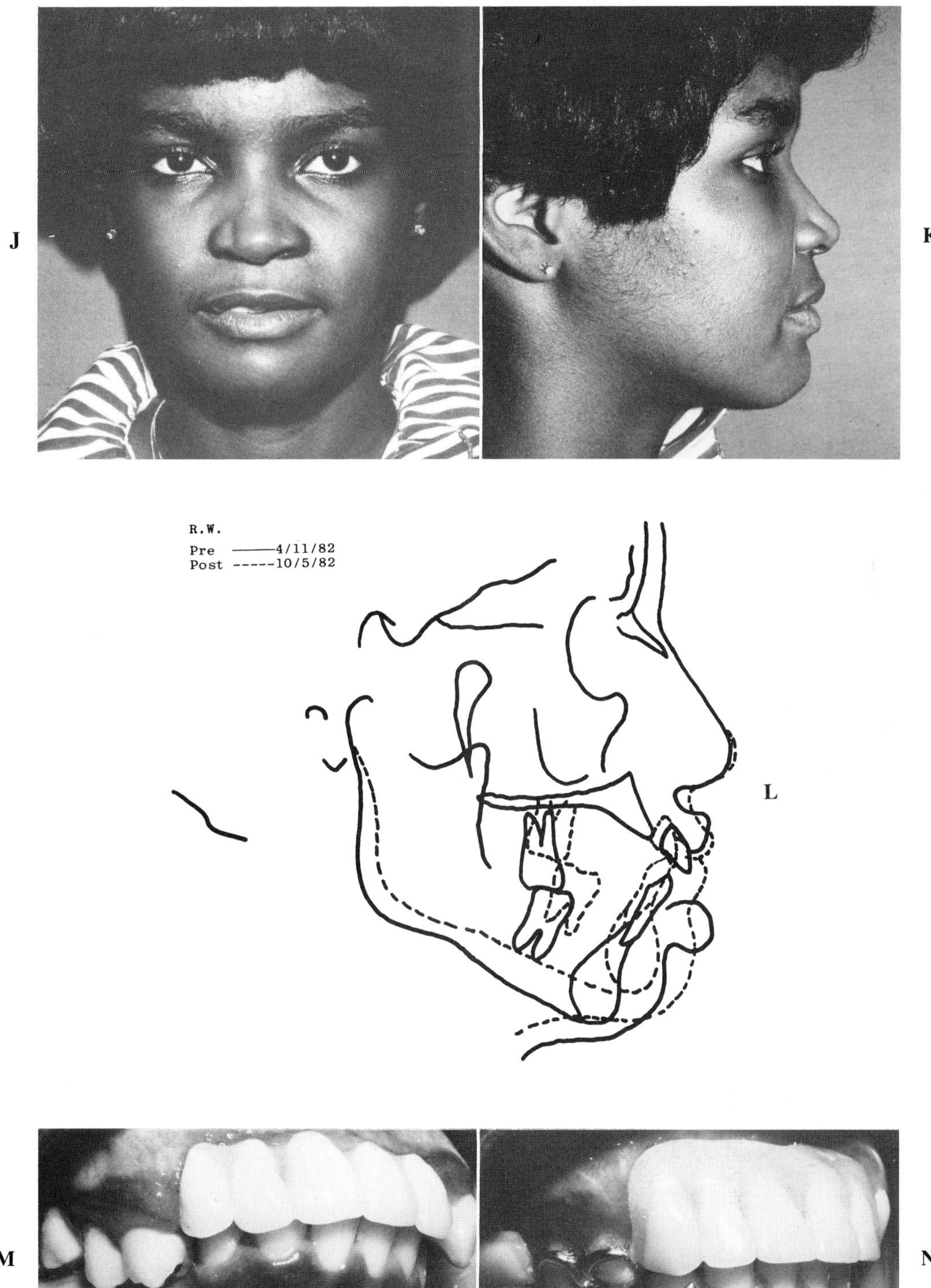

Fig. 6-5, cont'd. J to N.

Form F. Quantitative guide for surgical-prosthetic patients

Previous prosthetic history

Favorable _______✓_______________________________________

Unfavorable ____

None ____

Esthetic facial evaluation

Frontal objectives _*Increase fullness upper lip, decrease promi-*_
*nence chin, decrease wrinkles in upper lip*

Profile objectives _*Decrease prominence chin*_
____

Cephalometric evaluation

Anteroposterior jaw (ridge) disharmonies

Class III	1	2	3	(4)	5
Class II	1	2	3	4	5

Vertical jaw disharmonies

Excessive interarch distances	1	2	3	(4)	5
Insufficient interarch distances	1	2	3	4	5

Dental model evaluation

Transverse jaw disharmonies

Buccal cross-bite	1	2	3	4	5
Lingual cross-bite	1	2	(3)	4	5

Maxillary ridge disharmonies

Size of ridge	1	2	3	4	5
Labiobuccal vestibule	1	2	3	4	5
Palatal depth	1	2	3	4	5
Bony irregularities	1	2	3	4	5
Soft tissue disorders	1	2	3	4	5

Mandibular ridge disharmonies

Size of ridge	1	2	(3)	4	5
Labiobuccal vestibule	1	2	3	(4)	5
Floor of mouth	1	2	3	(4)	5
Bony irregularities	1	2	3	4	5
Soft tissue disorders	1	2	3	4	5

TMJ evaluation

Abnormal movements _None______________________________
____

Symptoms _____None________________________________
____

Signs _______None_________________________________
____

Probable diagnosis _______________________________________
____

CASE 5 (Fig. 6-6)

A and **B,** Pretreatment facial views. **C,** Pretreatment cephalometric tracing.

Treatment plan

Inferoanterior repositioning of the maxilla with interpositional autogenous bone graft. Mandibular staple implant. Posterior mandibular ridge augmentation with hydroxyapatite. Maxillary and mandibular full denture prostheses.

D and **E,** Model surgery to advance and inferiorly reposition the maxilla. **F** and **G,** Posttreatment facial views. **H,** Composite pre- and posttreatment cephalometric tracings. **I** and **J,** Pre- and posttreatment mandibular staple implant. **K** and **L,** Posttreatment occlusion.

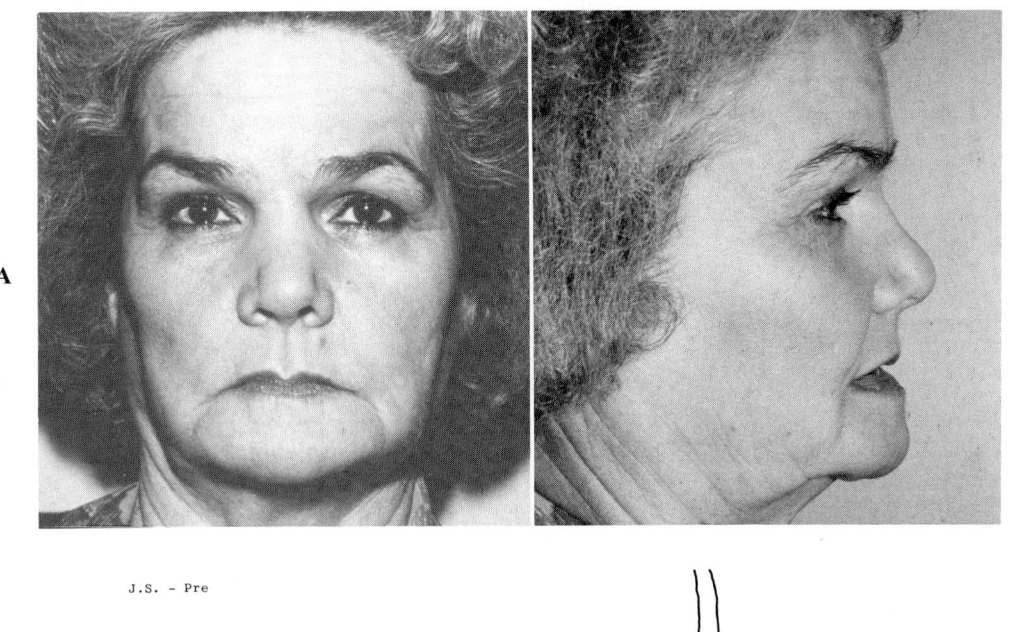

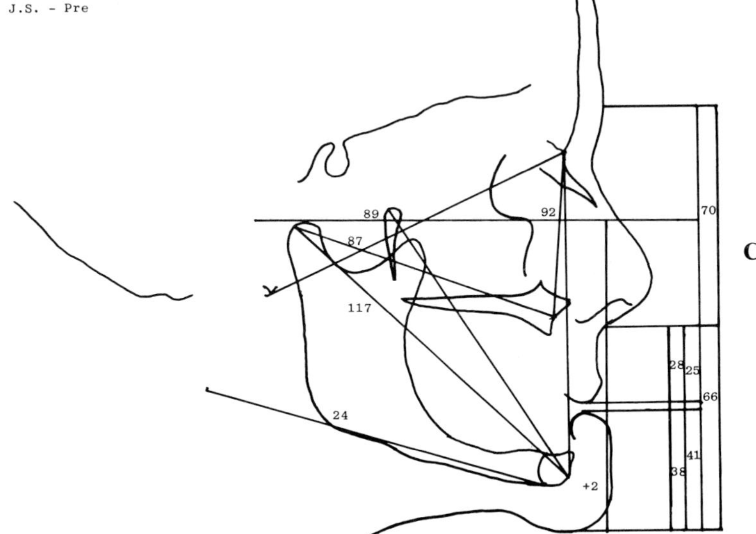

Fig. 6-6, A, B, and **C.**

Continued.

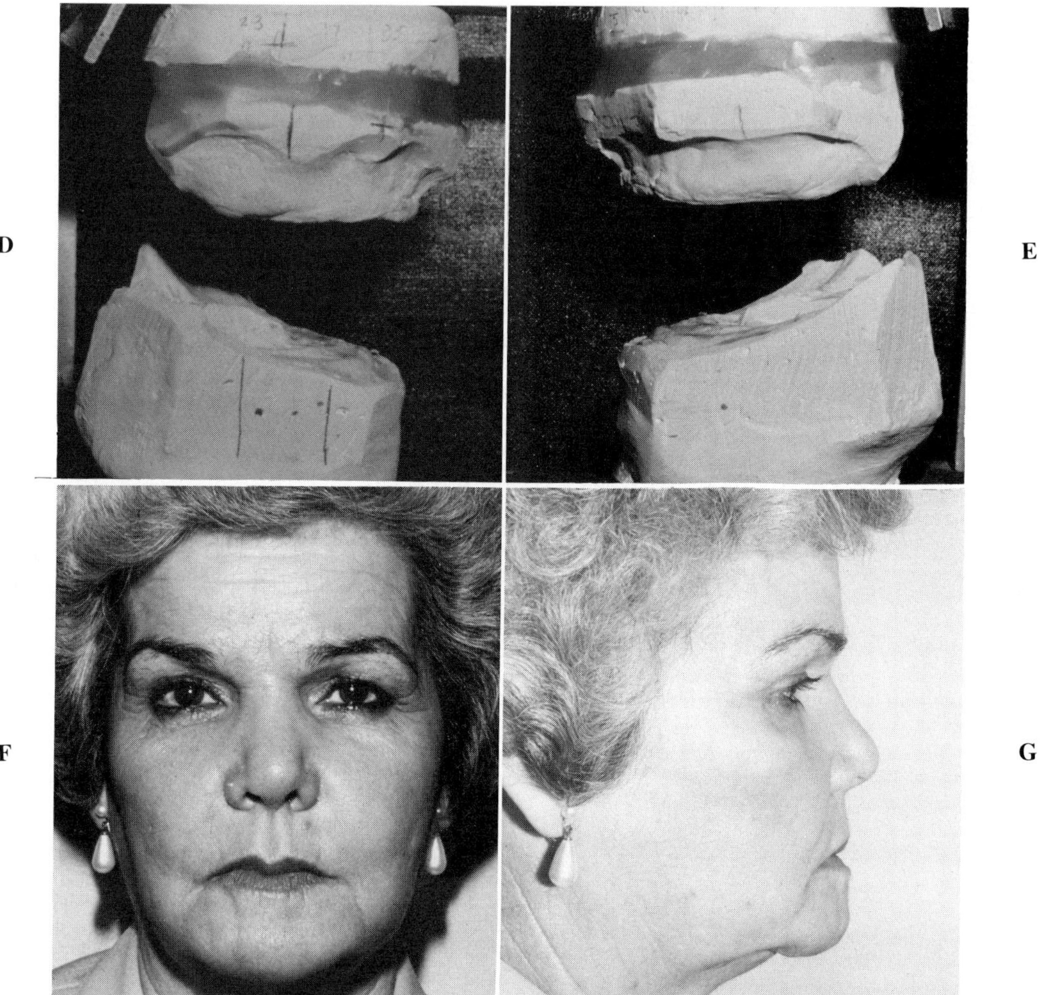

Fig. 6-6, cont'd. D to G.

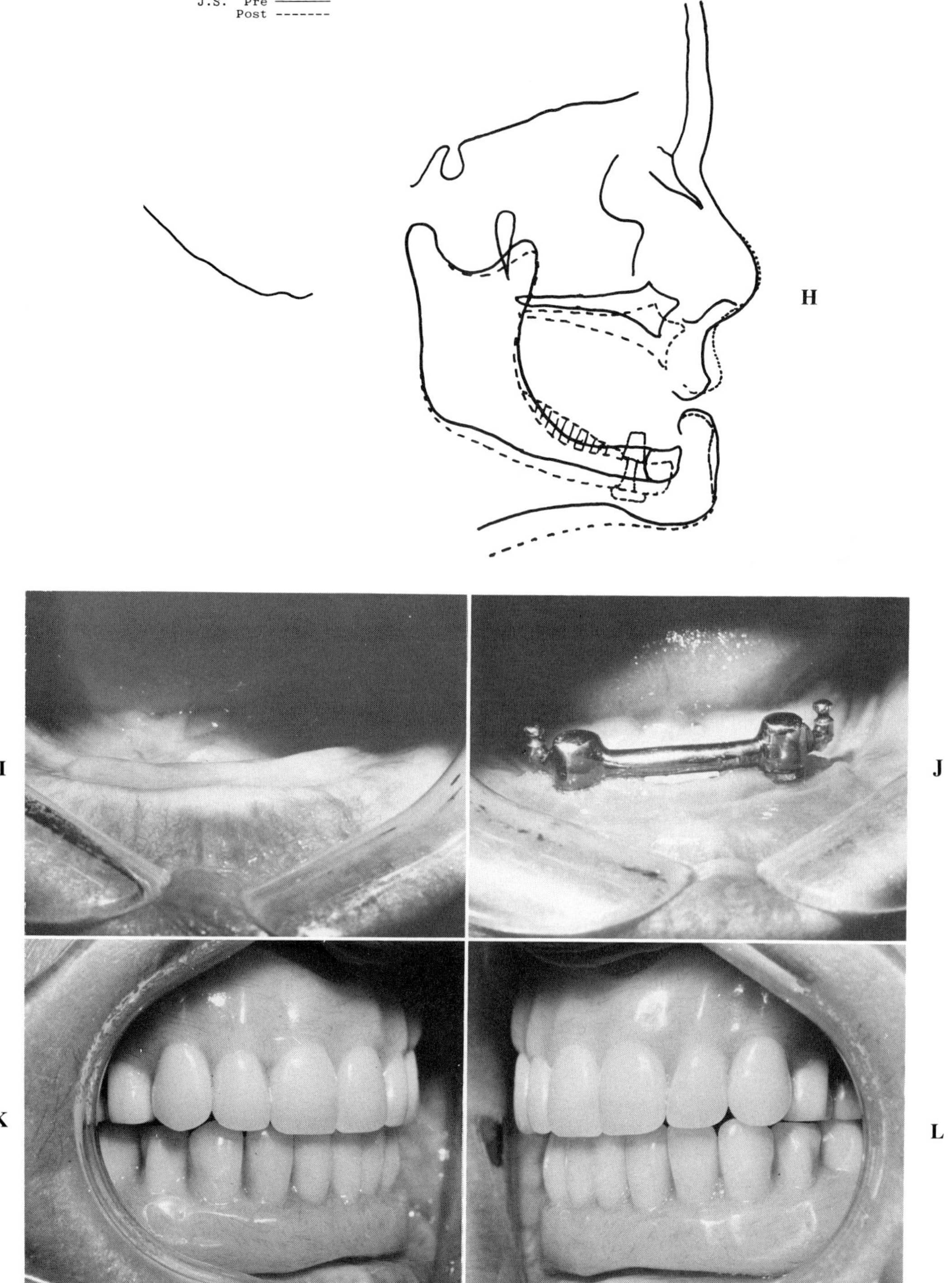

Fig. 6-6, cont'd. H to **L.**

CONCLUSIONS

A systematic approach utilizing a quantitative index for diagnosing and treatment planning the surgical-prosthetic patient has been presented. It helps to pinpoint deficiencies or disharmonies and, in an objective fashion, places a numerical value on their severity.

It, furthermore, initiates cooperation between the reconstructive dentist and the oral and maxillofacial surgeon—placing responsibility for treatment planning on the reconstructive dentist, who will be responsible for constructing the dental prosthesis from the relationships achieved by surgery. Nevertheless, it allows the surgeon to decide specifically how to achieve these prosthetic objectives, utilizing his technical expertise.

RECOMMENDED READINGS

1. Babbush, C.: Surgical atlas of dental implant techniques, Philadelphia, 1980, W.B. Saunders Co.
2. Burstone, C.J.: Lip posture and its significance in treatment planning, Am. J. Orthod. **53:**262, 1967.
3. Dolwick, M.F., et al.: Arthrotomographic evaluation of the temporomandibular joint, J. Oral Surg. **37:**793, 1970.
4. Epker, B.N., and Fish, L.C.: Dentofacial deformities: an integrated orthodontic-surgical atlas, St. Louis, 1985, The C.V. Mosby Co.
5. Fish, L.C., and Epker, B.N.: Diagnosis and treatment planning for the correction of dentofacial deformities, Fort Worth, 1981, Published by the authors.
6. Goldstein, R.E.: Esthetics in dentistry, Philadelphia, 1976, J.B. Lippincott Co.
7. Gugino, C.F.: An orthodontic philosophy, Denver, 1977, Rocky Mountain/Communications.
8. Heintz, W.D.: Removal partial orthodontics. Symposium on common failures in removable partial prosthodontics, Dent. Clin. North Am., vol. 23, no. 1, 1979.
9. Henderson, D., et al.: McCracken's removable partial prosthodontics, ed. 7, St. Louis, 1985, The C.V. Mosby Co.
10. Hulsey, C.M.: An esthetic evaluation of lip-teeth relationships present in the smile, Am. J. Orthod. **73:**132, 1970.
11. Masello, R., and Mercier, P.: Surgical and prosthodontic reconstruction of the severely handicapped edentulous patient, J. Prosthet. Dent. **50:**377, 1983.
12. Ricketts, R.M.: Esthetics, environment, and the law of lip relation, Am. J. Orthod. **54:**4, 1968.
13. Starshak, T.J., and Sanders, B.: Preprosthetic oral and maxillofacial surgery, St. Louis, 1980, The C.V. Mosby Co.
14. Wessberg, G., et al.: Preprosthetic management of severe alveolar ridge atrophy, J. Am. Dent. Assoc. **104:**464, 1982.

CHAPTER 7

Reconstruction of the maxillary alveolar cleft palate

H. ANTHONY NEAL

As we approach this area of residual alveolar cleft palate, it is necessary to have some knowledge of the entire complex of developmental defects associated with the cleft lip and cleft palate patient. All too often we fail to appreciate the tremendous handicap experienced by the person with cleft lip and cleft palate. The ability to have an acceptable appearance and speech apparatus is essential to achieving one's full potential in the world. Persons with these acceptable features may find it easy to forget their value. Our face is the way the world recognizes us at first glance, and it usually produces the first impressions on other people. When these facial features and the vocal apparatus are distorted, it can be a cruel and at times tremendous handicap.

Clefts of the lip and palate certainly constitute such a handicap. Clefts are the most common of orofacial deformities. More than a quarter-million people living in the United States today were born with a cleft lip, a cleft palate, or both.[24] The incidence of cleft lip and palate is one in every 600 to 700 births among whites, less among blacks (1 in every 2000).[24] Most persons who receive comprehensive treatment today are able to move into society and recognize their full potential.

The history of surgical repair of the cleft lip and palate dates to antiquity. The earliest reports come from a Chinese surgeon who successfully repaired a cleft lip in 390 A.D. One of the early successful repairs of a cleft palate was performed by Le Monnier, a dentist, in 1776.[90] Development of refinements in surgical treatment has led to a long list of procedures carrying the name of the surgeon—von Graefe,[110] Roux,[94] Mirault,[68] Dieffenbach,[28] von Langenbeck,[111] Hagedorn,[41] Veau,[109] Dorrance,[31] Wardill,[115] Le Mesurier,[58] and Millard.[66]

True expertise in oral and maxillofacial surgery and plastic surgery was late developing, with little prior to 1940. Before this time most of these surgical procedures were carried out by general surgeons who had little experience in working with the demanding environment of the oral cavity. This is an extremely difficult area within which to operate, especially in the cleft lip and palate patient in whom the anatomy has been distorted secondary to the developmental anomaly. Surgical intervention at the wrong time or too extensively can, as we know now, result in more damage to the growth centers and can make the establishment of normal mastication, swallowing, and speech impossible. Graber[39] was the first to call attention (in 1949) to the fact that surgery was a principal cause of the more severe defects seen in children with cleft lip and palate. This stimulated much controversy; and as Ross and Johnston[93] point out, "The result has been a tremendous interest in facial growth and development."

D. Bolinsky did the illustrations of the cleft deformities for this chapter.

The problem with this approach, however, is that it takes many years of follow-up to discover the defect in early surgical intervention as it relates to growth. It is imperative that those involved in the treatment of cleft lip and palate be willing to extend follow-up on their patients for long periods to determine the actual success of their reconstructive procedures. Anytime we do surgical procedures close to the centers of growth, we may be deceived with an early successful surgical repair but a long-term failure as we retrospectively look at growth and development. Much knowledge has been gained in the areas of growth and development and surgical technique in the treatment of the cleft lip and palate patient. However, we must guard against past mistakes.

The cleft lip and palate deformity represents a wide range of defects—from notching of the lip to bilateral complete cleft lip and palate (Fig. 7-1). The deformity carries with it a complexity not found in many other deformities. Because of this, in many centers a team approach to the problem has developed. One of the first clinics with such a treatment concept was the Lancaster Cleft Palate Clinic (Lancaster, Pennsylvania), which was started in 1938 by Dr. Herbert K. Cooper, a dentist with vision and concern for patients with this crippling deformity. Rehabilitation of the patient with cleft lip and palate requires consideration of the appearance, speech, occlusion, mastication, hearing, and deglutition as well as the emotional and social well-being of the child. To meet these many requirements, there must be a wide variety of disciplines involved in the decision-making process. An oral and maxillofacial surgeon, plastic surgeon, pediatrician, prostho-

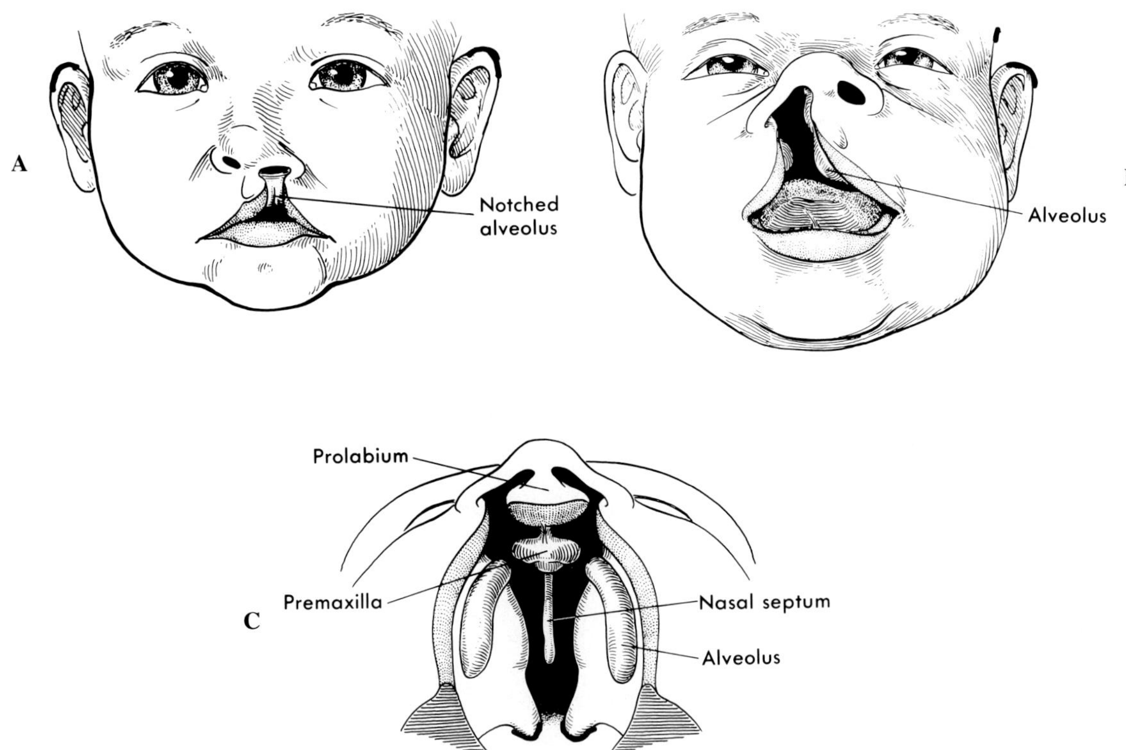

Fig. 7-1.
Range of defects. **A,** Simple notching of the alveolus. **B,** Unilateral complete cleft lip and palate. **C,** Bilateral complete cleft lip and palate.
Reprinted from Smith, H.: The atlas of cleft lip and cleft palate surgery, New York, 1983, Grune & Stratton, Inc.

dontist, orthodontist, general dentist, otolaryngologist, speech pathologist, audiologist, radiologist and geneticist as well as the social worker should all be included.

Generally the lip closure is accomplished at 1 to 3 weeks of age. If there is concern about other congenital problems, however, many surgeons will use the "rule of ten" as a guide. At this time the child has reached a body weight of 10 pounds and 10 weeks of age and has a hemoglobin count of 10 g with a white cell count of less than 10,000. Numerous techniques are advocated for lip closure, but their consideration is outside the scope of this chapter. The hard and soft palates are generally closed between 18 and 24 months. There is controversy as to staging of this procedure, with closure of the soft palate to be followed at a later date by hard palate closure.[46,82] Other authors* favor closure of both the soft and the hard palate simultaneously. The goals of the closure are as follows:

1. To help the child speak more clearly. This can be accomplished best if the closure is completed before the child's speech patterns develop. Also, to speak clearly requires a soft palate that is movable and of adequate length to gain a posterior pharyngeal seal.
2. To reestablish the palatal eustachian tube function.
3. To bring about normal dental and oral appearance and function.

Along with advances in surgical technique have come new diagnostic modalities, such as cineradiography and nasopharyngoscopy,[77] to aid in the diagnosis of velopharyngeal insufficiency, but these will not be discussed in further detail at this time. Approximately 25% of all clefts involve the alveolus or prepalate. Another 25% involve a portion or all of the palate. The remaining 50% represent a combination of alveolar and palatal clefts; and since these constitute 75% of all cleft deformities involving the alveolar or prepalatal segment, it is the purpose of this chapter to discuss their reconstruction.

---

*References 102, 108, 112.

DESCRIPTION OF THE DEFORMITY
Embryology

Some general statements can be related to the embryologic basis of the deformity, but much knowledge is still missing. The congenital defect of the cleft lip or cleft palate is established by the eighth week in utero.[78] There are many theories about its development.[36,84] It is believed to be due to failure of either mesodermal fusion or mesodermal penetration of the involved palatal and nasal processes. Failure of mesodermal penetration seems more likely at present. Even though the timing of the development of the defect is generally agreed on, the etiology remains obscure. Many medications have been shown to produce clefts in rats and have been implicated in humans.[30,95] Cortisone is one such medication, but no review has been able to show a causal relation.[116] It appears that a single factor cannot be attributed to the causation of cleft palate although hope continues that methods of prevention will in the future be developed. Environmental factors have also been suggested but, again, without clear evidence.

Incidence

The incidence of cleft lip and cleft palate varies with race: Orientals show the highest incidence (1.61 per 1000), whites are intermediate (0.90 per 1000), and American blacks the lowest (0.31 per 1000).[24(p. 113)] There are sex differences also. The ratios differ for various clefts. More boys are born with the combination of cleft lip and palate, and boys tend to have more severe defects when large numbers of cases are reviewed. Girls are more often afflicted with an isolated cleft palate. Meskin et al.[65] offer an interesting explanation of this variation. They suggest that there is a difference in the developmental time sequence between males and females, with males being more mature at any one moment in embryogenesis. If this is true and the teratogenic insult is transient, then the defect would have different presentations in boys and girls. Another interesting finding is that more clefts occur on the left than on the right.[24 (p.117)] There is also an increased incidence of associated abnormalities in the cleft lip and palate patient. Between 10% and

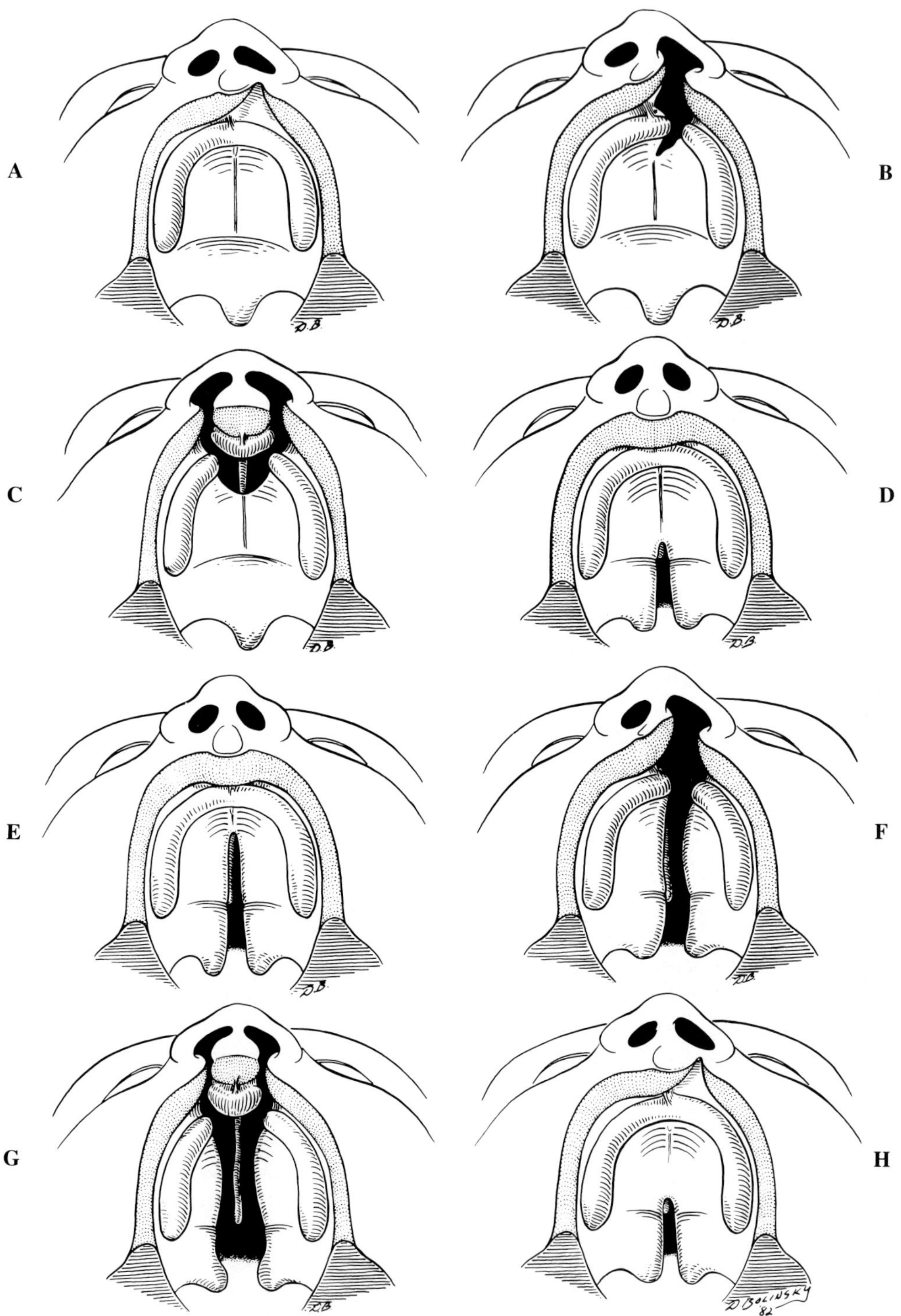

Fig. 7-2.
For legend see opposite page.

25% have abnormalities of other organ systems.[24 (p. 120)] Gorlin et al.[37,38] and Curtis[26] have reviewed this and they suggest close examination of these patients prior to surgery for associated defects.

Patients with a cleft lip and palate or parents with a child who has such deformity share a concern for the probability that the defect will be present in additional children. We are often called on to give advice in these areas. The statistics vary with each defect and with the presentation within the specific family. If both parents are normal and the first child is affected with a cleft lip with or without a cleft of the palate, the chances of the next child's being affected are 4%. If both parents are normal and they have two children with cleft lip with or without cleft palate, the chances of the next child's having the same deformity increase to 9%. If one parent has a cleft lip or cleft palate with no affected children, the chances of the next child's having a defect are 4%. If there is an affected child, the chances are 17%. If one parent has a cleft palate, the chances that the next child will be affected are 6% if there are no affected children; however, they increase to 15% if there is an affected child.

Classification

Several classifications exist for describing the cleft deformity. One, the Veau method,[109] divides the defect into clefts of the soft palate only, soft palate plus hard palate but not the alveolus, unilateral complete through the alveolus, and bilateral complete through the alveolus. A more comprehensive classification is presented by Kernahan and Stark[50] (Fig. 7-2).

Diagnostic features

Clefts of the alveolus can range from unilateral to bilateral and can have varying presenta-tions from simple notching of the alveolus (Fig. 7-3, *A*) to severe unilateral or bilateral complete cleft (Fig. 7-3, *B* and *C*). After closure of the hard and soft palates the residual alveolar cleft does not usually cause any severe problems early on. However, as the patient matures and the maxilla begins to show continued growth, the related problems become more noticeable and can contribute significantly to the difficulty of future surgical, orthodontic, or prosthetic treatment for this patient.

If the typical unilateral cleft (Figs. 7-4 and 7-5, *A*) extends into the nasal cavity, the patient will exhibit a flattening of the nasal bones and lower lateral and alar cartilages. This flatness is due in part to deflection toward the noncleft side but also to the deficiency of the maxilla on the cleft side. The columella is displaced to the noncleft side. The anterior nasal spine is deviated to the noncleft side and is more prominent in the buccal vestibule on the unaffected side. This position also contributes to the displacement of the columella.

Since there is no bony support along the alveolus, the posterior segment generally presents in malocclusion. The most common finding is a lingual cross-bite involving the posterior segment on the involved side. This segment is mobile to varying degrees and can usually be moved with digital pressure. The adjacent anterior teeth are often rotated superiorly into the labial defect. This causes the patient numerous difficulties in maintenance of proper oral hygiene. As a result rampant caries is not unusual in these patients. Congenitally missing anterior teeth are common, with the lateral incisor on the cleft side being the most often involved. Supernumerary teeth are also frequent in the area of the cleft. The decision regarding removal of these teeth should be made in consul-

Text continued on p. 239.

Fig. 7-2.
Classification: **A,** left incomplete cleft of the primary palate; **B,** left complete cleft of the primary palate; **C,** bilateral complete cleft of the primary palate; **D,** incomplete cleft of the secondary palate; **E,** complete cleft of the secondary palate; **F,** left complete cleft of the primary and secondary palate; **G,** bilateral complete cleft of the primary and secondary palates; **H,** left incomplete cleft of the primary palate and incomplete cleft of the secondary palate.
Reprinted from Smith, H.: The atlas of cleft lip and cleft palate surgery, New York, 1983, Grune & Stratton, Inc.

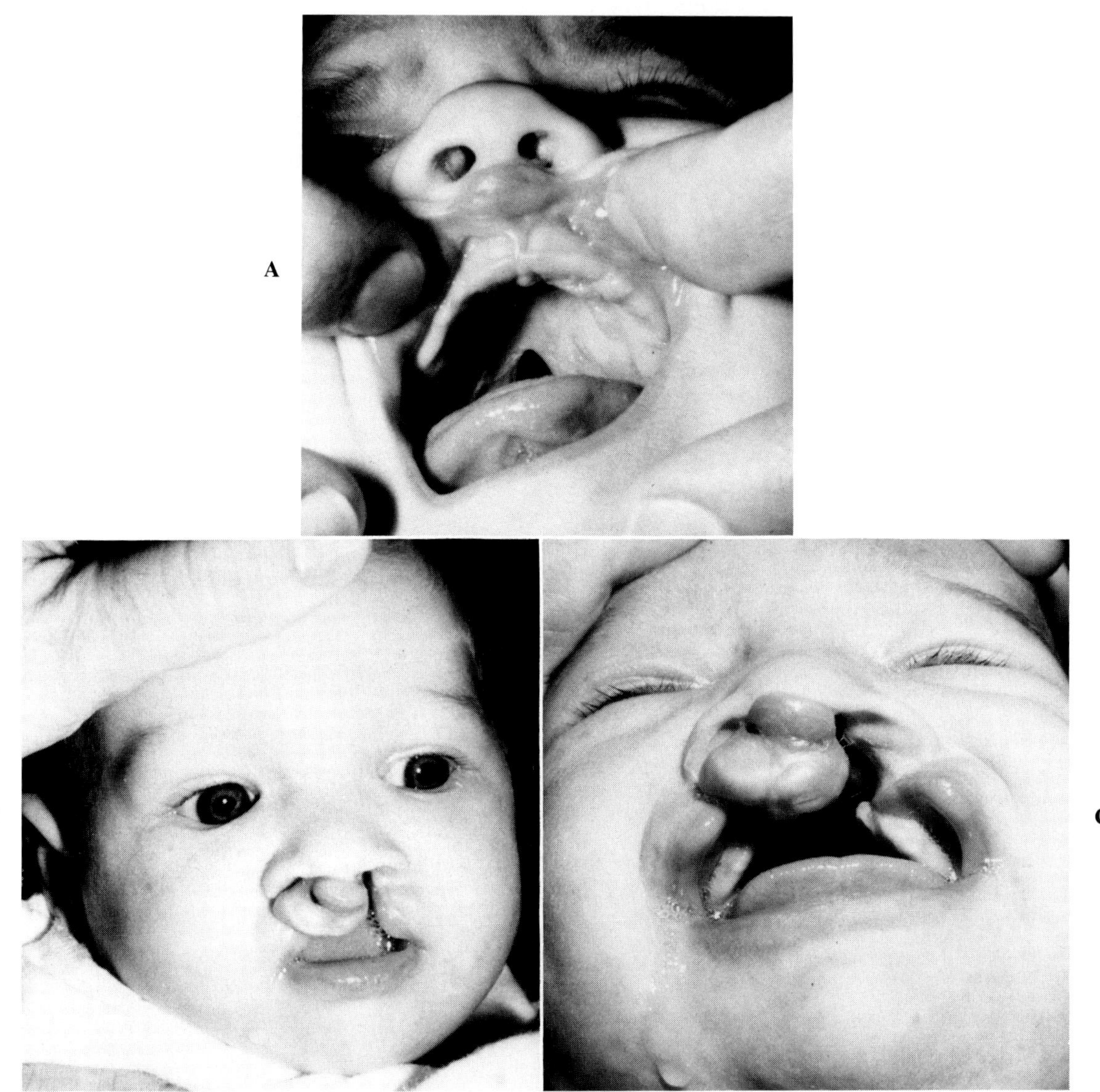

Fig. 7-3.
Clinical range of defects. **A,** Notching of the lip and secondary palate. **B,** Bilateral complete cleft of the lip and palate. **C,** Severe protrusion of the premaxilla and prolabium in a bilateral complete cleft lip and palate.

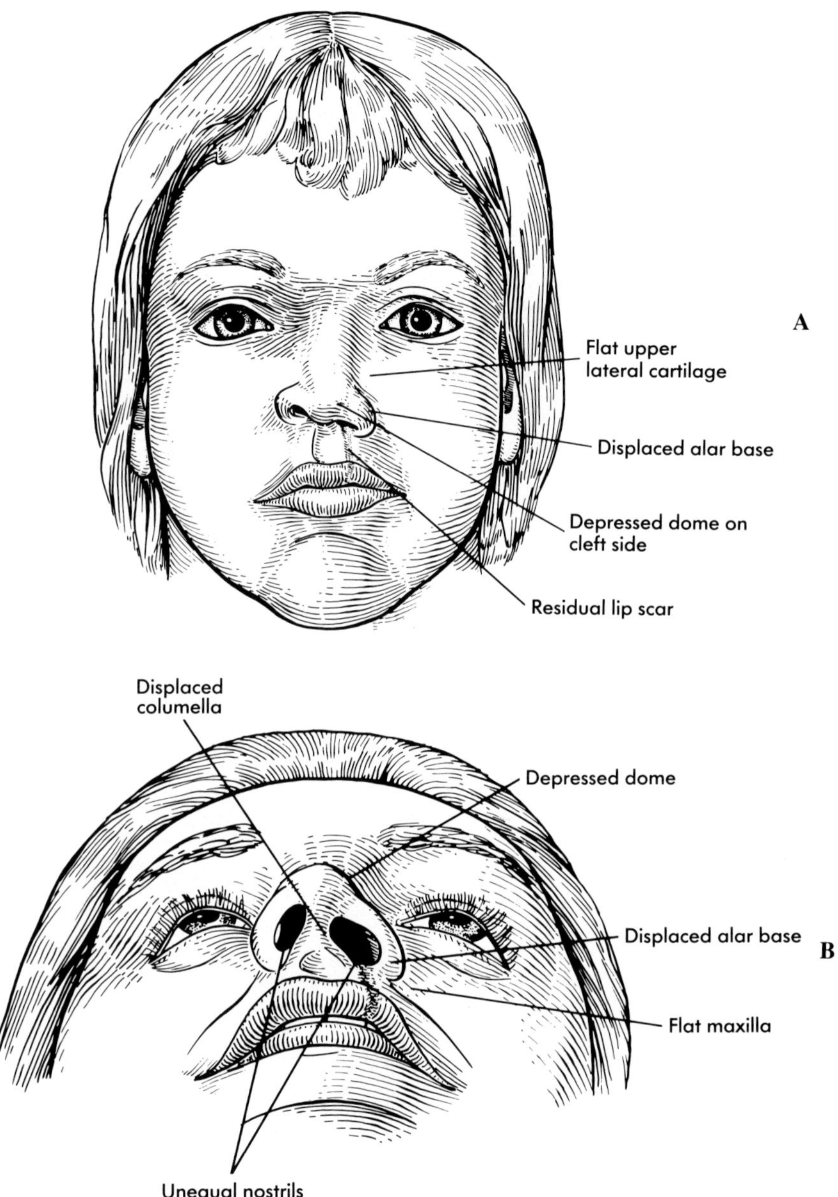

Fig. 7-4.
Facial features. **A,** Frontal and, **B,** basilar view.
Reprinted from Smith, H.: The atlas of cleft lip and cleft palate surgery, New York, 1983, Grune & Stratton, Inc.

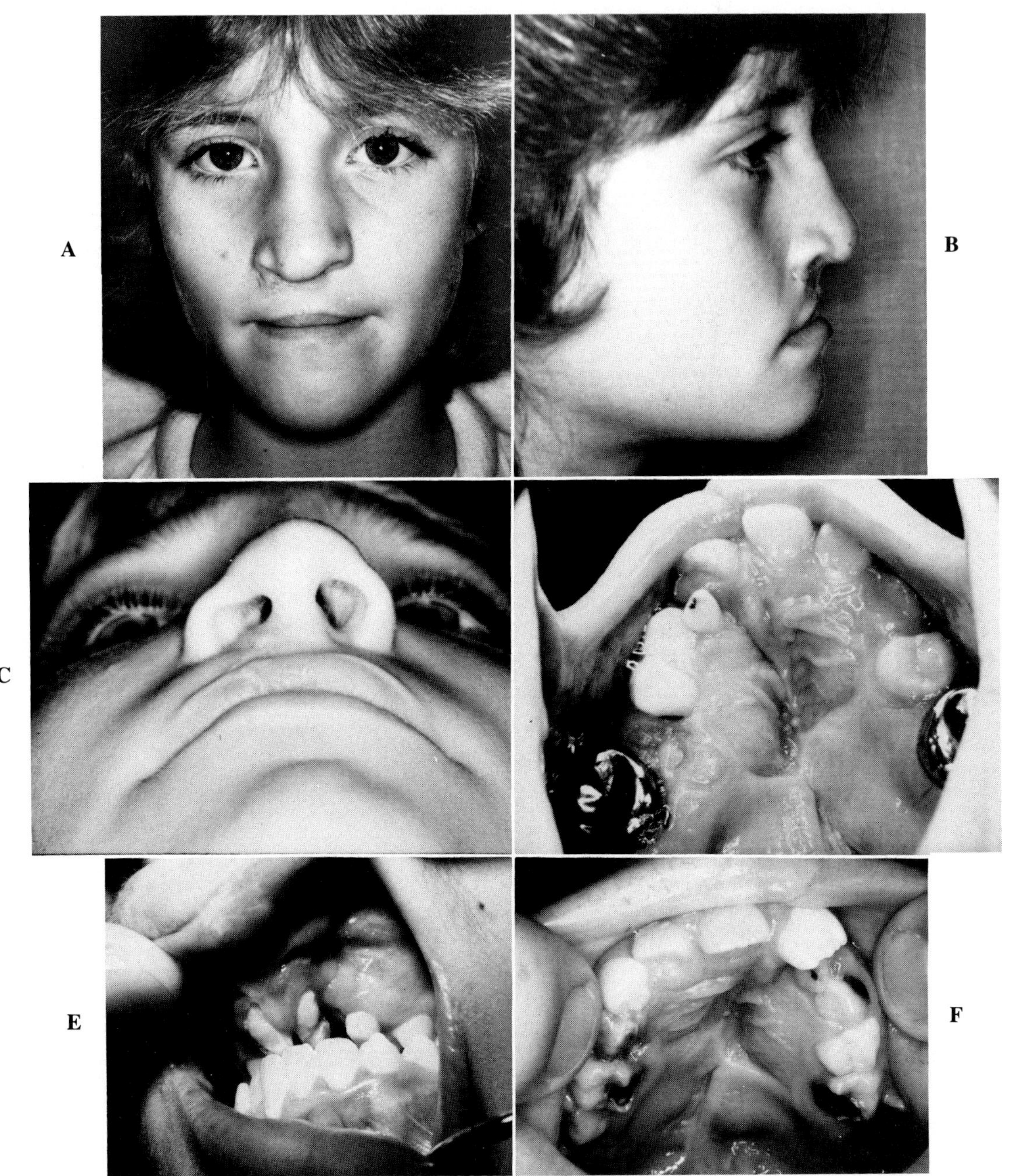

Fig. 7-5.
Diagnostic features. **A** to **C**, Facial characteristics. **D**, Collapse of the posterior segment.
E, Malposition of teeth. **F**, Dental caries.

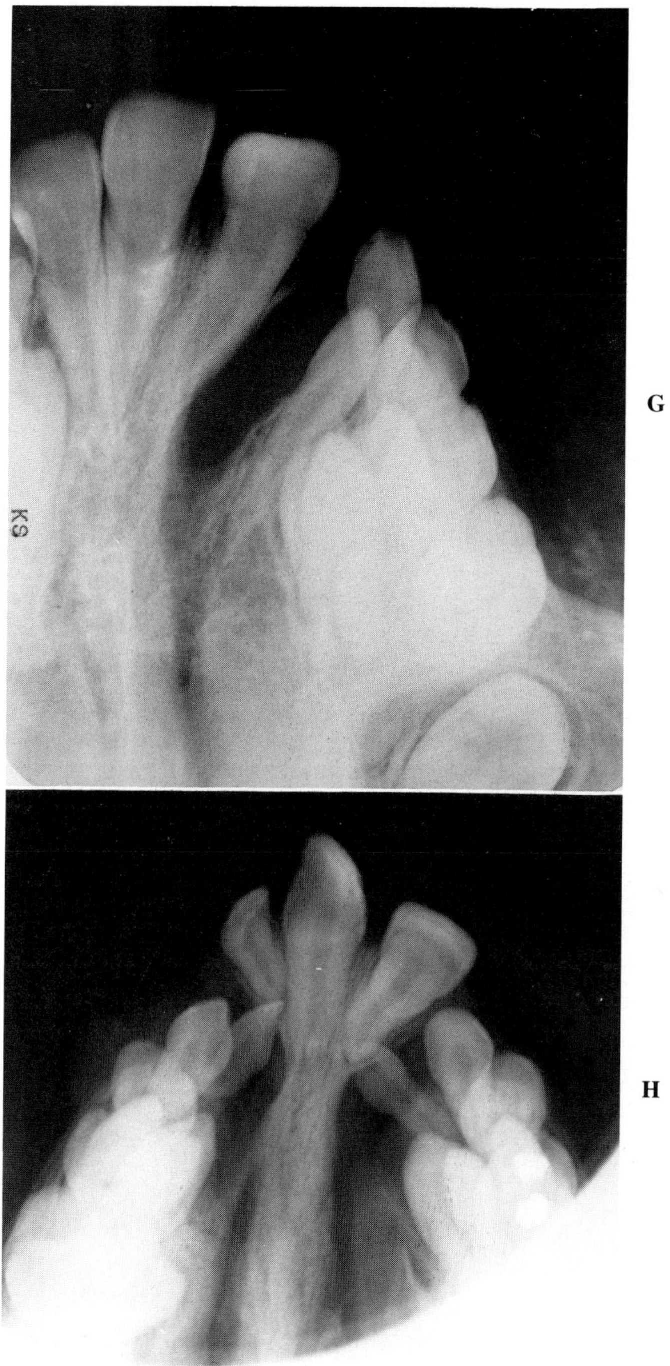

Continued.

Fig. 7-5—cont'd.
G, Lack of periodontal support. **H,** Mobile premaxillary segment.

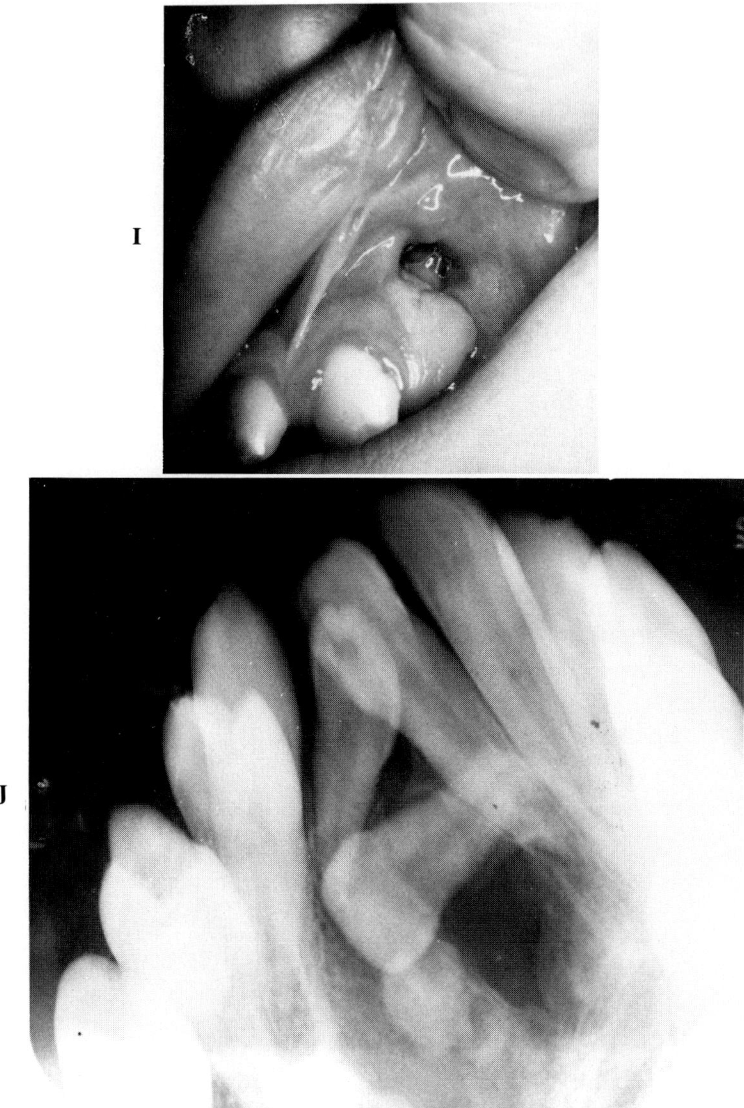

Fig. 7-5—cont'd.
I, Oronasal fistula. **J,** Rhinolith.

tation with the restorative dentist and orthodontist. If the tooth is structurally of little benefit or is in such a position as to offer little hope of being moved orthodontically into position, it should be removed. Generally such teeth are not removed until the time of the reconstructive procedure, so there will be the maximum amount of alveolar bone prior to grafting.

The permanent dentition adjacent to the cleft usually has minimal periodontal bone support. The permanent central incisor along the distal surface and the canine along its mesial aspect will have only a thin layer of bone overlying their root surfaces. The lateral incisor, if present, is generally rotated into the cleft, with often less than half its root surface covered by bone. As the canine erupts into the cleft site, there is no bone to support it. The cleft thus constitutes a chronic periodontal defect that continually worsens with time, eventually contributing to the further demise of these teeth.

The patient with a bilateral cleft lip and palate has a mobile premaxillary segment that is often severely displaced. The premaxilla is attached to the prolabium by a thin labial vestibule and to the facial skeleton only at the nasal septum. This segment is generally displaced anteriorly and inferiorly and at times shows severe linguoinclination. Since there is no attachment of the lateral palatal shelves to the vomer, bilateral collapse of the alveolar segments is present and usually results in a bilateral posterior lingual cross-bite.

The problem of mobile posterior segments is present in both the unilateral and the bilateral cleft and contributes to the generally unsatisfactory long-term prosthodontic restoration with a fixed appliance. It contributes also to further breakdown of the periodontal status of the abutment teeth along the margins of the cleft and, in addition, is a problem with removable appliances (which create further hygiene problems with the adjacent teeth and along the oronasal fistula).

The deficiency in the maxilla and the posterior segment collapse contribute to maxillary arch constriction. This deformation increases the difficulty with articulation. The narrow arch tends to restrict movement of the tongue and prevents precise articulation of certain sibilant sounds (/s/, /z/, /sh/, /ch/, /j/).

The residual oronasal fistula continues to be a problem in the cleft patient prior to closure. Normally the oral and nasal cavities are separated and perform separately their functions of mastication and deglutition along with humidification of the air and olfaction. When the two cavities communicate, neither is able to function properly or acceptably in the production of speech. Without a nasopharyngeal seal anteriorly and posteriorly, proper speech is unattainable. The soft palate normally acts as a valve to effect closure of the nasopharynx during speech. When an oronasal fistula is present, and with the increased oral pressure produced with consonant sounds, there results an abnormal and unacceptable nasal emission and hypernasality during speech. The residual fistula also contributes to hygiene problems insofar as fluids can reflux through the nose and food material can lodge within the tract. Rhinoliths in the fistulous tract are not uncommon and require removal. Additionally, crusting around the nostril secondary to chronic inflammation and secretion along the fistula is unacceptable.

CLEFT PALATE ORTHOPEDICS

There remains a great deal of controversy concerning the effectiveness and benefits of neonatal arch manipulation. The procedures were first introduced in the early 1950s by Kjellgren[54] and McNeil.[64] It is not so much whether the arches can be expanded as whether the benefits of such intervention justify the time, effort, and cost. Advocates tend to cite the normalization of feeding, improved tongue posture and swallowing, and guidance of growth of the palatal segments. Evidence seems inconclusive, however, although arguments can be developed on this side. Those who object to the procedures claim that too much clinical time is required in relation to the benefits obtained and that treatment is too complex to be carried out except in specialized clinics. Excellent reviews of this subject have been presented by Lubit[60] and Berkowitz.[6] It appears that most advocates of presurgical orthopedics have been in European countries and that it is less practiced in the United States. Hotz and Gnoinski[46] present a comprehensive plan for approaching neonatal orthopedics as performed at Zurich University over a number of years. We do not generally use maxillary orthopedics until the cleft patient is in the permanent dentition and ready for bone grafting or after the grafting is completed.

BONE GRAFTING IN THE CLEFT PALATE PATIENT
Terms

Much of the confusion associated with bone grafting in the reconstruction of residual alveolar cleft palates has to do with a consistent use of terminology. It is at times difficult to sort out the results of various studies because authors use the same term to mean an entirely different procedure. For the purposes of this chapter the following terms will be utilized to describe bone grafts[15]:

Primary When the graft material is placed in children less than 2 years of age.
Early secondary When the graft material is placed in children between ages 2 and 5.
Secondary The graft material is placed between ages 6 and 15.
Late secondary The graft material is placed in physically mature adults.

Primary bone grafting. Historically, primary bone grafting of the congenital cleft palate began in Europe. Drachter is credited with the first procedure in 1914.[83] Axhausen later reported use of bone grafting in 1952. Early primary grafting as part of the repair of cleft palates was enthusiastically endorsed in the 1950s and 1960s by many surgeons.* The advantages cited were (1) control or fixation of the maxillary arch with prevention of collapse, (2) unit growth of the maxilla with eruption and movement of teeth through the grafted material, and (3) proportional growth of the maxilla with the mandible to maintain proper dental occlusion. A wide variety of donor sites were used for these procedures. Pfeiffer and Schuchardt[83] employed autologous full-thickness rib in reconstruction of unilateral and bilateral cleft palates. Johanson and Ohlsson,[48] as well as Backdahl and Nordin,[3] utilized autogenous tibia for their primary repairs. Skoog[101] modified the technique using Surgicel between the periosteal flaps for closure and reported bone formation.

However, few surgeons were able to reproduce his results. Considerable discussion ensued and has continued on the efficacy of these procedures. Early clinical follow-up began to show less than satisfactory results, with much controversy as to the cause of failure. Pruzansky[85] was one of the first to speak out against the procedure at the 1963 American Cleft Palate Association meeting. He referred to primary bone grafting as "needless and sometimes barbaric." This was followed shortly by other unfavorable reports, the objections being related to the effect on maxillary growth. In general, these results have led to restriction of lateral maxillary growth and the development of a severe malocclusion, including cross-bite and other deformities. The results continue to be inconsistent, with some authors (Rosenstein et al.[92]) still advocating primary grafting and reporting acceptable results. Generally, however, primary grafting is not advocated at present.

Early secondary bone grafting. Review of this particular area is rather confusing, and it is difficult to evaluate the long-term reports because of variation in the technique or lack of information on the exact age at which the procedures were performed and the technique utilized. Successful grafting in the 2-to-5-year age group has been reported by Longacre.[59] Surgeons feel generally that early secondary grafting has the same advantages as mentioned for primary grafting, with the additional benefit of improving the nasal floor by prevention of distortion of the lower lateral nasal cartilages when their bases are elevated through placement of the material.

Secondary bone grafting. Most surgeons seem to agree that the optimum time for bone grafting is during the mixed dentition. In the 1970s, studies suggested that if bone grafting was delayed until the age of the mixed dentition (8 to 14 years) good function could result with less effect on growth and development. Boyne and Sands[14] in 1972 and Broude and Waite[17] in 1974 reported using iliac bone and marrow for reconstruction of alveolar cleft palate defects. Most surgeons utilizing secondary bone grafting[63,86] have in the past preferred to expand the palate prior to the grafting procedure. This primarily reflects the goal of the surgery, to "fix or

---

*References 73, 74, 96, 98.

stabilize'' the maxillary segments after orthodontic expansion, and takes a pessimistic view of the ability of the bone graft to respond to orthodontic forces.[15]

Late secondary bone grafting. With the further development of orthognathic surgery and progress in the utilization of bone grafting techniques, there has been renewed interest in the late secondary grafting in adult patients.* Many of these procedures are combined with orthognathic surgery for correction of the skeletal developmental deformity and simultaneously reconstructing the alveolar and palatal cleft defect with a bone graft.[35]

Types of bone grafts

Autogenous grafts. Autogenous bone has become the standard against which other materials are judged. Both cortical grafts and particulate cancellous marrow have been utilized for maxillofacial reconstructive and orthognathic procedures. Initially, cortical grafts were obtained from the long bones, rib, and ilium.[8,114,119] Mowlem[69,70] was the first to observe the advantages of cancellous bone over cortical bone in grafting maxillofacial defects. He specifically noted an increase in healing rate and a tolerance to infection not demonstrated by cortical grafts. It is outside the scope of this chapter to deal in depth with the numerous grafting systems available. Rather, the reader is referred to excellent treatment of the broader scope of bone grafting by Bloomquist[9] and Bays.[5]

In the reconstruction of cleft palate defects the use of autogenous rib grafts has led to equivocal results because of failure of the graft or inability of the graft to respond to postoperative orthodontic movement.[14,99] Composite grafts of solid one-piece iliac crest with cancellous marrow have also been used, but with orthodontic expansion having been accomplished prior to grafting.† Autogenous particulate marrow and cancellous bone (PMCB) has become the preferred grafting material for reconstruction of cleft palate defects primarily because Boyne[11,12] and Boyne and Sands[14,15] showed the practicality of using this material in

maxillofacial defects. The primary advantage of the PMCB graft is that it is an active osteogenic substance that produces desirable effects in the regeneration of osseous defects.[10] This appears to be due to its increased osteogenic inductive capacity[19,104] along with its ability to maintain viable cells that differentiate into osteoblasts.[80] It has also been shown that this graft system can respond to orthodontic movement of teeth into the grafted area.*

Homogenous grafts. Homogenous bone grafts have been in use for many years but have met with minimal success because of the high antigenic potential of the graft. However, with the development of newer methods of preservation, there has been an increased utilization in certain situations. Basically three types of homogenous bone are available: (1) freeze-dried, (2) decalcified bone, and (3) frozen bone.

A great deal of debate has gone on over the osteogenic inductive capacity of the homogenous bone graft. Urist et al.[107] and Burwell[20,21] provide the most extensive work in this area and believe that with proper preparation the homogenous bone graft does have some induction potential though rather weak. Urist[105] has demonstrated that bone induction is mediated through an acid-insoluble protein, which he calls bone morphogenic protein (BMP), and that this induces mesenchymal cells in the graft recipient bed to differentiate and form bone as functional osteoblasts. He has also confirmed[19] BMP and bone induction from allogeneic sources.

The concept of using homogenous bone in the treatment of cleft palate is not new. Backdahl and Nordin[4] used frozen bone in the 1950s until they converted to autogenous grafts. They reported a success rate of only 40% with the frozen bone but 100% with autogenous bone. Marx et al.[62] demonstrated autogenous particulate bone and marrow to be the superior graft material, although the allogeneic grafts showed bone formation through inductive change. However, they found that the allogeneic material did not induce sufficient bone formation by the host and they therefore could not recommend this graft system for alveolar cleft palates. It was felt that the grafts could not be expected

---

to respond to passive tooth eruption, orthodontic tooth movement, or orthopedic and growth forces.

Graft donor sites. Cortical bone grafts have in the past been obtained form the long bones, such as the femur, tibia, or fibula. However, these sources are limited in maxillofacial procedures. Therefore other sources have become more prominent. The mandible has served as a ready source of cortical bone and has minimized the need to go to another anatomic source.* The symphysis region of the mandible also offers a limited source of marrow for the oral and maxillofacial regions. However, this area does not generally offer the amount of particulate cancellous bone marrow needed for reconstruction of maxillary alveolar cleft palates. The primary source of this graft material is the ilium since all three types of autogenous graft material—cortical, cancellous, and corticocancellous—can be harvested.[29] Concerns related to this anatomic site have been that the iliac crest is one of the growth centers of the ilium and surgical intervention could produce undesirable alterations in growth of the hip. The second concern is related to the morbidity of the procedure itself.

When certain precautions are followed in the growing patient, concerns about damage to the growth centers have not proved to be a problem.[23,25] Care should be taken through the second decade of life since the epiphyseal cartilage tends to persist past puberty.[9] A surgical procedure that avoids damage to the epiphyseal cartilage is described later in this chapter. The problem with morbidity is primarily related to the elevation of the gluteal muscles at the time of harvesting the graft. This results in difficulty with early ambulation and prolonged discomfort after surgery.[57] Laurie et al.[57] reviewed donor-site morbidity after harvesting rib and iliac bone and showed that early morbidity with iliac bone grafts was greater than with rib donor sites. However, although hip symptoms largely resolved, a significant number of rib donor sites had persistent chest wall pain. Methods for modification of this adverse sequela at the iliac site include (1) minimal reflection of the gluteals when possible, (2) use of a lateral skin incision and approaching the crest medially when possible, and (3) if a full-thickness graft is required, raising the crest separately and replacing it. By following these rules we have seen very few problems in more than 60 grafts taken from the anterior iliac crest in patients ranging in age from 7 to 24 years. The patients are usually able to walk the day after surgery and generally require crutches for no longer than 2 days postoperatively.

Wolfe and Berkowitz[121] describe a procedure for obtaining cortical and cancellous bone from the cranium for use in alveolar and palatal clefts and list the following advantages of cranial bone as a donor source:

1. Rapid harvesting, with assurance of as much bone as needed
2. Donor area in the same operative field
3. Virtual absence of postoperative pain in the donor site and an invisible scar
4. Shorter length of hospitalization (1 to 2 days) as a result of less pain in the donor area

Disadvantages include the need to shave the head, elevation of a large scalp flap, bleeding from the diploic veins, and potential intracranial trauma.

Surgical approach to the anterior iliac crest

Numerous techniques have been reported for obtaining bone from the ilium.* These techniques are generally the same in soft tissue approach and vary mainly in the method of bone removal. When possible, the crest itself should be spared to decrease surgical morbidity rates and to avoid an unacceptable cosmetic result. By maintaining the contour of the crest, a more acceptable cosmetic result is obtained and the possibility of a "landslide" hernia is decreased. The skin incision should be placed lateral to the anterior crest rather than directly over the crest. This avoids problems with delayed early healing and later discomfort when the incision is rubbed by the clothing. Once the incision is placed, the skin and subcutaneous tissues are retracted medially to allow a direct approach to the iliac crest. This helps to avoid excessive muscle dissection, which contributes to in-

---

*References 2, 55, 103, 125.

*References 23, 25, 47, 49, 71, 89, 118, 122.

creased morbidity. It is also recommended that the graft be obtained from the medial ilium to avoid dissection of the gluteal muscles and tensor fasciae latae. By raising a "trapdoor" as described by Jackson et al.,[47] it is often possible to spare these muscles; and by removing the graft below the intact crest, late problems of resorption and irregular crest contour can be avoided.[23] This procedure also minimizes damage to the epiphysis in children.[25,71]

Technique. The patient is placed on the operating table in the supine position, and general anesthesia is induced. A sandbag under the patient's hip elevates and medially rotates the anterior iliac crest. The surgical sites are prepared and draped in the routine manner. Care is taken not to cross-contaminate the hip surgical site from the oral cavity. The oral cavity is isolated from the donor site by separate half sheets attached to IV poles. This can be done with either one or two surgical teams without cross-contamination. We generally utilize a two-team approach since it allows for more efficient use of general anesthesia and operating room time. The graft recipient site is prepared simultaneously with the obtaining of the bone graft.

Bony landmarks are identified and include the anterior superior iliac spine and the iliac crest, which curves superiorly and posteriorly from the spine. The anterior superior iliac spine should serve as the medial limit of the incision so the lateral femoral cutaneous nerve will not be damaged. The incision is placed approximately 1 cm lateral to the crest and follows the crest 6 cm. It is carried through skin and subcutaneous tissue to the fascia layer. The superior portion of the incision is then retracted medially to expose the crest of the ilium. The insertion of the gluteal and abdominal muscles is identified by a thick white periosteal attachment over the iliac crest. An incision is placed through this periosteum down to the crest. To avoid damage to the inguinal ligament, care should be taken to end the incision at least 1 cm from the anterior superior iliac spine. This attachment is carefully reflected with a periosteal elevator and carried medially into the iliac fossa.

A "trapdoor" is created[47] by making two vertical bony cuts through the crest with a straight chisel at the width of the incision. The medial cut is then accomplished with a curved osteotome, and the crest is fractured laterally with the periosteal and gluteal attachments intact. Cancellous marrow and particulate bone can be removed between the cortices with orthopedic goouges. To maintain viability of the cells and avoid drying, the marrow should be stored in a blood-soaked sponge. A corticocancellous graft can be taken at this time by carrying the vertical cuts along the medial surface of the ilium to the desired length with chisels, rotary burs, or reciprocating saw. The inferior cut can then be accomplished with the oscillating saw. An orthopedic chisel is used to separate the block graft from the lateral cortex.[9]

Hemostasis is accomplished with bone wax prior to closure. The trapdoor is repositioned, and the periosteum of the crest is sutured to the abdominal muscles with 2-0 chromic gut. The periosteum must be sutured tightly to ensure good position of the crest. The remaining layers are closed with 2-0 chromic for the fascia and fat. Subcuticular closure is obtained with 3-0 plain gut suture. The skin is then closed with a 3-0 nylon in a continuous fashion. The incision is dressed with Adaptic, and a pressure bandage is applied to prevent superficial hematoma formation. If hemostasis has been good, there is no need for drains. The patient is encouraged to walk on the day after surgery with the aid of crutches, if necessary, and is generally discharged on the second to third postoperative day with little need for ambulatory assistance.

Patients generally complain of more discomfort in the hip than in the maxillofacial area. However, even this has been minimal, requiring analgesics only on the day of surgery. The most frequent complication reported is paresthesia of the lateral femoral cutaneous nerve with retraction,[49] but usually this resolves without any long-term loss of sensation. Although thigh hypesthesia causes little inconvenience, meralgia paresthetica is a debilitating condition that is difficult to treat.[117] In our series of 60 grafts only one complication was related to the donor site, a seroma, which required aspiration and did not recur. There have been no incidences of infection at the donor site. Prophylactic antibiotics are given preoperatively and for 5 days postoperatively.

Advantages of bone grafting in the cleft palate patient

The basic goal of any reconstructive procedure should be to restore (1) function and (2) form. Bone grafting in the cleft palate patient allows restoration of function by stabilizing the maxillary segments to form a continuous arch for the proper occlusal relationship of the maxilla and mandible. This stability will decrease orthodontic relapse after expansion of the arches and create a more solid base for any prosthetic appliances, be they fixed or removable. The bone matrix will allow adequate osseous tissue for the eruption of teeth and orthodontic movement into the grafted area. The osseous matrix offers improved periodontal support for the teeth adjacent to the cleft. Restoration of the nasal floor and closure of the oronasal fistula will separate the nasal and oral cavities, allowing restoration of their normal functions. This also eliminates the hygiene problems of fluid and secretion reflux along the fistula. Restoration of the form of the maxillary arch allows for correction of the malocclusion and improvement of the patient's appearance. With a properly placed bone graft, it is possible to gain support for the alar base of the nose and improved facial esthetics.[67] This also gives a solid bony foundation for later secondary soft tissue revisions if required, all adding to the psychologic and physical well-being of the patient.

The goals of secondary grafting in the cleft palate patient between the ages of 6 and 15 are to allow for continued growth in the area grafted and to respond to the orthodontic demands of arch expansion and tooth movement.[15] However, in the physically mature patient the goals are quite different. Then it is desired to form a solid bone structure for prosthetic restoration and maintenance of good periodontal support.

PRESURGICAL CONSIDERATIONS

There continues to be disagreement as to the best time for undertaking reconstruction of the cleft palate defect. Some authors* have felt that the grafting should be undertaken at the time of primary palatal closure. Others have preferred to wait until lateral growth of the maxilla is complete. This is an effort to avoid some of the severe restriction of maxillary growth reported by Graber,[39] Pruzansky,[85] and others. Ideally one should wait until complete maxillary growth has taken place. However, the demands of nutrition, speech development, swallowing, esthetics, and psychologic well-being all play a part in determining the optimum timing of the reconstructive procedure.

In the 1970s, studies began to appear showing that secondary grafting procedures could be undertaken in the mixed dentition age group without adverse effects. Boyne and Sands[14] recommended surgery between the ages of 9 and 11 years. Waite and Kersten[113] also recommend this timing but state that chronologic age is probably not as important as the development and position of the teeth in relation to the cleft. There is general agreement that the permanent canine should be high in the alveolus with its root development one half to two thirds complete. As experience has been gained, I have tended to operate on the patient at a slightly younger age to avoid loss of the lateral incisor into the cleft. No adverse problems have been noted with this earlier intervention. The youngest patient in our series to have undergone a grafting was 7 years old at the time of surgery. The great majority of patients have been in the 8-to-12-year range.

The decision for surgical reconstruction should be a collaborated one. The complexities of the cleft lip and palate patient require that multiple disciplines be involved in the decision-making process. The need for a team approach is critical. The patient's general dental condition should be optimal, with elimination of gross caries and instruction in proper hygiene. Input is needed in the older-age patient as to possible prosthetic appliance fabrication after surgery. Orthodontic input is necessary for a decision as to which if any teeth should be removed and a definite plan of treatment both pre- and postoperatively.

Generally we have elected not to extract teeth in the cleft unless they were nonrestorable. The severely malpositioned teeth within the cleft are evaluated at the time of surgery. If they are in a position that precludes their eruption into the oral cavity through the graft or are inaccessible

---

*References 61, 75, 88, 91, 92, 97.

to later exposure and orthodontic movement, they are extracted. If a tooth may require exposure at a later time, its position is recorded in the operative notes for future reference. Supernumerary teeth are similarly evaluated. If they are not a hindrance to the procedure and may be of some use later, they are retained. It is easy to extract at a later time if they prove not to be needed.

In the past, with the use of autogenous rib grafts and cortical grafts, orthodontic movement of teeth into the reconstructed area was extremely difficult.[87] Therefore orthodontic tooth movement and arch expansion were accomplished prior to surgical intervention. With the use of autogenous particulate marrow and cancellous bone, teeth are now able to erupt into the grafted area and can respond to orthodontic movement into the grafted area. The maxillary arch can respond favorably to orthodontic expansion within 2 months of the grafting procedure.[15] Since using this graft system exclusively in the secondary bone graft patient, we have not routinely been expanding the maxilla prior to surgery. Orthodontic tooth movement and arch expansion have been undertaken as early as 2 months postoperatively. We have had no problems with this approach.

In the long-term evaluation of the patient with a unilateral or bilateral cleft palate defect, accurate records are extremely important. One problem we have seen in the past with cleft palate surgery has been early success which later gave way to the deleterious impact of the surgical procedure on the overall growth of the maxilla. For those involved in the treatment of the patient with cleft lip and palate, it is imperative that adequate records be maintained to document treatment and to allow long-term evaluation of results. A family history, study models, radiographs (periapical, occlusal, and cephalometric) as indicated, along with standardized clinical photographs, are necessary. Often these patients have a facial skeletal deformity that will require correction at a later date or, in older patients, may be corrected simultaneously. Orthognathic surgical correction of the skeletal or dental deformity may be performed at the time of grafting in this older group of patients.

SURGICAL TECHNIQUE

Numerous descriptions of surgical techniques have been reported in recent years. Boyne and Sands,[14] Waite and Kersten,[113] Hall and Posnick,[42] Epker and Wolford,[35] Bertz,[7] and others present techniques that have merit and offer variations that meet specific needs (which will be addressed later). In this series of patients I have utilized the technique described by Hall and Posnick[42] with only slight modifications.

The procedure is done under general anesthesia with nasoendotracheal intubation for the patient with a unilateral cleft. The patient with a bilateral defect is intubated orally because of difficulty with the nasal intubation and restriction of the operative field during reflection of the nasal mucosa. The patient is given antibiotics during the procedure and for 5 days postoperatively. An initial dose of 1 million units aqueous penicillin is administered intravenously at the beginning of the procedure and repeated every 2 hours during the procedure. This is followed by 250 mg orally every 6 hours for as much as 5 days. Dexamethasone (Decadron) is given perioperatively to decrease edema in the upper lip and infraorbital area.

The bone graft is harvested from the ilium simultaneously with preparation of the recipient graft site by a second surgical team. This better utilizes the operating room and minimizes the time under general anesthesia. Even in young patients there is little problem with the teams working simultaneously.

Unilateral alveolar cleft. The patient is positioned with the head in an extended position and a small sandbag under the neck for stability. The surgeon sits at the head of the patient and looks directly down on the palate and into the labial defect.

Initial attention is given to infiltration of local anesthetic with a vasoconstrictor along the labial and palatal tissues to aid in hemostasis during the procedure. The needle is also used to identify the bony margins of the cleft prior to placement of the incisions (Fig. 7-6). The labial incision is carried into the medial and distal cleft margins vertically and extended posteriorly along the free gingival sulcus for at least a distance of two teeth on each side of the cleft. These incisions extend to bone. The remaining

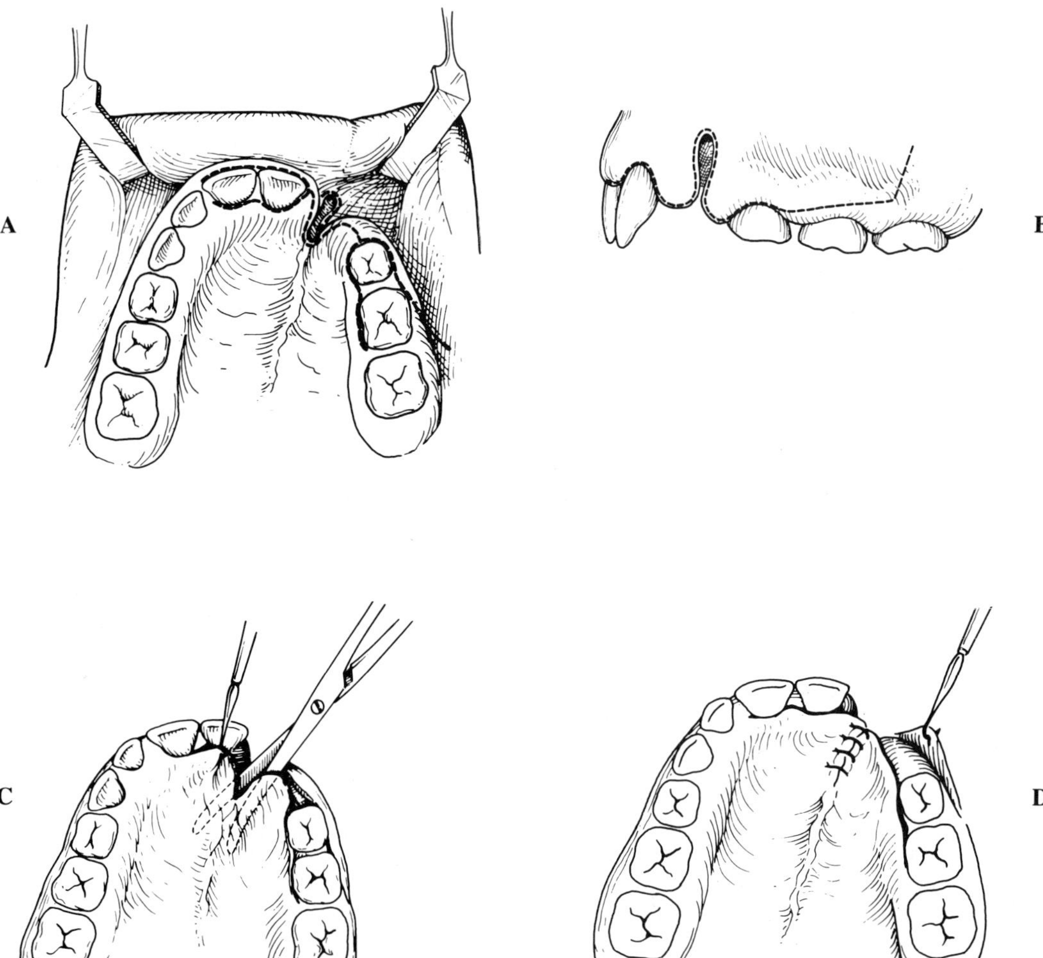

Fig. 7-6.
Basic reconstructive procedure for the unilateral alveolar cleft palate. **A,** Palatal and gingival incisions; **B,** labial mucosal incisions; **C,** division of the palatal and nasal mucosa; **D,** palatal closure.
Reprinted from Hall, D.H., and Posnick, J.C.: J. Oral Maxillofac. Surg. **41:**289, 1983.

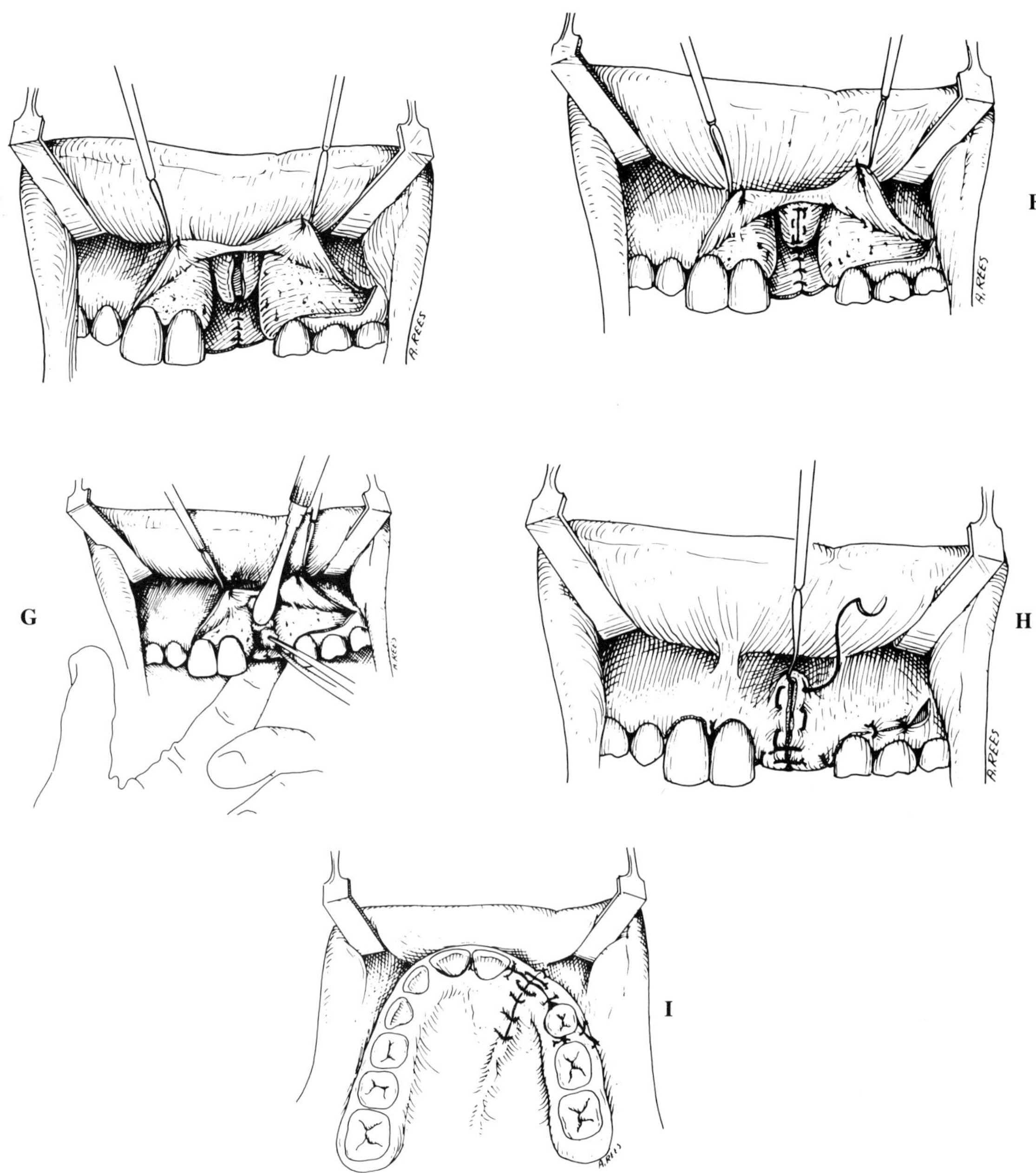

Fig. 7-6—cont'd.
E, Nasal mucosal flaps ready for closure; **F,** nasal mucosal flaps closed; **G,** insertion of the bone graft into the defect; **H,** labial closure after advancement of the labial flaps; **I,** all incisions closed (horizontal mattress suture closing the corners of the four flaps on the crest of the ridge).

portion of the incision in the depth of the vestibule will be split-thickness to allow development of a soft tissue flap continuous with the floor of the nasal cavity. The labial attached gingiva is reflected as a full-thickness mucoperiosteal flap to expose the bony margins of the cleft. Under direct visualization and with the Woodson elevator, subperiosteal dissection is carried superiorly to expose the anterior nasal spine, nasal septum, and floor of the nasal cavity medially. In a similar manner the lateral piriform rim is exposed. A Metzenbaum scissors is used to develop a split-thickness mucosal flap around the oronasal fistula. This is accomplished by both blunt and sharp dissection to separate the extension of the nasal floor into the upper lip. The nasal mucosa is reflected palatally to expose the walls of the cleft as they extend palatally.

A periosteal elevator is used to elevate a subperiosteal flap along the margins of the palatal defect. This creates a subperiosteal tunnel into which the blades of the Metzenbaum scissors can be inserted. The tissue between the blades is cut to allow further reflection of the nasal mucosa along the horizontal process of the palate. The palatal flaps are then approximated and closed with 4-0 Dexon. If the defect is wide, the

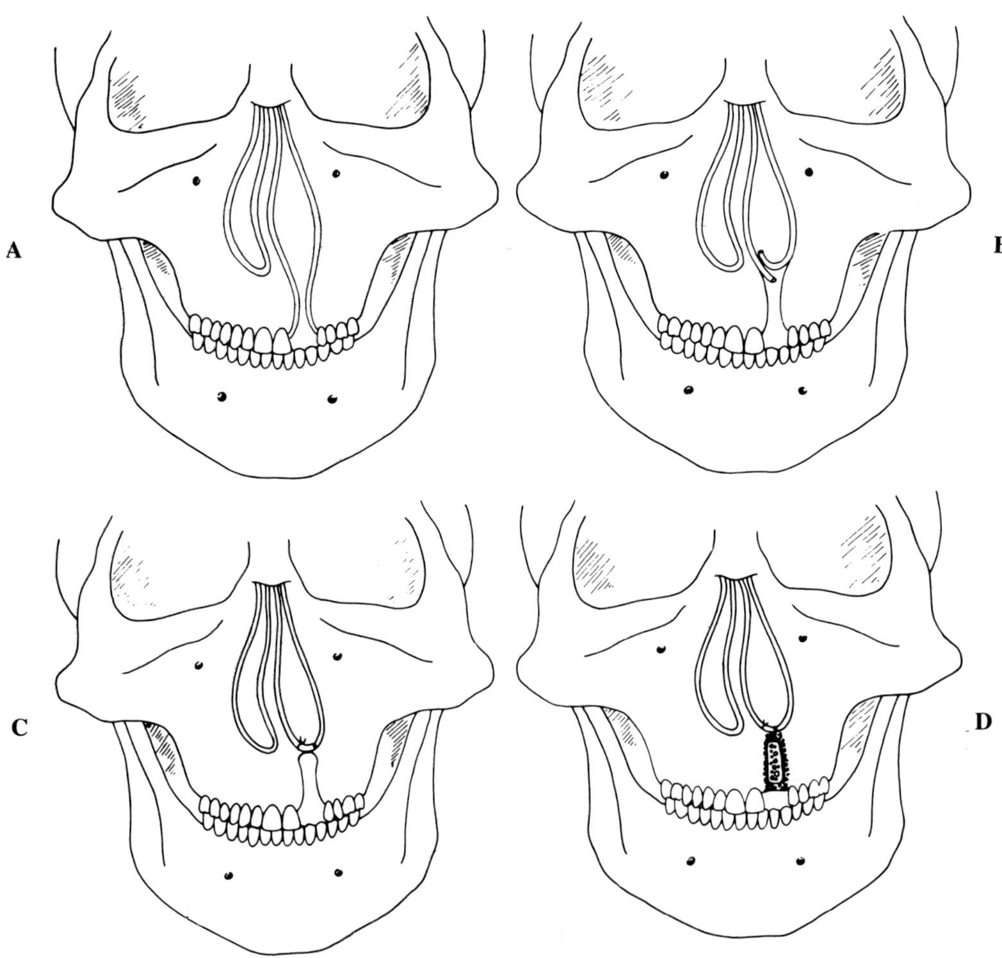

Fig. 7-7.
Nasal closure in a unilateral alveolar cleft palate. **A,** Prior to repair; **B,** elevation of the nasal flaps medially and laterally; **C,** closure of the flaps; **D,** insertion of the bone graft.
From Bell, W.H., et al.: Surgical correction of dentofacial deformities, Philadelphia, 1980, W.B. Saunders Co.

palatal flap can be released posteriorly to allow rotation but this has rarely been needed in my experience.

The reflected nasal mucosal flap is approached labially and excess tissue is excised to allow better visualization and room for the bone graft. Care must be taken not to remove too much tissue early in the procedure. Fig. 7-7 shows the concept of nasal closure. The nasal floor is then closed with a horizontal mattress suture (4-0 Dexon) on a small needle (PR-4 or S-2). A microsurgical needle holder is helpful in suturing this area.

The labial flap is released with an oblique

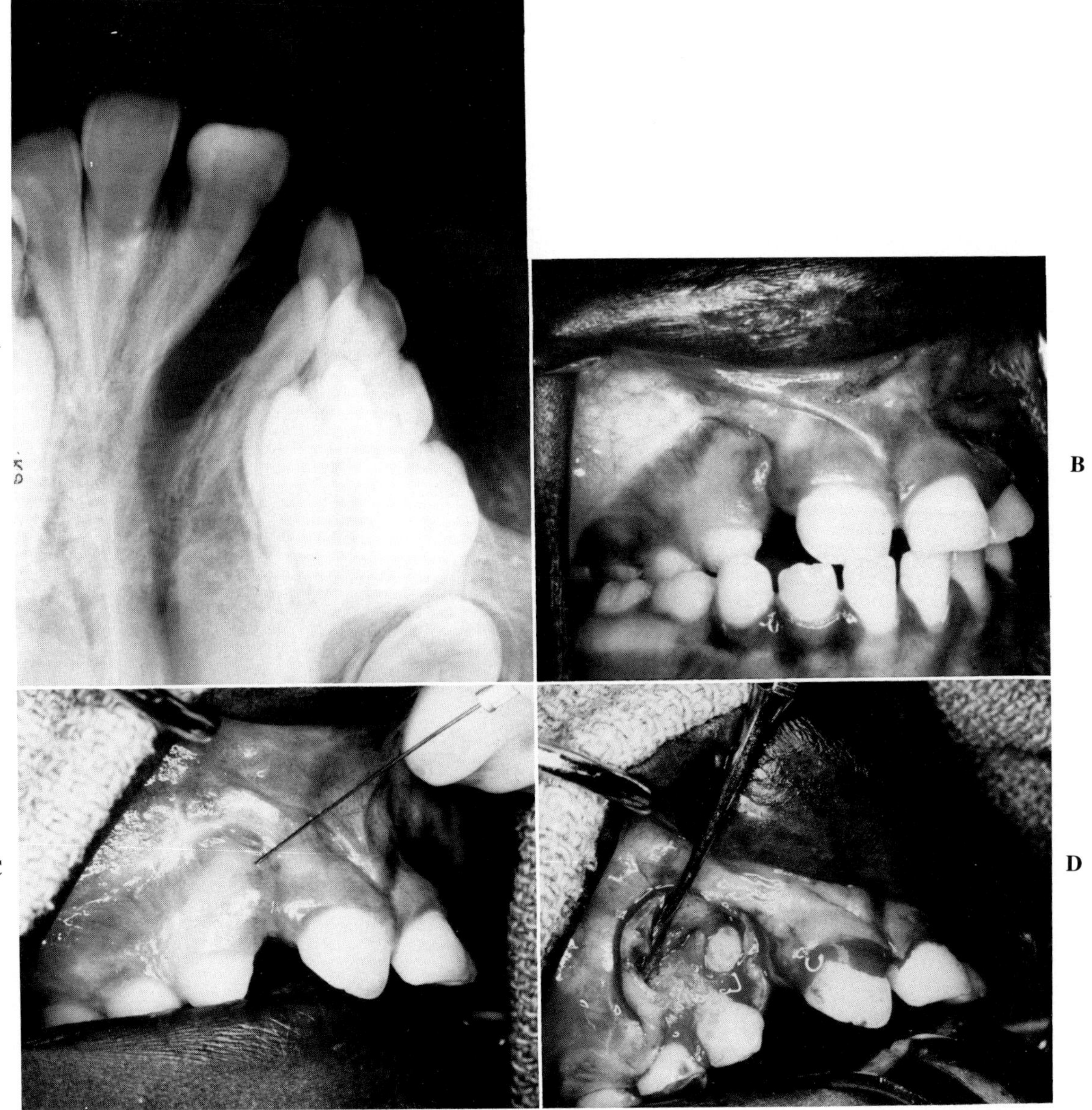

Continued.

Fig. 7-8.
Clinical reconstructive procedure for the unilateral alveolar cleft palate. **A,** Preoperative. **B,** Fistulous tract. **C,** Identifying the bony margins with a needle. **D,** Labial incision along the distal cleft margin with elevation of a mucoperiosteal flap.

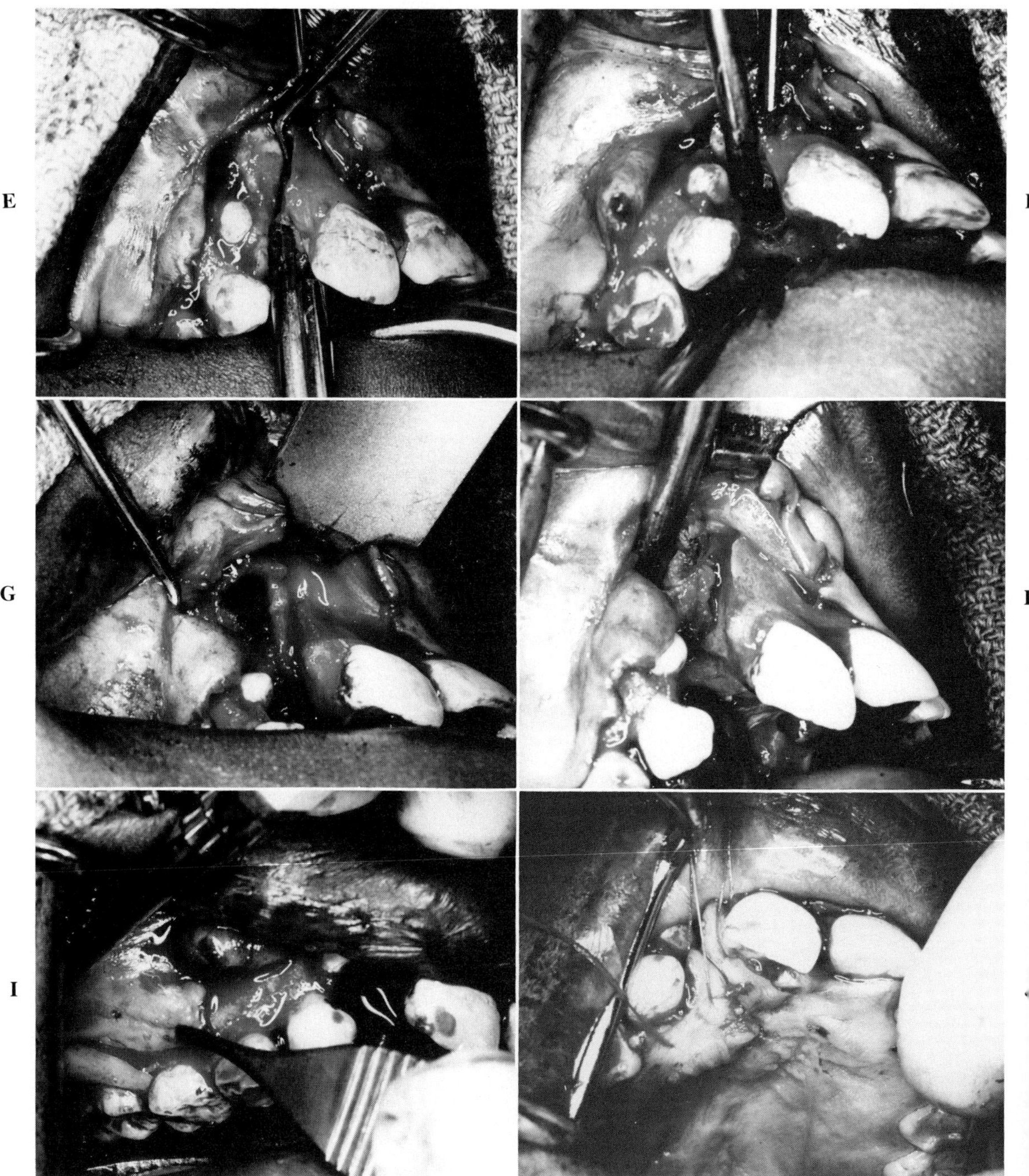

Fig. 7-8—cont'd.
E, Elevation of the nasal flap along the medial cleft surgery. **F,** Elevation of a palatal flap and nasal flaps. **G,** Oronasal fistula after elevation of the flaps. **H,** Closure of the nasal flaps. **I,** Release of the labial mucoperiosteal flap for advancement. **J,** Palatal closure with traction sutures in place.

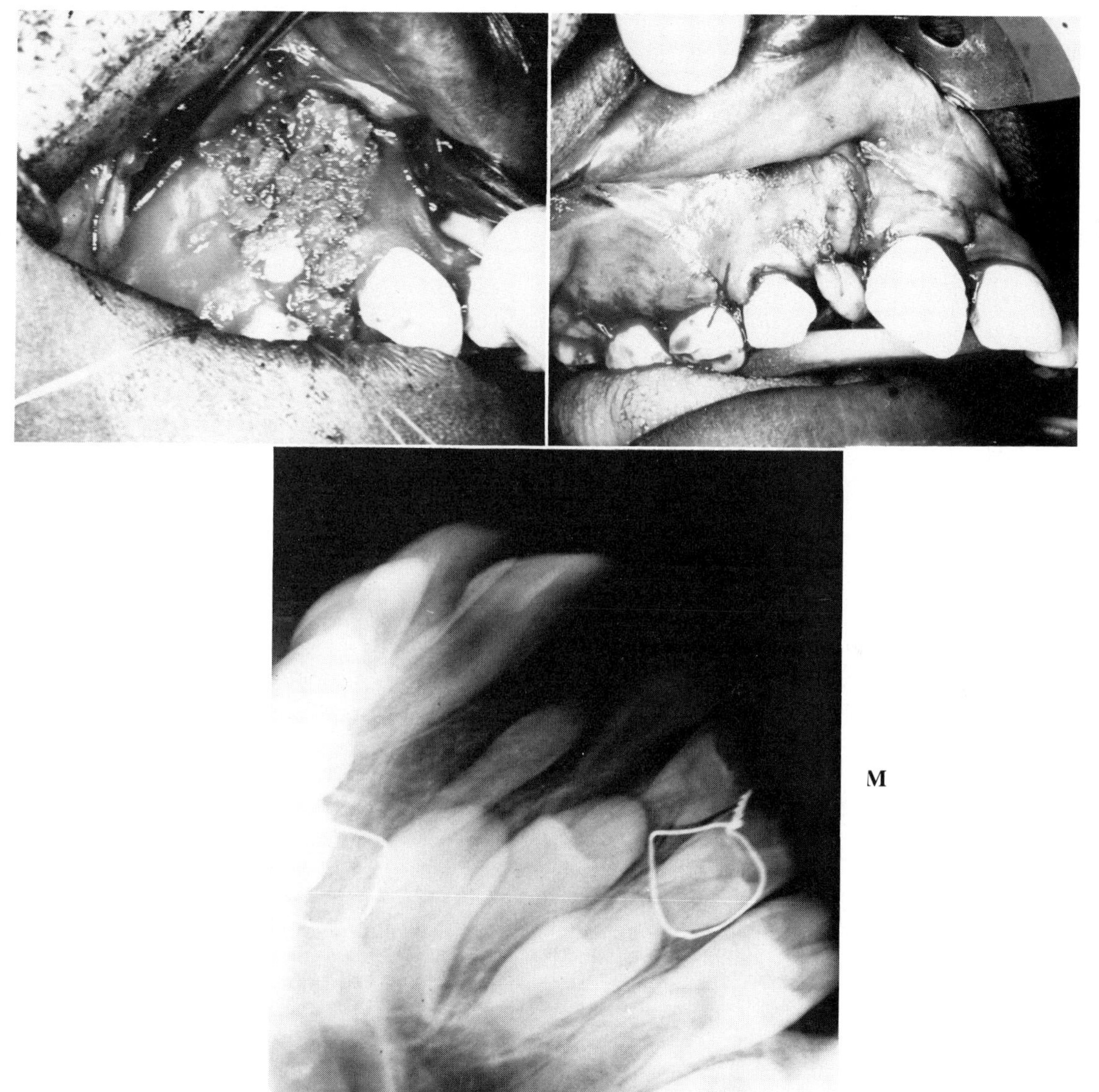

Fig. 7-8—cont'd.
K, Bone graft inserted into the defect and over an unerupted tooth. **L,** Advancement of the labial mucosal flaps and closure. **M,** Immediately postoperative, bone graft in place.

incision into the vestibule at the first molar. With the mucoperiosteal flap elevated the periosteum is incised vertically to allow further anterior and inferior positioning of the flap. A previously fabricated palatal acrylic splint is now placed and wired to the dentition to stabilize the maxillary segments and protect the surgical site. The strips of autogenous cancellous bone and marrow obtained earlier are cut into small particles that are then inserted into the cleft defect from palatal to labial. A periosteal elevator is used to pack the bone graft firmly against the palatal mucosa. The bone is placed over any unerupted teeth and layered along the piriform rim to gain additional soft tissue support.

The labial flaps are then advanced to cover the graft and closed with a 4-0 horizontal mattress suture. The labial flap is also secured to the palatal flap with a horizontal mattress suture. The lateral incisions are closed with interrupted suture. A periodontal dressing is then placed to maintain the flaps in position. Fig. 7-8 illustrates this surgical sequence.

Pedicle flaps. There are times when the alveolar defect is of such size as to make closure

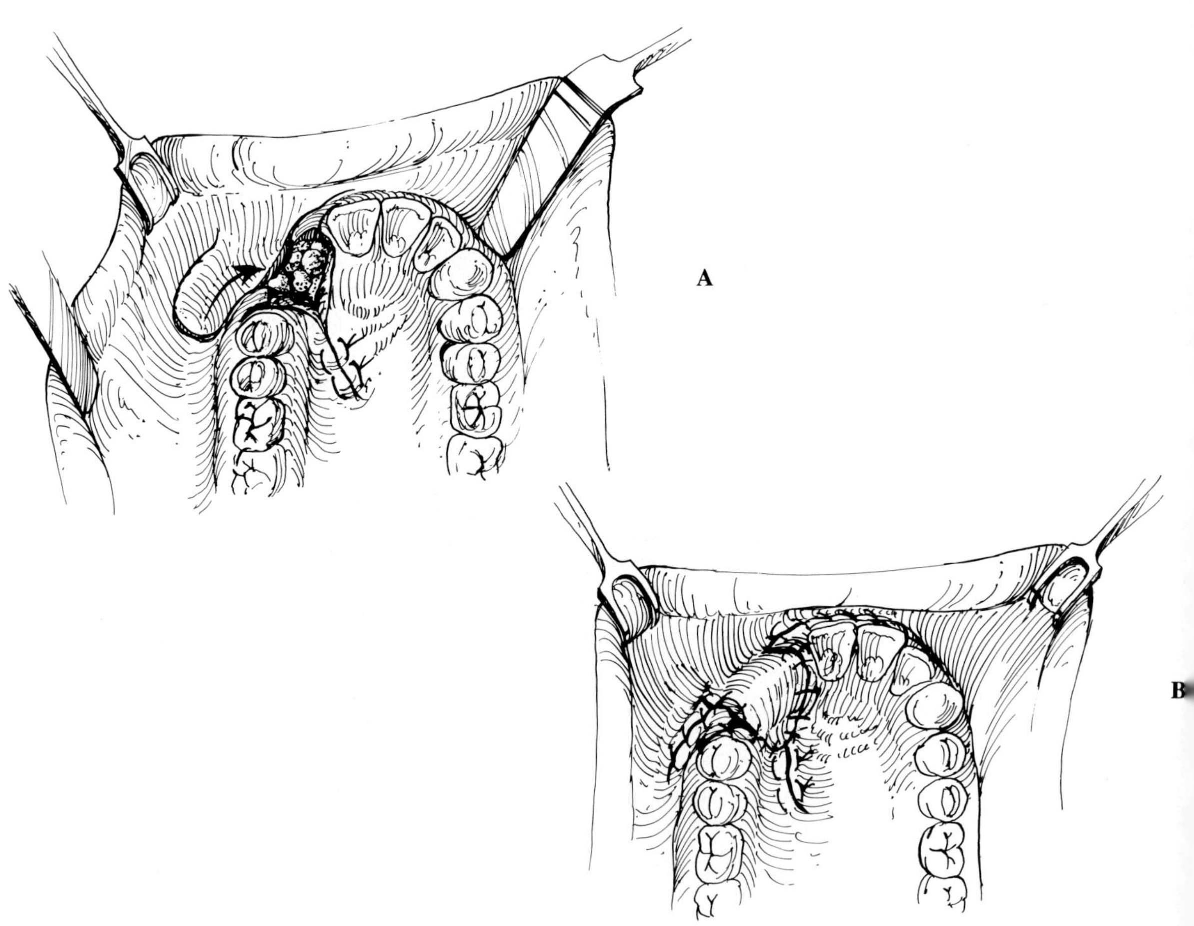

Fig. 7-9.
Finger flap. **A,** Elevation of the mucosal flap from the depth of the labial vestibule; **B,** rotation and closure of the flap over the bone graft and defect.
Reprinted from Epker, B.N., and Wolford, L.M.: Dentofacial deformities: surgical-orthodontic correction, St. Louis, 1980, The C.V. Mosby Co.

impossible with horizontally advanced flaps. This can usually be managed with development of a pedicle or "finger" flap with the labial vestibule (Fig. 7-9). The flap is long and narrow and is raised from the depth of the labial vestibule to be rotated over the bone graft and alveolar defect. Its blood supply is based superiorly, and its width should be at least one third its length. This rule must be followed carefully to avoid avascular necrosis of the distal portion of the flap. The pedicle flap can similarly be used if a soft tissue deficiency exists on the palate. It can be designed to extend into this area for coverage and is closed usually with horizontal mattress sutures.

Another pedicle-type flap that is of advantage is the trapezoidal lip flap (Fig. 7-10). This is developed full thickness to the orbicularis oris muscle with divergent vertical incisions into the labial vestibule. It is then advanced palatally to cover the bone graft. It has a wide based vascular supply, resulting in excellent viability, but it can result in shortening of the labial vestibule and it does not generally have attached mucosa adjacent to the neck of the teeth. Nevertheless it can be easily managed by release and the place-

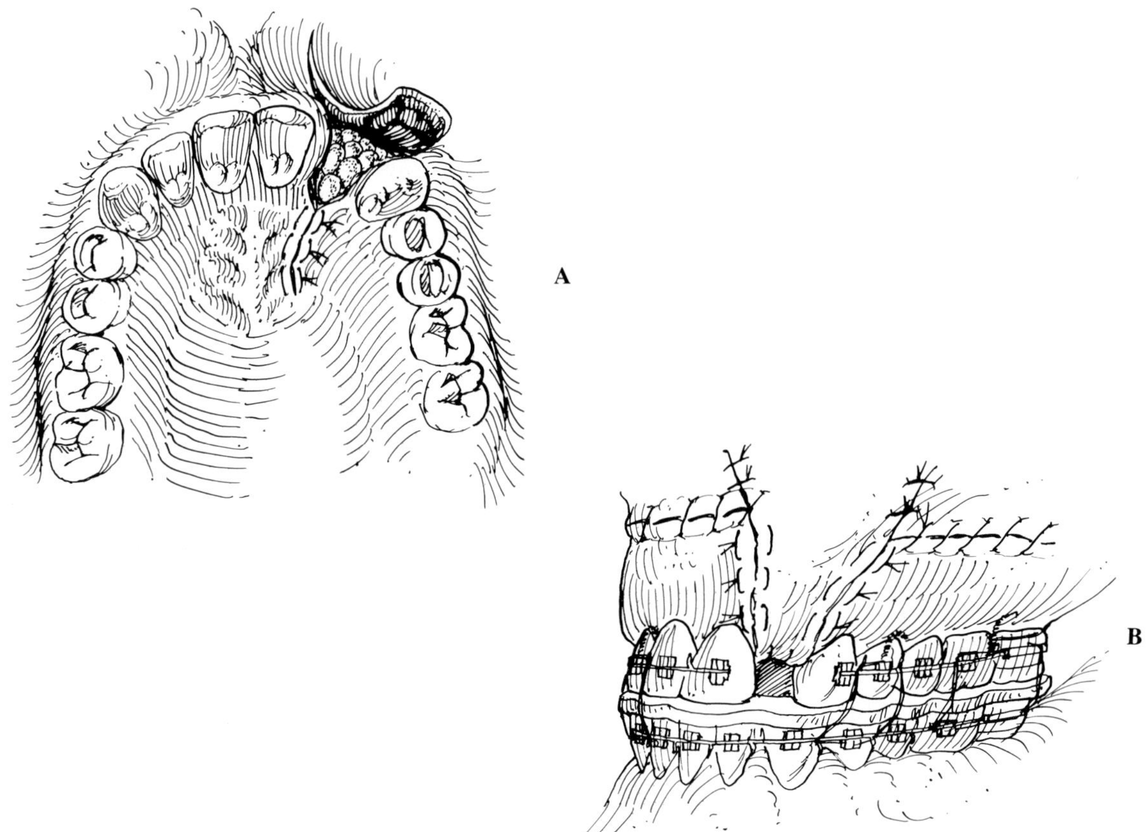

Fig. 7-10.
Trapezoidal flap. **A,** Elevation of mucosa from the lip; **B,** advancement and closure to cover the bone graft and defect.
From Epker, B.N., and Wolford, L.M.: Dentofacial deformities: surgical-orthodontic correction, St. Louis, 1980, The C.V. Mosby Co.

ment of a palatal mucosal graft 2 to 3 months after the bone grafting procedure. The release is accomplished by a supraperiosteal dissection with return of the flap to the lip. The palatal mucosal graft is then placed over the periosteum, sutured into position, and covered with a periodontal dressing (which is left in place for 1 week to maintain proper position). The donor site will granulate and reepithelialize in a short time. An acrylic splint has been used to protect the palate from tongue activity and to increase patient comfort.

Myomucosal flaps such as the hemi–tongue flap or variations offer additional soft tissue coverage when a very large defect exists. These flaps were described by Guerrero-Santos[40] in 1966 to close palatal fistulae and later in 1973 for coverage of bone grafts. Carlesso et al.[22] described the use of anteriorly based hemi–tongue flaps to close palatal fistulae. More recently Kinnebrew and Malloy[53] have used pos-

teriorly based lateral lingual flaps for primary coverage of alveolar cleft bone grafts. In the combined maxillary osteotomies and alveolar cleft bone grafts this technique avoids interrupting the segmental blood supply, as is often necessary with maxillary advancement and palatal flaps. The labial and palatal soft tissues frequently have considerable scarring from previous surgery, resulting in questionable vascularity. The introduction of new soft tissue is desirable to modify further scar formation and contracture and may help to reduce the amount of palatal collapse of the posterior segment after expansion. Kinnebrew and Malloy[53] report successful use and follow-up over a 5-year period.

Bilateral alveolar cleft. The surgical approach for reconstruction of the bilateral alveolar cleft palate is basically the same as for the unilateral cleft repair, with a few exceptions (Fig. 7-11).

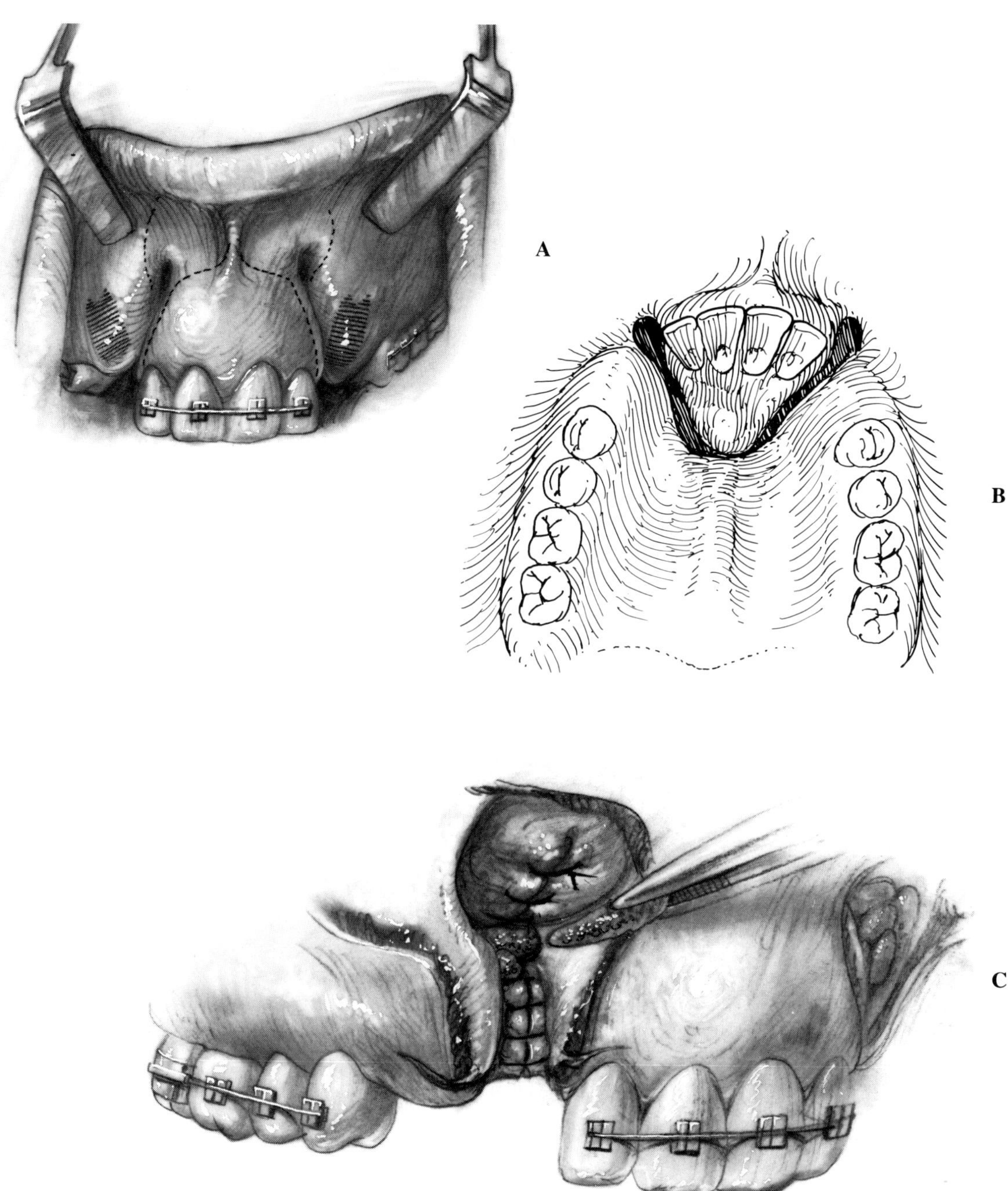

Fig. 7-11.
Bilateral alveolar cleft bone graft. **A,** The defect with oronasal fistulae and unerupted teeth; **B,** palatal view; **C,** elevation of palatal and nasal flaps with closure and insertion of the bone graft.

Fig. 7-11—cont'd.
D, Advancement of the labial flap for closure; **E,** palatal closure complete; **F,** advancement of a finger flap and a trapezoidal flap for closure of the defect when additional soft tissue coverage is needed.

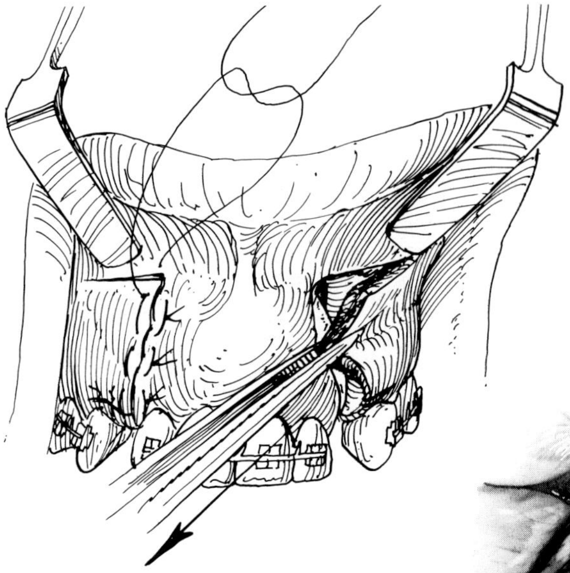

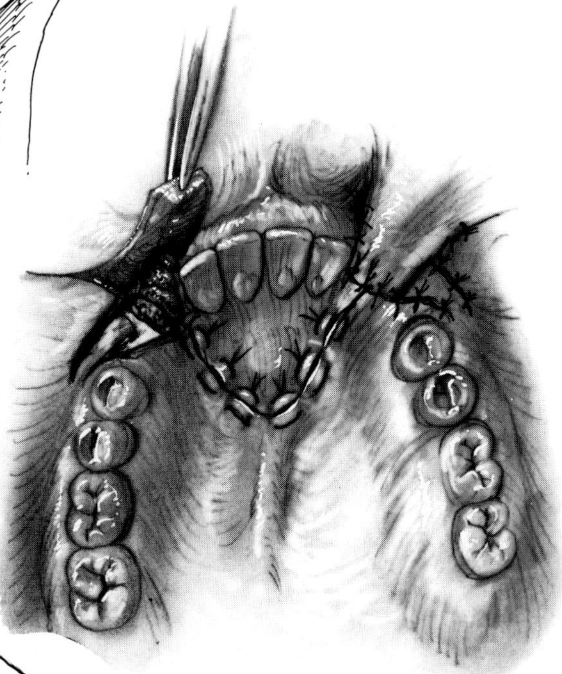

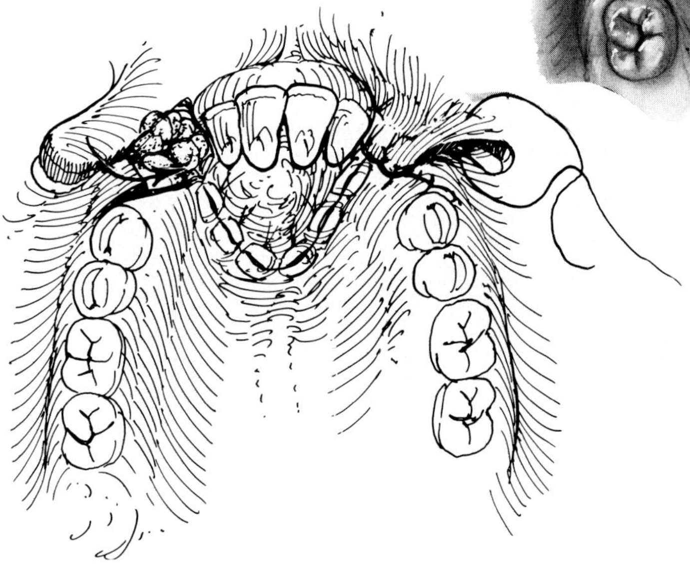

The labial incisions along the distal aspect of the cleft margins and the mucoperiosteal reflections are the same. However, care must be exercised in the reflection of tissue along the premaxillary segment. In bilateral alveolar cleft palate the premaxilla is usually moderately mobile and attached only to the vomer and cartilaginous nasal septum. The blood supply to this segment is primarily from the nasal septal mucosa and the labial mucosal pedicle. Therefore extreme care should be exercised in reflection of the nasal mucosal flap. There should be almost no labial reflection of tissue on the premaxillary segment. The incision extending palatally along the premaxilla will become continuous with the same incision on the opposite side. It is then carried palatally directly over the vomer to allow reflection of two separate vomerian flaps, one on each side. The palatal flaps are raised bilaterally and rotated medially to close the midline cleft and cover the exposed vomer. The lateral nasal and medial septal flaps

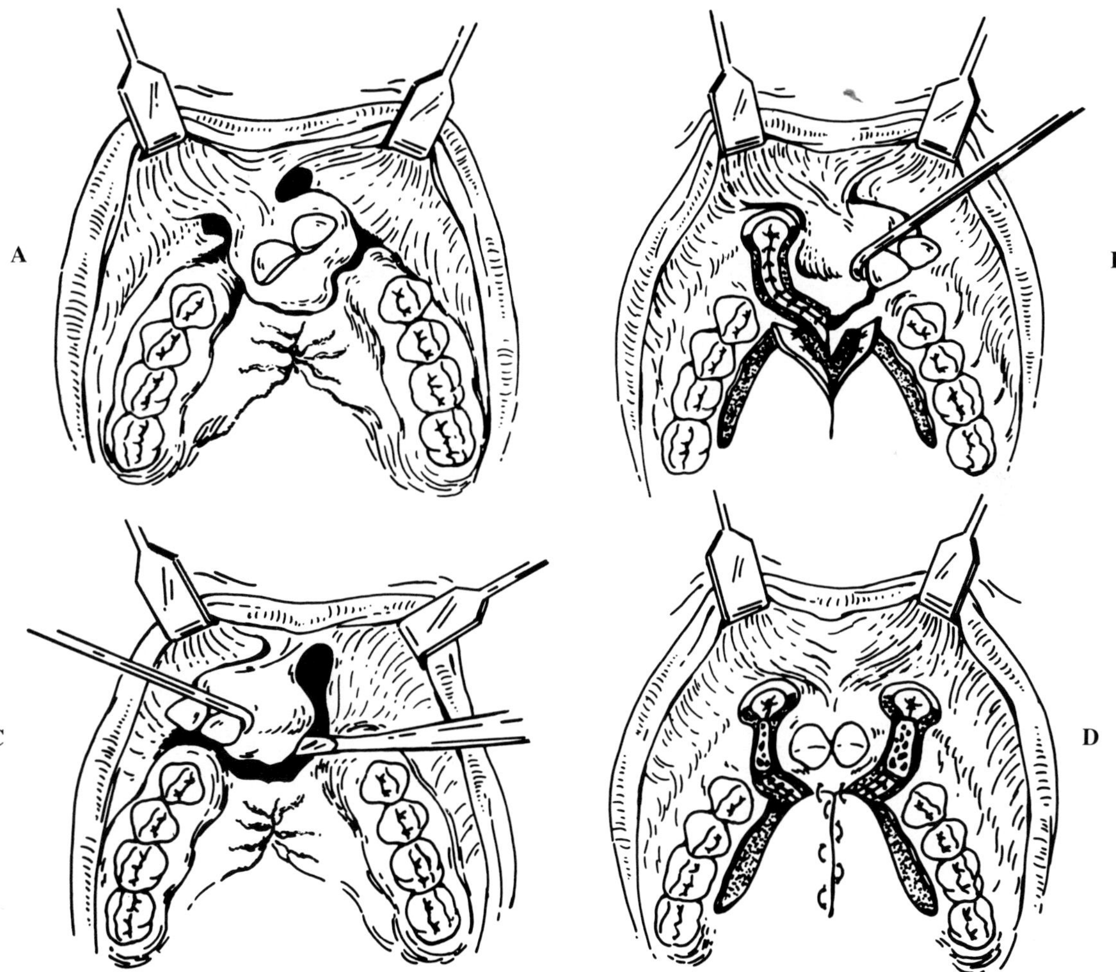

Fig. 7-12.
Retraction of the premaxilla in a bilateral cleft. The premaxilla can usually be retracted with a skin hook to gain additional access for elevation of flaps and closure.
Reprinted from Bell, W.H., et al.: Surgical correction of dentofacial deformities, Philadelphia, 1980, W.B. Saunders Co.

are approximated and sutured with a horizontal mattress suture. This can be aided by retraction of the semimobile premaxilla with a skin hook (Fig. 7-12).

Since the premaxilla is often mobile, a skin hook can be utilized to retract the segment slightly to aid in gaining additional access for closure. The palatal flaps are now closed in a similar fashion. It may be necessary to leave a small portion of exposed palatal bone laterally to gain adequate closure on the midline. This will cover with granulation tissue in a few days. The labial defects usually require development and rotation of a pedicle finger flap bilaterally so there will be adequate tissue to cover the bone-grafted defect. These flaps must be raised over the posterior segment, with their bases oriented anteriorly. It must be remembered that with the flaps developed in this technique, the entire vascular supply to the premaxillary segment is from the labial pedicle. No soft tissue must be raised from the labial portion of the premaxilla. With the nasal floor and palatal closure accomplished, the previously obtained bone graft is inserted bilaterally and posterior to the premaxilla. The pedicle flaps are rotated into position and sutured. These flaps must be long enough to extend posterior to the premaxilla without tension, since this is a common place for breakdown in bilateral repairs. If there is adequate palatal soft tissue, this flap may be sutured directly to the palatal aspect of the premaxilla.

Often the premaxilla will require surgical repositioning simultaneously with the bone grafting of the defect (Fig. 7-13). Once the soft tissue flaps are developed as just described, a curved osteotome is inserted palatally and a vertical osteotomy carried to the level of the nasal septum. The premaxilla is then fractured with digital pressure and rotated labially to allow direct visualization for removal of any bony or cartilaginous interferences to proper repositioning of the segment. Care must be exercised in protection of the labial vascular supply to the segment.

With the segment now mobilized, closure of the palatal and nasal flaps is accomplished. Closure of the nasal floor is greatly facilitated by rotation of the premaxilla labially, allowing direct visualization. The premaxilla is then positioned and secured. The bone graft is inserted and the labial closure is accomplished as previously described.

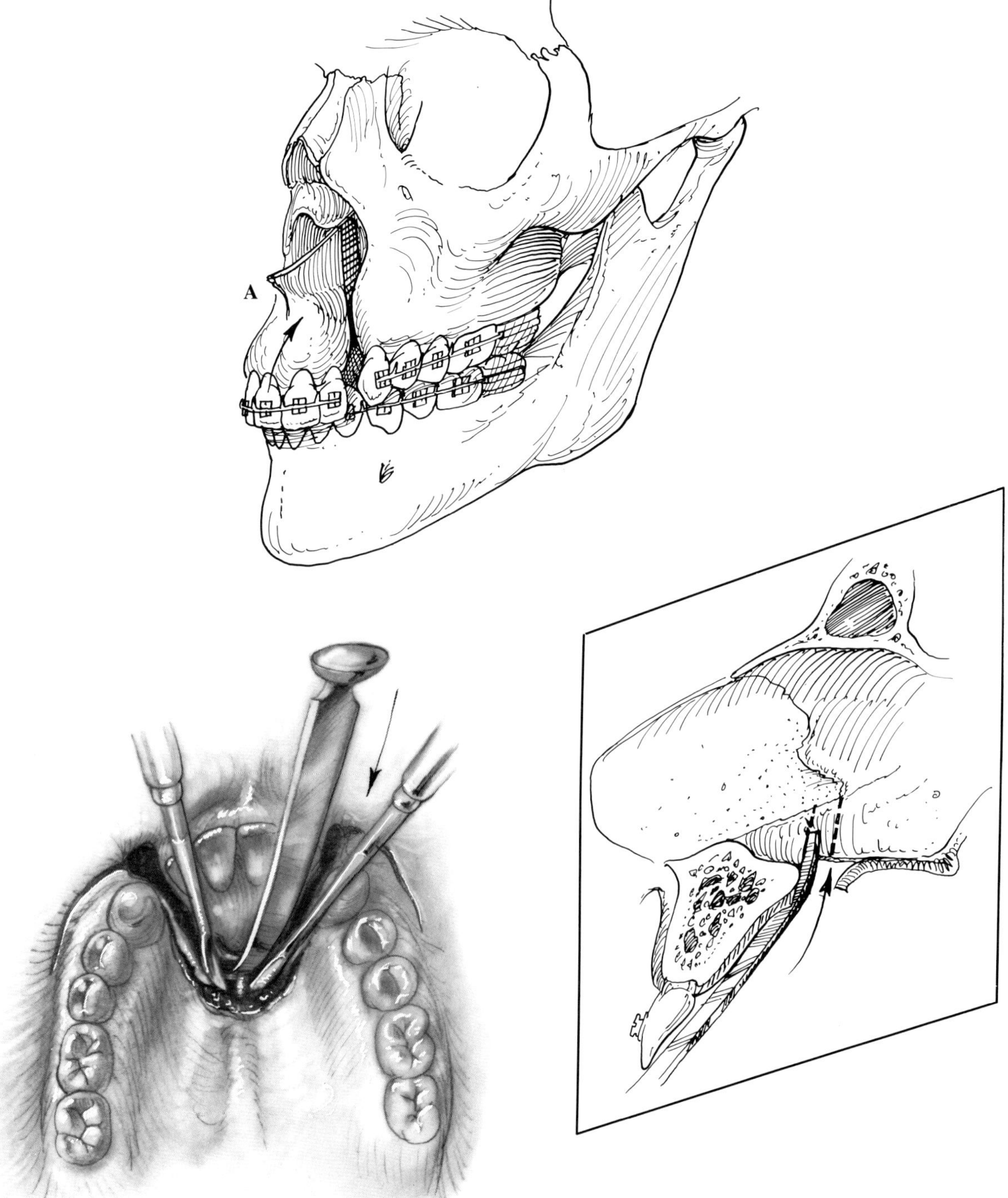

Fig. 7-13.

Simultaneous mobilization of the premaxilla with bone grafting. **A,** Often in a bilateral cleft the premaxilla will require repositioning; **B,** after elevation of the nasal and palatal flaps an osteotome is inserted and malleted to section the vomer to the level of the cartilaginous nasal septum.

A to **E** reprinted from Epker, B.N., and Wolford, L.M.: Dentofacial deformities: surgical-orthodontic correction, St. Louis, 1980, The C.V. Mosby Co.

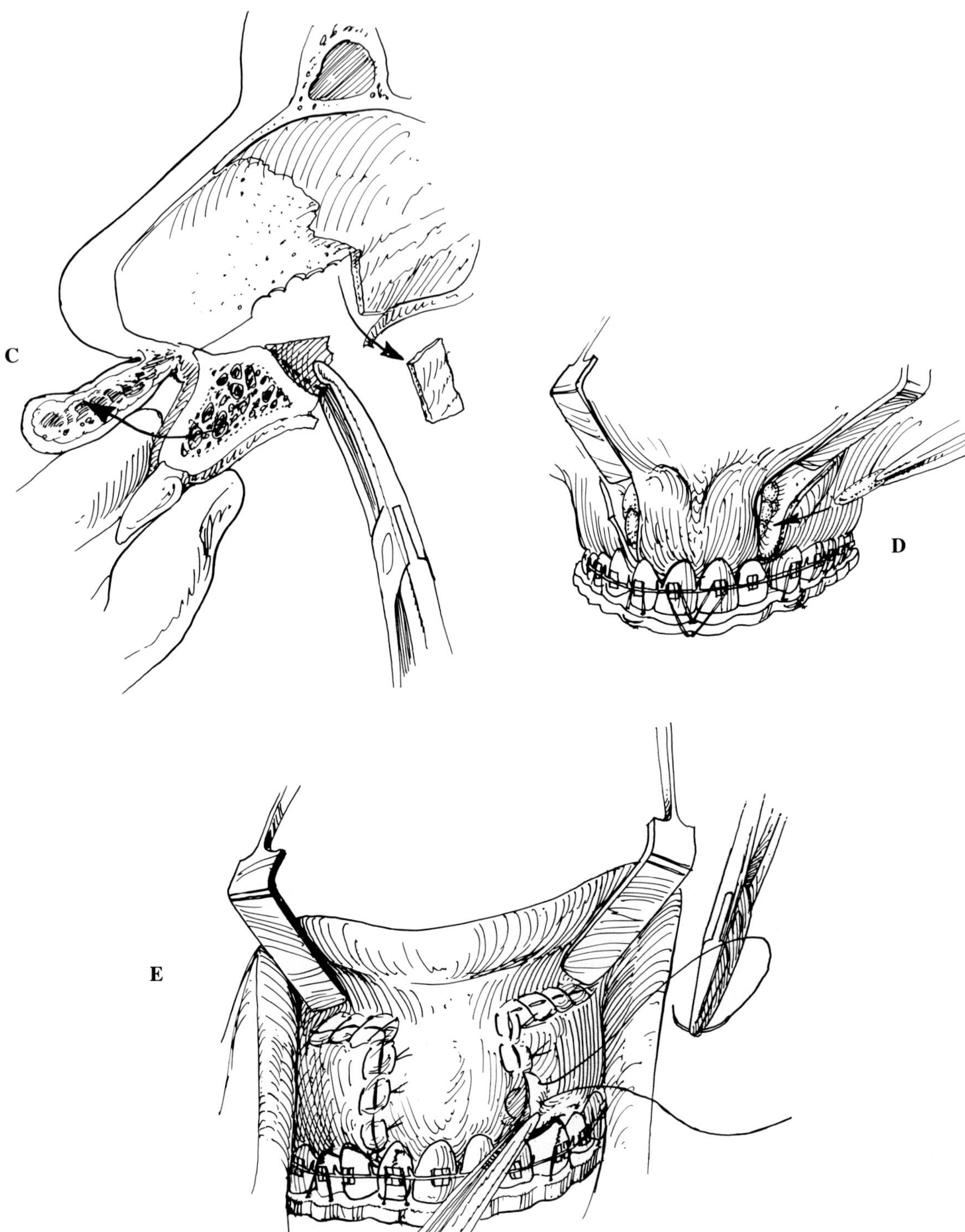

Fig. 7-13—cont'd.
C, The premaxilla is then out-fractured while pedicled to the labial mucoperiosteal flap; bony interferences can be removed from the vomer and nasal septum with a rongeur or bone bur; **D,** the segment is immobilized in a splint, and the bone graft is inserted; **E,** advancement of labial flaps and closure of the incisions.

POSTSURGICAL MANAGEMENT

Antibiotics are used routinely, beginning with the surgical procedure and continuing for 5 days postoperatively. For the nonallergic patient, penicillin is the drug of choice and a cephalosporin is second choice. Nasal decongestants are used for the first 2 days to decrease mucosal swelling and increase patient comfort. The patient is maintained on liquids for 1 week, semisoft for another week, and then a regular diet without use of the anterior teeth thereafter. The area is regularly irrigated with warm saline rinses after meals. The periodontal pack is removed at 1 week. The acrylic splint is maintained for 4 weeks to stabilize the segments and prevent exploration of the surgical site with the tongue.

The donor site dressing is changed usually on the day after surgery to Telfa and a light gauze bandage to protect the incision from direct contact with the clothing. The patient is ambulated on the morning after surgery, with instruction on crutches if necessary. Most patients will need crutches for only 1 or 2 days and can dis-card them by the third postoperative day, at the time of discharge. Generally younger patients (pre-teen) experience less discomfort from the donor site than do older patients. They also seem to have less limp and are walking without a limp by 2 weeks. The sutures from the donor site are removed at 10 days, and Steri-Strips are applied to prevent tension for another week. The patients are usually able to return to normal activities 8 to 10 days after surgery.

Orthodontic treatment can be instituted at 2 months postoperative with movement of teeth into the graft area or arch expansion. The unerupted teeth generally will erupt into the oral cavity through the graft if they are unimpeded. If not, then exposure and orthodontic assistance may be required, which can be undertaken at this time. Prosthodontic treatment in older patients can also be undertaken at this time. The pedicle flaps may heal leaving bulky coverage over the alveolar ridge, but this can be managed with a free palatal mucosal graft or a Z-plasty to create an optimum ridge for pontic or other appliance construction.

COMPLICATIONS

The complications associated with reconstruction of alveolar cleft palates using autogenous marrow and cancellous bone are few when the procedure is properly performed. In repair of alveolar defects, dehiscence of the wound may occur and is usually related to the creation of undue tension on or venous congestion in the flap. However, dehiscence of the wound has rarely resulted in complete loss of the graft. As reported by others,[17,42] it is usually only superficial and can be managed with irrigation and conservative debridement as bone spicules are sequestered. The entire graft is rarely lost, occurring in 2% or less of Hall and Posnick's cases.[42] The most common complication is development of an area of hyperplastic granulation tissue at 2 to 3 weeks after surgery (Fig. 7-14, *A*). This is easily treated by conservative excision, and usually there is no recurrence.

Breakdown of the nasal flaps can contribute to failure of the graft but has not been a major problem in most series. It can be minimized by use of oral intubation in bilateral cases or intubation on the noncleft side in the unilateral deformity. Nasal suction on the surgical side should be minimized or avoided if possible. It can be performed, however, by use of a nasal speculum and direct visualization to avoid damage to the suture line. Nasal decongestants will also aid in patient comfort and avoid initiating problems with excessive blowing in an effort to clear the nasal passages. Nasal hemorrhage is infrequent and can be managed with pressure or (rarely) a nasal pack.

As mentioned, shortening of the vestibule can occur with pedicle flaps but can be managed with free mucosal palatal grafts or Z-plasty.

Failure of teeth to erupt into the graft can occur. Broude and Waite[17] reported that 78% of unerupted canines at the time of grafting erupted into the graft. Hinrichs et al.[44] have reported that of 56% of unerupted canines in their series required surgical exposure for eruption and 44% of those then required orthodontic assistance, in addition, to move into position. They also concluded that osseous grafting of alveolar cleft defects resulted in clinically satisfactory periodontal support for cleft-associated canines up to 8 years following surgery.

Root resorption has been associated with autogenous cancellous bone marrow grafts in direct contact with root surfaces[18,32] (Fig. 7-14, *B*) and may be related to mechanical instrumentation of the root surface. Other reports,[34] however, show inconsistent results. Boyne[13] has recommended that although placing autografts in contact with teeth to reconstruct cleft defects is acceptable in children, it is not recommended in adults. There is usually a thin layer of bone overlying these teeth in the cleft site, which might explain the low incidence of root resorption in cleft patients. Care should be taken in reflection of mucoperiosteal flaps along the margins of the cleft to avoid inadvertent elevation of this thin layer of bone, best accomplished by beginning the reflection high in the cleft and working inferiorly to the alveolar crest.

El-Deeb et al.[33] have reported almost complete resorption of a bone graft in a reconstructed alveolar cleft secondary to a dental follicle of an unerupted canine in the cleft. This case emphasizes the importance of early detection of any abnormal radiologic changes and surgical intervention to prevent destruction of the grafted bone.

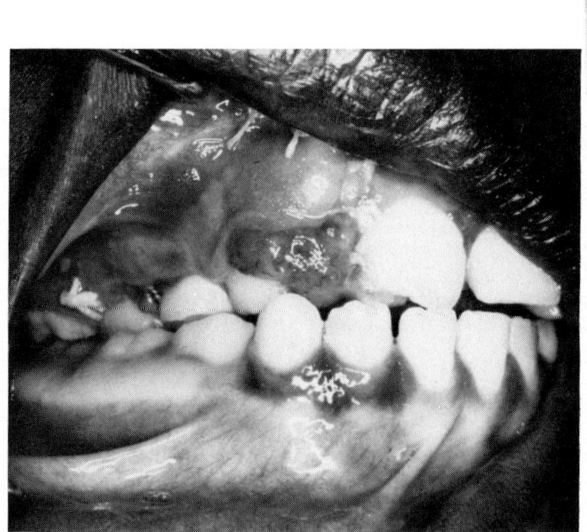
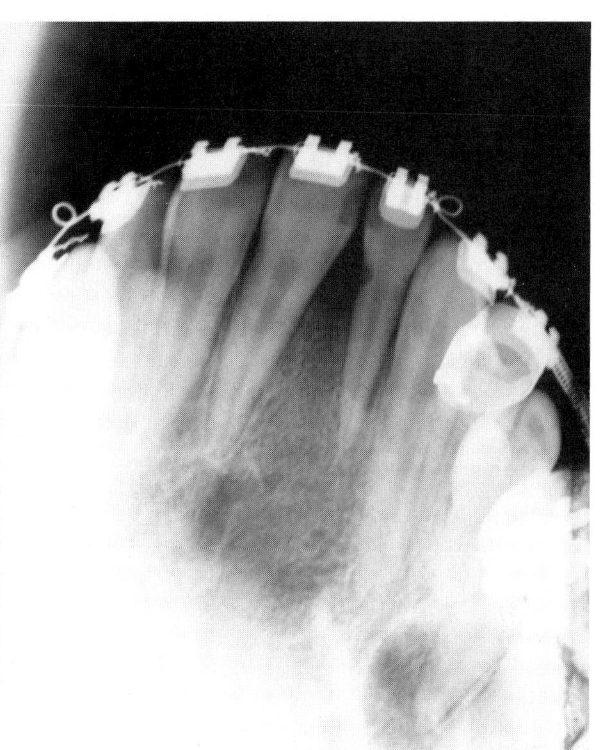

Fig. 7-14.
Complications: **A,** hyperplastic granulation tissue; **B,** external root resorption 6 months postoperative.

ORTHOGNATHIC MANAGEMENT

Orthognathic surgical correction is an integral part of the overall treatment of the cleft lip and palate. In most cases skeletal dentofacial developmental deformities also will require treatment. These procedures are usually done after orthodontic treatment and reconstruction of the alveolar cleft defect, during the late teenage years. However, in older patients simultaneous late secondary bone grafting may be successfully incorporated with orthognathic correction of the skeletal deformity.

Prior to surgical intervention, segmental orthodontic alignment should be accomplished to allow for proper positioning of the dentition in basal bone. Various techniques have been described to correct the skeletal deformity associated with the cleft anomaly. Obwegeser[76] introduced the concept of simultaneous correction of the skeletal and cleft defects. Henderson and Jackson[43] reported simultaneous cleft lip revision, bone grafting of the alveolar defect, and advancement of the maxilla utilizing a LeFort I osteotomy. Pederson and Blaho,[79] Tideman et al.,[104] Westbrook et al.,[120] and others have described various techniques for simultaneous management of the maxillary deficiency and bone grafting of the cleft defect.

The basic flap design must allow an adequate vascular pedicle to the major and minor segments. The design must also allow for adequate mobilization of a soft tissue pedicle to cover the alveolar defects along with the bone graft. Epker and Wolford[35] describe a complete circumvestibular incision with minimal reflection inferiorly to allow maximum vascular pedicle to the major and minor segments (Fig. 7-15). The lateral osteotomies are carried in a horizontal fashion on both the greater and the lesser segments. The medial antral wall is sectioned, allowing for mobilization of the lesser segment after separation from the pterygoid plate. This is accomplished on the greater segment with further reflection of the nasal mucoperiosteum and separation of the nasal septum and vomer. The greater segment is then down-fractured. As the maxilla is further mobilized, care must be taken to split the soft tissue between the nasal floor on the cleft side and the palate. With the maxillae down-fractured, the nasal floor can be closed under direct visualization. The palate is closed and the arch is expanded and advanced as necessary. The bone graft is now inserted, and a labial pedicle flap is mobilized to close the defect. This pedicle should be long enough to cover the alveolar and palatal defects along with the bone graft. The length should not be more than three times the width of the flap.

Fig. 7-15.
Simultaneous advancement and grafting in the unilateral cleft. **A,** Such a cleft with retrusion of the maxilla; **B,** circumvestibular incision passing through the superior aspect of the fistula; elevation of the mucoperiosteal flaps to expose the lateral maxilla and floor of the nasal cavity; lateral osteotomies are accomplished, and the nasal septum is separated from the maxilla with an osteotome; **C,** if a separate anterior segment is needed in the unilateral cleft, a labial pedicle should be maintained to ensure an adequate vascular supply to the segment.

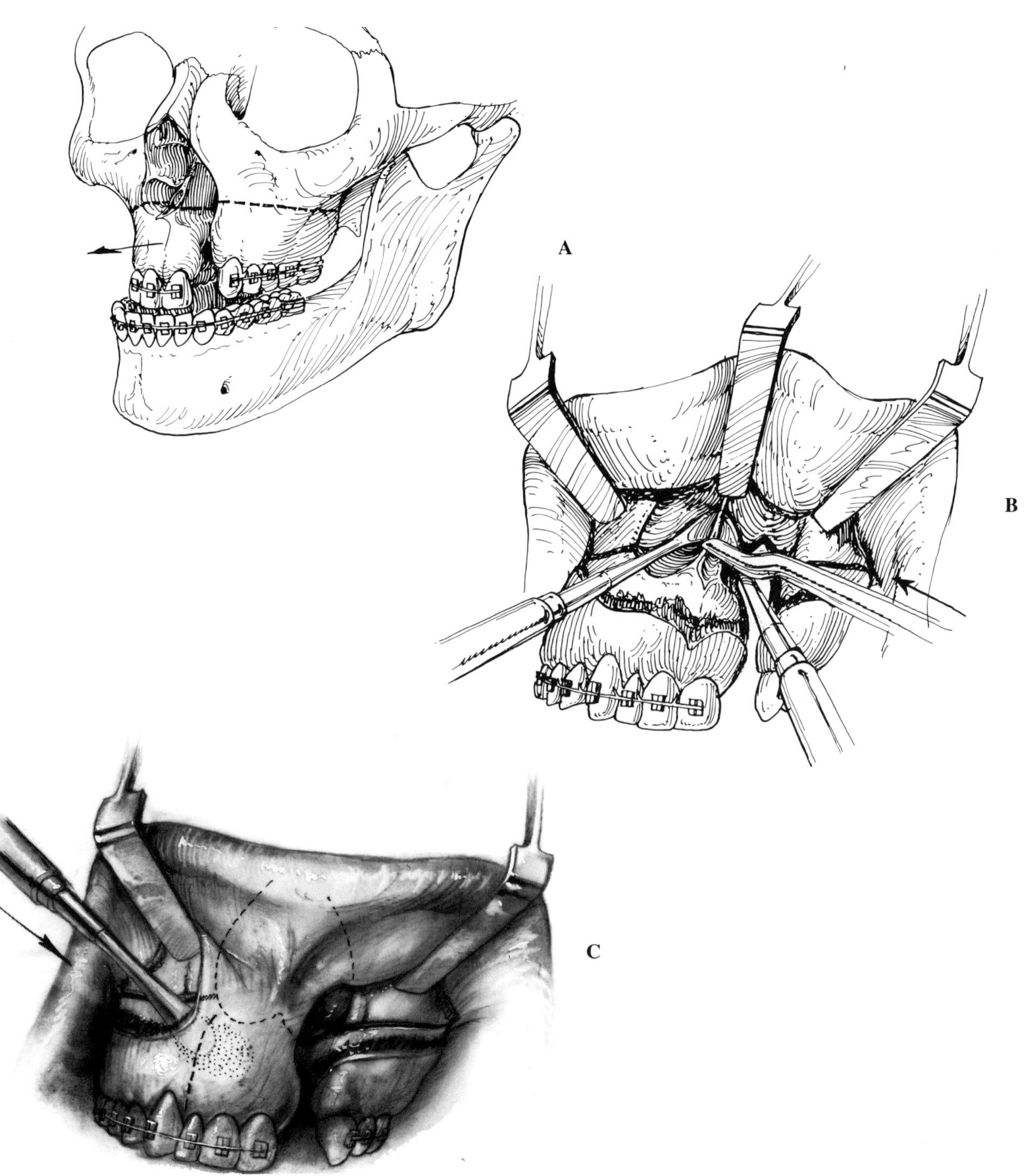

Fig. 7-15.
For legend see opposite page.

Continued.

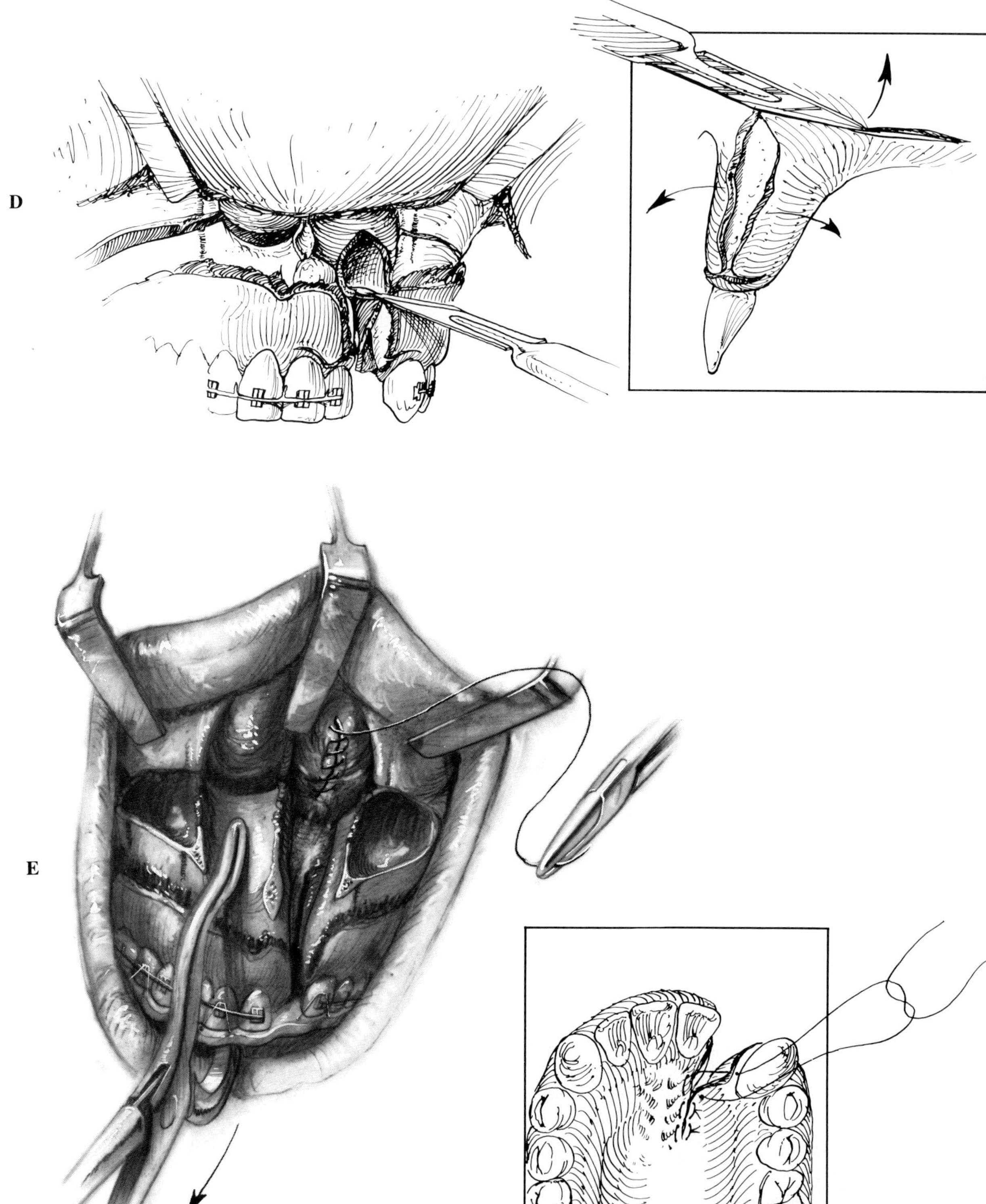

Fig. 7-15—cont'd.
D, The nasal mucosa is incised at the level of the nasal floor; to avoid tearing the mucosa in the cleft, this should be accomplished prior to the down-fracturing of the maxilla; **E,** the maxillary segments are down-fractured and mobilized; the nasal floor is closed by suturing the medial and lateral nasal flaps; the palatal mucoperiosteal flaps are closed; and the occlusal splint is inserted.

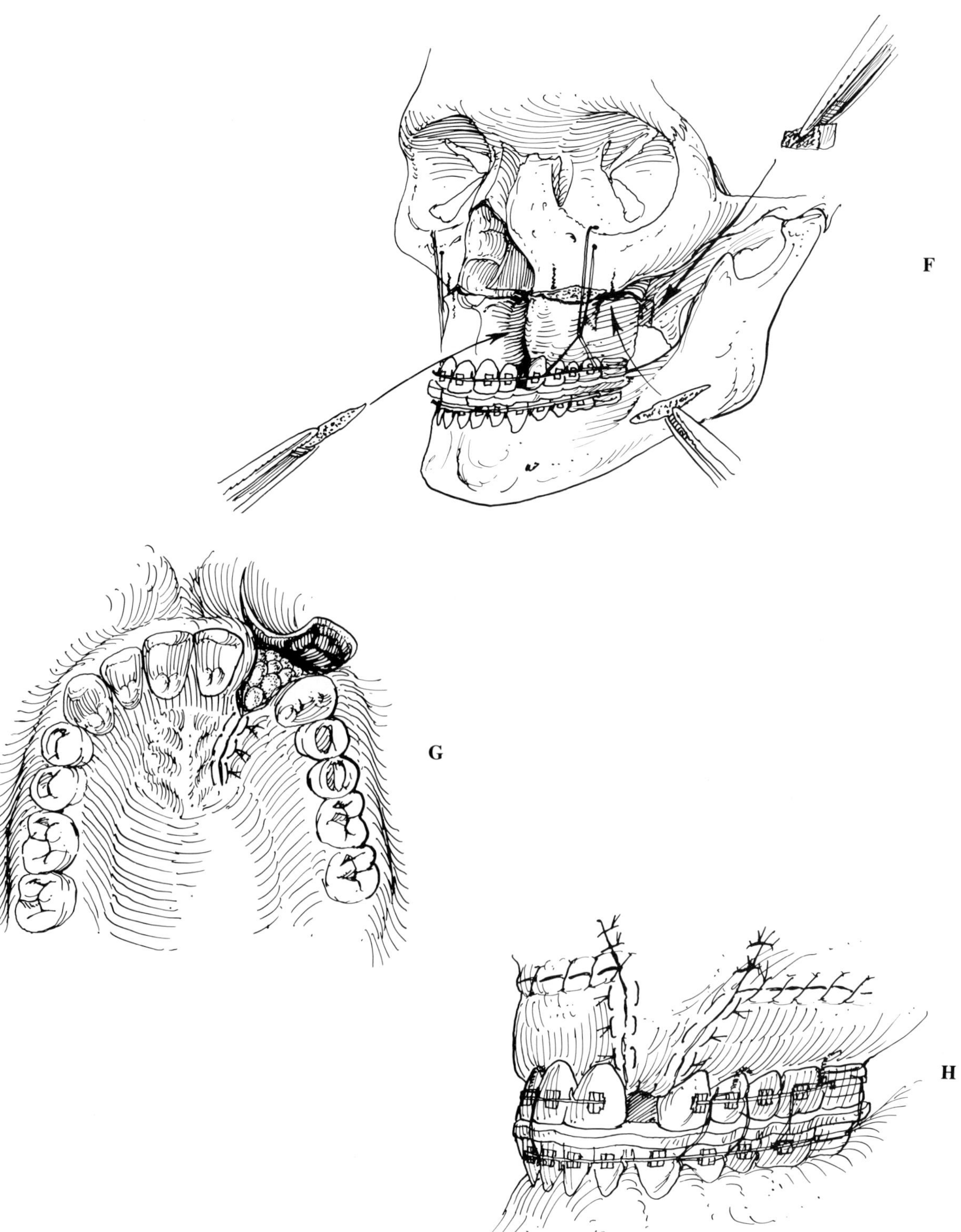

Fig. 7-15—cont'd.
F, The maxilla is advanced and secured with skeletal suspension from the infraorbital rims; bone grafts are placed in the tuberosity area, lateral antral walls, and alveolar cleft defect; **G,** a trapezoidal or finger flap is used to close the labial defect and bone graft; **H,** the circumvestibular incision is closed.

The bilateral cleft palate can be simultaneously reconstructed with a bone graft and the maxilla advanced with few modifications to the aforementioned procedure (Fig. 7-16). The flaps along the premaxillary segment are developed as previously described for repositioning of the anterior segment alone. The principles of the Wunderer[124] osteotomy are applied to mobilize the premaxilla, following which the LeFort I level osteotomy can be approached in a coronal plane. Care must be exercised to maintain the vascular pedicle to the premaxilla. The osteotomy of the posterior segments can be accomplished through horizontal circumvestibular incisions bilaterally extending to the anterior cleft margins.[35] The osteotomy can also be accomplished through multiple vertical incisions utilizing a tunneling technique and thereby maintaining an additional vascular pedicle to the posterior segments.[120] This technique is valuable when the blood supply to the segments may be questionable secondary to severe scarring with multiple surgical procedures. The segments are sectioned from the pterygoid plates and mobilized individually. The premaxilla is sectioned from the vomer and nasal septum and then "out-fractured." The posterior segments are expanded and advanced as indicated. The nasal floor can be closed under direct visualization. The palatal flaps are closed and the segment secured with splints. The osteotomy sites are bone grafted and wired into position. The cleft defect is grafted and pedicle flaps advanced to close the anterior defect and cover the bone graft as previously described. The horizontal or vertical posterior incisions are similarly closed.

Choice of procedure

The cleft palate patient will usually demonstrate a maxillary hypoplasia and retrusion, presenting as a Class III appearance and occlusion. The procedure of choice to correct the deformity is the LeFort I maxillary advancement osteotomy. However, the patient should be evaluated as to the amount of scarring of the palate and previous pharyngeal flaps, which may contribute to increased tendency toward relapse. In the patient with severe scarring and dense fibrotic palatal tissue a mandibular setback may offer a more stable result when the esthetic changes are within acceptable limits. In patients requiring large moves to correct the deformity consideration should be given to a bimaxillary procedure. This would avoid the entire movement in the same jaw and decrease the potential relapse.

Orthodontic expansion

The need for orthodontic expansion is almost universal in the cleft palate patient. In most instances this can be accomplished without difficulty by a number of orthodontic appliances. However, in the patient with a severely scarred and inelastic palatal soft tissue it may be difficult. The soft tissue can be released to a certain degree by making a releasing incision at the palatoalveolar junction on the major segment. The mucoperiosteum is elevated to the midline to allow expansion of the minor segment. This will leave an area devoid of soft tissue on the major segment, which will granulate and reepithelialize.

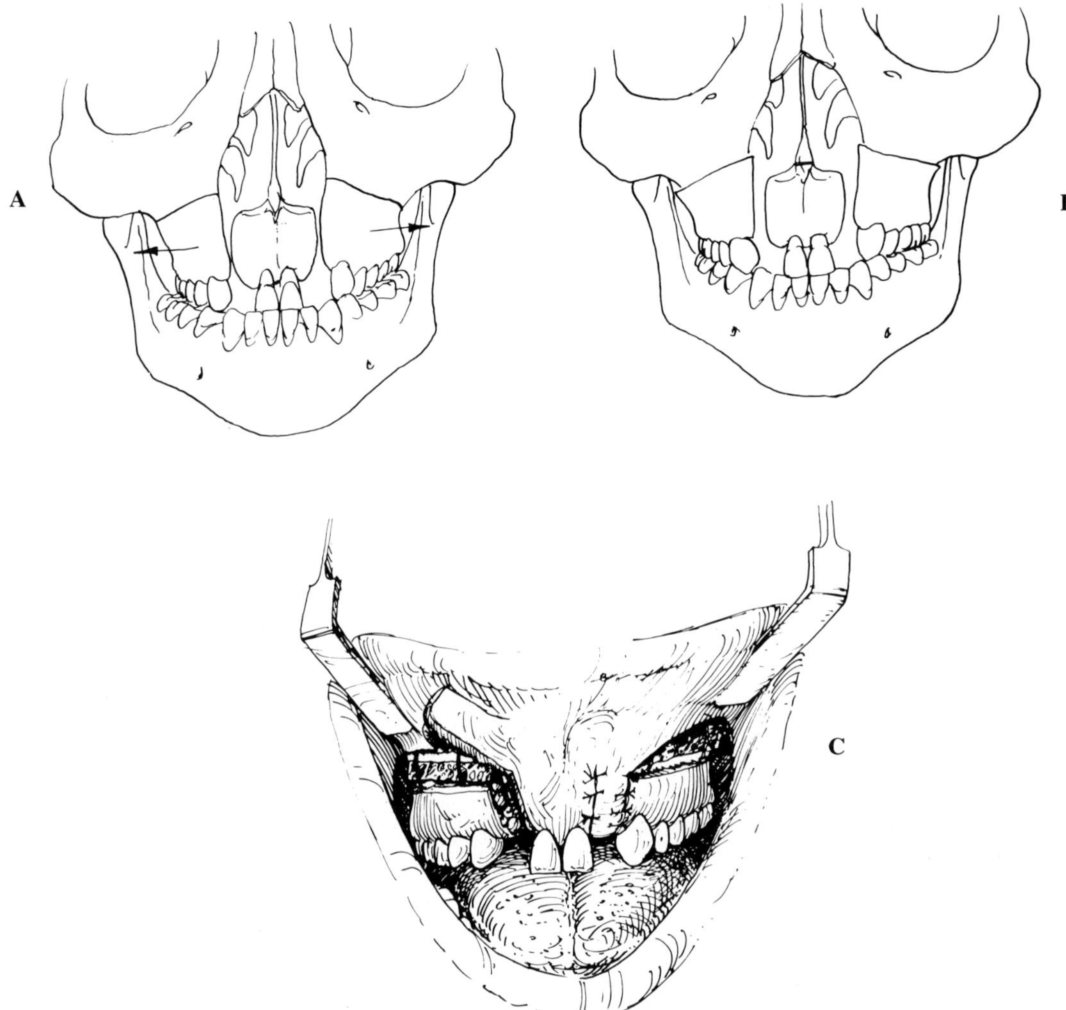

Fig. 7-16.
Simultaneous advancement and grafting in the bilateral cleft. The elevation of soft tissue flaps in the bilateral defect is similar to that in the unilateral except for maintenance of a labial mucoperiosteal pedicle to the anterior segment. **A,** Lateral osteotomies are accomplished, and the segments are separated from the pterygoid plates. The posterior segments are mobilized. **B,** The premaxilla is out-fractured and mobilized. The segments are placed in the splint, and the nasal floor is closed. **C,** Bone grafts are placed in the tuberosity area, lateral antral wall, and alveolar cleft defect. Finger flaps are developed bilaterally and rotated into position to cover the bone graft and defect. It is often necessary to use these flaps to complete the palatal closure. The vestibular incision is then closed horizontally.

Reprinted from Bell, W.H., et al.: Surgical correction of dentofacial deformities, Philadelphia, 1980, W.B. Saunders Co.

SOFT TISSUE REVISIONS

It is outside the scope of this chapter to address the numerous procedures related to the secondary revisions often necessary in the cleft palate patient. However, for completeness it is important to recognize that 10% of patients with a unilateral cleft lip will have an unacceptable result after the first repair. Approximately 30% will require additional surgery for correction of the nasal deformities. Approximately 25% of bilateral cleft lips will have an unacceptable result after the primary repair, requiring a secondary revision.[124] Kinnebrew and Kent[52] give an overview of this particular subject. Revisions may range from simple scar release to rotation of tissue utilizing an Abbe flap or other regional flaps.[51] Most of these patients will also require nasal revision to correct the nasal septal deviation and the distortion of the lateral nasal cartilages* (Fig. 7-17).

---

*References 27, 52, 124.

RESULTS

The characteristics of this series of patients[72] are represented in Table 7-1 and are fairly consistent with those in other series. Approximately 80% of this group had unilateral defects, with two thirds of the defects occurring on the left. Males represented a higher percentage, in both groups.

The average age at the time of surgery was 11.6 years in the unilateral group and 12.1 in the bilateral group (Table 7-2). Between 70% and 80% of the patients had symptomatic oronasal fistulae, represented usually by reflux of liquids under certain conditions. The range of age for patients operated on was 7 to 24 in the unilateral group and 9 to 17 in the bilateral group.

The overall success rate for grafting of the alveolar cleft defect with autogenous particulate cancellous marrow was 98.3%, with failure of only one defect in the 60 reconstructed. The complications are listed in Table 7-3. Minor

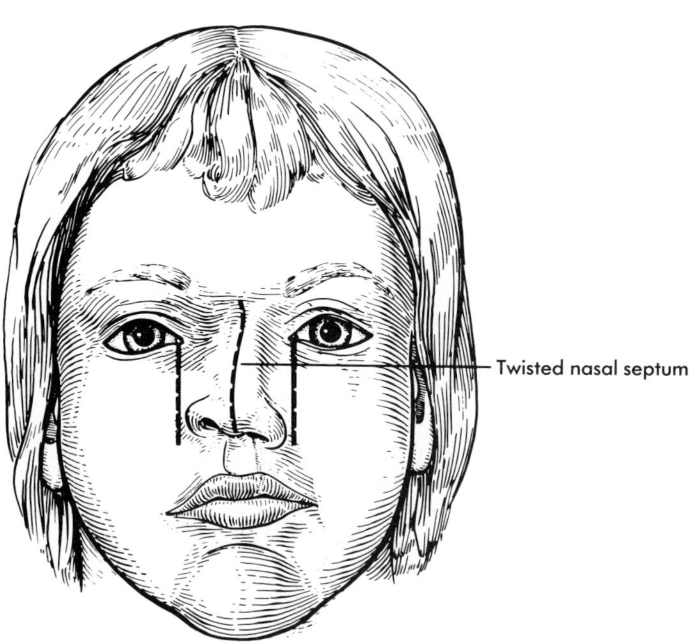

Fig. 7-17.
Secondary revisions. The twisted nasal septum and distorted nasal cartilages will require secondary procedures for correction.
Reprinted from Smith, H.: The atlas of cleft lip and cleft palate surgery, New York, 1983, Grune & Stratton, Inc.

soft tissue dehiscence occurred in 3.3% of the cases, usually in the earlier ones, and may have represented failure to mobilize the soft tissue flaps adequately for closure of the defects. However, even in these cases, it remained superficial, with only minimal loss of bone graft. The grafts seemed to show a resistance to infection and breakdown. There were no infections, and the most common complication was the development of hyperplastic granulation tissue at about 2 to 3 weeks (occurring in 11.7% of our cases). This was easily managed with conservative excision and was sometimes associated with the sequestration of a bony spicule (5% of the cases). Root resorption was seen in one case, on the lateral incisor in an adult patient. The only complication related to the donor site was a seroma, which required aspiration but caused no other problem. The worst complication was complete loss of the bone graft (in one defect). This occurred in a patient with bilateral clefts that were repaired simultaneously. The

patient's hospital course was uneventful, but he failed to return for 6 weeks. When we saw him, he had removed his palatal splint and the graft was exposed on one side, with evidence of refistulization. The bone graft was eventually lost. On the opposite side the graft took but did not result in as high a level of bone as we would have desired. This failure could represent a technical error but was more likely due to lack of patient cooperation.

Most patients received orthodontic treatment (Table 7-4), 25% of the unilateral and 40% of the bilateral groups receiving it presurgically. A higher percentage received it postsurgically, and we found no increased problem with arch expansion in these patients.

There were no significant bleeding problems in the series, and no patient required blood transfusion. The average hospitalization was 3.5 days, with a slight increase for bilateral procedures. Generally the length of operation was 2 hours for a unilateral and 3 hours for a

Table 7-1.

Analysis of 50 cleft palate patients

Type of cleft	Race (% Caucasian)	Sex (%)		Location of cleft (%)	
		Male	Female	Right	Left
Unilateral (n = 40)	60.5	55	45	30	70
Bilateral (n = 10)	80	70	30	100	100
TOTAL DEFECTS, 60					

Table 7-2.

Age at operation (symptomatic oronasal fistula)

Type of cleft	Average age at operation (yr)	Symptomatic oronasal fistula (%)
Unilateral	11.6 (7 to 24)*	80
Bilateral	12.1 (9 to 17)*	70

*Range of age.

Table 7-3.

Complications

	Number	Percent
Minor soft tissue dehiscence	2	3.3
Hyperplastic granulation tissue	7	11.7
Bony spicule sequestered	3	5.0
Root resorption	1	1.7
Seroma of hip	1	1.7
Complete loss of graft	1	1.7

Table 7-4.
Orthodontic treatment

Type of cleft	Before surgery (%)	After surgery (%)	Planned for later (%)
Unilateral	25	62.5	12.5
Bilateral	40	50	10

bilateral procedure (including the simultaneous obtaining of the bone graft by a second surgical team).

Stability of the reconstructed alveolar cleft palate is yet to be determined in a predictable manner. Overall it seems good, but with long-term follow-up we see a tendency toward collapse of the minor segment without permanent retention. It would seem unlikely that we could expect less when we try to expand a palate that is deficient and has been subjected to multiple surgical procedures that scar and increase the tension on those tissues. Although the stability gained and the improvement in functional and esthetic parameters certainly justify the procedure, bone grafting is not the total solution for long-term stability.

The following case studies represent the principles and techniques discussed (Figs. 7-18 to 7-21).

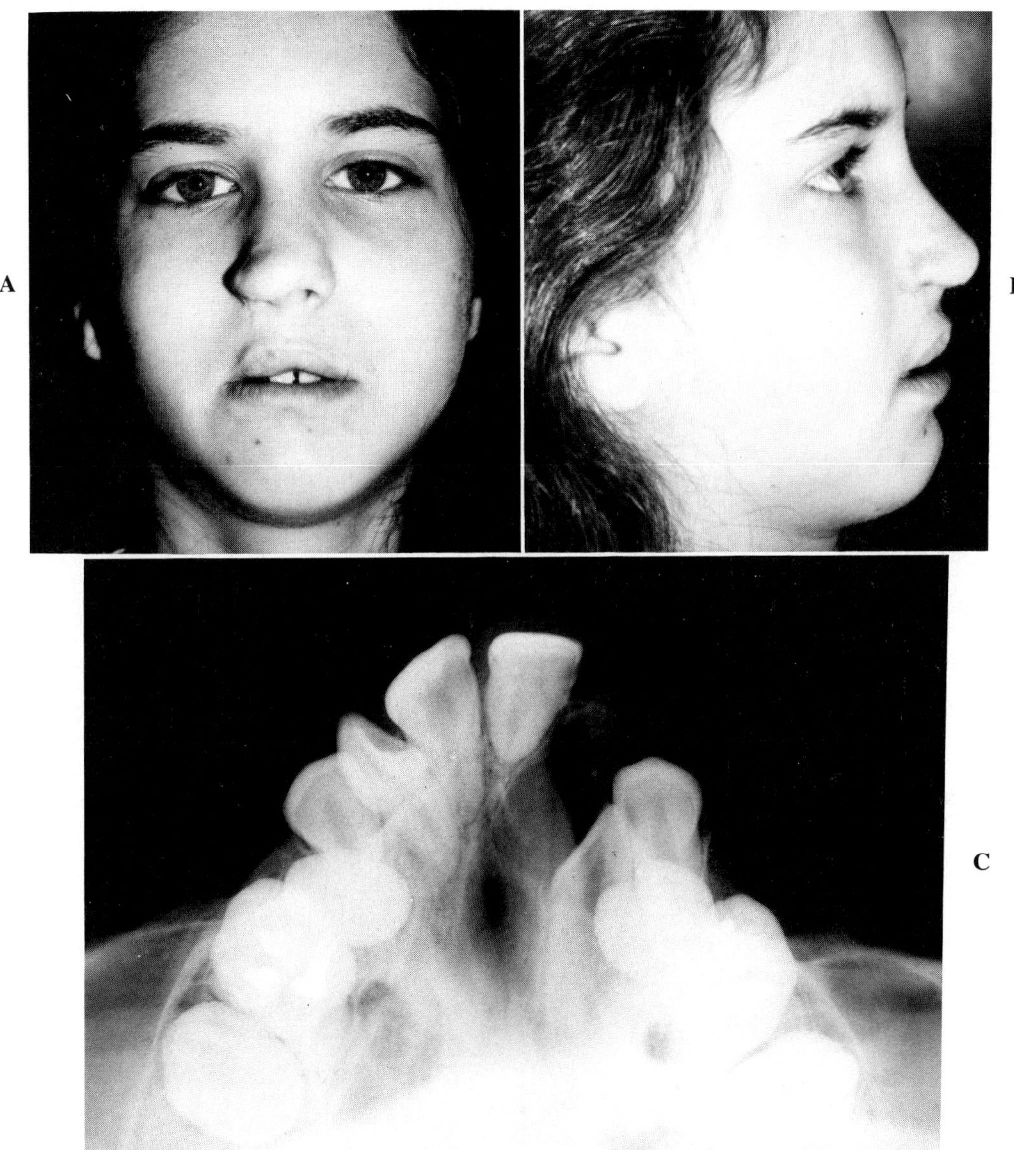

Continued.

Fig. 7-18.
Unilateral alveolar cleft. **A** to **C,** Preoperative appearance.

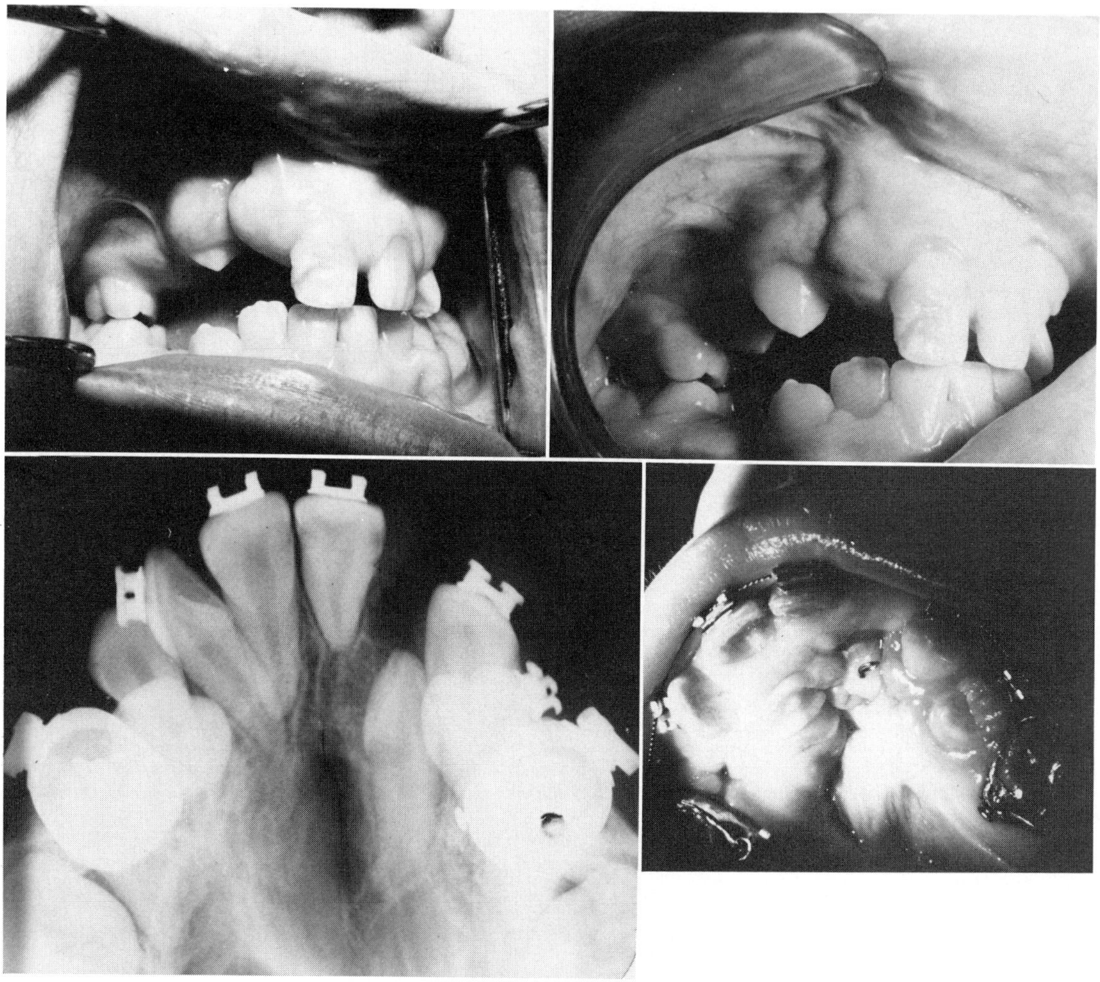

Fig. 7-18—cont'd.
D, The alveolar defect with oronasal fistula. **E,** Six weeks postoperative. Good labial contour. A tooth is erupting through the graft. **F,** Three months postoperative. Good bone fill. **G,** Four months exposure of the lateral incisor.

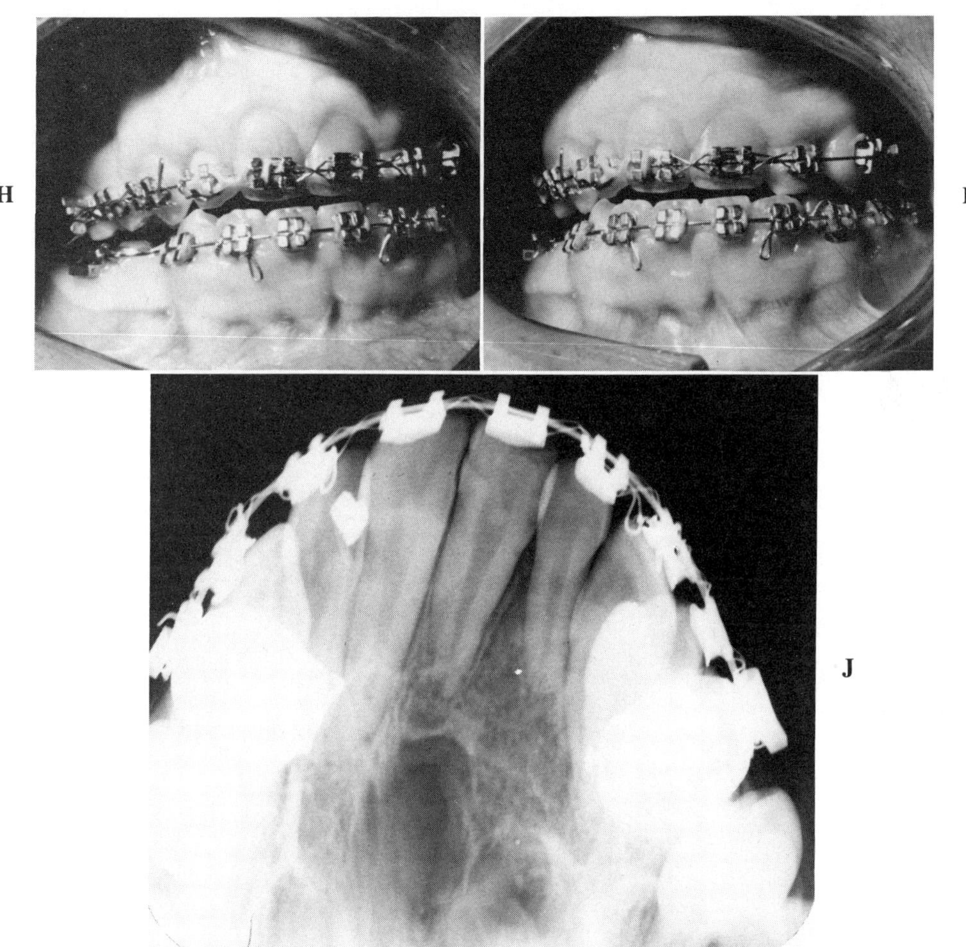

Continued.

Fig. 7-18—cont'd.
H to **J,** One year postoperative. Movement of the lateral incisor into position and an adequate level of attached gingiva.

K L M

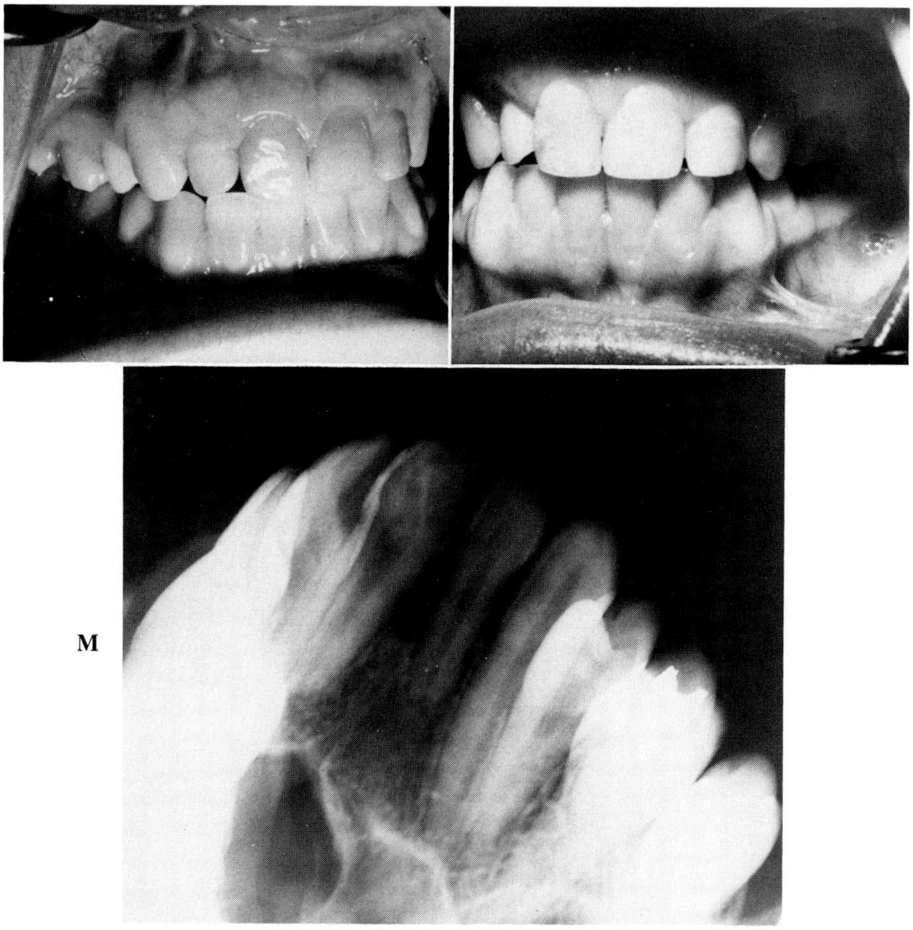

Fig. 7-18—cont'd.
K to **M,** Three years postoperative. Maintenance of a good bone level and periodontal support.

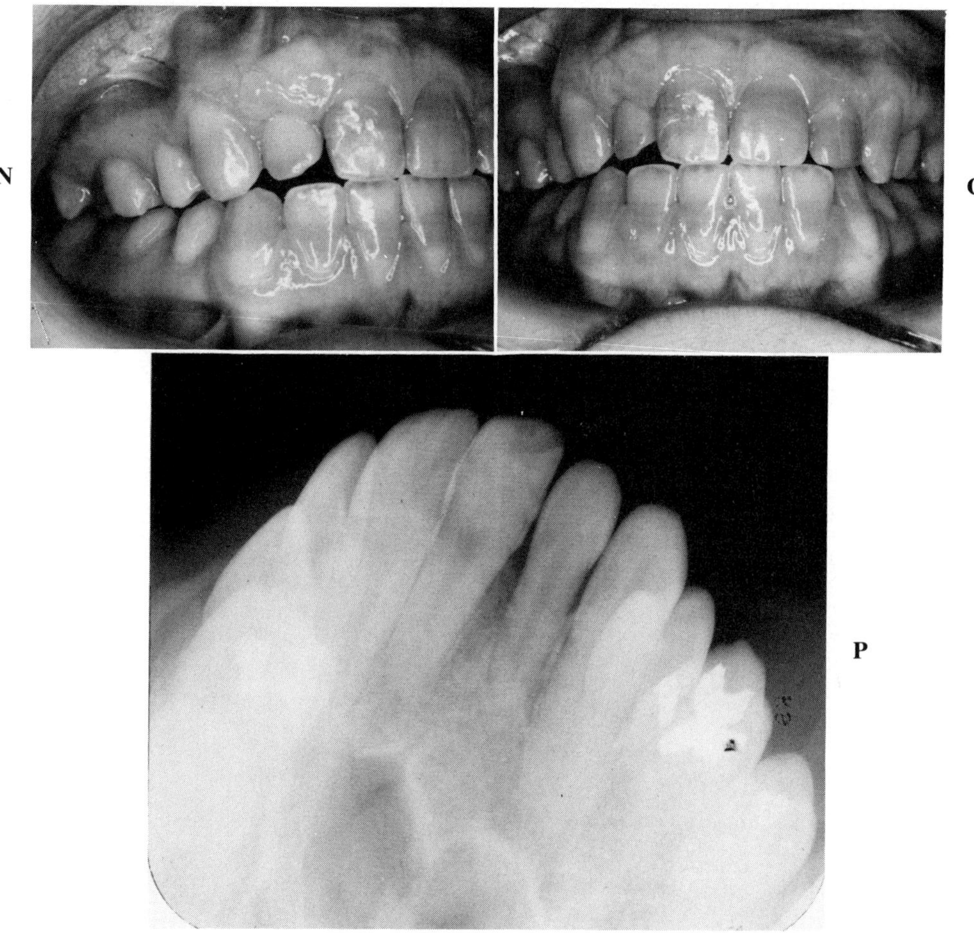

Fig. 7-18—cont'd.
N to **P,** Five years postoperative. Some relapse of the lateral incisor but good stability of the minor segment and overall occlusion. Note the slight loss of bone height on the radiograph.

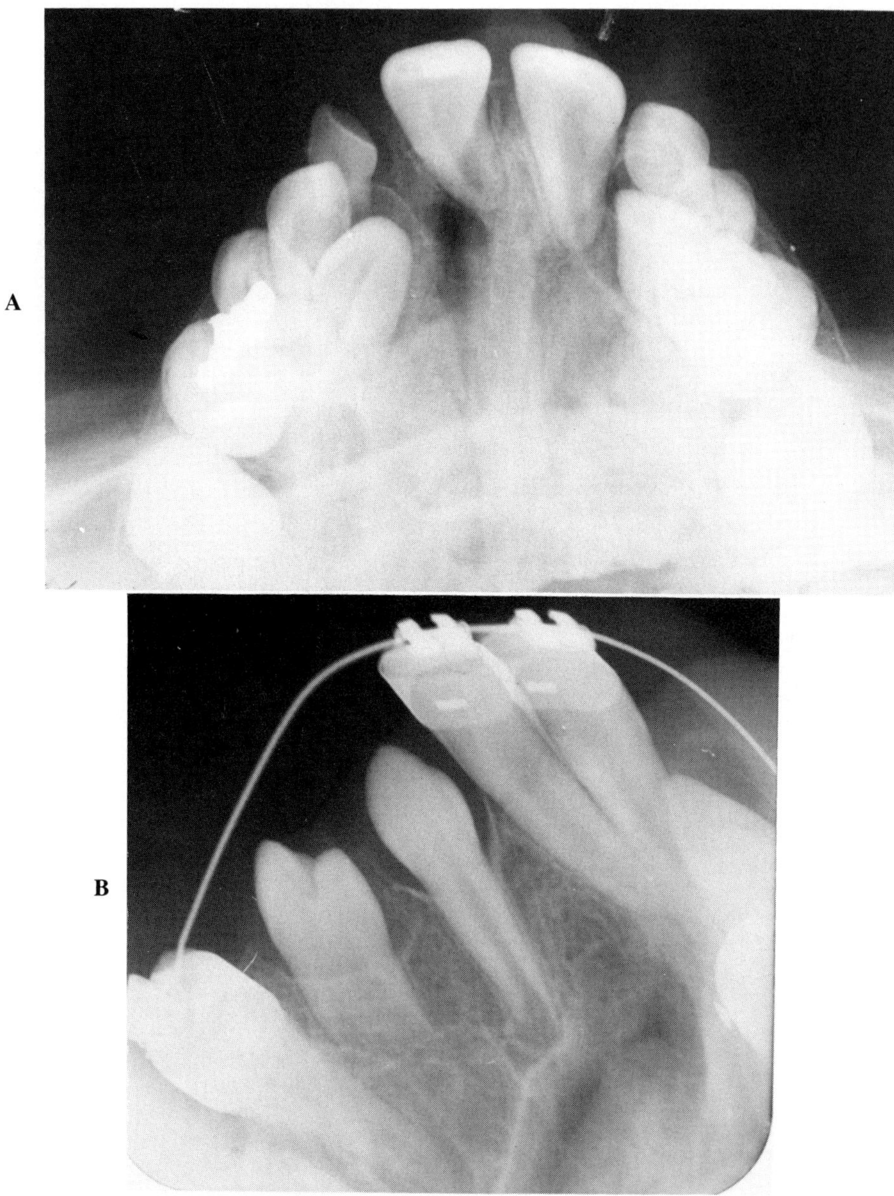

Fig. 7-19.
Canine eruption through a bone graft. **A,** Preoperative appearance. **B,** Two years postoperative. Good bone height and mineralization of the graft.

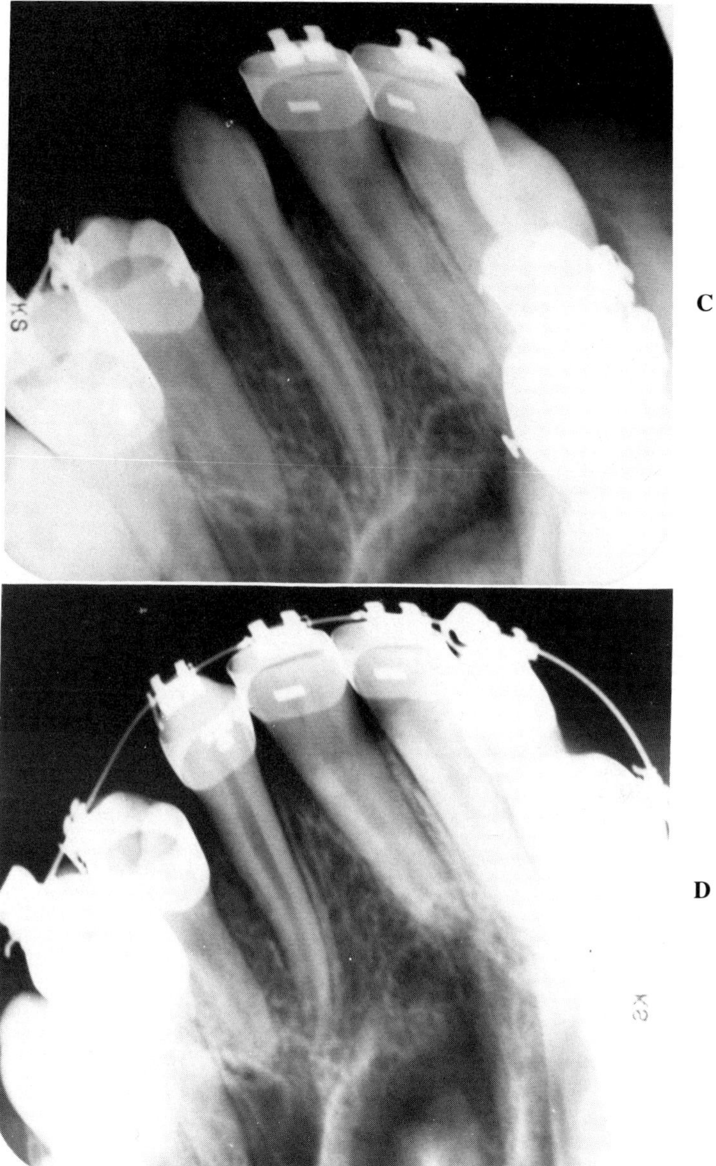

Fig. 7-19—cont'd.
C, Four years postoperative. The canine has erupted into the oral cavity without orthodontic assistance. **D,** Five years postoperative. Full orthodontic appliances with maintenance of good bone height and periodontal support.

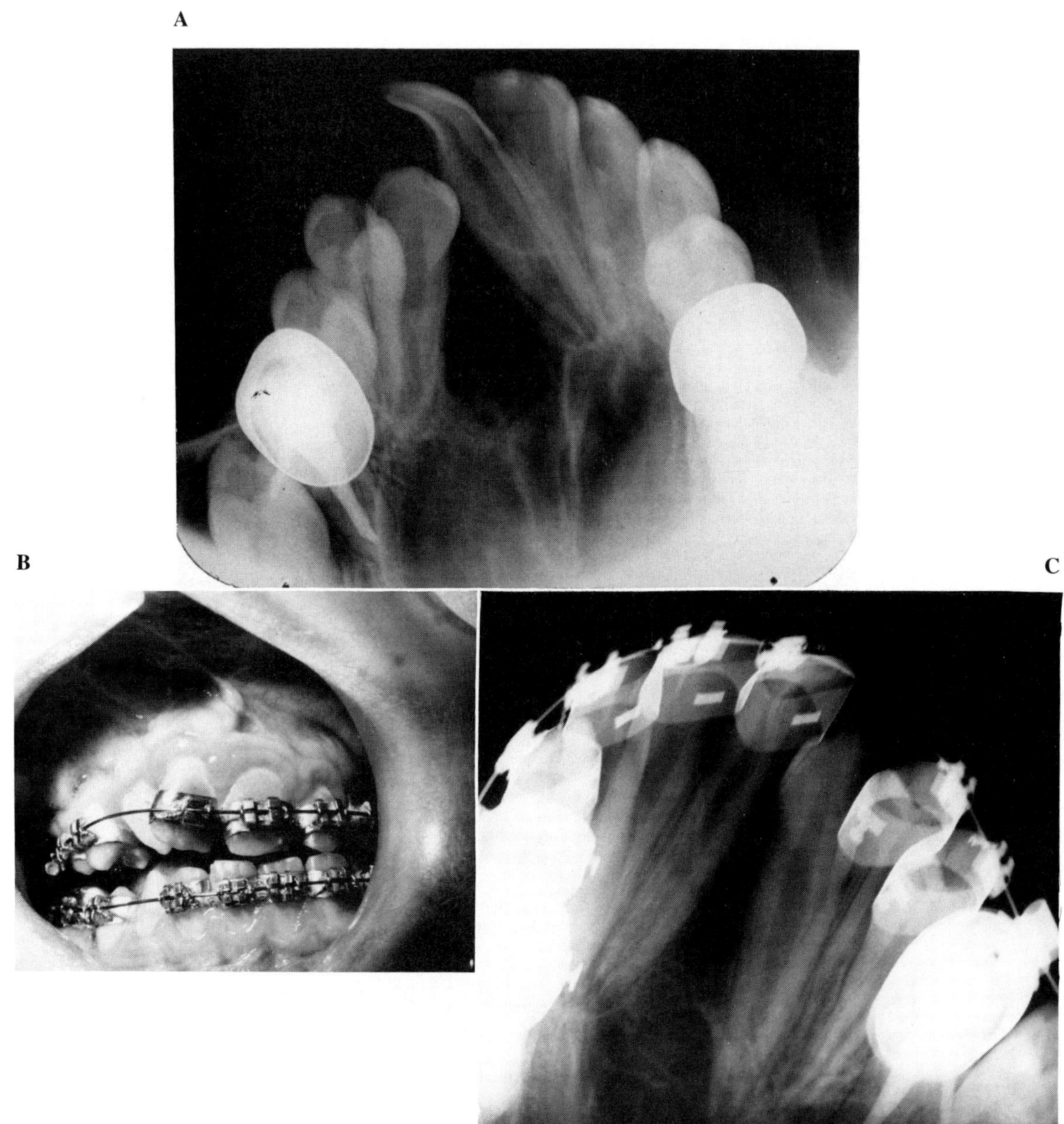

Fig. 7-20.
Unilateral alveolar cleft. **A,** Preoperative appearance. Bony defect with malposition of teeth along the margins of the cleft and minimal periodontal support. **B** and **C,** One year postoperative. Orthodontic treatment has been initiated. Good bone height and periodontal support.

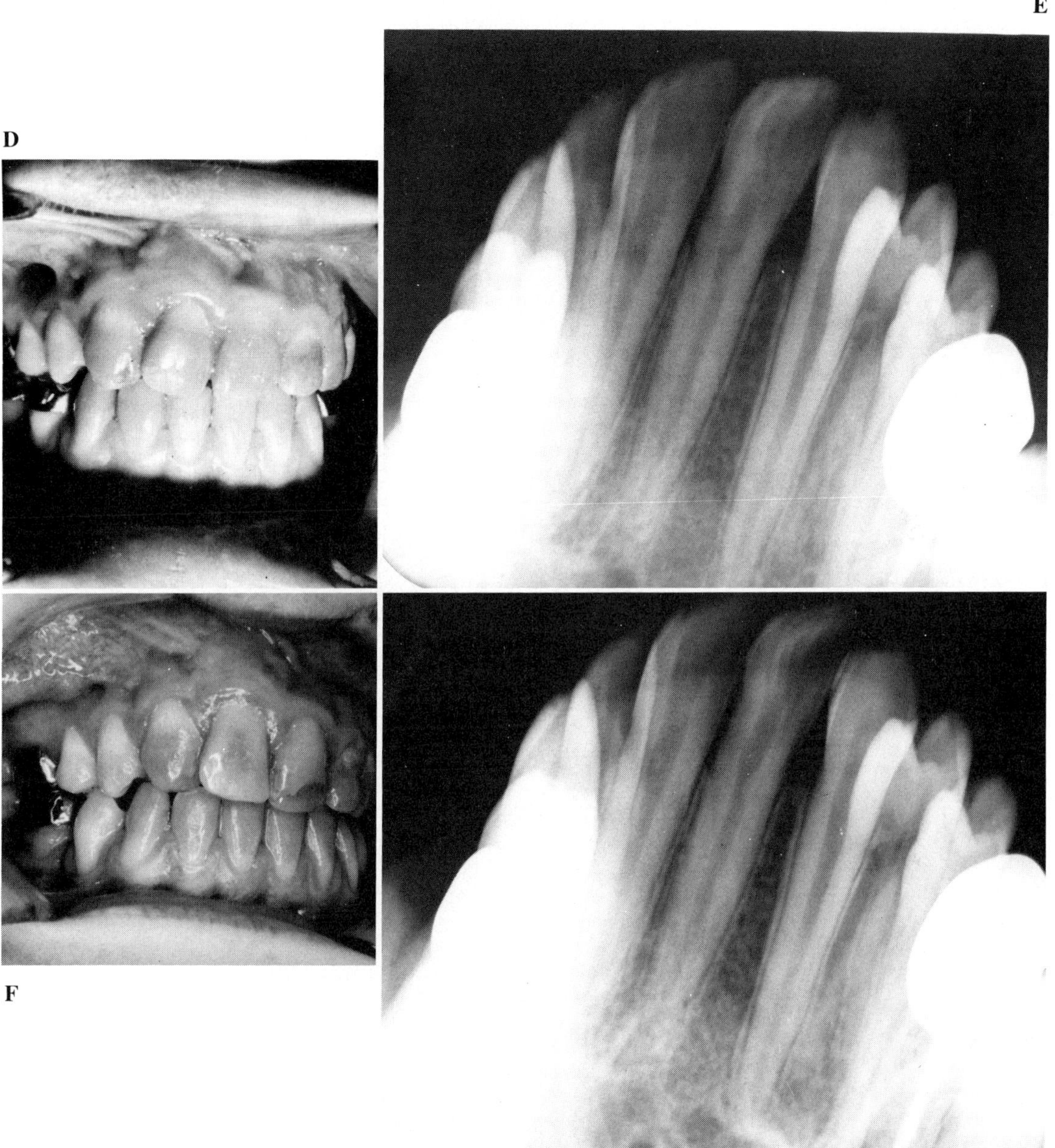

Fig. 7-20—cont'd.
D and **E,** Two years postoperative. Good position of the canine. The roots have been aligned orthodontically into the graft. **F** and **G,** Five years postoperative. Good stability of the minor segment and dentition. The bone height between the canine and central incisor is excellent.

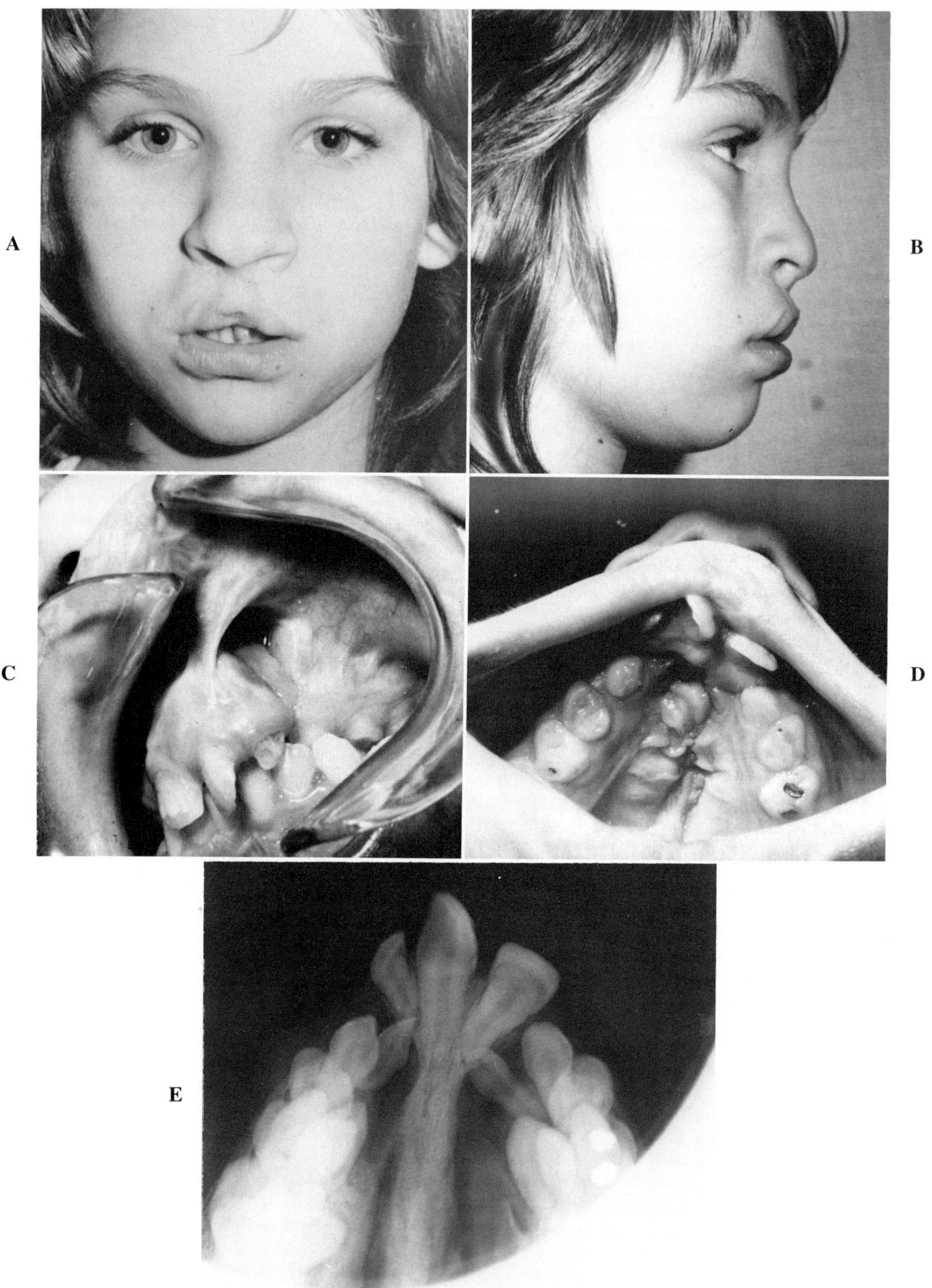

Fig. 7-21.
Bilateral alveolar cleft. **A** and **B,** Typical facial characteristics. **C,** Large oronasal fistula with severe rotation and malposition of the teeth. **D,** Bilateral collapse of the posterior segments and severe rotation of the incisors. **E,** Preoperative. Bone defect with teeth erupting into the cleft bilaterally.

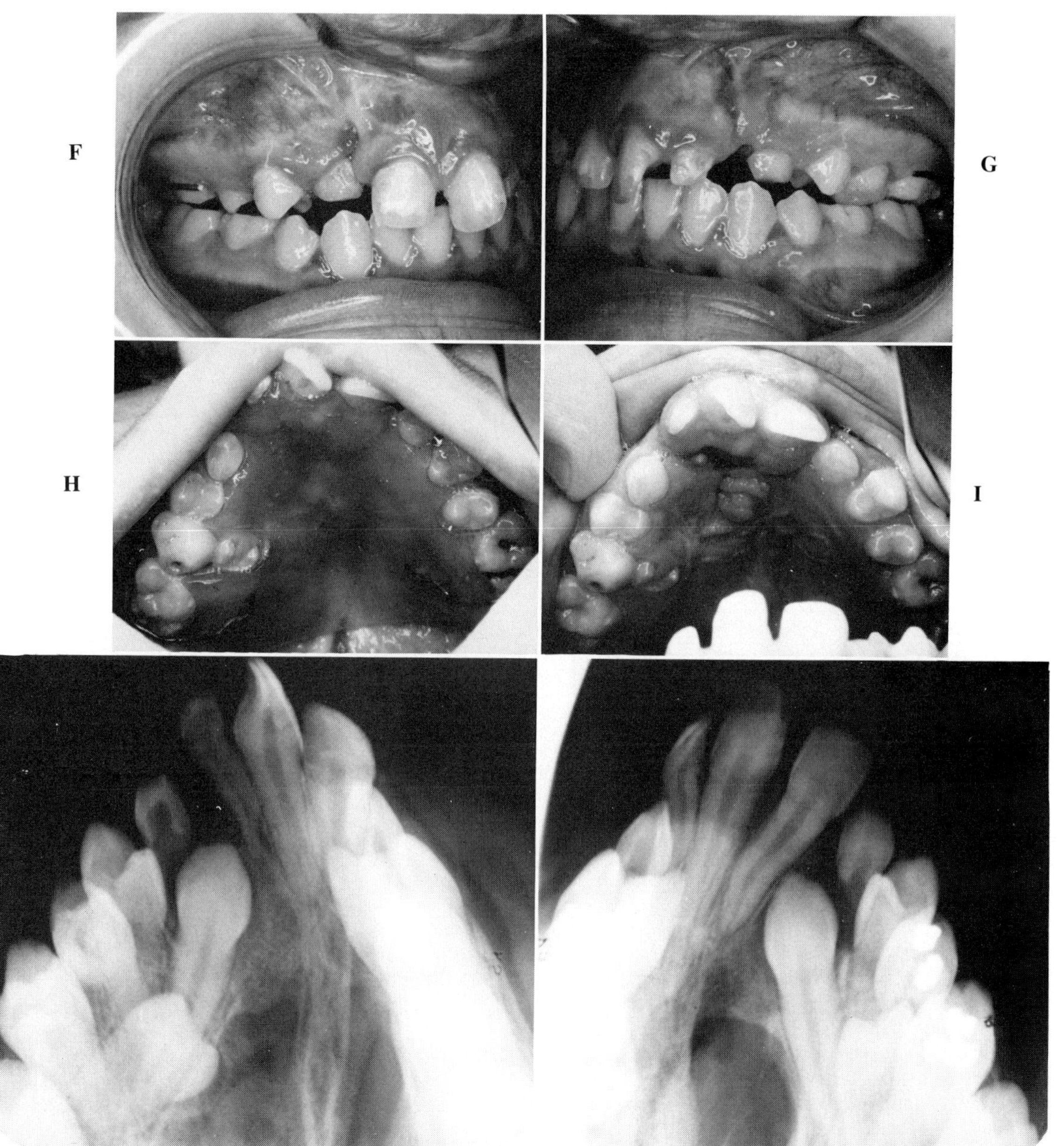

Fig. 7-21—cont'd.
F to I, Three years postoperative. There is good labial contour, and the oronasal fistulae have been eliminated. Expansion of the posterior segments was achieved and the premaxilla aligned. The canine can be seen erupting palatally into the graft site. **J** and **K,** Mineralization of the bone graft. Full orthodontic treatment is not shown in this case since the principles have already been demonstrated in previous cases.

REFERENCES

1. Ames, J.R., and Maki, K.A.: The autogenous particulate cancellous bone marrow graft in alveolar defects, Oral Surg. **51:**588, 1981.
2. Aslanian, R.A., et al.: Use of mandibular bone for revision of malunion of the maxilla: a report of a case, J. Oral Surg. **29:**825, 1971.
3. Backdahl, M., et al.: Bone grafting to the maxillary defect in cleft lip and palate by the method of Backdahl and Nordin. In Transactions of the Third International Congress of Plastic Surgery. International congress series no. 66, New York, 1964, Excerpta Medica Foundation.
4. Backdahl, M., and Nordin, K.E.: Replacement of the maxillary bone defect in cleft palate: a new procedure, Acta Chir. Scand. **122:**131, 1961.
5. Bays, R.A.: Current concepts in bone grafting. In Irby, W.B., and Shelton, D.W., editors: Current advances in oral and maxillofacial surgery, vol. 4, St. Louis, 1983, The C.V. Mosby Co.
6. Berkowitz, S.: State of the art in cleft palate orofacial growth and dentistry, Am. J. Orthod. **74:**564, 1978.
7. Bertz, J.E.: Bone grafting of alveolar clefts, J. Oral Surg. **39:**874, 1981.
8. Billington, W., et al.: Bone-grafting in gunshot fractures of the jaw, Proc. R. Soc. Med. **12:**41, 1919.
9. Bloomquist, D.S.: Bone grafting in dentofacial defects. In Bell, W.H., et al., editors: Surgical correction of dentofacial deformities, Philadelphia, 1980, W.B. Saunders Co.
10. Boyne, P.J.: Autogenous cancellous bone marrow transplants, Clin. Orthop. **73:**199, 1970.
11. Boyne, P.J.: Osseous grafts and implants in the restoration of large oral defects, J. Periodontol. **45:**378, 1974.
12. Boyne, P.J.: Use of marrow–cancellous bone grafts in maxillary alveolar and palatal clefts, J. Dent. Res. **53:**821, 1974.
13. Boyne, P.J.: Tissue transplantation. In Kruger, G.O., editor: Textbook of oral and maxillofacial surgery, ed. 5, St. Louis, 1979, The C.V. Mosby Co.
14. Boyne, P.J., and Sands, N.R.: Secondary bone grafting of residual alveolar and palatal clefts, J. Oral Surg. **30:**87, 1972.
15. Boyne, P.J., and Sands, N.R.: Combined orthodontic-surgical management of residual palatoalveolar cleft defects, Am. J. Orthod. **70:**20, 1976.
16. Braun, T.W., and Sotereanos, G.C.: Alveolar reconstruction in adolescent patients with cleft palates, J. Oral Surg. **39:**510, 1981.
17. Broude, D.J., and Waite, D.E.: Secondary closure of alveolar defects, Oral Surg. **37:**829, 1974.
18. Burnette, E.W., Jr.: Fate of an iliac crest graft, J. Periodontol. **43:**88, 1972.
19. Burwell, G.R.: Studies in the transplantation of bone: treated composite homografts of cancellous bone. An analysis of inductive mechanisms in bone transplantation, J. Bone Joint Surg. **48B:**532, 1966.
20. Burwell, G.R.: The fate of bone grafts. In Apley, A.G., editor: Recent advances in orthopedics, London, 1969, J.&.A. Churchill, Ltd.
21. Burwell, G.R.: The fate of freeze-dried bone alloplasts, Transplant. Proc. **8**(suppl. 1):95, 1976.
22. Carlesso, J., et al.: Hemi-tongue flaps, Plast. Reconstr. Surg. **66:**4, 1980.
23. Converse, J.M., et al.: Bone grafts in surgery of the face, Surg. Clin. North Am. **34:**375, 1954.
24. Cooper, H.K., et al.: Cleft palate and cleft lip: a team approach to clinical management and rehabilitation of the patient, ed. 1, Philadelphia, 1979, W.B. Saunders Co.
25. Crockford, D.A., and Converse, J.M.: The ilium as a source of bone grafts in children, Plast. Reconstr. Surg. **50:**270, 1972.
26. Curtis, E.J.: Genetical and environmental factors in the etiology of the cleft lip and cleft palate, J. Can. Dent. Assoc. **23:**576, 1957.
27. Dibbell, D.G.: Cleft lip nasal reconstruction: correcting the classic unilateral defect, Plast. Reconstr. Surg. **69:**264, 1982.
28. Dieffenbach, J.F.: Die operative Chirurgie, Leipzig, 1845, F.A. Bockhaus.
29. Dingman, R.O.: The use of iliac bone in the repair of facial and cranial defects, Plast. Reconstr. Surg. **6:** 179, 1950.
30. Doig, R.K., and Coltman, O.M.: Cleft palate following cortisone therapy in early pregnancy, Lancet **2:** 270, 1956.
31. Dorrance, G.M.: Lengthening of the soft palate operation, Ann. Surg. **82:**205, 1925.
32. Dragoo, M.R., and Sullivan, H.C.: A clinical and histologic evaluation of autogenous iliac bone grafts in humans. II. External root resorption, J. Periodontol. **44:**614, 1971.
33. El-Deeb, M., et al.: Alveolar bone graft resorption associated with abnormal dental follicle, Cleft Palate J. **21:**22, 1984.
34. Ellegaard, B., and Löe, H.: New attachment of periodontal tissue after treatment of intrabony lesions, J. Periodontol. **42:**648, 1971.
35. Epker, B.N., and Wolford, L.M.: Dentofacial deformities: surgical-orthodontic correction, St. Louis, 1980, The C.V. Mosby Co.
36. Ferguson, M.W.J.: Developmental mechanisms in normal and abnormal palate formation, with particular reference to the aetiology, pathogenesis, and prevention of cleft palate, Br. J. Orthod. **8:**115, 1981.
37. Gorlin, R.J., and Pindborg, J.J.: Syndromes of head and neck, New York, 1964, McGraw-Hill Book Co.
38. Gorlin, R.J., et al.: Facial clefting and its syndromes, Birth Defects **7:**3, June 1971.
39. Graber, T.M.: Craniofacial morphology in cleft palate and cleft lip deformities, Surg. Gynecol. Obstet. **88:**359, 1949.
40. Guerrero-Santos, J., and Altamirand, J.: The use of lingual flaps in repair of fistulas of the hard palate, Plast. Reconstr. Surg. **38:**123, 1966.

41. Hagedorn, H.C.: Über eine Modifikation der Hasen-schartenoperation, Zentralbl. Chir. **11**:756, 1884.
42. Hall, D.H., and Posnick, J.C.: Early results of secondary bone grafts in 106 alveolar clefts, J. Oral Maxillofac. Surg. **42**:289, 1983.
43. Henderson, D., and Jackson, I.T.: Combined cleft lip revision, anterior fistula closure, and maxillary osteotomy: a one stage procedure, Br. J. Oral Surg. **13**:33, 1975.
44. Hinrichs, J.E., et al.: Periodontal evaluation of canines erupted through grafted alveolar defects, J. Oral Maxillofac. Surg. **42**:717, 1984.
45. Hogman, K.E., et al.: Secondary bone grafting in the cleft palate: a follow-up of 145 patients, Cleft Palate J. **9**:39, 1972.
46. Hotz, M., and Gnoinski, W.: Comprehensive care of the cleft palate children at Zurich University: a preliminary report, Am. J. Orthod. **70**:481, 1976.
47. Jackson, I.T., et al.: Atlas of craniomaxillofacial surgery, St. Louis, 1982, The C.V. Mosby Co.
48. Johanson, B., and Ohlsson, A.: Bone grafting and dental orthopedics in primary and secondary cases of cleft lip and palate, Acta Chir. Scand. **122**:112, 1961.
49. Kazanjian, V.H., and Converse, J.M.: The surgical treatment of facial fractures, ed. 2, Baltimore, 1974, The Williams & Wilkins Co.
50. Kernahan, D.A., and Stark, R.B.: A new classification for cleft lip and cleft palate, Plast. Reconstr. Surg. **22**:435, 1958.
51. Kinnebrew, M.C.: Use of the Abbe flap in revision of the bilateral cleft lip-nose deformity, Oral Surg. **56**:12, 1983.
52. Kinnebrew, M.C., and Kent, J.N.: Late definitive correction of the orofacial cleft, Am. J. Orthod. **84**:104, 1983.
53. Kinnebrew, M.C., and Malloy, R.B.: Posteriorly based, lateral lingual flaps for alveolar cleft bone graft coverage, J. Oral Maxillofac. Surg. **41**:555, 1983.
54. Kjellgren, B.: Bettbehandling: gomspaltfall, Sven. Tandlak. Tidskr. **45**:207, 1951.
55. Kline, S.N., et al.: Use of autogenous bone from the symphysis for treatment of delayed union of the mandible: report of a case, J. Oral Surg. **28**:540, 1970.
56. Kwon, J.K., et al.: The management of alveolar cleft defects, J. Am. Dent. Assoc. **102**:848, 1981.
57. Laurie, S.W.S., et al.: Donor-site morbidity after harvesting rib and iliac bone, Plast. Reconstr. Surg. **73**:933, 1984.
58. Le Mesurier, A.B.: The treatment of complete unilateral harelip, Surg. Gynecol. Obstet. **95**:17, 1952.
59. Longacre, J.J.: Cleft palate deformation, Springfield, Ill., 1970, Charles C Thomas, Publisher.
60. Lubit, E.C.: Cleft palate orthopedics: why, when, how, Am. J. Orthod. **69**:562, 1976.
61. Lynch, J.B., et al.: Cephalometric study of maxillary growth five years after alveolar bone grafting of cleft palate infants, Plast. Reconstr. Surg. **46**:564, 1970.
62. Marx, R.E., et al.: A comparison of particulate allogeneic and particulate autogenous bone grafts into maxillary alveolar clefts in dogs, J. Oral Maxillofac. Surg. **42**:3, 1984.
63. Mathews, D.N.: Infant orthopedics and bone grafting. Presented at the International Congress on Cleft Palate, Houston, 1969.
64. McNeil, C.K.: Oral and facial deformity, London, 1954, Sir Isaac Pittman & Sons, Ltd.
65. Meskin, L.H., et al.: An epidemiological investigation of the factors related to the extent of facial clefts. I. Sex of patient, Cleft Palate J. **5**:23, 1968.
66. Millard, D.R.: Refinements in rotation-advancement cleft lip technique, Plast. Reconstr. Surg. **33**:26, 1964.
67. Millard, D.R.: Early correction of the unilateral cleft lip and nose, Plast. Reconstr. Surg. **70**:64, 1982.
68. Mirault: Lettre sur le bec-de-lièvre, Malgaigne J. Chir. **2**:257, 1964.
69. Mowlem, R.: Bone and cartilage transplants, their use and behaviour, Br. J. Surg. **29**:182, 1941.
70. Mowlem, R.: Cancellous chip bone-grafts. Report of 75 cases, Lancet **2**:746, 1944.
71. Mrazik, J., et al.: The ilium as a source of autogenous bone for grafting: clinical considerations, J. Oral Surg. **38**:29, 1980.
72. Neal, H.A.: Reconstruction of maxillary alveolar cleft palate: report of fifty cases. Submitted for publication.
73. Nordin, K.D.: Treatment of primary total cleft palate deformity. Preoperative orthopaedic correction of the displaced components of the upper jaw in infants followed by bone grafting to the alveolar process clefts. Transactions of the European Orthodontic Society, The Hague, 1957.
74. Nordin, K.D., and Johanson, B.: Frei-Knocken-transplantation bei Defekten im Alveolar-kam nach Kieferortopädisher Einstellung der Maxilla bein Lippen-Kiefer-Gaumen spalten, Fortschr. Kiefer. Gesichtschr., vol. 1, 1955.
75. Nylen, B., et al.: Primary, early bone grafting in complete clefts of the lip and palate. A follow-up study of 53 cases, Scand. J. Plast. Surg. **8**:79, 1974.
76. Obwegeser, H.L.: Surgical correction of small or retrodisplaced maxilla. The "dish-face deformity," Plast. Reconstr. Surg. **43**:351, 1969.
77. Osberg, R.E., and Witzel, M.A.: The physiologic basis of hypernasality during connected speech in cleft palate patients: a nasoendoscopic study, Plast. Reconstr. Surg. **67**:1, 1981.
78. Patten, B.M.: Foundations of embryology, ed. 2, New York, 1964, McGraw-Hill Book Co.
79. Pederson, G.W., and Blaho, D.M.: Total maxillary osteotomy for cleft palate rehabilitation, Oral Surg. **39**:669, 1975.
80. Peer, L.A.: The fate of autogenous human bone grafts, Br. J. Plast. Surg. **3**:233, 1950.
81. Perko, M.: Surgical correction of the position of the premaxilla in secondary deformities of cleft lip and palate, International congress series no. 174, Rome, 1967, Excerpta Medica.

82. Perko, M.A.: Two stage closure of cleft palate, J. Maxillofac. Surg. **7:**76, 1979.
83. Pfeiffer, G., and Schuchardt, K.: Growth of the nose, upper jaw, and teeth after primary osteoplastic completion of the cleft alveolar ridge in patients with cleft lip and palate. Transactions of the Third International Congress of Plastic Surgery. International congress series no. 66, New York, 1969, Excerpta Medica Foundation.
84. Poswello, D.: Mechanisms of congenital deformity, J. Dent. Res. **45:**584, 1966.
85. Pruzansky, S.: Pre-surgical orthopedics and bone grafting for infants with cleft lip and palate: a dissent, Cleft Palate J. **2:**7, 1965.
86. Rehrmann, A., et al.: Late results of cleft palate repair in patients with primary or secondary bone grafting. Presented at the International Congress on Cleft Palate, Houston, 1969.
87. Ritter, R.: Early orthodontic care in alveolar and palate clefts. In Schuchardt, K., editor: Treatment of patients with clefts of lip, alveolus, and palate. Second Hamburg International Symposium, Stuttgart, 1964, Georg Thieme Verlag.
88. Robinson, F.: Primary bone grafting in the treatment of cleft lip and palate with special reference to the alveolar collapse, Br. J. Plast. Surg. **22:**336, 1969.
89. Robinson, M., et al.: A method of treatment of chronic infective osteitis, J. Bone Joint Surg. **28:**19, 1946.
90. Rogers, B.O.: Palate surgery prior to von Graefe's pioneering staphylorrhaphy (1816): an historical review of the early causes of surgical indifference in repairing the cleft palate, Plast. Reconstr. Surg. **39:**1, 1967.
91. Rosenstein, S.W.: Orthodontic and bone grafting procedures in cleft lip and palate series: an interim cephalometric evaluation, Angle Orthod. **45:**227, 1975.
92. Rosenstein, S.W., et al.: The case for early bone grafting in cleft lip and cleft palate, Plast. Reconstr. Surg. **70:**297, 1982.
93. Ross, R.B., and Johnston, M.C.: Cleft lip and palate, Baltimore, 1972, The Williams & Wilkins Co.
94. Roux, J.: Observation sur une division congénitale du voile du palais et de la luette, guérie au moyen d'une opération analogue à celle du bec-de-lièvre practiqué par M. Roux, J. Univ. Sci. Med. J. **15:**356, 1819.
95. Safra, M.J., and Oakley, G.P.: Valium: an oral teratogen? Cleft Palate J. **13:**198, 1976.
96. Schmidt, E.: Die Annäherung der Kieferstumpfe bie Lippen-Kiefer-Gaumen spalten. Ihre schädlichen Folgen und Vermeidung, Fortschr. Kiefer. Gesichtschir., vol. 1, 1955.
97. Schmidt, E., et al.: The development of the cleft upper jaw following primary osteoplasty and orthodontic treatment, J. Maxillofac. Surg. **2:**92, 1974.
98. Schuchardt, K.: Discussion Zum Vortrag von A. Rehrmann: Ästhetische Moment in der Lippenspalten Chirurgie (Nase und Lippe), Fortschr. Kiefer. Gesichtschir., vol. 7, 1961.
99. Spriestersbach, D.C., et al.: Clinical research in cleft lip and palate. The state of the art, Cleft Palate J. **10:**113, 1973.
100. Skoog, T.: The management of the bilateral cleft of the primary palate, Plast. Reconstr. Surg. **35:**140, 1965.
101. Skoog, T.: The use of periosteum and Surgicel for bone restoration in congenital clefts of the maxilla, Scand. J. Plast. Surg. **1:**113, 1967.
102. Skoog, T.: Plastic surgery, Philadelphia, 1974, W.B. Saunders Co.
103. Szmyd, L., et al.: Anterior ramus graft of the mandible: report of a case, J. Oral Surg. **27:**132, 1969.
104. Tideman, H., et al.: LeFort I advancement with segmental palatal osteotomies in patients with cleft palates, J. Oral Surg. **38:**196, 1980.
105. Urist, M.R.: Isolation and characterization of bone morphogenetic protein. In Bone grafting: biology and application. Course sponsored by the Plastic Surgery Research Foundation of San Diego and The Bone and Joint Disease Foundation, December 1981.
106. Urist, M.R., et al.: Genetic potency and new bone formation by induction transplants to the anterior chamber of the eye, J. Bone Joint Surg. **36A:**443, 1952.
107. Urist, M.R., et al.: Inductive substrates for bone formation, Clin. Orthop. **59:**59, 1968.
108. Veau, V.: Operative treatment of complete double hare lip, Ann. Surg. (Paris) **76:**143, 1922.
109. Veau, V.: Division palatine, Paris, 1931, Masson and Cie.
110. von Graefe, C.F.: Kurze Nachrichten und Auszuege, J. Prakt. Arzneik. Wundarztk. **44:**116, 1817.
111. von Langenbeck, B.R.K.: Operationen der angeborenen totalen Spaltung des harten Gaumens nach einer neuen Methode, Dsch. Arch. Klin. Med. **13:**231, 1861.
112. von Langenbeck, B.R.K.: Die Uranoplastik mittels Ablösung des Mokös-Periostalen Gaumenüberzuges, Arch. Klin. Chir. **2:**205, 1861.
113. Waite, D.E., and Kersten, R.B.: Residual alveolar and palatal clefts. In Bell, W.H., et al., editors: Surgical correction of dentofacial deformities, Philadelphia, 1980, W.B. Saunders Co.
114. Waldron, C.W.: Mandibular bone-grafts, Proc. R. Soc. Med. **12:**11, 1919.
115. Wardill, W.E.M.: Cleft palate, Br. J. Surg. **16:**127, 1928.
116. Warkany, J.: Congenital malformations, Chicago, 1971, Year Book Medical Publishers, Inc.
117. Weikel, A.M., and Habal, M.B.: Meralgia paresthetica: a complication of iliac bone procurement, Plast. Reconstr. Surg. **60:**572, 1977.

118. Weinstein, I.R.: Bone grafting after mandibular resection, J. Oral Surg. **26:**17, 1978.
119. West, C.E.: Experiences with transplant grafts in ununited fracture of the mandible, Proc. R. Soc. Med. **12:**26, 1919.
120. Westbrook, M.T., et al.: Simultaneous maxillary advancement and closure of bilateral alveolar clefts and oronasal fistulas, J. Oral Maxillofac. Surg. **41:**257, 1983.
121. Wolfe, S.A., and Berkowitz, S.: The use of cranial bone grafts in the closure of alveolar and anterior palatal clefts, Plast. Reconstr. Surg. **72:**659, 1983.
122. Wolfe, S.A., and Kawamoto, H.K.: Taking the ilium bone graft: a new technique, J. Bone Joint Surg. **60A:** 411, 1978.
123. Wray, R.C.: Secondary correction of nasal abnormalities associated with cleft lip, J. Oral Surg. **34:**113, 1976.
124. Wunderer, S.: Die Prognathie Operation mittels frontal gesteltem Maxillafragment, Oester. Z. Stomatol. **59:**98, 1962.
125. Youmans, R.D., et al.: The coronoid process: a new donor source for autogenous bone grafts, Oral Surg. **27:**422, 1969.

CHAPTER 8

Analysis and treatment of hemifacial microsomia

LEONARD B. KABAN
CARLA EVANS
JOHN B. MULLIKEN
JOSEPH E. MURRAY

Hemifacial microsomia (HFM) is a variable congenital anomaly involving first and second branchial arch structures. It is the second most common facial anomaly (after cleft lip and palate) and occurs as a spontaneous event during embryogenesis.[4,6,18]

In the past, treatment of hemifacial microsomia has been characterized by an emphasis on the jaw or ear depending on patient and family concerns and the primary surgeon's area of expertise and interest. Treatment of the skeletal defect was usually delayed until the child ceased growing and end-stage deformity was present.[3,13,16] Based on our experience with 80 hemifacial microsomia patients, we have developed an approach to analysis and treatment of this deformity that emphasizes early correction to maximize growth potential, minimize secondary distortion, and aid body image development.[8,14,15]

CLASSIFICATION OF DEFORMITY

The deformity of HFM consists of skeletal, subcutaneous soft tissue, auricular, and neuromuscular components. It is variable, and no two patients have the same pathologic anatomy.

For purposes of analysis and discussion, a classification system is useful. It should be understood that our knowledge of the pathogenesis of hemifacial microsomia is poor; thus classification of the deformity is somewhat arbitrary and utilitarian.

The skeletal deformity is classified into three types, focusing primarily on the anatomy of the mandible and temporomandibular joint[8,14,15,17] (Fig. 8-1):

Type I consists of a miniature mandible and temporomandibular joint. All structures are present, normally shaped, but hypoplastic.

Type II is characterized by a functioning temporomandibular joint. However, it is hypoplastic and usually displaced anteriorly and medially. The ramus is short and abnormally shaped.

Type III is manifested by complete absence of the mandibular ramus and glenoid fossa. The mandible on the affected side ends abruptly in the first or second molar region.

Soft tissue defects (Fig. 8-2) are also variable and are classified[15] as *mild* (minimal deformity and no ear or cranial nerve involvement), *severe* (major soft tissue bulk deficits associated with ear distortion, nerve deficits, and clefts of the face), or *moderate* (deformities between these extremes).

There is a wide spectrum of external ear anomalies, ranging from a normal ear to complete absence of the external ear (Fig. 8-3). Ab-

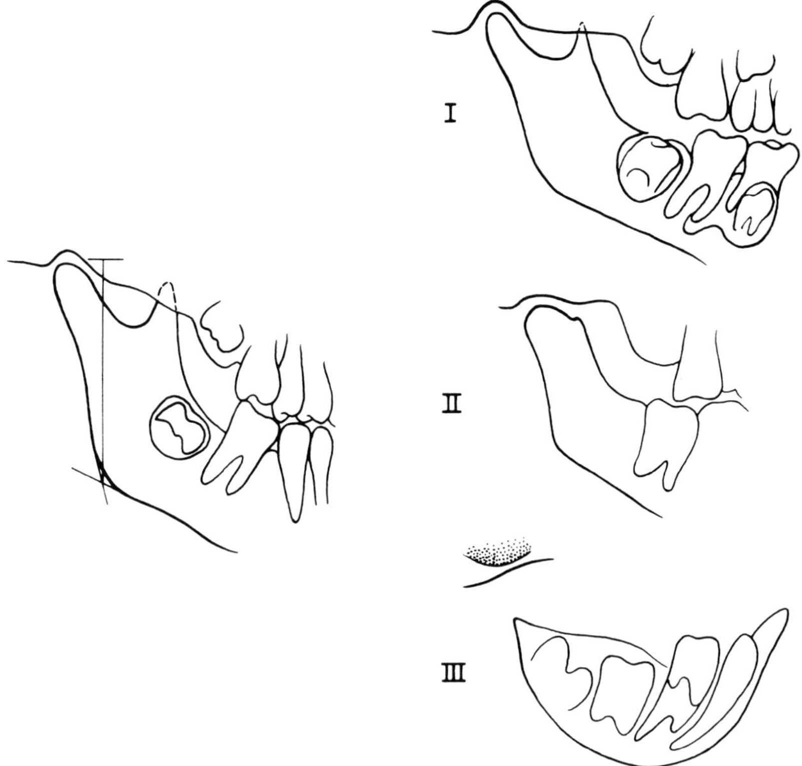

Fig. 8-1.
Three skeletal types of hemifacial microsomia (normal mandible and TMJ on the *left*). Note in Type III the inferior position of the temporal lobe and the thin temporal bone.

normalities of the middle ear also are common. The inner ear, which is not a first or second branchial arch structure, is unaffected. External ear defects are classified according to the system of Marx[9] as modified by Meurmann[11]:

Grade 1. Hypoplasia exists with mild cupping and some external auditory stenosis. All structures are present.

Grade 2. The external auditory canal is absent, and there is variable hypoplasia of the concha.

Grade 3. The auricle is missing, and the lobule is abnormally shaped and malpositioned.

The grade of ear deformity correlates with the facial nerve deficit; that is, the patient with a more severe ear defect is more likely to have seventh nerve paresis. However, the grade of ear defect and seventh nerve abnormalities do not correlate with the severity of skeletal deformity.

SKELETAL GROWTH PATTERNS IN HEMIFACIAL MICROSOMIA

Although hemifacial microsomia is usually considered a unilateral defect, 20% to 30% of those affected have bilateral anomalies.[15,18] However, the deformity is always asymmetric, with more severe skeletal and soft tissue involvement on one side of the face. The less severely affected side may exhibit a mild external ear abnormality or preauricular skin tag, but the skeleton is initially normal. The maxilla, nose, orbit, and zygoma may all be involved in hemifacial microsomia; but mandibular deformity is the earliest clinically evident skeletal defect. Asymmetric mandibular growth seems to play a pivotal role in the progressive distor-

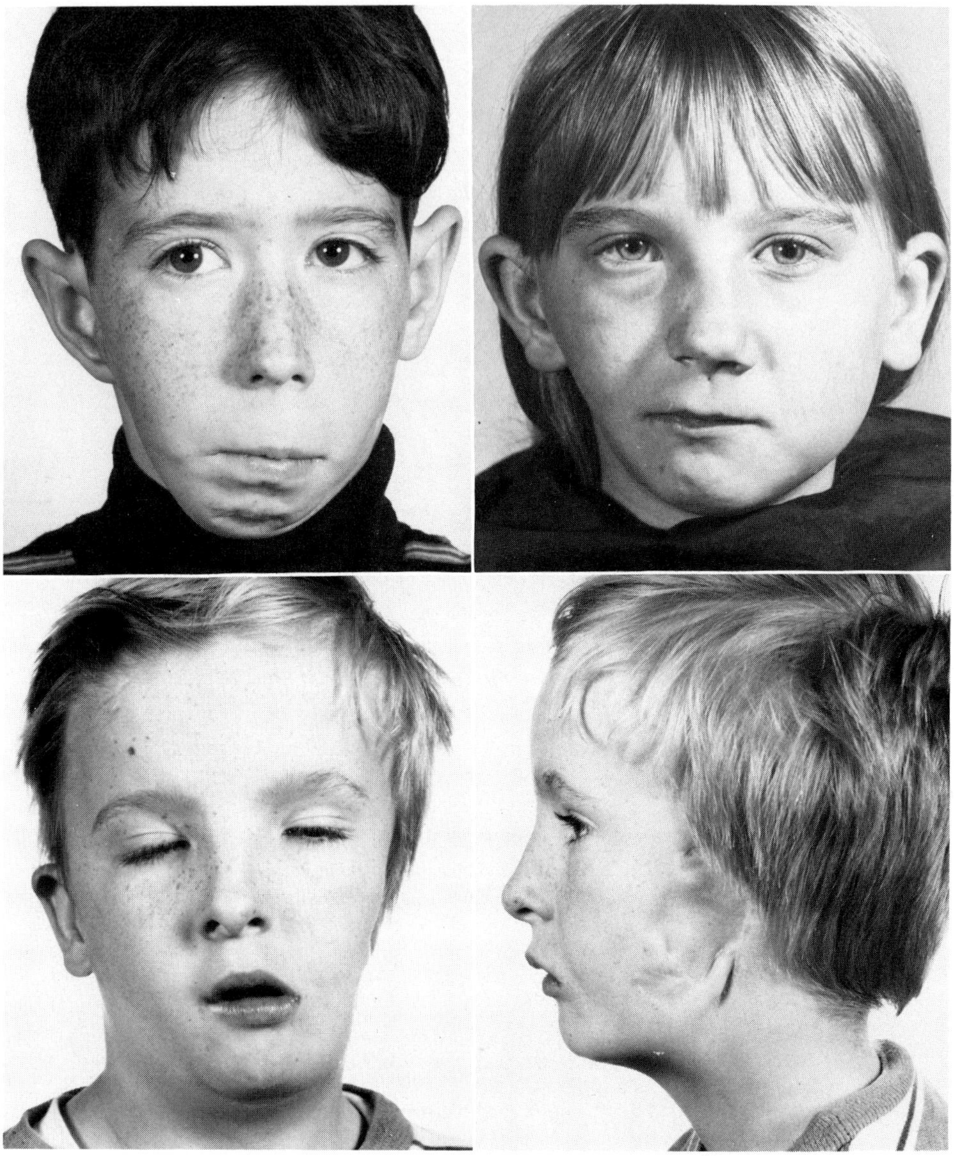

Fig. 8-2.
Spectrum of soft tissue defects in hemifacial microsomia. **A,** Mild soft tissue bulk defect and a normal ear. **B,** Moderate soft tissue defect. **C and D,** Severe soft tissue bulk defect and absence of the ear.

Fig. 8-3.
Spectrum of ear deformities. **A and B,** Type III hemifacial microsomia with a normal ear and preauricular skin tags. Note the absence of a mandibular ramus and condylar head and the poorly developed lateral pterygoid muscle on the axial CT scan. **C,** Grade II ear deformity with a cheek skin tag. **D,** Grade III ear deformity, that is, absence of the external ear except for a small lobule. Several procedures have been undertaken on this girl to construct a helix. **E,** Correlation of facial nerve palsy and the grade of ear defect. This patient has a Type I skeleton.

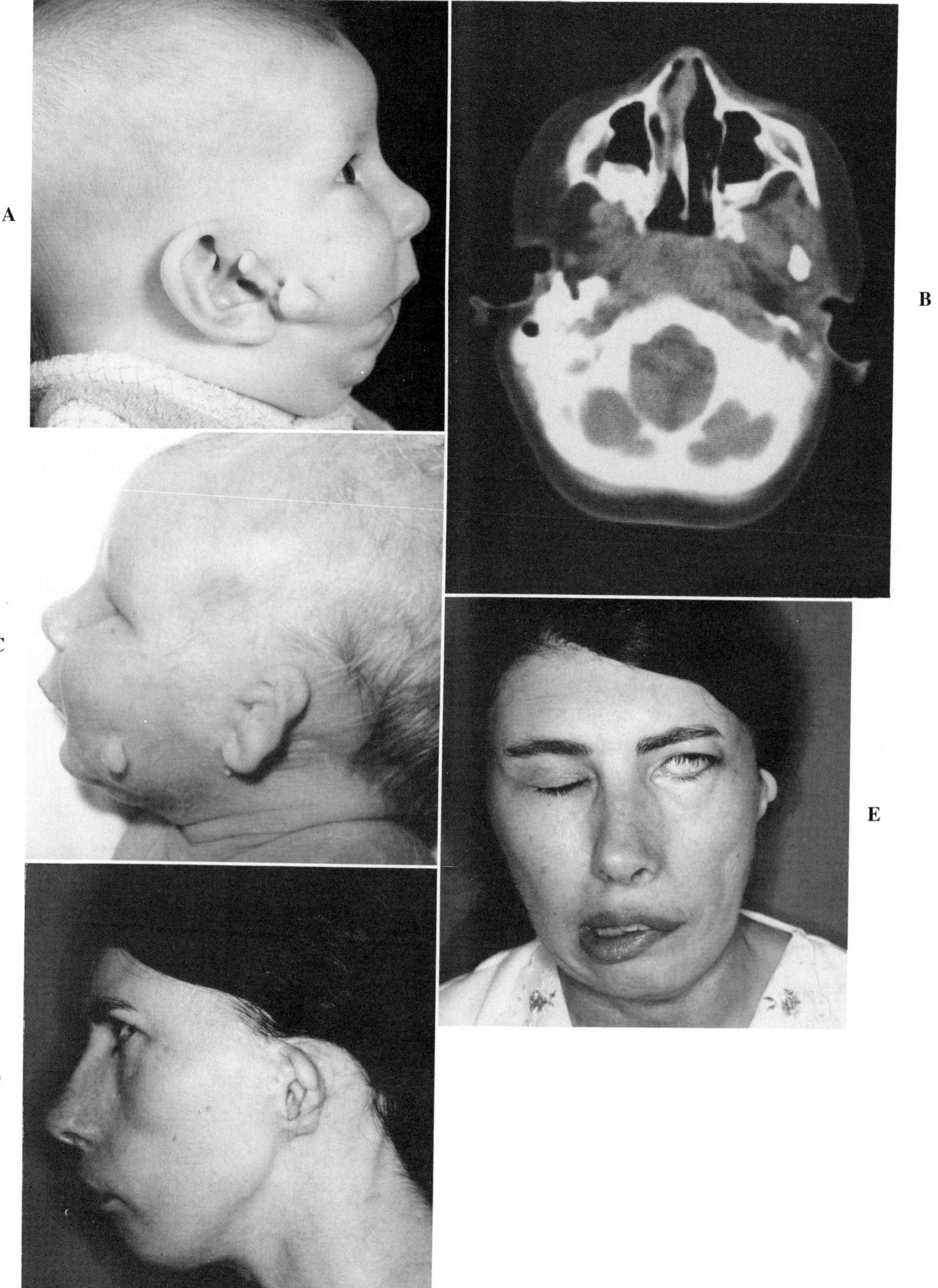

Fig. 8-3.
For legend see opposite page.

tion of both ipsilateral and contralateral facial skeletal structures.[8] The temporal bone and glenoid fossa are usually displaced medially and anteriorly; the zygomatic arch may be small or absent; and the orbit may be underdeveloped and inferiorly displaced. The maxilla becomes hypoplastic with an oblique occlusal plane. The piriform opening is elevated on the affected side, reflecting decreased distance (vertical growth) between the infraorbital rim and the maxillary occlusal plane (Fig. 8-11, *E*).

Normal mandibular growth involves bone deposition and resorption on the periosteal and endosteal surfaces. These processes determine the ultimate mandibular size and shape as well as its location with respect to the maxilla and base of the skull.[5] With unilateral growth impairment in hemifacial microsomia the mandibular skeletal midline is progressively displaced toward the affected side by unopposed growth of the ''normal'' mandible. Failure of remodeling in the transverse plane results in a narrow body and medially displaced ramus of the mandible.

The maxilla normally grows inferiorly and anteriorly, the result of bone resorption on the anterior and superior (nasal) surfaces with concomitant deposition on the posterior and inferior (palatal) surfaces.[5] As the nasomaxillary region grows downward and forward (away from the cranium), there is expansive growth of the overlying soft tissue. In turn, soft tissue mass and muscle function affect skeletal growth.[12]

On the affected side downward growth of the maxilla is restricted by the short mandible. This restriction of vertical maxillary growth prevents the usual progressive separation of the orbit from the maxillary alveolar ridge and piriform region of the nose. The distance between the orbital rim and maxillary alveolus is therefore decreased, resulting in an oblique occlusal plane.[8] In some patients the orbit is in-

feriorly displaced and the zygoma may be hypoplastic.

This hypothesis of growth dynamics in hemifacial microsomia has evolved from serial observation of patients from infancy through adulthood. Supportive evidence is derived from patients whose mandible is so narrow that it does not occlude with the maxillary arch. In these patients lack of restriction of the short mandible on the midface is evident. They have a horizontal maxillary occlusal plane and do not have decreased distance from the infraorbital rim to the piriform aperture or the maxillary alveolar ridge.[8]

The combination of early restriction of mandibular growth and its secondary effects on midface growth ultimately results in the end-stage skeletal deformity of hemifacial microsomia. It is helpful to understand the mandibular defect in three planes—coronal, sagittal, and transverse[8,15] (Figs. 8-4, 8-6, and 8-11):

In the *coronal* plane the affected mandible is short. The ramus is medially displaced and mandibular chin point is deviated toward the affected side. A plane through the dental midline superiorly and chin point inferiorly describes an axis deviated toward the affected side at the chin point and normal side at the dental midline (Fig. 8-4, *A* and *B*).

In the *sagittal* plane the mandible may be retruded and the chin small (microgenia) (Fig. 8-11, *C* and *D*).

In the *transverse* or horizontal plane the mandible is narrow and the TMJ is medially and anteriorly displaced (Fig. 8-6, *D* and *E*).

As noted, HFM is either a unilateral or an asymmetric bilateral defect (16% to 20%). Fifty-six percent of our patients have had a predominantly right-sided defect, and 44% a left-sided deformity. The pattern of skeletal types in our 80 cases is as follows: Type I, 47%; Type II, 34%; Type III, 19%.

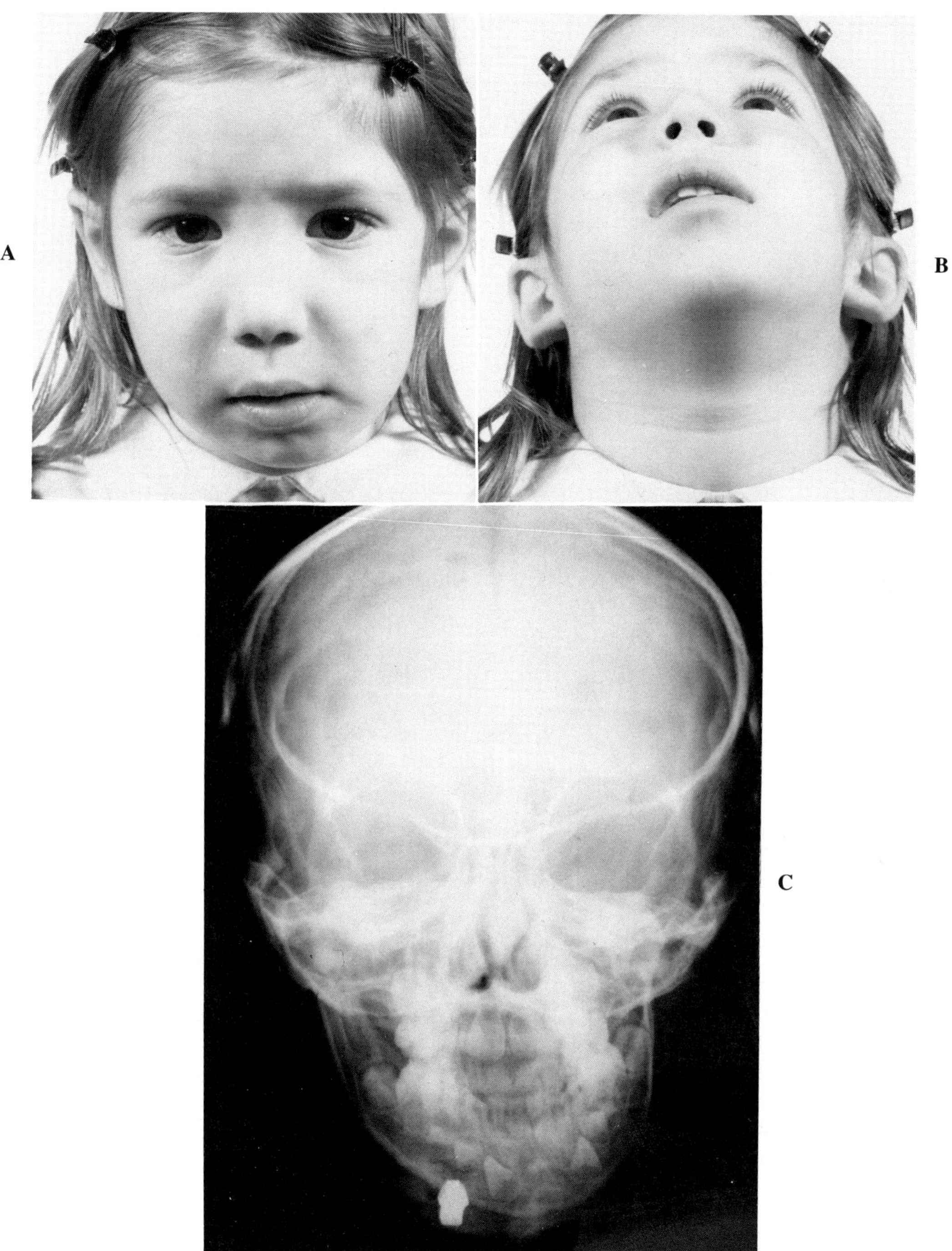

Continued.

Fig. 8-4.
Severe Type I left hemifacial microsomia. **A** and **B,** Deviation of the chin point, slight flatness of the left side of the face, and short ramus on the left side. **C,** Skeletal deviation of the chin point with a short ramus.

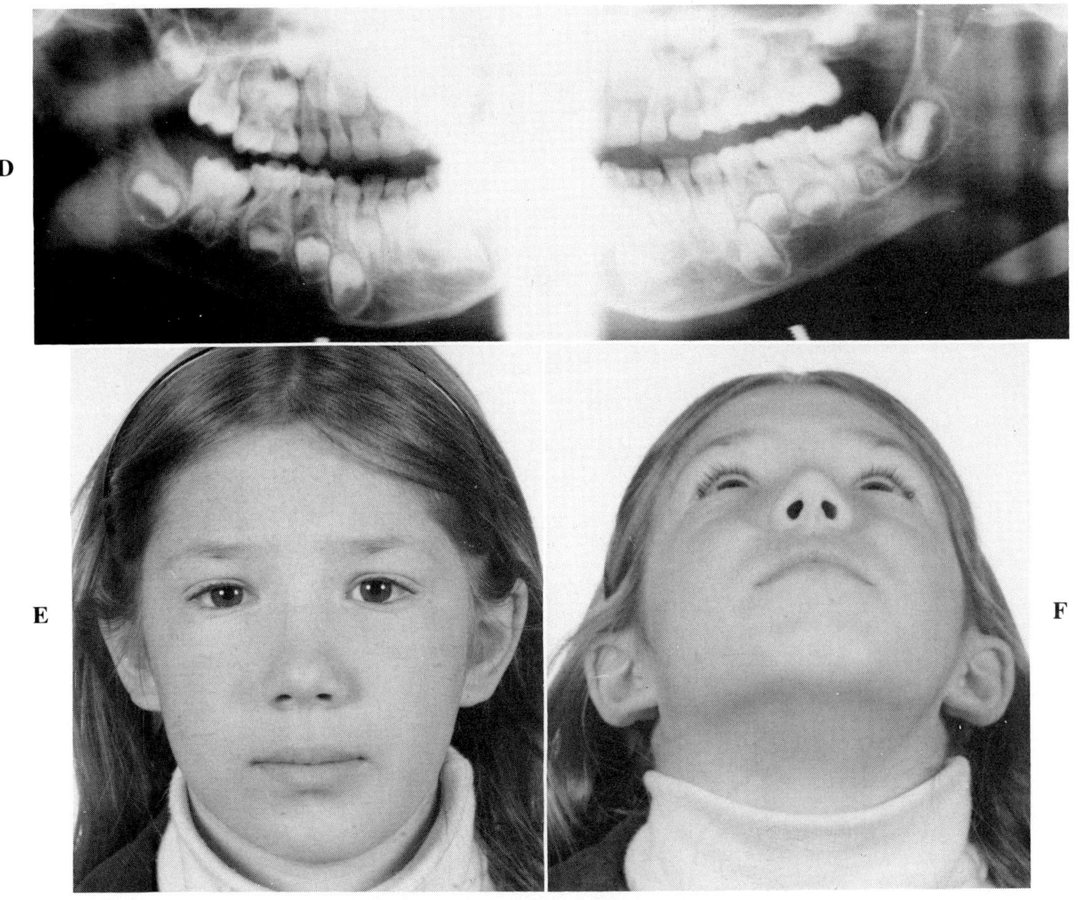

Fig. 8-4—cont'd.
D, Small left ramus. The temporomandibular joint, condyle, and coronoid all serve to classify this as a Type I deformity. **E** and **F,** Five years after elongation and rotation of the mandible with creation of an open-bite. Note the symmetry of the chin and the equal ramal height.

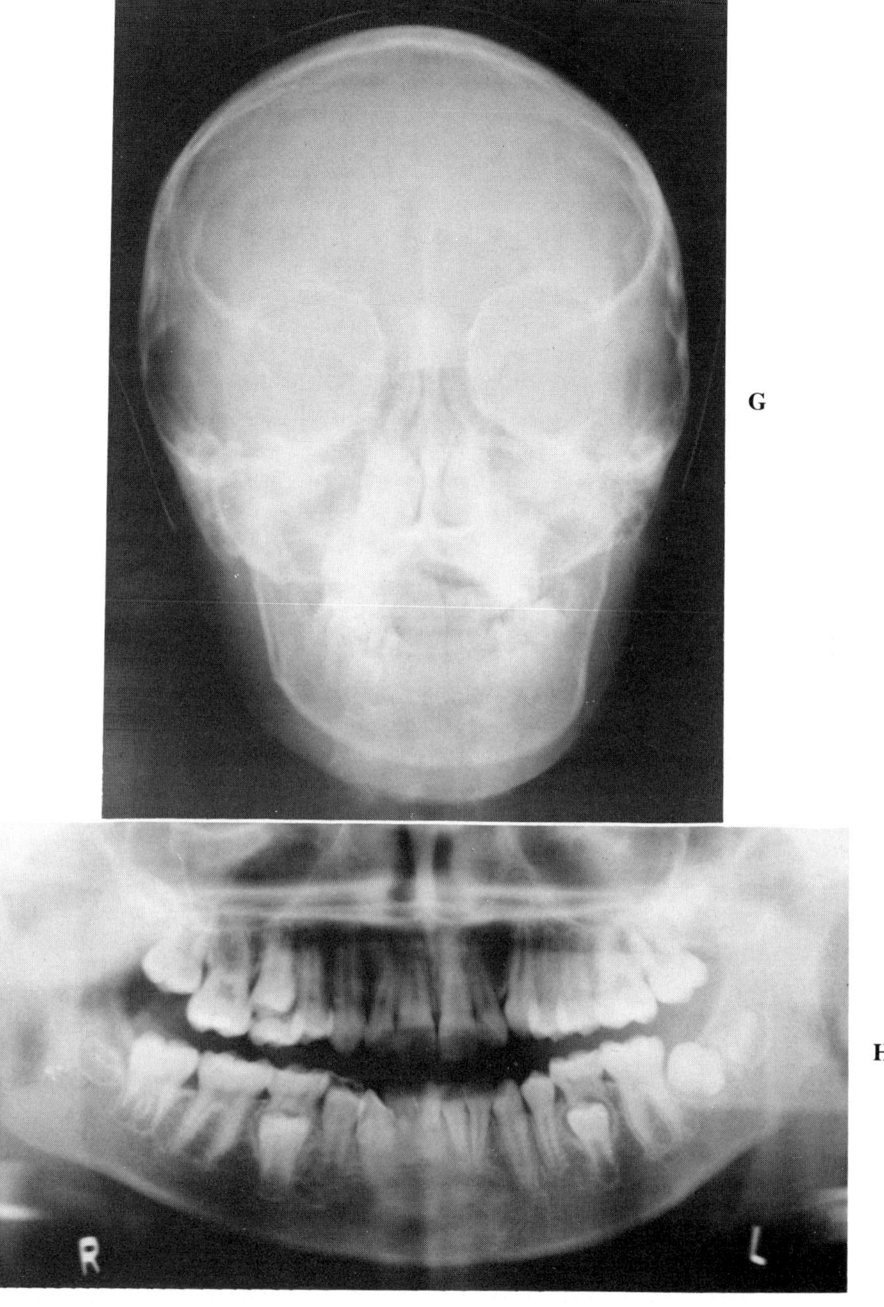

Fig. 8-4—cont'd.
G, Mandibular ramal symmetry, correct positioning of the midline, and level piriform apertures. **H,** Note the symmetric ramal height.

SOFT TISSUE DEFECT

The soft tissue defect has been mild in 50% of our patients, moderate in 40%, and severe in 10%. One third of the patients have had a normal ear on the affected side, 19% a Grade I deformity, 19% a Grade II, and 27% a Grade III deformity. Thirty-seven percent have had cranial nerve involvement that included most commonly seventh nerve palsy. In patients with seventh nerve palsy, involvement of the marginal mandibular branch or frontal branch was most common. In addition, 16% of patients have had deviation of the palate upward toward the normal side with motion. Cranial nerve involvement and grade of ear defect have not correlated with the skeletal type. However, cranial nerve involvement has correlated with the severity of the ear deformity, those with the most severe ear deformities having a greater incidence of cranial nerve deficit.

TREATMENT PLANNING
Skeletal analysis

Although cranial base asymmetry is often present, it is disregarded in planning therapy because the area is not accessible to operative correction. Management is based on analysis of the facial skeletal radiographs in frontal, sagittal, and transverse planes (Figs. 8-4, 8-6, 8-9, and 8-11).

The frontal (coronal) plane is evaluated by a posteroanterior (PA) cephalogram. This demonstrates asymmetry of the mandible, maxilla, piriform apertures, and orbits. Obliquity and rotation of the plane formed by the mandibular dental and skeletal midlines are also demonstrated.

The sagittal (lateral) plane is evaluated by a lateral cephalogram. This shows the ramal height discrepancy as a superimposed contour asymmetry. It also demonstrates the relationship of maxilla and mandible to each other and to the cranial base. Standard orthodontic measurements are used to determine the need for orthodontic treatment and/or advancement of the mandible.

The transverse plane is evaluated by a submentovertex radiograph. This demonstrates the shape and width of the mandibular body. It also shows asymmetry in the zygomatic arches, medial and anterior displacement of the TMJs, and deviation of the chin point to the affected side.

Soft tissue analysis

Soft tissue analysis is qualitative and consists of clinical examination and evaluation of standardized facial photographs in four views (frontal, lateral, oblique, and submental). Contour deficiency on the affected side of the face is truly a combination of skeletal and soft tissue hypoplasia. Once the skeletal deformity is corrected, the soft tissue defect often becomes more obvious. Computed tomography is a technique currently being used to assess the bulk of soft tissues and to document the presence or absence of the temporalis, masseter, and medial and lateral pterygoids. In the future it will be helpful in quantifying soft tissue defects for treatment planning and follow-up.

Neuromuscular analysis

The muscles of the first and second branchial arches are variably hypoplastic. In patients with Type III skeletal deformity the lateral pterygoid may be absent and the temporalis, masseter, and medial pterygoid markedly hypoplastic or absent. The muscles of the palate are also poorly developed.

Deviation of the mandible on opening is caused by a combination of the skeletal asymmetry and hypoplastic weak muscles on the affected side. Deviation of the palate to the normal side with function is a result of hypoplastic muscle and seventh nerve deficit.

Rarely the patient will have absence of sensation in the fifth nerve (sensory nerve of the first branchial arch), which may result in trophic or pressure ulcers.

TREATMENT

The timing and procedures outlined in this section have evolved over a 25-year period and experience with over 80 patients. Because the error of morphogenesis that results in hemifacial microsomia cannot be treated, the purpose of operative correction is to create an environment that potentiates normal facial growth and minimizes secondary distortion. Timing and procedures are constantly being reevaluated. In this chapter we present the most current concepts that guide our treatment protocols.

The first essential step in planning treatment is to determine the patient's skeletal type.[8,14,15] Severity of mandibular and TMJ deformity predicts the rate of secondary distortion of adjacent facial structures. For example, in patients with Type II HFM, obliquity of the occlusal plane and shortening of midface height develop at an earlier age than in those with Type I deformity. Patients with Type III deformity have the greatest inherent growth defect, and obliquity of the occlusal plane develops at an earlier age than in Type I or Type II patients.

The first objective is to correct the mandibular deformity by rotating and elongating the jaw to place it in normal position in three planes: frontal, sagittal, and transverse. It is crucial to determine the proper position of the TMJ and the two mandibular midlines (dental and skeletal). The vertical height of the ramus is increased on the affected side, the mandibular midline is rotated, and anteromedial displacement of the ramus is corrected. The specific operative plan is based on the type of deformity, the patient's age, and an analysis of photographs, radiographs, and dental models. In Table 8-1 nine possible treatment plans are shown based on age and skeletal type.[15]

In patients with a Type I skeletal deformity seen at an early age, treatment is begun by construction of a functional orthodontic appliance ("activator"). This is used to guide the mandible into a more physiologic position. By positioning the affected side of the jaw downward, forward, and to the midline, the activator places tension on the affected soft tissues.[7] The stretching of surrounding soft tissue may lead to appositional bone growth.[10] If the orthodontic appliance does not prevent obliquity of the occlusal plane, an operation is indicated (Figs. 8-4 and 8-5). The first operation is usually performed during the late mixed dentition; it consists of a vertical mandibular ramal osteotomy for elongation and rotation. A compensatory subcondylar osteotomy on the normal side is necessary if the mandible does not passively move into the new position. No operation is performed on the maxilla. The created openbite on the affected side is maintained by an orthodontic appliance, which controls eruptive forces to allow optimal vertical maxillary growth (Figs. 8-4 and 8-5).

Table 8-1.

Treatment of hemifacial microsomia based on age (dentition) and anatomic type

	0 to 5 years (deciduous)	*6 to 12 years (mixed)*	*12 years (adult)*
Type I	Activator may stimulate mandibular growth	If activator ineffective, mandible should be advanced, rotated, and elongated; open-bite purposely produced, will be regulated with occlusal spacer	Mandibular elongation and maxillary osteotomy, either segmental or LeFort I, necessary; orthodontic alignment may be required
Type II	Activator less likely to stimulate mandibular growth	Operation will usually be necessary to advance, rotate, and elongate mandible; open-bite will be regulated by occlusal spacer; critical decision is selection of site for TMJ if existing one is in poor anatomic position	Three-plane mandibular repair required; maxillary osteotomies, segmental or LeFort I, usually necessary; selection of fulcrum or rotation of maxilla (i.e., elongation or impaction of the maxillary occlusal plane) crucial; pre- or postoperative orthodontia must be considered
Type III	Full construction of zygoma, glenoid fossa, condyle, ramus, angle, and body of mandible required; postoperative activator needed	Activator use continued; if ineffective, repeat operation required; if patient first seen at this stage, total construction required	Full reconstruction of all structures indicated; selection of site of TMJ, fulcrum of rotation of maxilla, and extent of orthodontia must be individualized

From Murray, J.E., et al.: Plast. Reconstr. Surg. **74:**186, 1984.

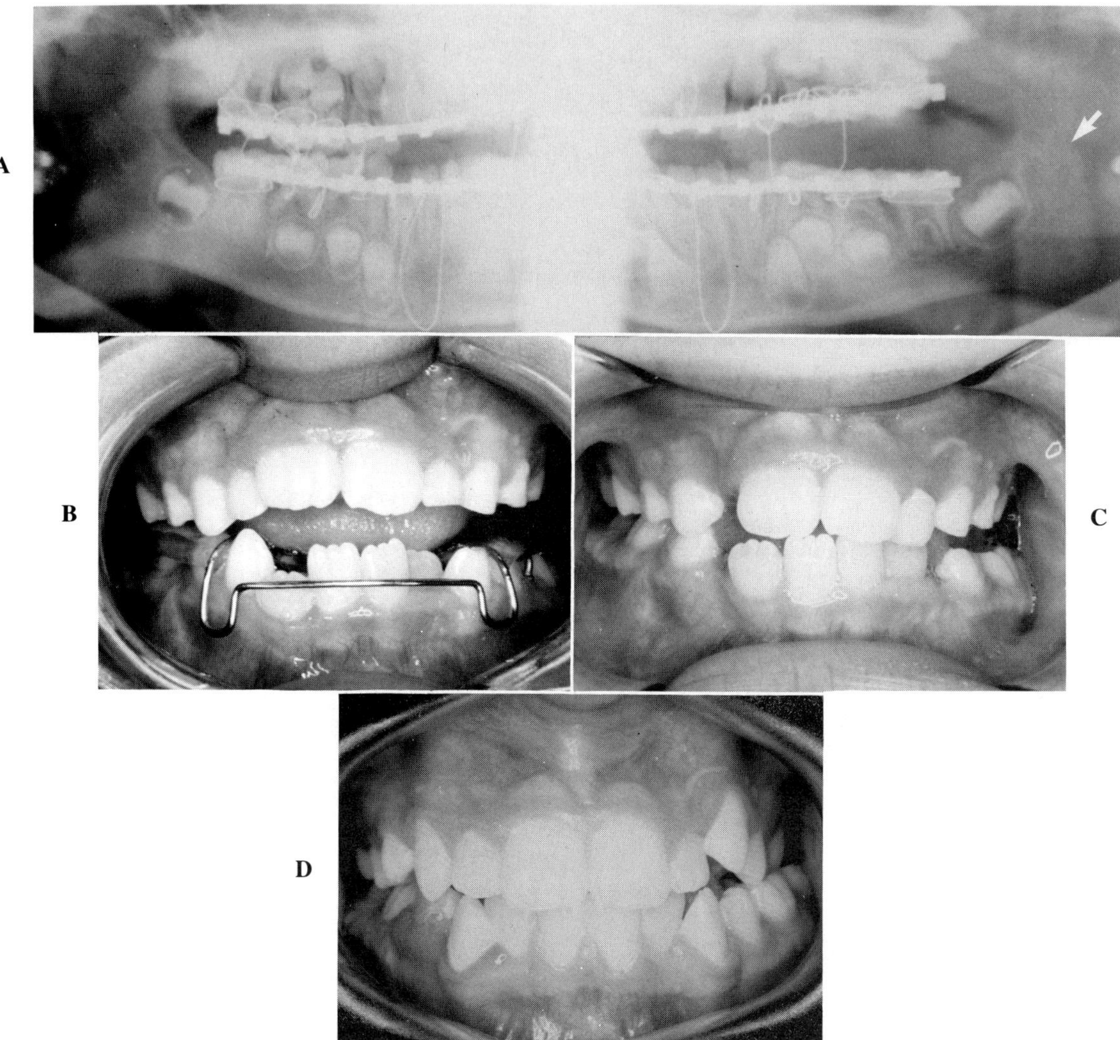

Fig. 8-5.
A, Immediately postoperative Panorex, same patient as in Fig. 8-4. Note that a vertical osteotomy was done and the proximal fragment was positioned in the glenoid fossa and then doweled into a notch on the cut segment of the ramus *(arrow)*. Notice also the surgically created open-bite on the patient's left side. **B,** One year postoperative. Remaining open-bite on the patient's left side maintained by the orthodontic appliance. **C,** Two years postoperative. Small remaining open-bite. **D,** Four and one half years postoperative. Midlines of the maxilla and mandible aligned. The patient now has crowding and a cross-bite on the left side. She will receive conventional orthodontic treatment because her jaws are compatible and the skeleton is symmetric.

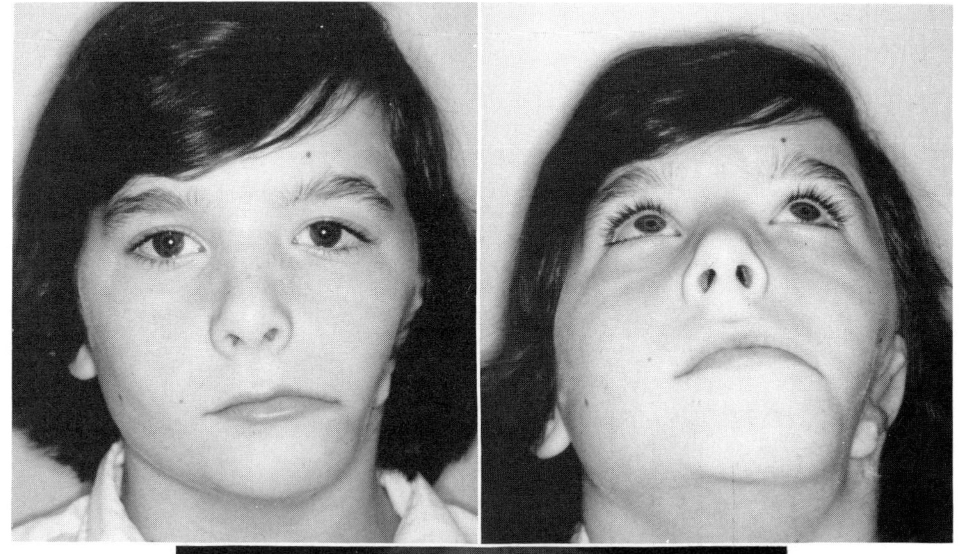

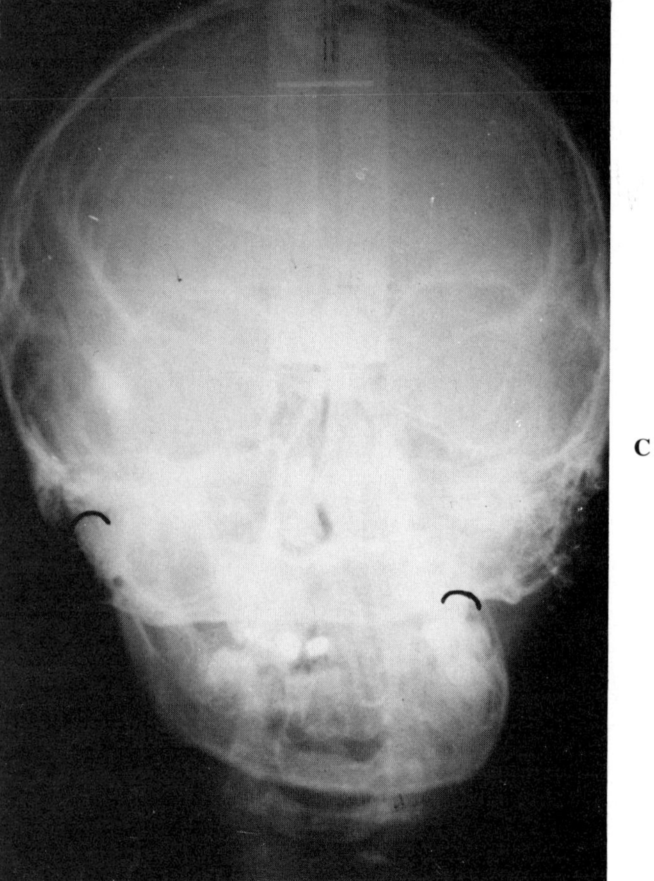

Fig. 8-6.

Continued.

Severe Type II hemifacial microsomia. **A** and **B,** Note deviation of the chin point, flatness of the left side of the face, the soft tissue bulk defect and ear deformity, and the macrostomia. Notice also that the piriform apertures and commissures tilt upward toward the affected side. **C,** Tilting of the piriform apertures, marked deviation of the mandibular chin point, and abnormal location of the rudimentary temporomandibular joint and condyle.

A to **E** from Murray, J.E., et al.: Plast. Reconstr. Surg. **74:**186, 1984.

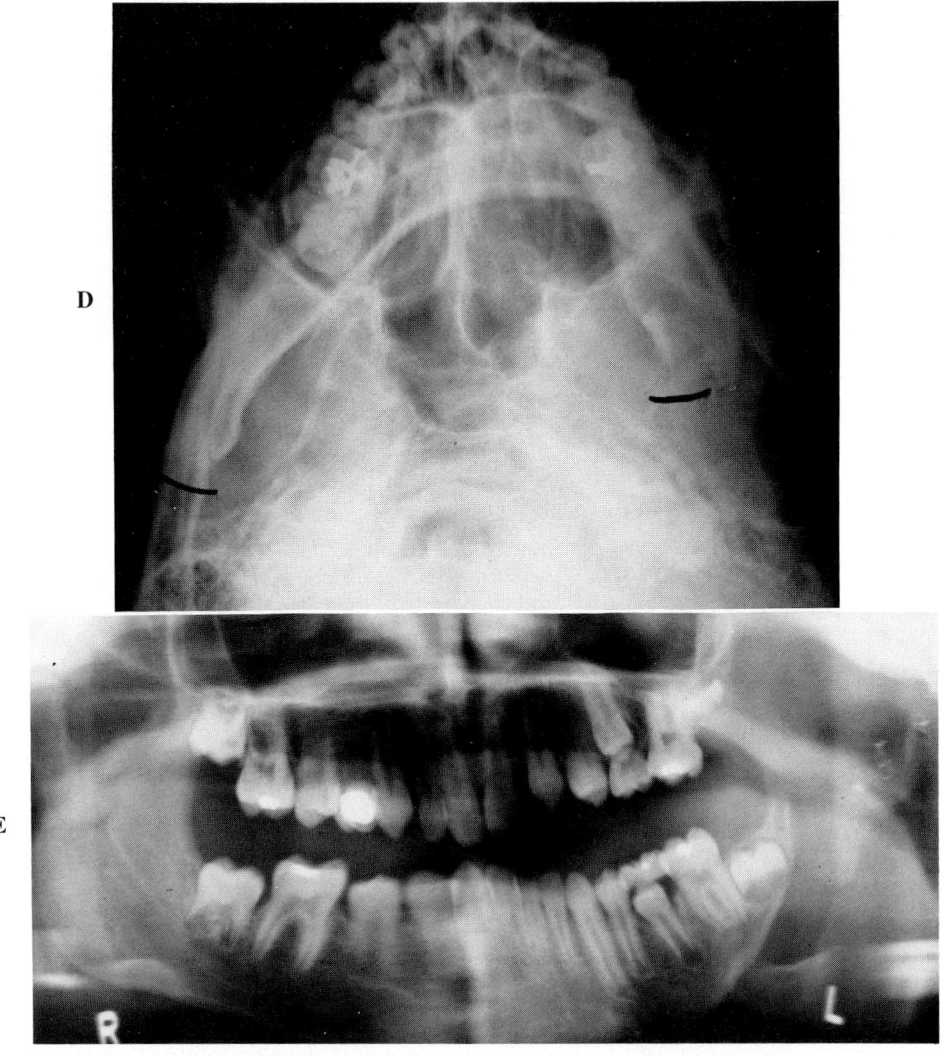

Fig. 8-6—cont'd.
D, Deviation of the chin point and anteromedial displacement of the rudimentary TMJ. **E,** The rudimentary ramus and TMJ. Wires on the left side are from a previous ear construction done elsewhere.

Type I patients may require a second ramal lengthening procedure after completion of growth. If proper orthodontic appliances are used sequentially and if adequate lengthening of the mandible and midface occurs, no further surgical treatment is necessary. With unimpeded downward growth the maxilla will maintain a normal horizontal occlusal plane.

In patients with Type II skeletal deformity seen at an early age, treatment can also begin with a functional activator appliance. However, these patients are less likely than Type I patients to respond to it; nevertheless, the stretching effect on skin, subcutaneous tissue, and muscle is beneficial.[7] As with a Type I patient, time for surgical correction in Type II is determined by the occurrence of secondary deformities (such as shortening of the midface, manifested by an oblique occlusal plane). This usually becomes significant at an earlier age in Type II patients. Operation, when indicated, is performed during the early mixed dentition.

The major decision with Type II patients, contrary to that with Type I, is site selection for the temporomandibular joint (Fig. 8-6). If the existing TMJ is in a normal anatomic location, the mandible is osteotomized and placed in its proper location in three dimensions. If the TMJ is medially and/or anteriorly displaced to an unfavorable location, it is excised and a new one constructed at a location symmetric with the normal side (Fig. 8-7). Only then can proper mandibular function, with symmetric motion, be achieved. Once the TMJ is properly located, the mandible is osteotomized as described for Type I patients. An open-bite is created on the affected side and maintained with an orthodontic appliance. Compensatory osteotomy of the opposite ramus is almost always required in Type II patients. Furthermore, in some patients, the ramus and condyle are so hypoplastic as to be of no use. Then the ramus, condyle, and disc remnants are excised and reconstructed with iliac crest and costochondral junction for the condylar head. The constructed TMJ is lined with perichondrium (Fig. 8-7). Again, in the mixed dentition, no surgery is done on the maxilla.

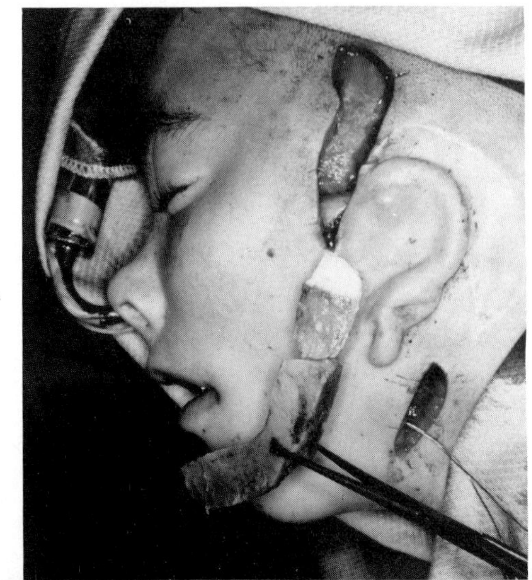

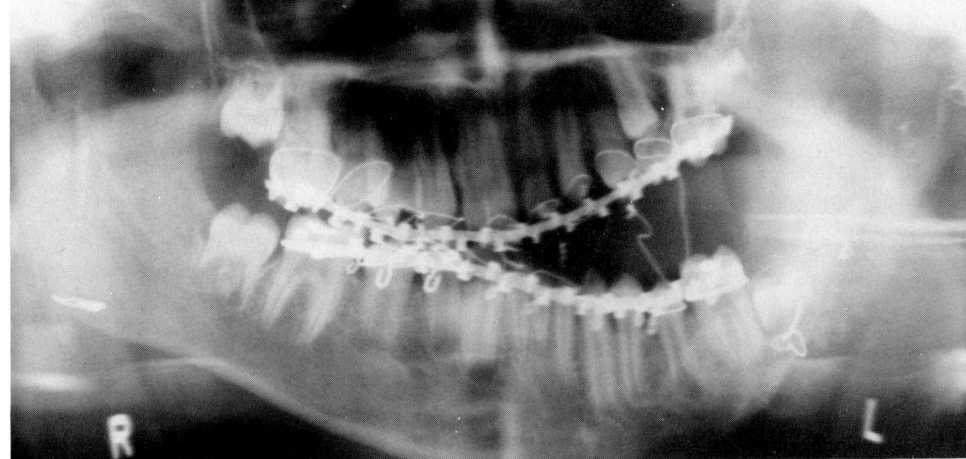

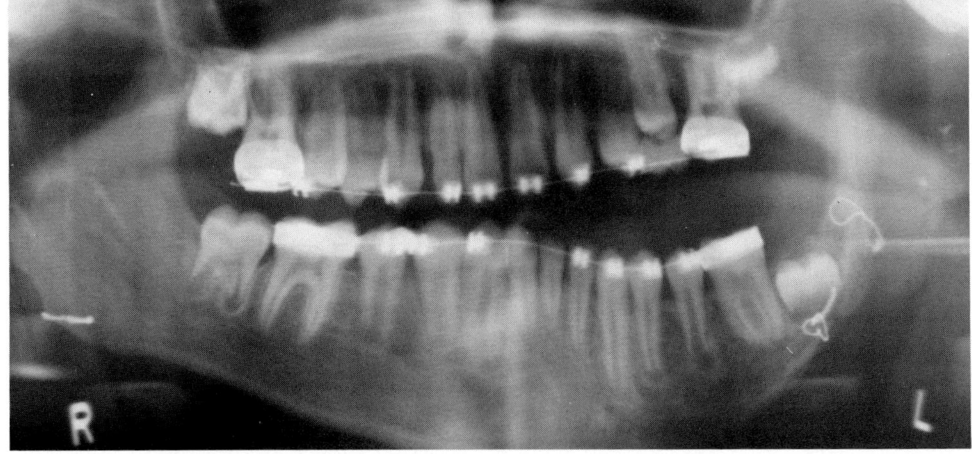

Fig. 8-7.
Same patient as in Fig. 8-6. **A,** The temporomandibular joint was in an unacceptable anteromedial position and was not useful. A new one was created with perichondrium-lined iliac bone. The mandibular ramus, angle, and body were constructed from the iliac crest, and the costochondral junction was doweled to make a condylar head. **B,** The surgically created open-bite. Note that a compensatory osteotomy was needed on the right side. **C,** One year postoperative. The open-bite is being regulated by an orthodontic appliance.

B, C, and **E** from Murray, J.E., et al.: Plast. Reconstr. Surg. **74:**186, 1984.

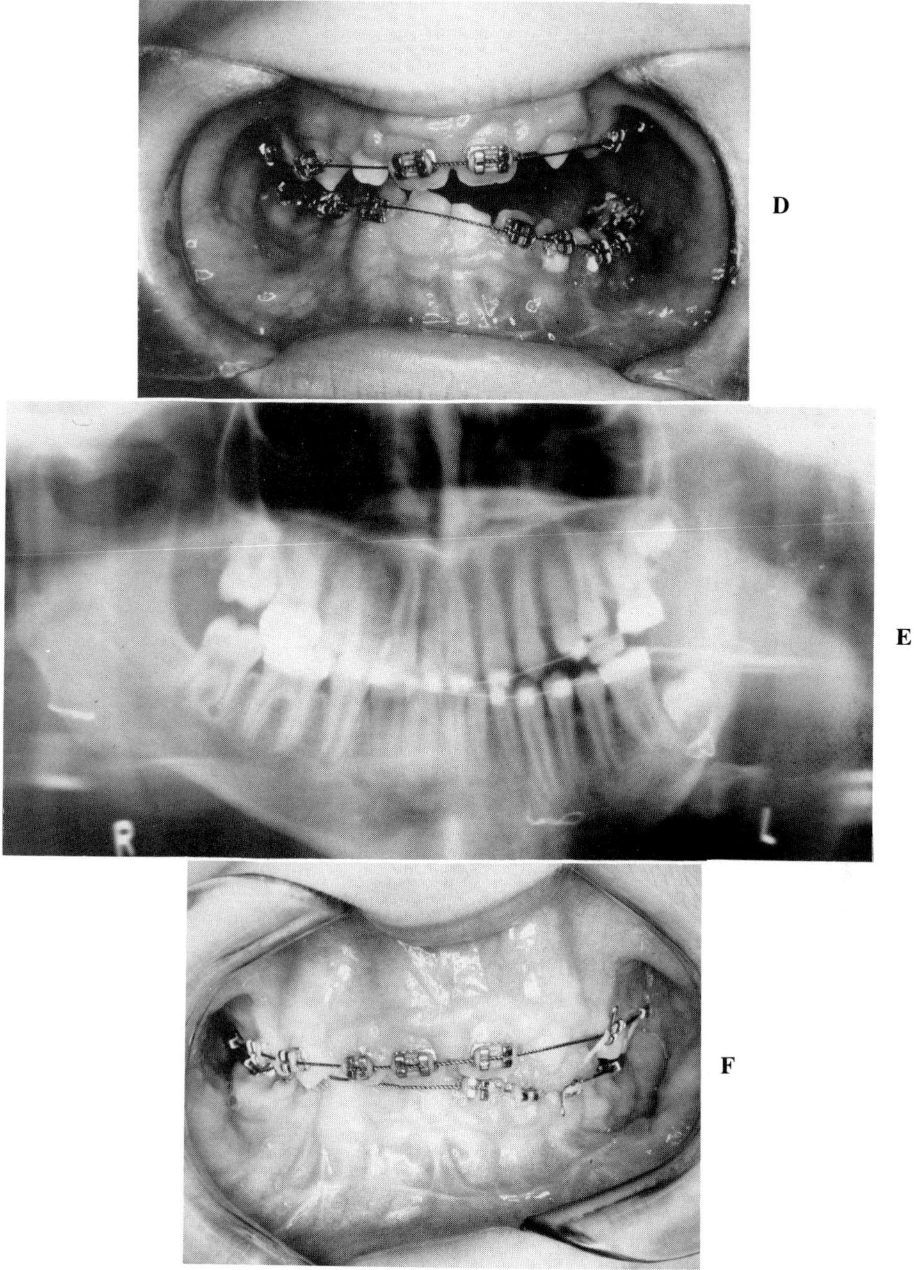

Fig. 8-7—cont'd.
D, Clinical correlation with **C. E,** Two years postoperative. Open-bite almost totally closed. Note the constructed ramus on the left side. **F,** Clinical correlation with **E.**

In operations during the mixed dentition a unilateral or bilateral posterior open-bite is deliberately created. If bilateral open-bite is necessary, it is always larger on the side with the greater deformity. The surgically created open-bite requires selective differential splinting postoperatively to optimize eruption of the maxillary teeth and allow inferior growth of the maxilla. This is the same as described for Type I patients (Fig. 8-8).

In patients with untreated Type III skeletal deformity the result is a displaced, flattened, and distorted maxilla, mandible, and zygoma, often with a concavity of the midface on the affected side (Fig. 8-9). The orbit may be displaced inferiorly, and the vertical distance between the infraorbital rim and piriform aperture is decreased. In these patients construction of a glenoid fossa, ramus, TMJ, zygomatic arch, and mandibular body is performed as early as 2 to 4 years of age, or whenever the patient has enough deciduous teeth for fixation (Fig. 8-9). Selection of a glenoid fossa site may be difficult in the absence of anatomic landmarks. It should be constructed as lateral and posterior as possible to correspond to the contralateral zygomatic process of the temporal bone. A preoperative guide to positioning the glenoid fossa is obtained by first drawing a vertical line from the crista galli to the anterior nasal spine. Then a horizontal line is drawn perpendicular to this at the level of the normal glenoid. The site for the new TMJ can be selected by measurements on the radiographs. Corresponding markings can be made in the operating room with the patient anesthetized and properly positioned.

Total construction of the TMJ requires a new glenoid fossa, best made using a cortical graft of ilium or rib anchored to the preselected site. This is hollowed inferiorly to create a concave surface to which the constructed condyle can be fitted. The new glenoid fossa is placed lateral and posterior to any preexisting joint and lined with perichondrium (Fig. 8-9).

The zygomatic arch is made with rib or cranial bone. The ramus may be constructed with a full-thickness rib graft or iliac graft, or by a combination (doweling a costochondral junction into the iliac graft). The condylar head is constructed of costal cartilage or a perichondral graft wrapped over iliac bone (Fig. 8-9).

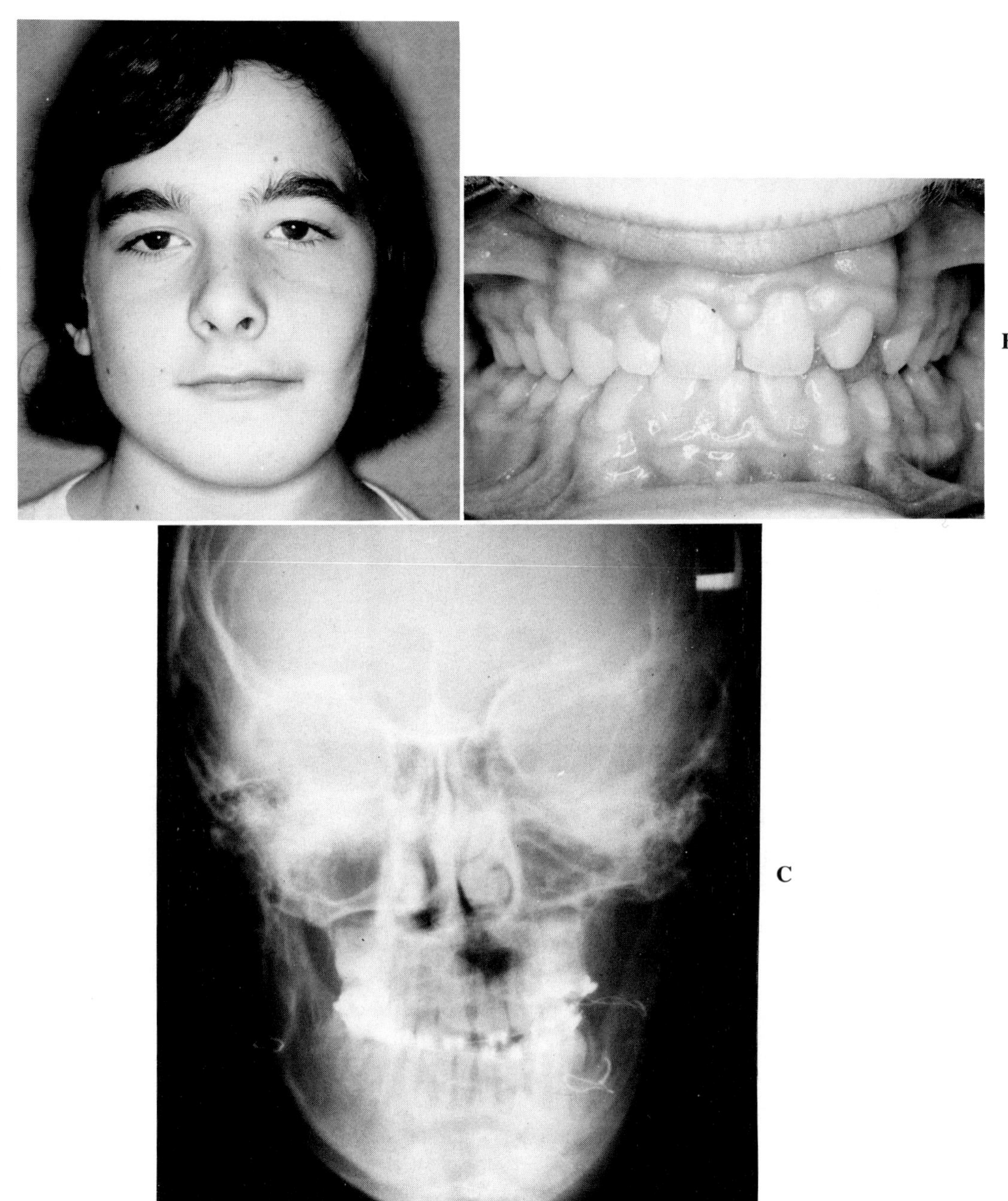

Fig. 8-8.
Same patient as in Figs. 8-6 and 8-7. **A** and **B,** Appearance 3 years postoperative. The contour of the left mandible was augmented with an onlay bone graft approximately 1½ years after the first operation. **C,** Cephalogram 3 years postoperative. Symmetry of the mandible and lateral location of the temporomandibular joint.

A and **C** from Murray, J.E., et al.: Plast. Reconstr. Surg. **74:**186, 1984.

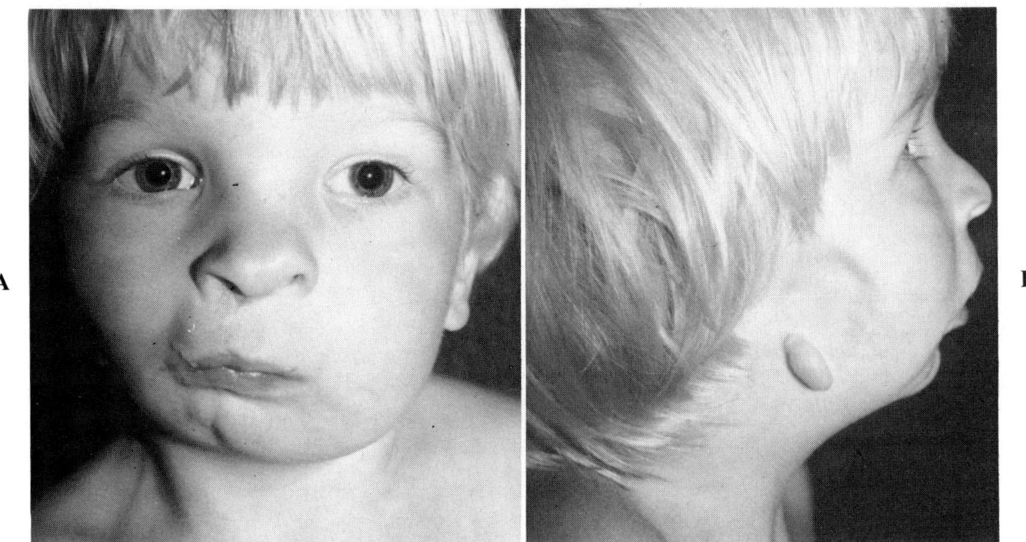

Fig. 8-9.
Type III hemifacial microsomia, 18-month-old child. **A** and **B,** The right unilateral cleft lip was previously repaired. Note the Grade III ear deformity.
A to **E** from Murray, J.E., et al.: Plast. Reconstr. Surg. **74:**186, 1984.

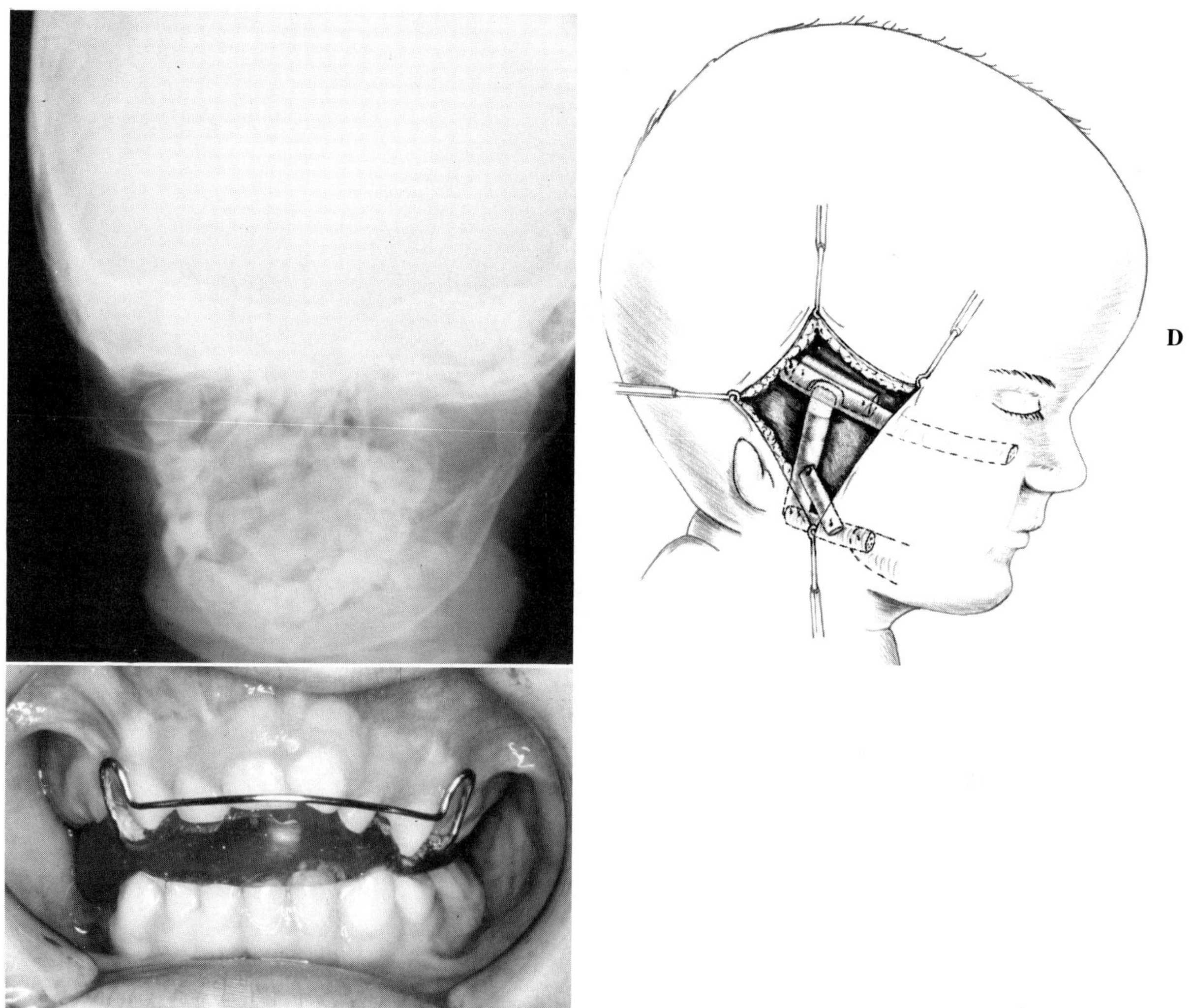

Fig. 8-9—cont'd.
C, Absent ramus and temporomandibublar joint. **D,** The operation used to construct the zygomatic arch, glenoid fossa, and ramus of the mandible in Type III hemifacial microsomia. In this particular patient the L-shaped angle was not constructed and the rib graft was simply wired into the existing angle. **E,** Orthodontic appliance for maintaining the surgically created open-bite.

In young patients (deciduous dentition) with Type III deformity, compensatory osteotomy of the normal ramus is not required because of the flexibility and remodeling potential of the normal TMJ. An open-bite is created on the affected side and maintained with an orthodontic activator appliance (Fig. 8-9). The patient may require another operation during the mixed dentition. In reality, such a patient has been converted to a Type II deformity by this procedure and is thereafter treated as such.

It is important to remember that the fixation period for pediatric patients who have received total construction should be no longer than 3 to

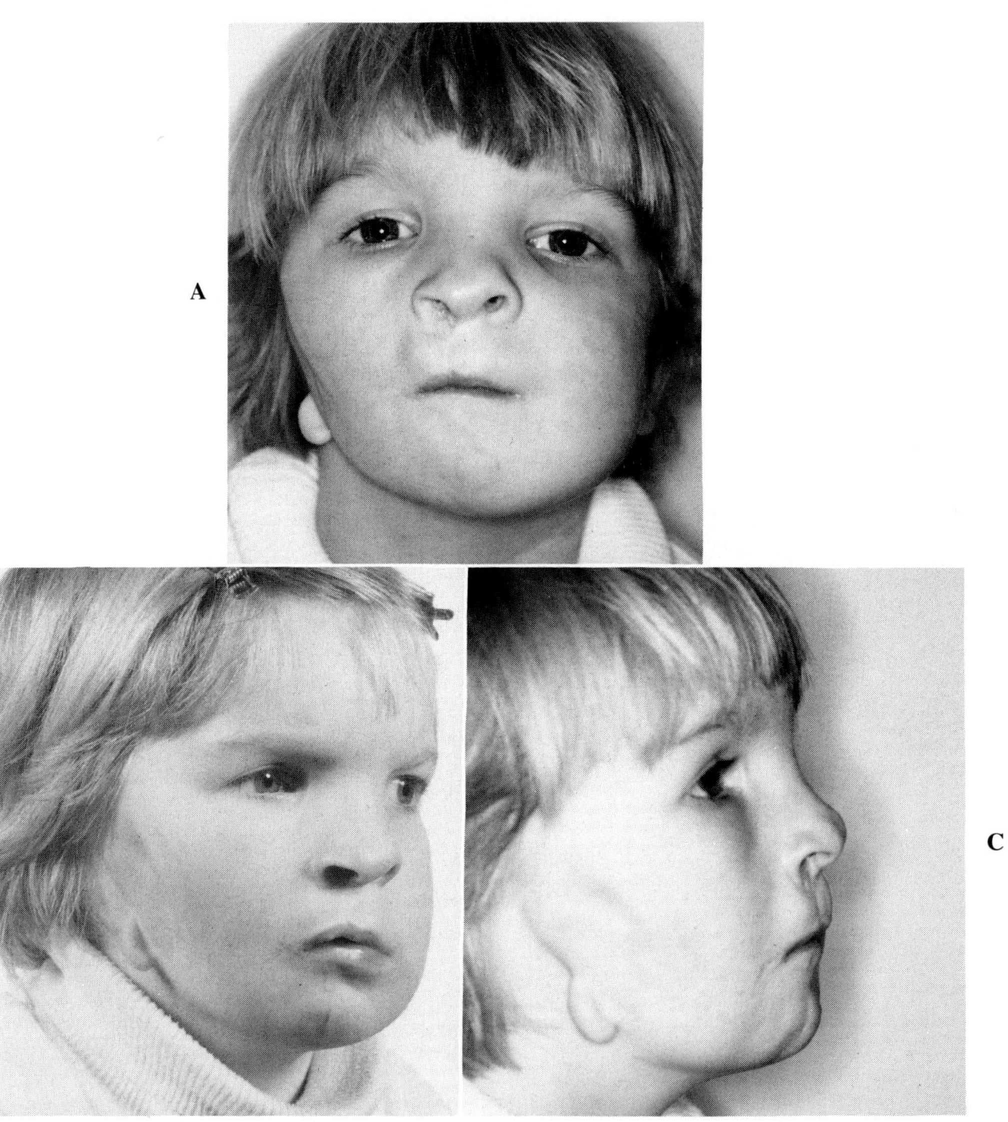

Fig. 8-10.
Same patient as in Fig. 8-9. **A** to **D,** Two years postoperative. Note the mandibular symmetry, angle of the jaw, and forward movement of the chin point with growth. **E,** Panoramic radiograph showing the constructed ramus.
A, C, D, and E from Murray, J.E., et al.: Plast. Reconstr. Surg. **74:**186, 1984.

4 weeks. The child is anesthetized 3 weeks postoperatively, and healing of the ramus graft and joint motion are examined. If the ramal graft is united to the mandible, the patient is left out of fixation. If the graft is not united, fixation is replaced for another week. No patients have

required longer then 4 weeks of intermaxillary fixation. This protocol of early motion has eliminated the problem of postoperative ankylosis (Fig. 8-10).

• • •

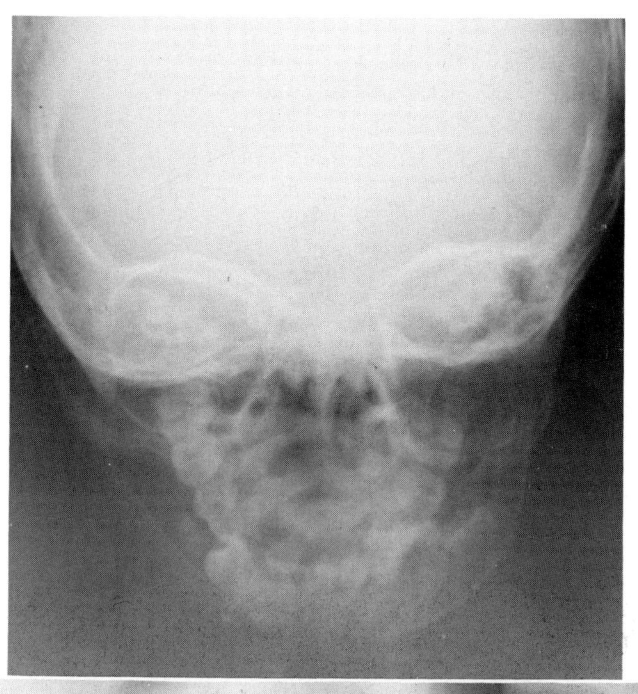

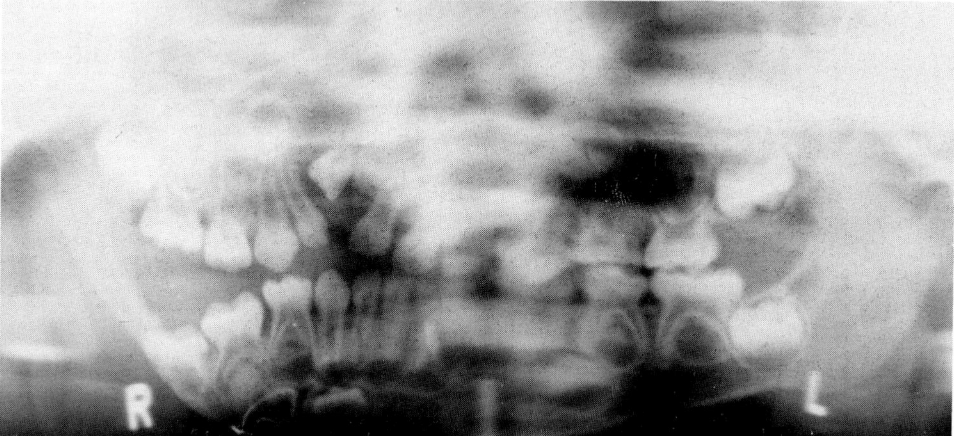

Fig. 8-10—cont'd.
For legend see opposite page.

The previous discussion considered treatment of hemifacial microsomia in the growing child. The goal of therapy was to create an environment that allowed full growth potential and minimized secondary distortion of adjacent structures. The following paragraphs relate to treatment of (nongrowing) adult patients with hemifacial microsomia.

The Type I patient who is first seen as an adult may often be treated with mandibular elongation, rotation, and advancement. At this age mandibular repositioning always requires compensatory osteotomy of the opposite ramus to prevent abnormal forces from acting on the normal TMJ. When the mandible is narrow, segmental osteotomy or orthodontic treatment may be needed to widen the dental arch. If the maxillary occlusal plane is oblique (in other words, midface short on the affected side), a concurrent LeFort I osteotomy is also necessary.

The adult with a Type II deformity always has obliquity of the occlusal plane, indicating a short midface on the affected side (Fig. 8-11). This patient must undergo a LeFort I osteotomy to create a symmetric maxilla. When a LeFort I osteotomy is planned, the fulcrum of rotation is determined by the desired postoperative length of the midface. If maximum midface lengthening is planned, the point of rotation should be the molar area on the normal side. If minimal to moderate lengthening is required, the fulcrum of rotation should be at the piriform aperture or nasal septum, with impaction of the maxilla superiorly on the normal side and elongation of the affected side. If exposure of the maxillary incisors below the upper lip is excessive, the rotational fulcrum should be the molar region of the abnormal side, or above, to produce maximum impaction of the normal side (Figs. 8-11 and 8-12).

The adult with a Type III deformity requires not only full construction of the zygoma, mandible, and TMJ but also a LeFort I osteotomy and in some instances orbital correction. The selection of LeFort I fulcrum is as indicated for the Type II deformity. We usually do this operation in one stage.

When the LeFort I and orbital osteotomies are completed and the maxilla is in its correct

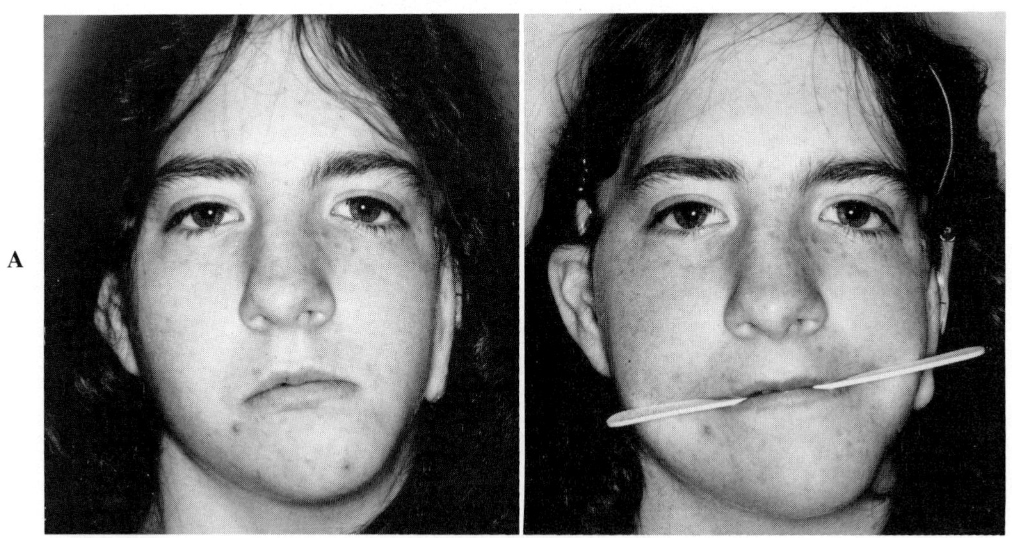

Fig. 8-11.
Type II hemifacial microsomia. **A** and **B,** Flatness of the left side of the face, deviation of the chin point to the left, and tilting of the piriform apertures, commissures of the lip, and occlusal plane. The patient's ear was previously constructed elsewhere.

position, the zygomatic arch and TMJ are constructed. The mandibular remnant on the affected side is then exposed. The appropriate osteotomy on the "normal" side is done—either an oblique or a sagittal split osteotomy (if advancement of the mandible is going to be part of the correction). The mandible is moved into fixation with the maxilla and immobilized. The mandibular ramus is then constructed and wired in place. An advancement genioplasty may be required to complete the correction of chin symmetry. Finally, onlay bone grafts are placed to augment the mandibular contour if necessary.

Construction of the external ear is deferred, whenever possible, until mandibular and zygomatic osseous frameworks have been established. The earliest age for repair of isolated microtia has been 6 to 8 years with the techniques described by Tanzer[20] and Brent.[1] Some patients are referred having already undergone ear reconstruction. If the ear framework has been placed in an unfavorable site, repositioning of the constructed ear complex is deferred until skeletal symmetry is obtained. In other cases it has been necessary to remove the framework completely.

Marked deficiencies of subcutaneous fat and facial musculature are corrected by an omental free flap placed in specially designed subcutaneous pockets.[21] In patients with mild deficiencies onlay bone grafts to the mandible and the zygoma or subcutaneous dermal fat grafts can be used effectively.

Although many patients present with seventh nerve paresis or palsy, especially frontalis and mandibular branches, neuromuscular transfers and nerve grafts are just beginning to be used in these cases.

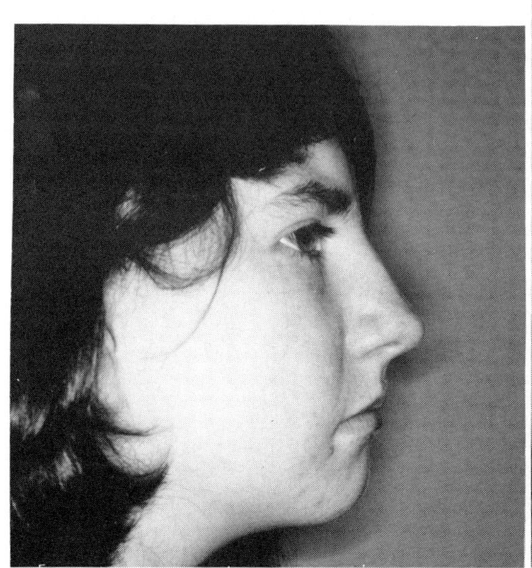

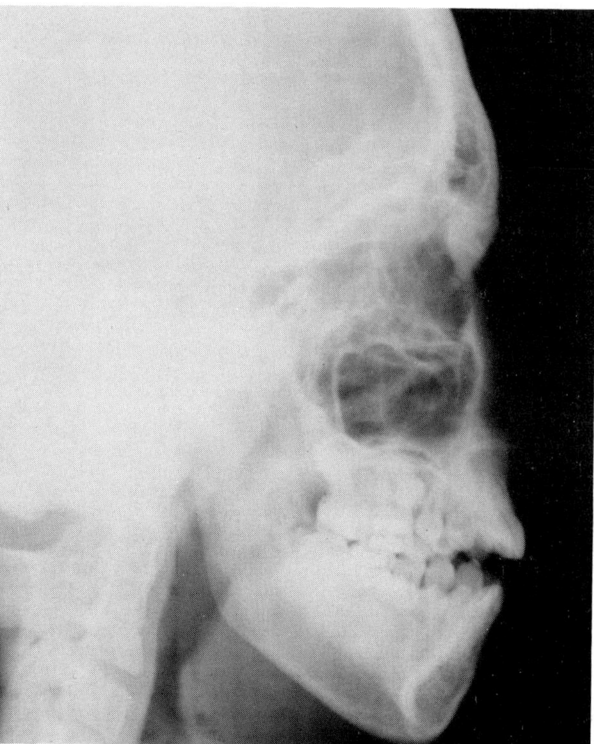

Continued.

Fig. 8-11—cont'd.
C and **D,** Retrusion of the mandible and a slight open-bite. Note the mandibular ramal and body height discrepancy as a double-contour shadow on the cephalogram.

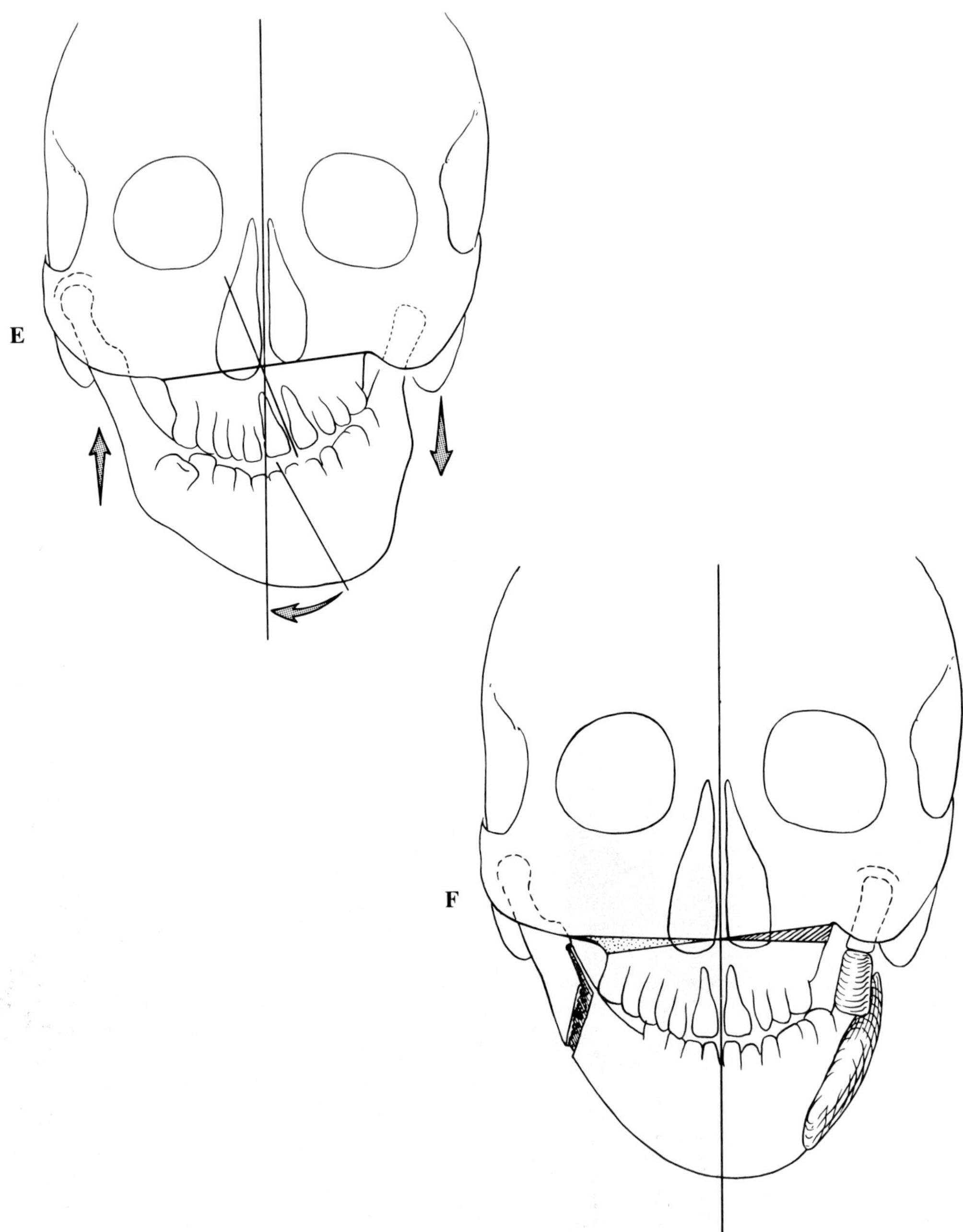

Fig. 8-11—cont'd.
E, Tilting of the occlusal plane with deviation of the maxillary and mandibular midlines and mandibular chin point. The plane described by a line connecting the dental and skeletal mandibular midlines is deviated toward the normal side at its upper end (incisors) and toward the abnormal side at its lower end (chin point). *Arrows,* Path of rotation to correct the skeletal deformity. **F,** The operation, including creation of a fulcrum for the LeFort I osteotomy.

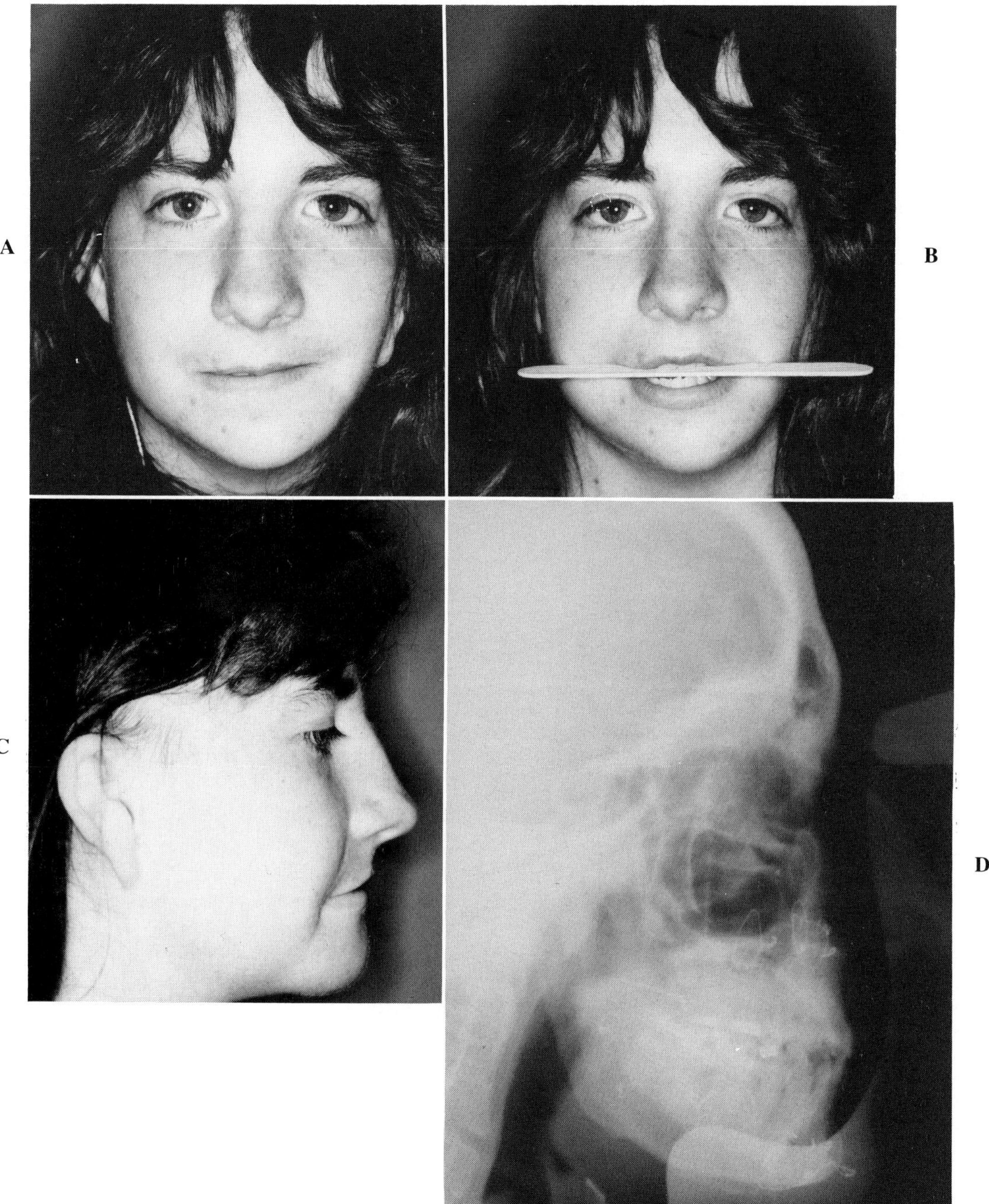

Fig. 8-12.
Same patient as in Fig. 8-11. **A** and **B,** Two years postoperative. Symmetry of the chin, fullness of
the left side of the mandible (accomplished with onlay bone grafts at the time of osteotomies), and a
level occlusal plane. **C** and **D,** An advancement genioplasty was part of this patient's treatment.
A and **D** from Murray, J.E., et al.: Plast. Reconstr. Surg. **74:**186, 1984.

DISCUSSION

Historically the earliest operations for hemifacial microsomia dealt with the external ear anomaly. Operations on the facial skeleton were avoided for fear of disturbing "growth centers." However, serial observation of children with hemifacial microsomia demonstrated that skeletal distortion progresses and secondary anomalies develop with age[8,15] because of diminished growth on the affected side. Therefore, in an effort to create a milieu for vertical midface growth, we began to operate on the mandible in growing children.

Our current management of patients with HFM deformities is three-dimensional. The mandible is elongated and rotated to the proper midline in the frontal plane. When necessary, the mandible and/or chin are advanced in the sagittal plan as well as widened in the transverse plane. The purpose of this is to create space for vertical midface growth and, in that way, to prevent secondary distortion.

The evolution of treatment of Type III deformity has been gradual, and our current one-stage construction has unfolded over the last 12 years.

In the early cases, at the first operation, a bone graft to the terminal end of the deformed mandibular body was placed to preserve tooth buds and to create a "handle" for subsequent osseous fixation. The second stage, 6 months to 2 years later, included construction of the glenoid fossa and the zygomatic arch. The third procedure was performed to bridge the defect between the constructed glenoid fossa and the augmented mandibular body. For this purpose we used rib grafts with attached costochondral junction. The cartilage was inserted into the previously constructed glenoid fossa. This three-stage total mandibular TMJ construction has evolved into the single-stage procedure described in the present chapter.

Comparison of adult defects with those in infants, however, suggested that adjacent normal structures were not growing optimally. In fact, it seemed that the mandible was restricting growth of the maxilla, the zygoma, and even the orbits. Although this hypothesis could not be proved, it seemed reasonable to try to prevent development of the adult end-stage defect.

Integrating these two paths of experience, we currently correct Type III deformities as early as safety allows, usually around 24 months of age. Complete construction of the mandible, TMJ, and zygoma is done in one stage. Our working hypothesis is that restoration of a symmetric "functional matrix" will unlock growth potential and minimize secondary distortion. Early correction also provides maximal psychologic benefit to the patient.[14]

It is difficult to prove that the constructed mandibular ramus is growing in these young patients. We have indirect evidence of this, in that symmetry is maintained as the child gets older. We are currently investigating the use of skeletal scintigraphy[2] to analyze normal and abnormal condylar growth, and we plan to apply this technique to document growth of the constructed mandible. There is no doubt, however, that early correction of the mandibular defect permits improved vertical growth of the midface and decreases secondary distortion in the maxilla, nose, and orbits.[15]

Finally, psychologic studies have documented that early correction aids in normal body image development.[14] We have found that patients with asymmetric facial deformities have greater psychologic difficulties than do those with symmetric defects. Perhaps, they compare the two sides (normal versus abnormal) everyday. We have documented that the earlier surgical correction is carried out the greater will be the improvement in body image development. This may be the most important benefit to the patient.

In the future, efforts will be directed to understanding the pathogenesis of HFM and possibly providing a means of preventing the deformity. From a surgical standpoint, now that skeletal malformation and soft tissue deformity are correctable, the next major breakthrough will be in the treatment of the neuromuscular defects.

REFERENCES

1. Brent, B.: The correction of microtia with autogenous cartilage grafts. I. The classic deformity, Plast. Reconst. Surg. **65:**1, 1980.
2. Cisneros, G., and Kaban, L.B.: Computerized skeletal scintigraphy for assessment of mandibular asymmetry, J. Oral Maxillofac. Surg. **42:**513, 1984.
3. Converse, J.M., et al.: The corrective treatment of the

skeletal asymmetry in hemifacial microsomia, Plast. Reconstr. Surg. **52:**221, 1973.

4. Converse, J.M., et al.: Clinical aspects of craniofacial microsomia. In Converse, J.M., et al., editors: Symposium on diagnosis and treatment of craniofacial anomalies, St. Louis, 1979, The C.V. Mosby Co.

5. Enlow, D.H.: Handbook of facial growth, p. 140, Philadelphia, 1975, W.B. Saunders Co.

6. Gorlin, R.J., et al.: Syndromes of the head and neck, New York, 1976, McGraw-Hill Book Co.

7. Harvold, E.P.: Treatment of hemifacial microsomia, New York, 1983, Alan R. Liss, Inc.

8. Kaban, L.B., et al.: Three-dimensional approach to analysis and treatment of hemifacial microsomia, Cleft Palate J. **18:**90, 1981.

9. Marx, H.: Die Missbildungen des Ohres: sekundäre Ohrmissbildungen. In Henke, F., and Lubarsch, O., editors: Handbuch der speziellen pathologischen Anatomie und Histologie, Berlin, 1926, Springer-Verlag.

10. McNamara, J.A.: Neuromuscular and skeletal adaptation to altered function in the orofacial region, Am. J. Orthod. **64:**578, 1973.

11. Meurmann, Y.: Congenital microtia and meatal atresia, Arch. Otolaryngol. **66:**443, 1957.

12. Moss, M.L.: Twenty years of functional cranial analysis, Am. J. Orthod. **61:**479, 1972.

13. Munro, I.: One stage reconstruction of the temporomandibular joint in hemifacial microsomia, Plast. Reconstr. Surg. **66:**699, 1980.

14. Murray, J.E., et al.: Twenty-year experience with maxillocraniofacial surgery: an evaluation of early surgery on growth, function, and body image, Ann. Surg. **190:**320, 1979.

15. Murray, J.E., et al.: Analysis and treatment of hemifacial microsomia, Plast. Reconstr. Surg. **74:**186, 1984.

16. Obwegeser, H.L.: Correction of skeletal anomalies of otomandibular dysostosis, J. Maxillofac. Surg. **2:**73, 1974.

17. Pruzansky, S.: Not all dwarfed mandibles are alike, March of Dimes **5:**120, 1969.

18. Ross, R.B.: Lateral facial dysplasia (first and second branchial arch syndrome, hemifacial microsomia), Birth Defects **11:**51, 1975.

19. Swanson, L.T., and Murray, J.E.: Asymmetries of the lower part of the face. In Whitaker, L.A., and Randall, P., editors: Symposium on reconstruction of jaw deformities, p. 171, St. Louis, 1978, The C.V. Mosby Co.

20. Tanzer, R.C.: The total reconstruction of the auricle. The evolution of a plan of treatment, Plast. Reconstr. Surg. **47:**523, 1971.

21. Upton, J. et al.: Restoration of facial contour using free vascularized omental transfer, Plast. Reconstr. Surg. **66:**560, 1980.

CHAPTER 9

Applications of high midface procedures in the management of dentofacial deformities

JOHN J. DANN

For two decades in the United States, surgical procedures have evolved for correction of high midfacial deformity in parallel with the development of orthognathic procedures for the correction of maxillomandibular deformity. Diagnostic considerations for the former emphasized etiologic, neurologic, ophthalmologic, and psychosocial considerations. By contrast, diagnostic concerns for the latter emphasized three-dimensional anatomic evaluation and close surgical-orthodontic coordination. A composite diagnostic approach that considers the etiology and anatomy as well as a comprehensive overview of associated disabilities lends itself to the application of high midface surgical procedures within the context of comprehensive patient rehabilitation. This chapter will discuss diagnostic stratagems and applications of subcranial high midface procedures for dentofacial deformity.

Craniofacial dysjunction, nasoorbitomaxillary osteotomy, was first described in the 1950s.[10] The initial technical difficulties encountered with it, however, delayed more sophisticated applications of nasoorbitomaxillary repositioning until the late 1960s and early 1970s.* Since the early 1970s multiple patterns of osteotomy in the nasoorbitomaxillary region

have been described.[1,7,25,27] These procedures appear to be adaptable to a wide variety of clinical malformations. Nevertheless, the literature describing them is somewhat confusing because the procedures are often based on the LeFort fracture classification. This classification is, in fact, a misnomer since elective osteotomies are generally not performed along the classic fracture lines. I prefer to discuss high midface osteotomies in terms of the anatomic regions of the midfacial skeleton to be mobilized.

Fig. 9-1 illustrates the regions of the midface skeleton amenable to en bloc mobilization. Considerable variation in the design of the osteotomy is possible within the stippled areas.

DIAGNOSTIC EVALUATION OF HIGH MIDFACIAL DEFORMITY

General considerations. As the expression of osseous deformity progresses into the upper portions of the middle third of the face, somewhat more extensive diagnostic considerations are necessary than are called for in routine orthognathic surgery. Generally, specific attention must be directed to consideration of the etiology and anatomy of the deformity and the functional disability posed by it. Each of these considerations bears specifically on the choice of a surgical procedure and the timing of surgery.

---

*References 12, 20, 22, 28, 29.

316

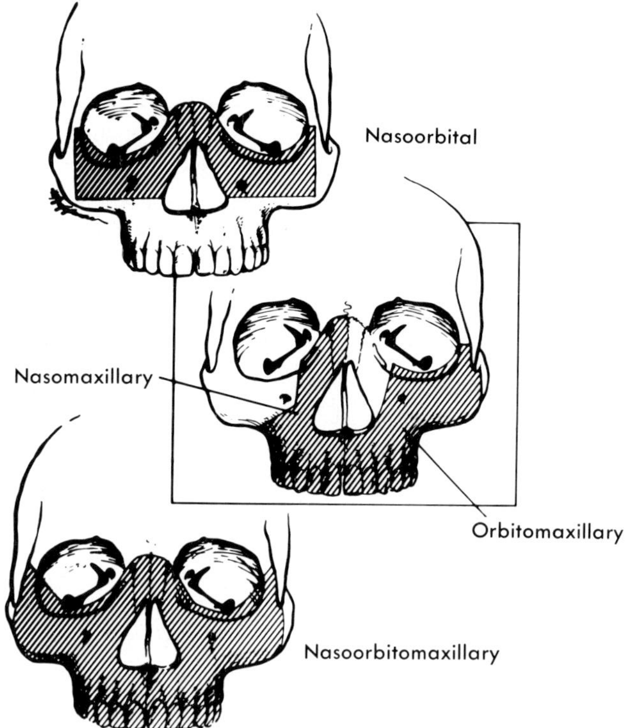

Fig. 9-1.
Classification of high midface osteotomies.

Etiologic considerations. In general, the etiology of midfacial deformity can be congenital, developmental, or acquired. The assignment of a deformity to each of these categories brings with it pertinent information for the management of the individual patient.

By definition, *congenital* malformations are present at birth. It should be remembered that in approximately 45% of the patients with three or more major structural malformations it is possible to identify a malformation syndrome diagnosis.[26] Such a diagnosis is significant because several of the malformation syndromes will demonstrate a predictable pattern of evolution of midfacial deformity to its end-stage and, therefore, allow the surgeon accurately to sequence reconstructive surgery. Certainly for patients with a heritable malformation aspects of genetic counseling should not be overlooked.

Late-onset midfacial malformations are gen-erally considered to be *developmental* in etiology. The majority will be mild to moderate in severity. They are considered to represent expressions of polygenic heritance. The assignment of developmental etiology, however, is often done by exclusion. The fact should not be overlooked that congenital heritable malformation with variable penetrance and expressivity may be subtle and inapparent to the inexperienced clinician. The diagnostic team must therefore be well aware of the concept of microforms of multiple malformation syndromes.

Finally, the patient with *acquired* midfacial malformation probably represents the most difficult challenge for surgical reconstruction. Malformation resulting from a pathologic process or prior radiation therapy, trauma, or ablative surgery generally presents with a composite soft tissue and osseous deformity. The soft tissue aspects of an acquired deformity should not be overlooked, for they may place discrete limitations upon the prognosis for overall rehabilitation. Similarly the psychosocial implications of acquired deformity cannot be overlooked. The treatment expectations of patients with acquired deformity frequently exceed the capabilities of the treatment team.

Anatomic evaluation. Anatomic characterization of high midfacial deformity is critical to the actual planning of specific surgical procedures. A systematic anatomic evaluation also yields information that is helpful in confirming the etiology of a given deformity and in determining the relationship of a given pattern of deformity to specific functional disability in the patient.

Our approach to the anatomic evaluation of a patient with high midfacial deformity is similar to the basic concepts of "systematic evaluation" of the orthognathic surgical patient.[6] We proceed from *clinical anatomic evaluation* to *radiographic correlation* and finally to integration of the *occlusal relationships* with the *osseous anatomic characteristics* of the deformity. For patients with a high midfacial deformity the clinical evaluation is generally extended to include neurologic and ophthalmologic considerations.

Clinical evaluation proceeds from qualitative description of vertical, sagittal, and transverse relationships in the upper, middle, and lower third of the face to specific consideration of anatomic structures including the cranium, nasal and orbital structures, and maxillary and mandibular structures.

Extensive cranial malformation rarely presents an indication for cosmetic reconstruction. The size and shape of the cranium, however, must be carefully considered in making a determination of the role of neurocranial influences on the expression of midfacial deformity. The anterior basicranium can be looked upon as a boundary across which neurocranial development influences midfacial growth. Conversely, specific patterns of midfacial malformation may index the presence of structural malformations in the central nervous system.[5]

Minimum clinical assessment of cranial structures should include documentation of the occipitofrontal circumference, the shape and dimensions of the fontanels in younger patients, the presence of focal contour malformations, and the overall pattern of cranial development (including the calculation of a cranial index). When significant cranial abnormalities exist, particularly in conjunction with specific patterns of midfacial malformation such as frontonasal dysplasia, consideration should be given to detailed neurologic assessment.

Specific neurocranial malformations will contraindicate subcranial correction of midfacial deformity. These include inferior prolapse of the cribriform plate, nasoorbital encephalocele, and anterior displacement of the temporal lobe into the lateral orbit. The surgeon should also be familiar with the anatomy and clinical presentation of "atypical" craniofacial clefting.[14] Coronal CT scanning is generally undertaken for preoperative assessment of craniomidfacial anatomy.

Nasal evaluation entails assessment of external morphology and airway patency. The osseous and cartilaginous nasal skeleton demonstrates significant normal variation. Ongoing development of nasal structures into adulthood compounds the problem of attempting rigorous quantitative nasal evaluation. We have begun to correlate cephalometric nasal norms with findings on clinical examination.[30] Preliminary data suggest that identifiable patterns of nasal deformity are frequently associated with maxillary and midfacial deformity. In addition, predictable changes in nasal morphology appear to occur with midface osteotomy.

The clinical nasal examination includes attention to the size, shape, and position of the following structures: frontonasal angle, nasal dorsum, tip structures, alar base, columella, and septum. Isolated deformities of each of these structures can occur, as can identifiable patterns of deformity affecting multiple nasal structures. Finally, particular attention is directed to assessment of the relative nasal height and depth and the projection of dorsum and tip.

The preoperative nasal evaluation also focuses on factors affecting nasal airway patency. Significant septal deformity, abnormal turbinates, and choanal hypoplasia or atresia must be evaluated in planning surgery for midfacial hypoplasia. Clinical and radiographic evaluation of the septum, turbinates and choanal region are routinely undertaken prior to planning intraoperative and postoperative airway management.

Deformity in the orbital region may involve the osseous orbit, globe, lids, and adnexal structures. Each of these must be considered in isolation and in relation to each other. Osseous orbital malformation is a clinical diagnosis amenable to semiquantitative radiographic confimation. Orbital hypoplasia will be evident clinically with varying degrees of exophthalmos, prominence of the lid structures, and inadequate malar body contour.

The osseous orbit cannot be considered without concomitant evaluation of the globe and orbital adnexal structures.[32] Specifically the differential diagnosis of exophthalmos extends well beyond a consideration of just the osseous orbital deformity.[11] Abnormal patterns of extraocular motion may also be associated with identifiable patterns of osseous orbital deformity. Finally, atypical craniofacial clefting may extend into the globe structures, including the iris and retina. For these reasons a detailed ophthalmologic assessment, including acuity, visual fields, globe motility, funduscopic evaluation, and determination of intraocular pressures is a routine part of our preoperative workup for patients with orbital malformation.

The position of the globe in the vertical and sagittal planes may present discrete limitations for planning correction with nasoorbitomaxillary osteotomies. As discussed elsewhere,[8,32] an exophthalmometer may be used to provide a quantitative assessment of relationships of the superior, lateral, and inferior orbital rims to the globe as well as the relationship of the globe to the nasal bridge.

The relationships that we routinely measure are illustrated in Fig. 9-2. In attempting a quantitative exophthalmometric evaluation one needs to be aware of the role of lateral rim deformity. Sufficient orbital protection for the globe is present if the convexity of the cornea lies on or approximately 1 to 2 mm anterior to a tangent to the superior and inferior orbital rims. Normal values for the measurements are presented.

The anatomic evaluation of maxillomandibular structures proceeds as for the patient with suborbital deformity. After a thorough examination of the specific nasal, orbital, and maxillomandibular structures, the relationship of these to each other is rigorously assessed. En bloc osteotomy of the midfacial complex is suc-

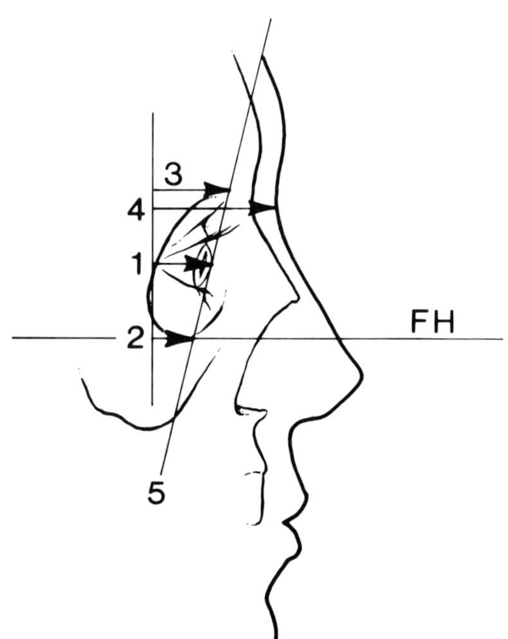

Fig. 9-2.
Clinical assessment of relationships of the nose, orbit, and globe. *FH,* Frankfort horizontal.

Normal range of projections from the lateral orbital rim (mm)
1, Exophthalmos 10 to 14
2, Inferior rim 0 to 4
3, Superior rim 8 to 16
4, Nasal dorsum 15 to 24
5, Tangent to superior and inferior orbital rims

cessful only when a similar magnitude of deformity of congruent structures exists. Otherwise, the osteotomy simply yields a new pattern of deformity.

Cephalometric assessment can be helpful in determining the magnitude and relative severity of deformity in adjacent midfacial structures. It should be noted, however, that cephalometric values are frequently derived from cranial base referents, which are themselves deformed with increasing severity of midfacial deformity.

Fig. 9-3 illustrates measurements that we find helpful in assessing orbital morphology.[4,18] Cranial base length (measurement *1*) is assessed as an index of cranial base deformity. Orbital height (measurement *2*) is measured and compared to norms, since the design of an osteotomy and the intended pattern of movement of the inferior orbital rim constitute important surgical planning considerations. The angle sella-nasion-orbitale is normally 65 degrees and approximates relative sagittal positioning of the inferolateral orbital rim to the frontonasal junction. The distance between orbitale and the N-A line (measurement *4*) is generally on the order of 15 mm and can provide a semiquantitative estimate of relative magnitude of an inferior orbital and maxillary sagittal deformity. The sub-

mentovertex cephalometric projection supplements PA and lateral studies for ortibal asymmetry.

Finally, anatomic evaluation is directed to an *assessment of malocclusion relative to the position of the maxilla and mandible within the maxillofacial complex.* Although several authors state that high midfacial surgery is not undertaken primarily for occlusal rehabilitation, at least one prominent craniofacial surgeon[13] believes that definitive occlusal adjustment must be undertaken to allow successful stable repositioning of the midfacial complex. It has been our experience that an integrated sequence of orthodontic and surgical management is critical to obtaining a stable functional and esthetic result for patients with high midfacial deformity.

The anatomic evaluation directs itself to an assessment of the size and position of various elements of the maxillofacial complex. Clinical examination with radiographic correlation establishes the presence, site, and magnitude of deformity. It cannot be overstated that the shape of the various elements of the maxillofacial complex must be taken into account in planning definitive reconstructive surgery. The diagnosis of significant contour deformity rests with clinical esthetic judgment. The surgeon cannot un-

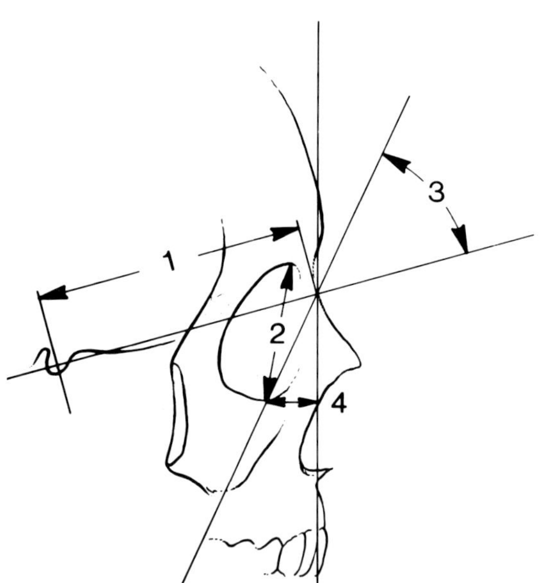

Fig. 9-3.
Cephalometric orbitomaxillary relationships.

dertake a simple en bloc mobilization of contour-deformed bones and hope to obtain definitive esthetic reconstruction. The correction of contour deformity of the maxillofacial skeleton is generally undertaken either at the first stage with onlay bone grafting or secondarily with alloplastic implants.

Assessment of functional disability. Anatomic diagnostic evaluation requires detailed knowledge of nasoorbitomaxillary anatomy and physiology. Although the maxillofacial surgeon should have sufficient expertise to characterize anatomic deformity, comprehensive patient evaluation includes a thorough assessment of the functional disability associated with a given pattern of deformity. Therefore diagnostic evaluation is performed within the context of a multidisciplinary team. Attention is directed equally to an evaluation of the anatomy-related disability and the concomitant psychosocial disability.

The makeup of our multidisciplinary diagnostic and treatment team is as follows:

> Primary care
> > Pediatric
> > Family practice
> Surgical
> > Oral and maxillofacial
> > Plastic
> > Otolaryngologic
> > Anesthesiologic
> Dental
> > Orthodontic
> > Pediatric dental
> > Prosthetic
> Consultative
> > Radiology
> > Ophthalmology
> > Neurology
> > Psychology
> > Neurosurgery
> > Clinical psychology
> > Genetics, dysmorphology
> Paraprofessional
> > Nursing
> > Speech pathology
> > Audiology
> > Social services
> > Physical therapy
> > Dietary counseling

Thorough multidisciplinary diagnostic evaluation is then followed by appropriate specialty treatment within the context of an overall plan and sequence for rehabilitation of the individual patient.

SURGICAL MANAGEMENT OF MIDFACIAL DEFORMITIES

Basic considerations. Success in surgical management of the high midfacial deformity is predicated on a thorough diagnostic assessment and detailed planning of the surgical procedure. Several problems are addressed in planning surgical reconstruction: choosing the sites to be operated on, determining the type of procedure to be employed, planning the conduct of a given surgical procedure, and determining whether surgery is to be undertaken in stages.

Detailed clinical examination correlated with radiographic evaluation provides the data base that the surgeon uses in determining which sites of deformity are to be operated on. Determination also must be made as to whether deformities are of sufficient severity to warrant consideration for surgical reconstruction in view of the potential complications with a given procedure.

Choice of procedure. In general, en bloc osteotomy, alloplastic implants, and/or onlay grafting are used for correction of midfacial deformity. En bloc osteotomy can address the definitive management of abnormal size or position of facial bones. Where significant contour deformity coexists, consideration is also directed to definitive alloplastic contour augmentation.

Design of the osteotomy. The actual design of a midface osteotomy is predicated on quantitative plans for osseous repositioning in three planes, with provision for adequate stabilization of the midface complex. Most frequently an en bloc osteotomy involves combined vertical and sagittal repositioning. The design of orbital osteotomy is critical to allow accurate repositioning and provide an interlocking bone interface for secure stabilization.

Fig. 9-4 illustrates designs for orbital osteotomy that permit combined sagittal and vertical transposition. For purposes of anatomic reference the central illustration labels the inferior orbital fissure and the lacrimal fossa.

In general, inferolateral orbital osteotomy

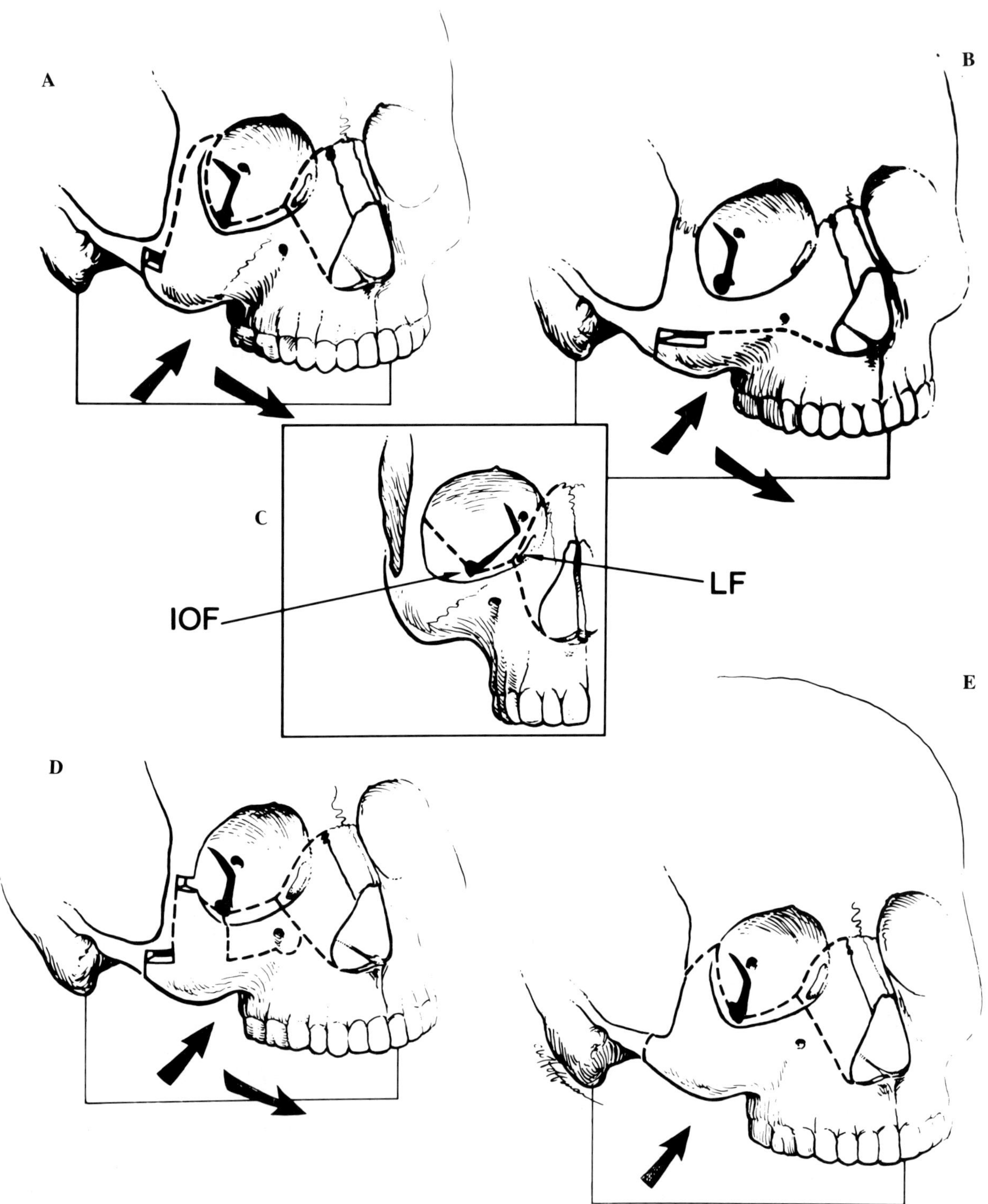

Fig. 9-4.
Variations of nasoorbitomalar osteotomy. *IOF,* Inferior orbital fissure; *LF,* lacrimal fossa.

will extend to the inferior orbital fissure (IOF) and then to the desired height in the lateral orbit and inferiorly along the posterolateral maxilla to the pterygomaxillary fissure. Medial to the IOF the osteotomy extends to the lacrimal fossa. At this point it may proceed inferiorly to the anterior maxilla when nasal repositioning is not indicated. Extension of the orbital osteotomy onto nasal structures proceeds either anterior or posterior to the medial canthal tendon depending upon lid and globe morphology at the medial canthus. The lateral or medial canthal tendons may be repositioned by canthopexy at the time of osteotomy.

Fig. 9-4, *A* and *C*, illustrates designs for stepped malar–lateral orbital osteotomy to provide sliding-interlocking bone interfaces and sites for graft stabilization. A modification of these stepped osteotomies for suborbital simultaneous correction of vertical maxillary excess and orbitomaxillary hypoplasia is illustrated in *B*. This procedure is described in detail elsewhere.[2] The pattern of zygomaticoorbital osteotomy illustrated in *D* renders precise stabilization of vertical and sagittal repositioning more difficult than does the stepped osteotomy.

It should be noted that dissimilar vectors of orbital, nasal, and maxillary movement can be obtained by planning ''rotational'' midface movement[15]; and, again, it has been my experience that such complex patterns of movement are facilitated by the design of stepped malar osteotomy.

In all midface osteotomies involving the inferior orbital rim, particular attention is directed to planning the vertical vector of inferior rim movement. Significant increase in the vertical orbital dimension is generally avoided since this decreases support for the lower lid, with resultant ''scleral show.'' By contrast, 3 to 4 mm of superior repositioning will augment the support of lid structures.

Whatever the design of lateral, inferior orbital, and nasomaxillary osteotomy, it is important also to attend to the design of the osteotomy of the lateral nasal wall. A significant potential for disruption of normal nasolacrimal and sinus physiology exists with uncontrolled down-fracturing in the lateral nasal wall.[17] It is preferable to design lateral nasal wall osteotomies in such a fashion that they traverse from the most superior aspect of the nasal or orbital osteotomy down the anterior aspect of the lateral nasal wall and then below the inferior turbinate, traversing proximally to the perpendicular plate of the palatine bone.

Surgical access and adjunctive procedures. Once the design of the midface osteotomy is complete, the surgeon considers surgical access and indications for adjunctive procedures.

A coronal scalp flap is preferred for access to nasal structures and to the superior, superomedial, and lateral orbit. A subconjunctival or infraciliary approach is used for the orbital floor. Oral incisions provide access to the posterolateral maxillae and pterygomaxillary fissures.

Adjunctive procedures undertaken at the time of midface osteotomy include medial or lateral canthopexy, decompression of orbital fat, and correction of frontal contour deformity. Definitive procedures involving the lids, extraocular muscles, nasolacrimal apparatus, and nasal cartilaginous skeleton are generally deferred to a second stage.

Intraoperative management. Intraoperative management is planned with attention to airway maintenance, anesthetic management, and organization of the surgical team.

Nasotracheal intubation is preferred when possible. In the presence of significant nasal obstruction, surgery is begun with orotracheal intubation followed by nasal intubation after surgical management of the obstruction, which may entail actual mobilization of the midface. The postoperative airway is secured with endotracheal intubation. Elective tracheostomy is seldom necessary.

Deliberate hypotensive anesthesia may be considered in complicated and lengthy cases, particularly in young patients. In adolescents and young adults sufficient hypotension can usually be maintained with a combined inhalation-narcotic technique without resorting to vasoactive agents. We attempt to have autogenous blood available for transfusion requirements.

Training and direction of the surgical team are undertaken by the primary surgeon. Thorough preparation is necessary for nursing and medicodental personnel. For lengthy procedures provision is made to spell members of the team. The availability of on-call surgical specialty consultants is assured prior to the operation in the event of unanticipated complications. This team concept is extended into the postoperative period and includes provision for training house staff and nursing, ICU, physical therapy, and respiratory therapy personnel.

EN BLOC MIDFACE OSTEOTOMY

En bloc osteotomy is indicated for the correction of clinically significant abnormal size and position of midfacial anatomic structures. With high midface osteotomy we attempt to avoid segmentalization of the maxillary dentoalveolus. When indicated, segmental osteotomy is undertaken as a second procedure.

The nasoorbitomaxillary osteotomy, or so called "LeFort III" osteotomy, is preferred for a variety of clinical situations.[13,29] Although sagittal hypoplasia of the midfacial complex involving nasal structures is most often evident with a saddle-nose deformity, vertical hypoplasia of midfacionasal structures represents a far more common indication for nasomaxillary or nasoorbitomaxillary osteotomy. The majority of saddle-nose deformities without vertical nasal hypoplasia can be corrected without extension of the osteotomy to the nasal pyramid. It should also be borne in mind that the variability of osseous and nasal cartilaginous morphology often does not allow definitive esthetic nasal correction by simple nasomaxillary or nasoorbitomaxillary osteotomy.

In Fig. 9-5, *A*, a rather typical vertical nasal hypoplasia exists in conjunction with a tip and supratip deformity of the nasal skeleton. This patient has a skeletal Class III malocclusion with moderate exophthalmos indicative of inadequate osseous support for the lower lid by the inferior orbital rim. A one-stage nasoorbitomaxillary osteotomy with bone graft stabilization and genioplasty was undertaken. The pattern of movement of the midfacial complex was rotational, with differential nasal, orbital, and maxillary movement. Note in *B* that the one-stage en bloc nasoorbitomaxillary osteotomy did not definitively address the tip or supratip nasal deformity nor did it correct the columellar base retraction. These composite contour deformities of the cartilaginous and osseous nasal skeleton must be addressed by a second-stage procedure. Also note that whereas sagittal augmentation of the nasal dorsum has attenuated the degree of tip and supratip deformity this may be accompanied by a tendency to obliteration of the frontonasal angle. The composite soft tissue changes observed with simultaneous nasoorbitomaxillary osteotomy and genioplasty are illustrated in *C*.

En bloc orbitomaxillary repositioning represents perhaps the most versatile of all midface osteotomies. The orbital aspects of the procedure may be extended to varying levels within the lateral orbital rims depending on the conformation of the deformity (Fig. 9-4). A degree of rotation of the orbitomaxillary complex is also possible to allow the surgeon to address both vertical and sagittal deformities. Finally, mild to moderate asymmetry correction in the orbitomaxillary complex is feasible as long as systematic planning of the osteotomies is performed.

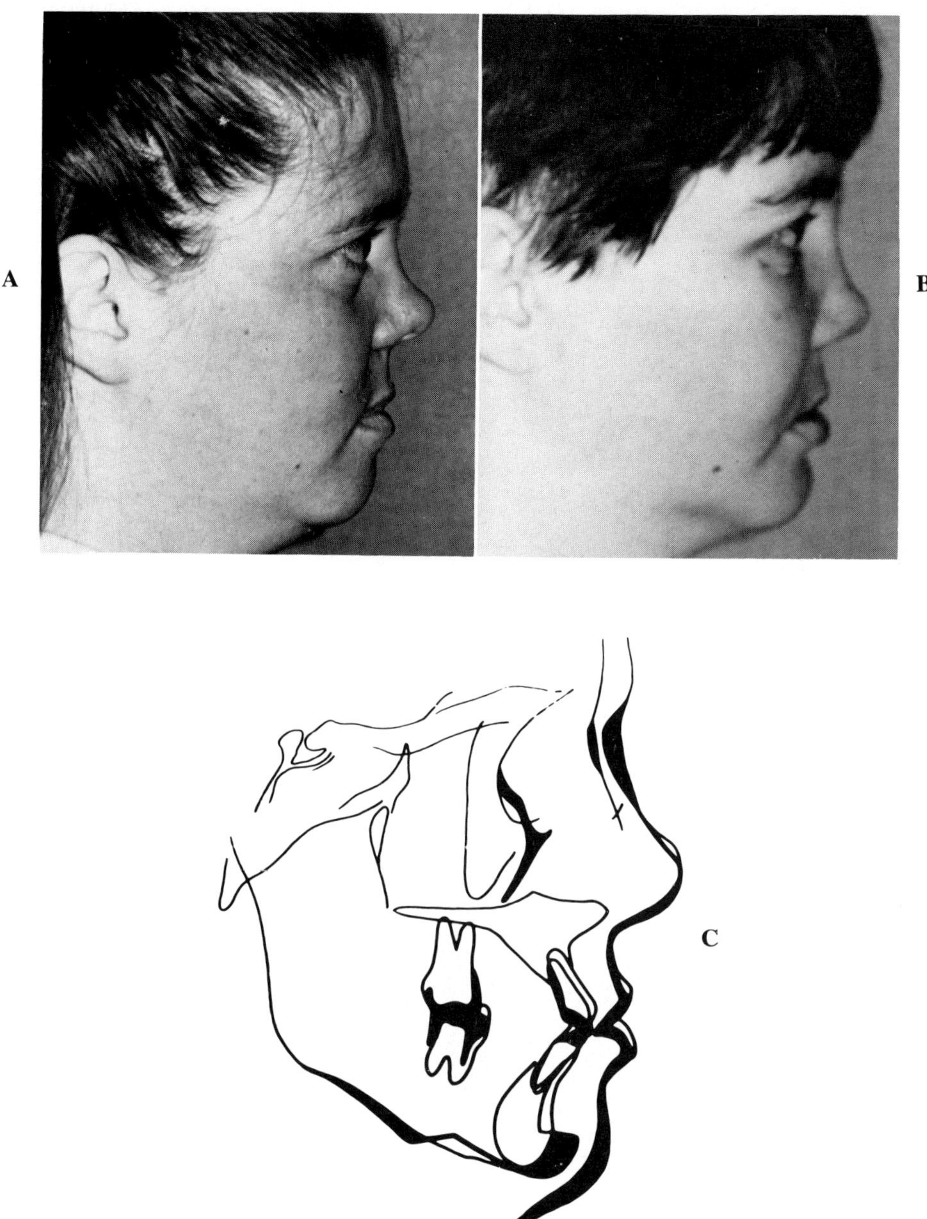

Fig. 9-5.
Nasoorbitomaxillary hypoplasia. **A,** Preoperative appearance and, **B,** after nasoorbitomaxillary osteotomy. **C,** Composite cephalometric changes.

Fig. 9-6 demonstrates the treatment of orbitomaxillary hypoplasia following childhood midfacial trauma. In *A* an inferior orbital and anterior maxillary contour deformity is accompanied by a decrease in the width of the alar base. In *B* the hypoplasia with lack of osseous protection of the globe is evident. There is also a relatively normal nasal dorsum with a slightly drooped tip. In *C* the skeletal Class III open-bite malocclusion is partially edentulous secondary to the avulsive trauma.

Preoperative orthodontic leveling and align-

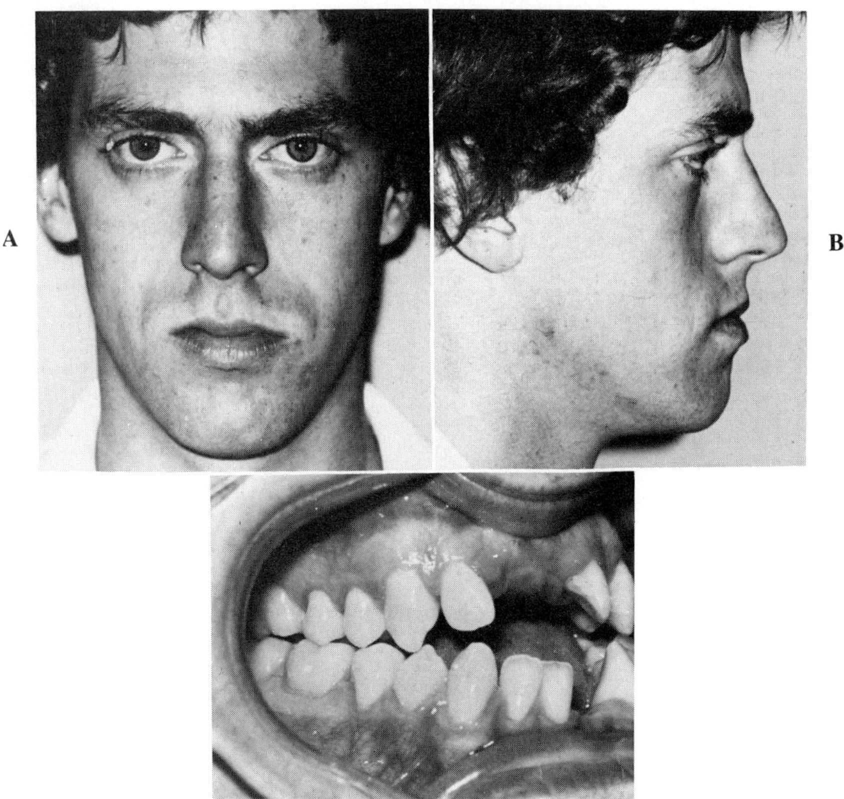

Fig. 9-6.
Orbitomaxillary hypoplasia. **A** to **C,** Preoperative appearance.

ment in both arches was followed by orbito-maxillary osteotomy. Postoperatively (Fig. 9-6, *D* to *F*), note the improved contour in the infra-orbitomalar regions as well as the provision of osseous protection for the globe. Some tip ele-vation of nasal structures has occurred in con-junction with a widening of the alar base and subtle changes in the perinasal contour. This 9 mm rotational orbitomaxillary advancement has been stable for 6½ years postoperatively.

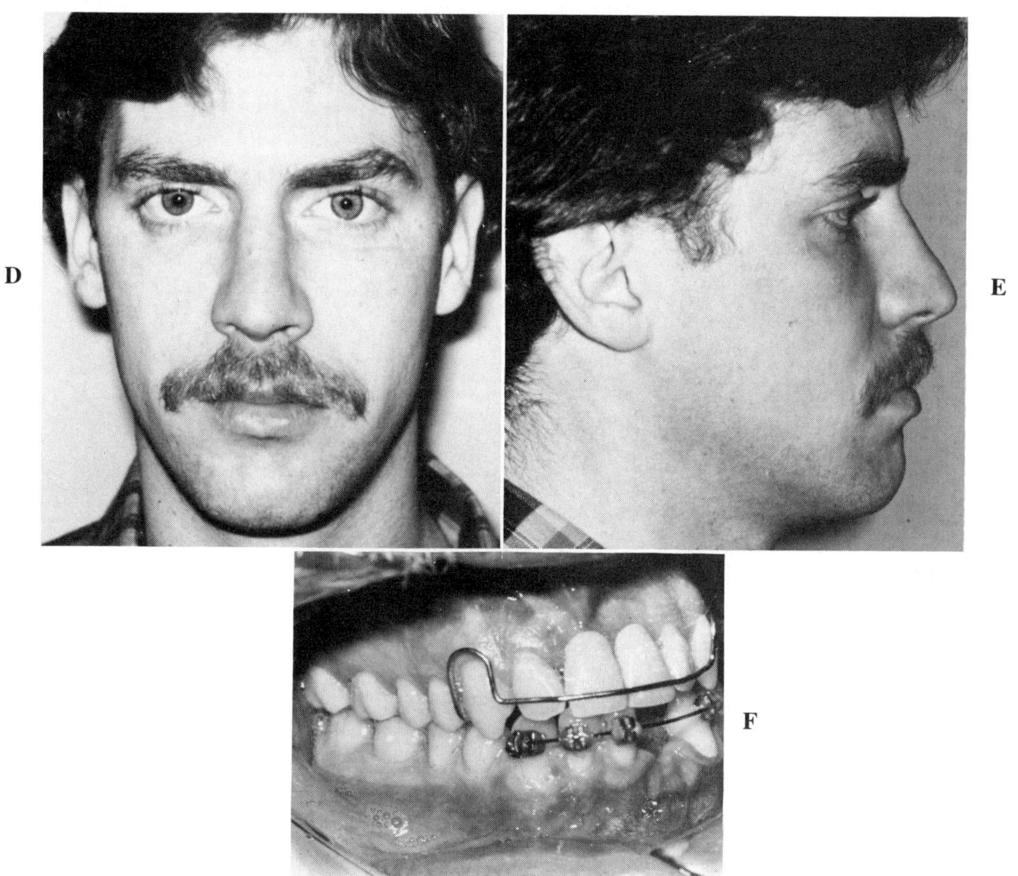

Fig. 9-6—cont'd.
Orbitomaxillary hypoplasia. **D** to **F**, Postoperative appearance.

Although it is versatile, orbitomaxillary osteotomy does not allow the simultaneous definitive correction of complex contour and positional abnormalities. Staging may be necessary for composite correction. Fig. 9-7, *A* and *B,* demonstrates an instance of Saethre-Chotzen syndrome, a variant of craniofacial synostosis. Note the complex asymmetry of the middle and lower facial thirds—involving the nose, palpebral fissures, maxillary dentoalveolus, and mandible. In profile the nasal dorsal projection is adequate if not excessive. A tip droop is present in conjunction with retraction of the columellar base. Relative and absolute sagittal mandibular excesses are noted. First-stage orbitomaxillary osteotomy with bone graft stabilization, lateral canthopexy, superolateral orbital rim augmentation, and mandibular ramal osteotomy resulted in the changes illustrated in *C* and *D*. Note in the frontal view that the previously subtle nasal dorsal asymmetry is now more apparent as normalization in the symmetry and width of the alar base structures has occurred. In profile the nasal tip has been significantly elevated. However, residual contour deformity of the nasal tip remains, as does asymmetry of the nasal dorsum, and there is an improved but still notable columellar base retraction. It is of interest that this patient had severe unilateral preoperative airway obstruction. The airway was successfully managed by left-sided nasoendotracheal intubation. Subsequent surgery consisted of nasoseptal reconstruction and genioplasty.

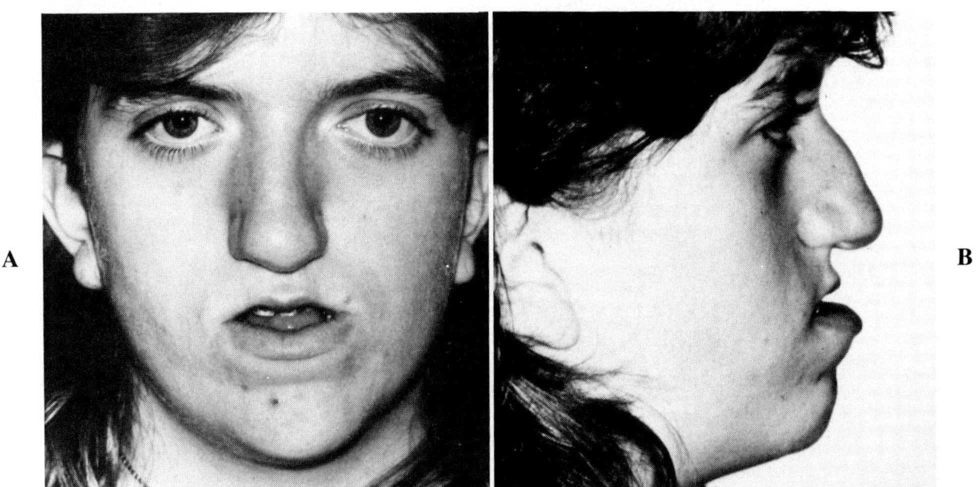

Fig. 9-7.
For legend see opposite page.

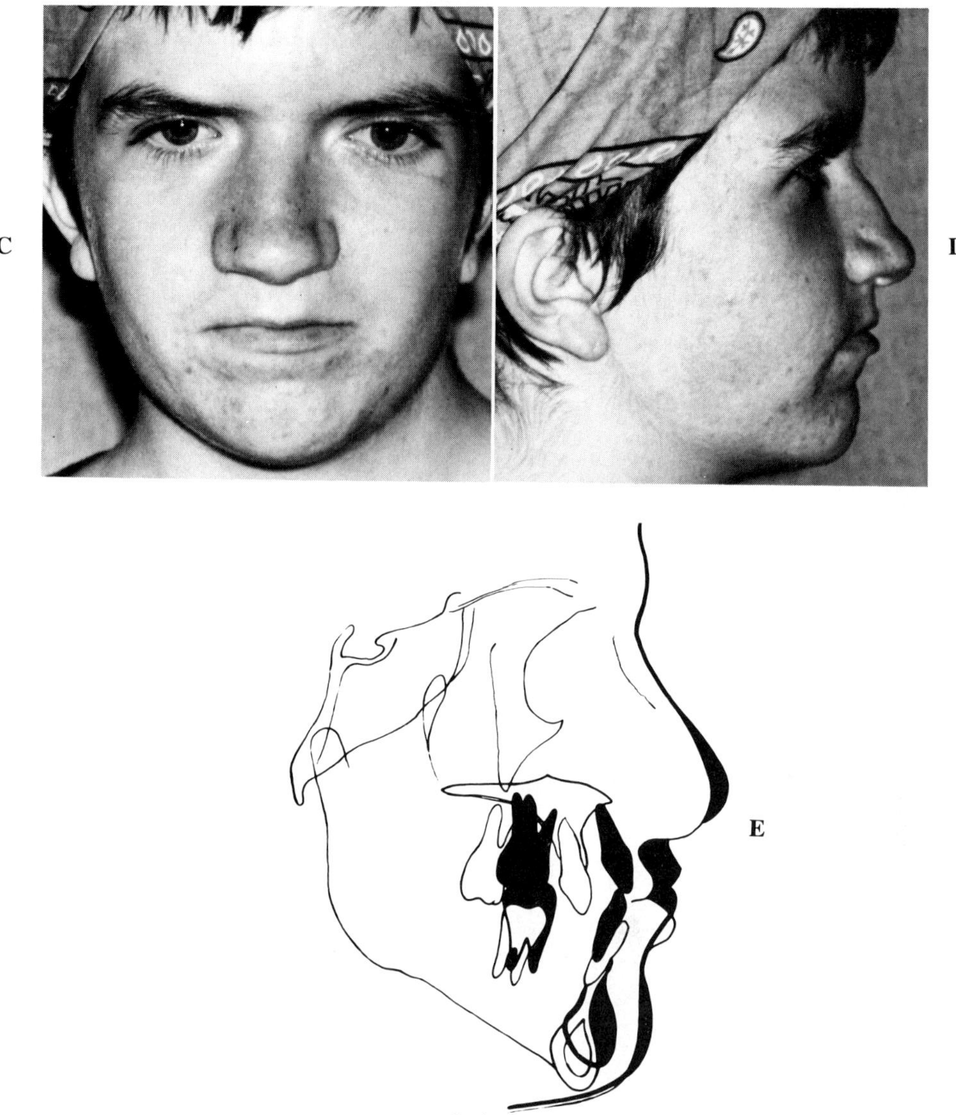

Fig. 9-7.
Orbitomaxillary hypoplasia and asymmetric prognathism (Saethre-Chetzen syndrome). **A** and **B,** Preoperative and, **C** and **D,** postoperative Stage I orbitomaxillary osteotomy. **E,** Composite cephalometric changes (centric occlusion).

On occasion, unilateral orbitomaxillary osteotomy will be indicated in conjunction with a LeFort I osteotomy. Fig. 9-8 demonstrates facial findings consistent with complex asymmetric orbitomaxillomandibular asymmetry secondary to Romberg's syndrome (hemifacial atrophy). One-stage en bloc surgical reconstruction consisted of segmental mandibular osteotomy in conjunction with segmental LeFort I osteotomy. An inferolateral orbital "wing" was attached to the right posterior maxillary segment. In this instance of complex segmentalized maxillomidfacial surgery, particular attention was devoted to the issue of providing adequate stabilization. As previously noted, however, we generally attempt to avoid high midface and segmental osteotomy at one stage.

In summary, the en bloc osteotomy is indicated for correction of significant positional deformities in the middle third of the face; but it does not successfully address simultaneous correction of positional and contour deformity in the setting of complex facial asymmetries and maxillary dentoalveolar irregularity, and thus its applications are limited by the surgeon's ability to provide secure stabilization.

Isolated orbital deformity is not uncommon, particularly in the posttraumatic setting. Fig. 9-9 illustrates such a case. Deformity of the right orbital contour, *A* and *B,* existed secondary to a malunited zygomaticomaxillary complex fracture. Note the lack of inferolateral lid support preoperatively corresponding to the inferomedial displacement of the zygomatic complex. For patients with noncomminuted malunited malar fractures, osteotomy with bone graft stabilization is the preferred approach to surgical reconstruction.[24] The clinical diagnosis of simple malposition versus combination malposition and contour deformity may be difficult. At a minimum, posteroanterior, lateral, and submentovertex cephalometric studies are indicated (*C* and *D*). Accurate repositioning of the malar complex cannot be obtained from direct anthropometric measurement without precise radiographic correlation. Care must also be taken to perform an evaluation of the position of the globe and obtain preoperative ophthalmologic evaluation and assessment of the function of orbitoadnexal structures. Goals of isolated orbital osteotomy are to obtain (1) correct position of the malar bone, (2) a reconstituted nor-

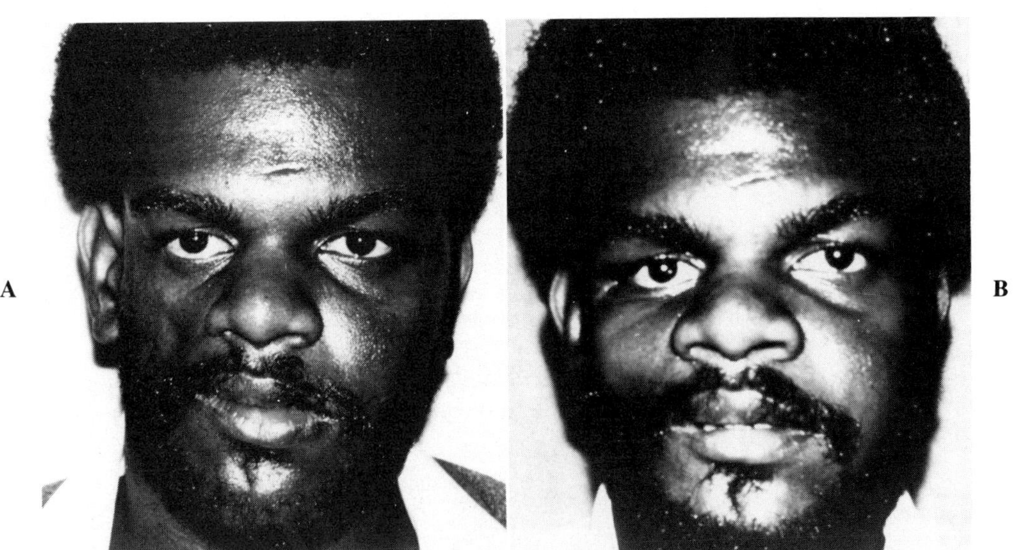

Fig. 9-8.
Unilateral orbitomaxillary osteotomy. **A,** Preoperative and, **B,** postoperative appearance.

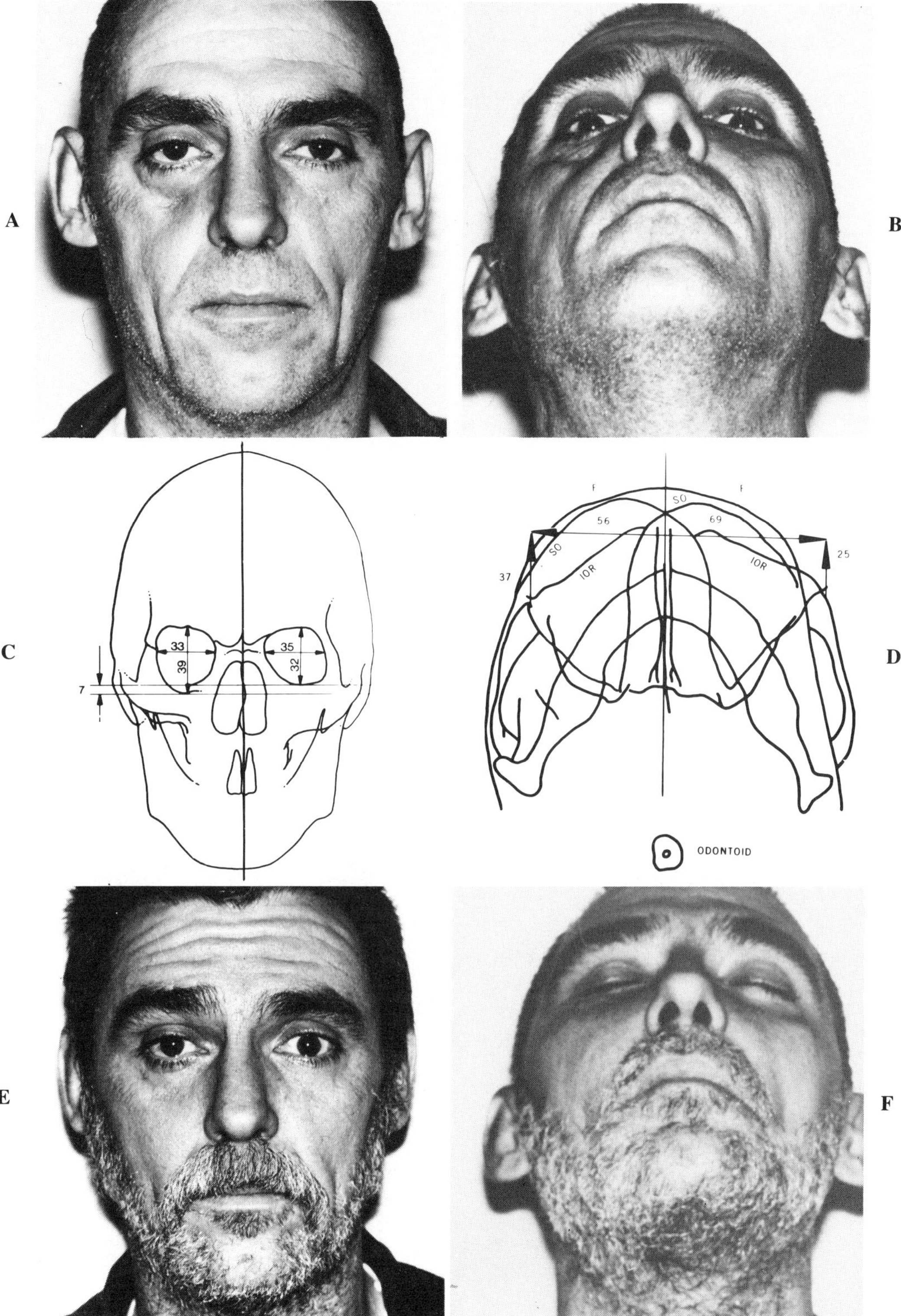

Fig. 9-9.
Isolated orbital deformity with malunion of the zygomatic complex. **A** and **B,** Preoperative appearance and, **C** and **D,** cephalometric assessment. **E** and **F,** After zygomatic osteotomy with bone graft.

mal vertical position of one globe relative to the other, (3) an improvement in the enophthalmos, and (4) better globe motility. Detailed preoperative evaluation is essential since lid deformity, ptosis, and nasolacrimal problems are not addressed by simple malar osteotomy.

Fig. 9-9, *E* and *F,* demonstrates the typical clinical result obtained by osteotomy and surgical repositioning of the orbital complex with bone graft stabilization. Note the provision of orbital rim continuity and the restoration of normal intraorbital volume for correction of vertical dystopia and enophthalmos by the or-

bital bone graft. In this patient both the orbital floor and the lateral orbit were grafted.

If there is significant soft tissue damage, orbital osteotomy or bone grafting is not uniformly successful in the correction of composite orbital deformities. Fig. 9-10 illustrates a post-traumatic enophthalmos, ptosis, and malunion of a right zygomaticomaxillary complex fracture. Right orbital ostectomy with inferior orbital floor augmentation did not provide definitive correction of the severe ptosis or enophthalmos occasioned by the periorbital scar contracture and residual ptosis.

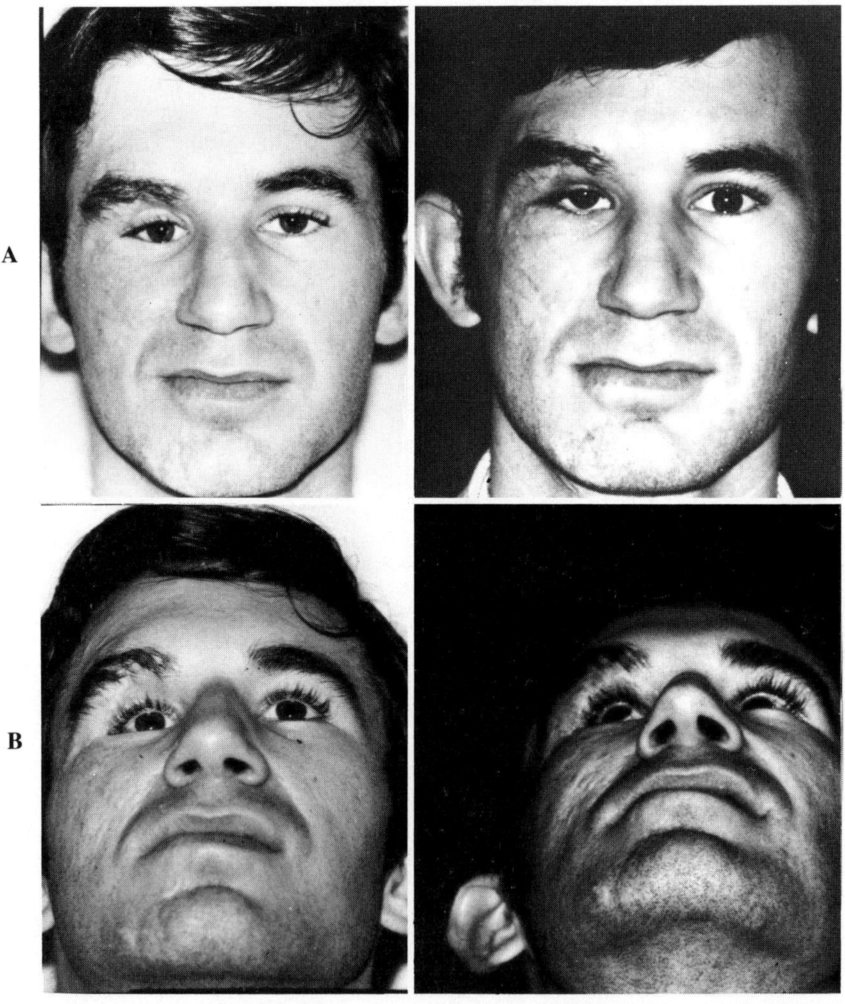

Fig. 9-10.
Residual enophthalmos with ptosis after osseous orbital reconstruction. **A,** Preoperative and, **B,** postoperative views.

CONTOUR DEFORMITY IN THE MIDFACE

Significant contour deformity in the midfacial skeleton, or composite contour and moderate positional deformity in the midfacial skeleton without significant maxillary dentoalveolar deformity, constitutes an indication for alloplastic and/or graft augmentation. In general, we consider positional deformities of less than 6 to 8 mm to be correctable with alloplastic material. Contour deformity is best addressed by an alloplastic implant. Although several graft augmentation procedures with autogenous and allogeneic materials have been described, long-term follow-up is lacking. In addition, several patients under our care who have previously undergone such procedures demonstrate extremely variable absorption of graft materials. Therefore, despite the long-term prospects of alloplastic extrusion and infection, we undertake the correction of midfacial contour and mild to moderate positional deformities using an alloplastic material (Proplast).

As previously stated, isolated nasal deformity is extremely common. Its coexistence with other maxillomandibular deformities is also common. When significant vertical nasal hypoplasia is absent but a significant sagittal nasal dorsal hypoplasia exists, alloplastic augmentation of the nasal dorsum may be indicated in conjunction with other reconstructive procedures. Fig. 9-11 illustrates a developmental maxillomandibular deformity consisting of maxillary vertical excess, maxillary sagittal excess, and mandibular sagittal excess. Nasal dorsal hypoplasia was also evident. Simultaneous segmented LeFort I osteotomy was performed in conjunction with bilateral mandibular ramal osteotomies, anterior segmental mandibular osteotomy, genioplasty, and nasal dorsal alloplastic augmentation. Note that increased nasal dorsal contour was obtained along with subtle nasal lengthening.

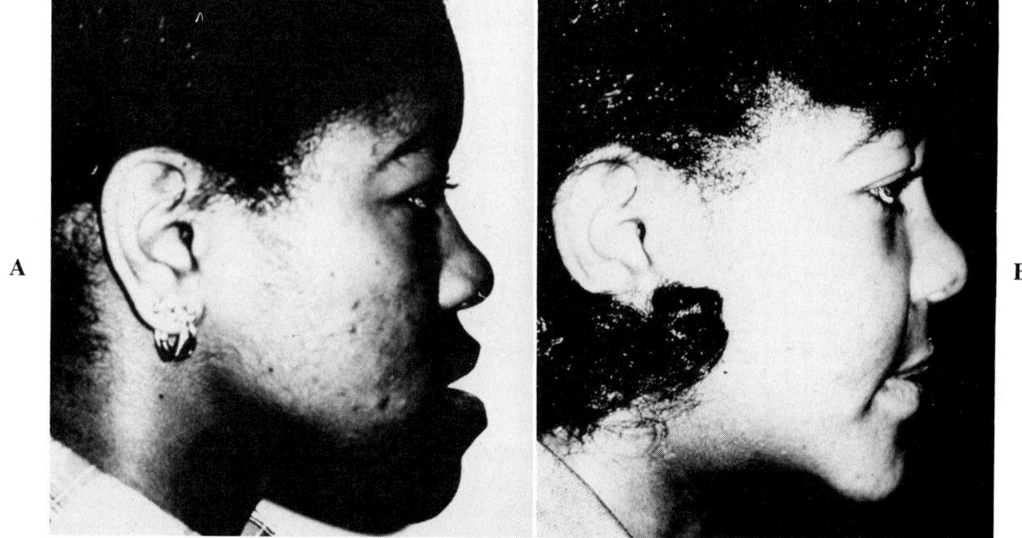

Fig. 9-11.
Saddle-nose defect treated by alloplastic augmentation in conjunction with orthognathic surgery.
A, Preoperative and, **B,** postoperative views.

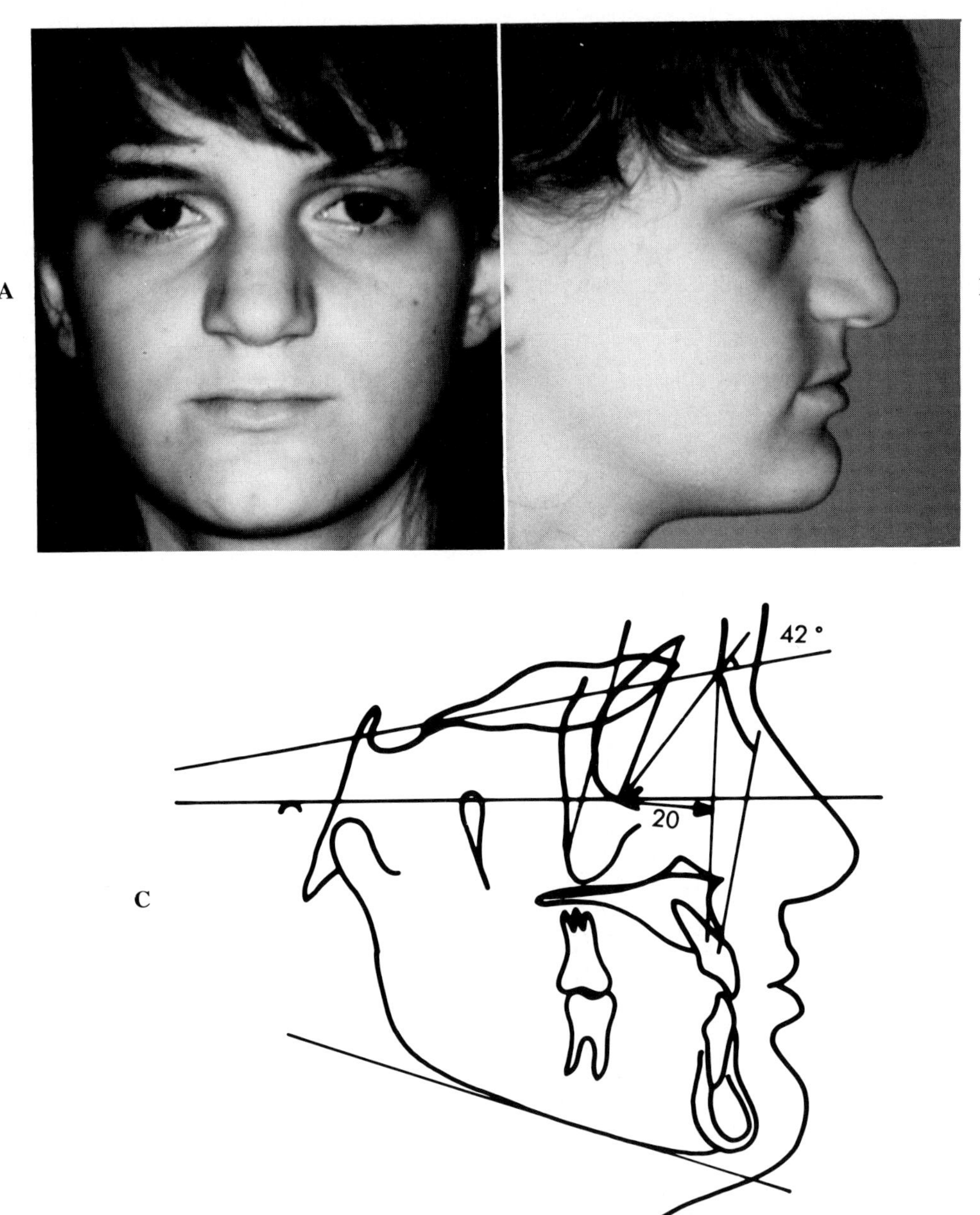

Fig. 9-12.
Isolated infraorbitomalar hypoplasia treated by alloplastic augmentation. **A** and **B,** Preoperative appearance and, **C,** diagnostic cephalometrics.

Correction of focal midfacial deformity by alloplastic implants may similarly be considered for patients with mild to moderate orbital deformity. This is particularly the case when nasomaxillomandibular relationships are normal. Fig. 9-12 illustrates a focal hypoplasia of the inferior orbital rim and malar body. In *A* and *B* contour deformity of the inferior orbital rim and malar body was present with inadequate osseous protection of the globe. This was documented by cephalometrics *(C)*. A Class I (bilateral) cross-bite secondary to minimal transverse maxillary hypoplasia was present and orthodontically correctable. Bilateral infraorbitomalar implants were placed and have been stable for 8 years *(D* and *E)*.

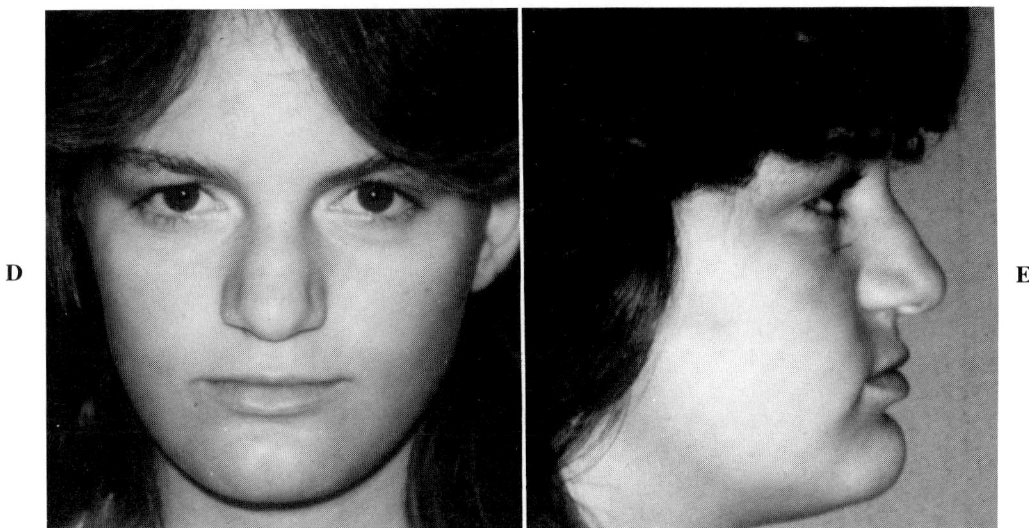

Fig. 9-12—cont'd.
D and **E,** Postoperative appearance.

COMPOSITE OSTEOTOMY AND ALLOPLASTIC RECONSTRUCTION

Occasionally the anatomic indications for en bloc osteotomy will be contraindicated by other clinical findings. Fig. 9-13, *A* and *B,* illustrates a rather marked orbitomaxillary hypoplasia accompanied by strong nasal projection, tip droop, subcolumellar retraction, and macrogenia. Previous trauma had resulted in retinal detachment and blindness of the right eye. Therefore a high LeFort I osteotomy with bone graft stabilization was undertaken in conjunction with alloplastic inferior and lateral orbital augmentation and rotational reduction genioplasty.[3] Adequate orbitomaxillary augmenta-

tion was obtained (*C* and *D*). Correction of the tip droop and improvement in the columellar retraction were also obtained. In addition, the preoperatively pinched alar base width was expanded. The composite preoperative and postoperative cephalometric soft tissue–osseous changes are illustrated in *E*.

We do not often undertake simultaneous en bloc osteotomy with alloplastic augmentation. The reason is that we fear contamination and infection around the implant (although to date we have not observed such an occurrence). However, staged alloplastic augmentation at the time of skeletal stabilization wire removal is eminently practical and feasible.

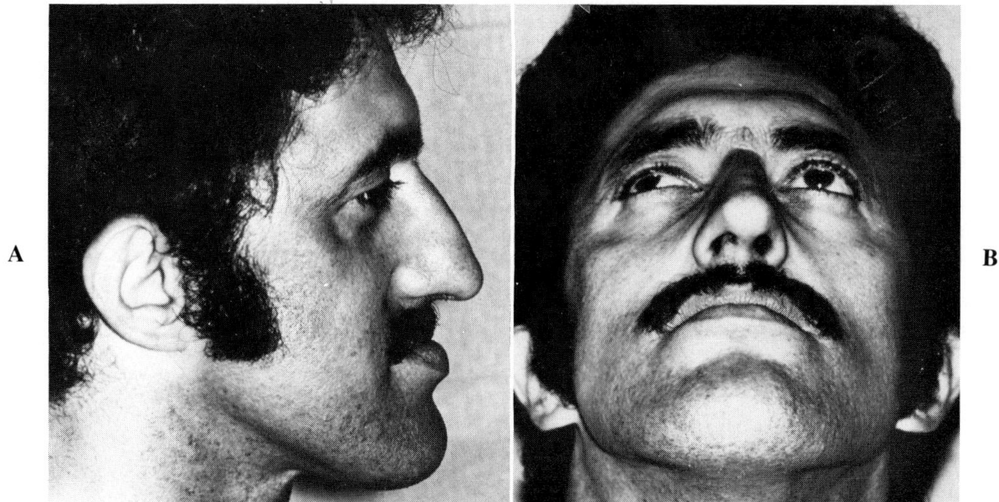

Fig. 9-13.
Orbitomaxillary hypoplasia and macrogenia treated by LeFort I osteotomy, alloplastic orbital augmentation, and rotational genioplasty. **A** and **B,** Preoperative appearance.

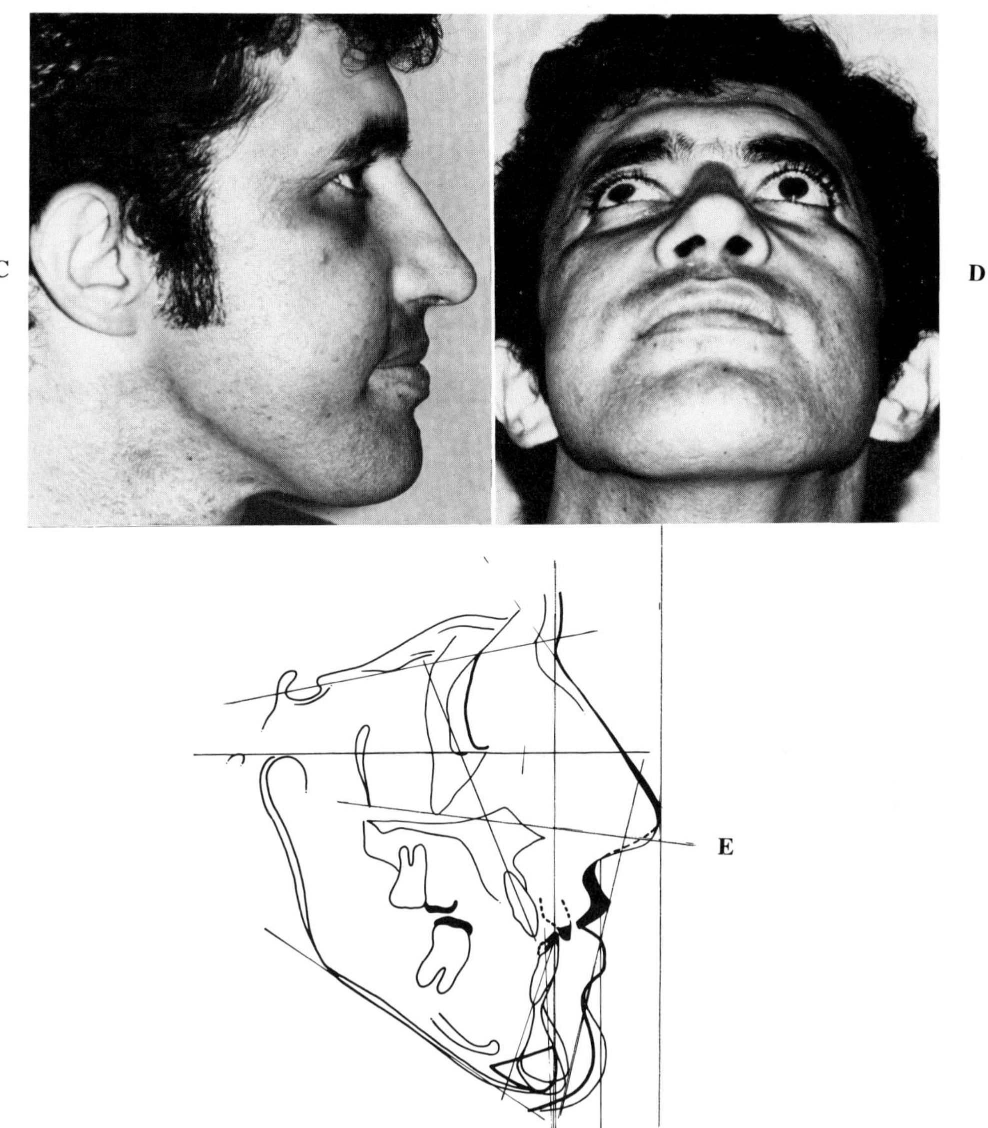

Fig. 9-13—cont'd.
C and **D,** Postoperative appearance. **E,** Composite cephalometric changes.

STAGED AND MIDFACIAL RECONSTRUCTIVE PROCEDURES

Severe positional deformity of variable severity across anatomic boundaries, concomitant significant contour deformity, and complex positional asymmetry with or without contour deformity are all indications for staged reconstruction. We disagree with statements regarding absolute indications for staged surgery in which both midfacial and mandibular structures are involved.[23] In our experience detailed attention to planning, passive surgical mobilization, and secure stabilization yield generally stable surgical results for bimaxillary procedures.

Fig. 9-14, *A* and *B,* illustrates the discrete indications for staged surgery: bilateral incomplete paramedian craniofacial clefting, ocular and orbital dystopia, and unilateral complete clefting of the left maxillary dentoalveolus with skeletal Class III malocclusion. In addition, this patient had a rather broad nasal root with asymmetry typical of the unilateral cleft lip–nasal deformity. Of particular importance, note the sagittal orbit and globe dystopia in the "worm's eye" view. Vertical malposition of the globe was correctable by osseous repositioning and bone grafting. In the majority of instances, however, sagittal dystopia of the globe is predictably more difficult to correct. Therefore a surgical plan was oriented toward fashioning the illusion of symmetry based on particular structures (the globes) whose sagittal position would not be altered by the surgery.

The procedure for this young woman was staged and consisted of the following:

1. Simultaneous LeFort I osteotomy with bone graft closure of the alveolar cleft
2. Anterior mandibular segmental osteotomy and normalization of the lateral and inferior orbital segments of the right orbit to a position symmetric with the globe itself
3. Cleft lip–nasal revision and a nasal dorsal implant

Second-stage surgery was undertaken with the goal of rotating the transverse nasal axis to match the axis of the globes, thereby creating the illusion of overall maxillofacial symmetry (Fig. 9-14, *C* and *D*).

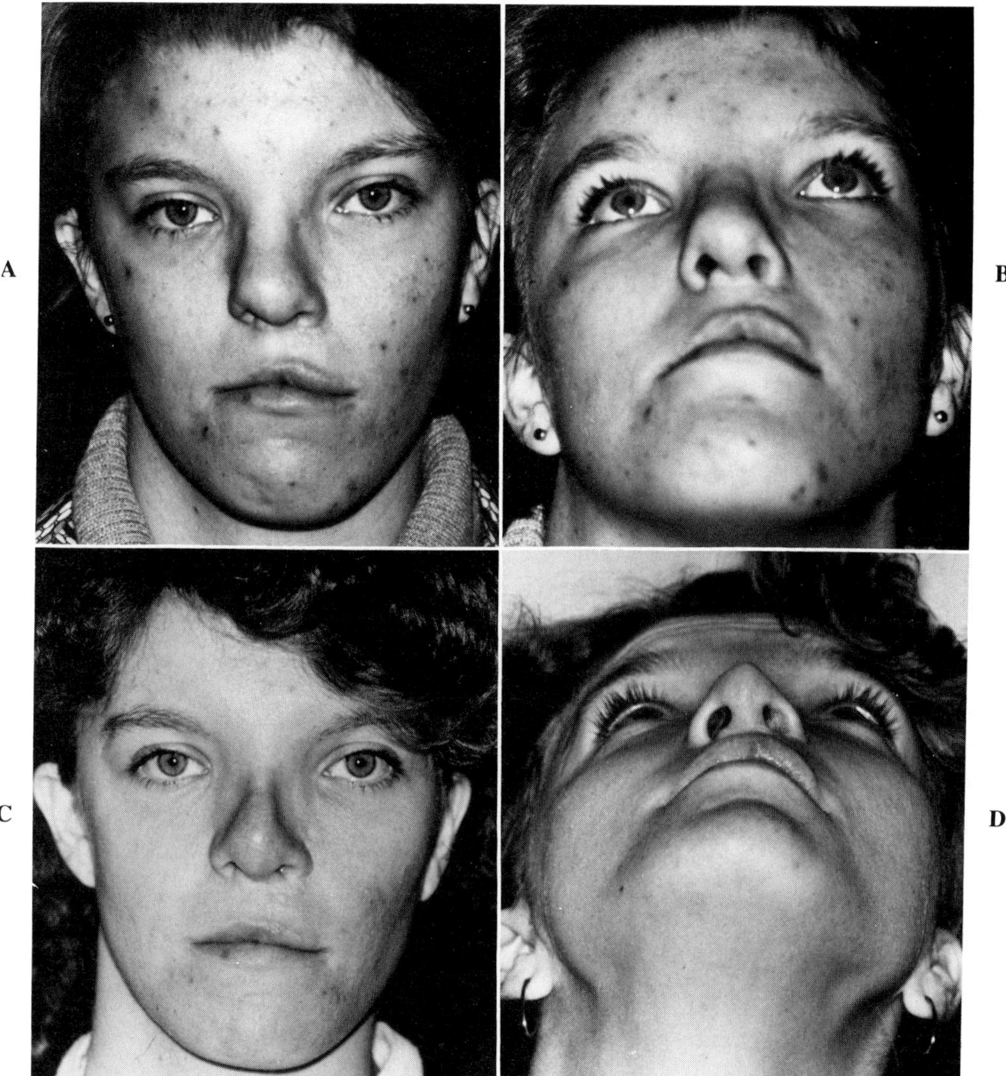

Fig. 9-14.
Atypical craniofacial cleft treated by staged reconstruction. **A** and **B,** Preoperative and, **C** and **D,** postoperative appearance.

Frequently disparate severity of deformity across anatomic boundaries coexists with significant contour deformity. Fig. 9-15 demonstrates the treatment of Crouzon's syndrome (craniofacial synostosis). Preoperatively *(A)*, note the significant orbitomaxillary hypoplasia with asymmetric exophthalmos. In *B* a typical "polly beak" deformity is present with increased nasal projection, prominence of the nasal tip structures, and some columellar retraction. In the frontal view mild alar base pinching also is evident. A severe, greater than 20 mm, Class III open-bite was present with significant transverse maxillary hypoplasia.

First-stage surgery consisted of the following:

1. Orbitomaxillary advancement (17 mm) with bone graft stabilization
2. Unilateral decompression of orbital fat
3. Bilateral lateral canthopexy and skeletal stabilization.

After this stage (*C* and *D*) the residual deformity consisted of first-degree hypertelorism, a skeletal Class III malocclusion with cross-bite, and a nasal contour deformity.

Subsequent surgery then entailed

1. LeFort I osteotomy for correction of the transverse maxillary hypoplasia
2. Bilateral ramal osteotomy for correction of the residual prognathism
3. Genioplasty and rhinoplasty

The end-stage result of reconstruction is illustrated in Fig. 9-15, *E* and *F*. Residual first-degree hypertelorism persists, although marked improvement in the composite deformity has been obtained. Such correction would not have been possible through the use of a one-stage surgical correction.

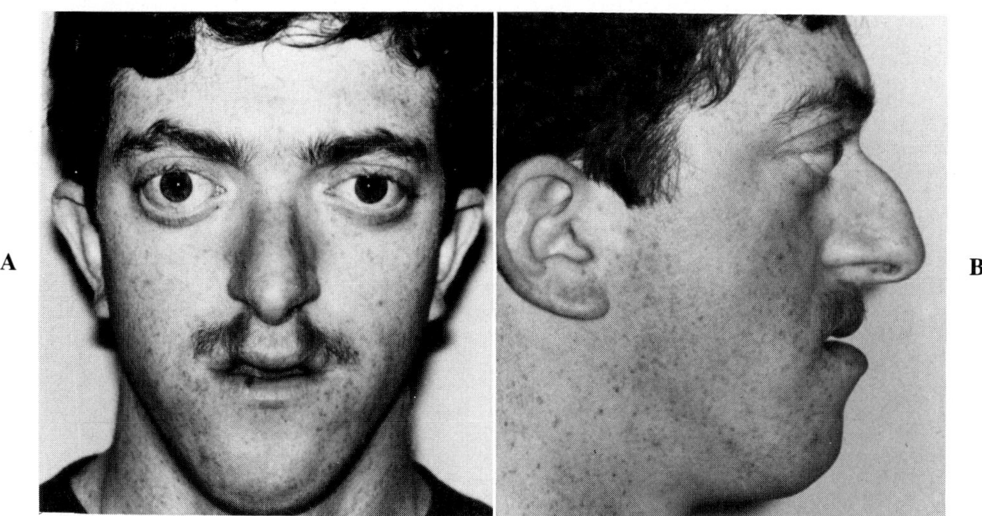

Fig. 9-15.
Craniofacial synostosis. **A** and **B,** Preoperative appearance.

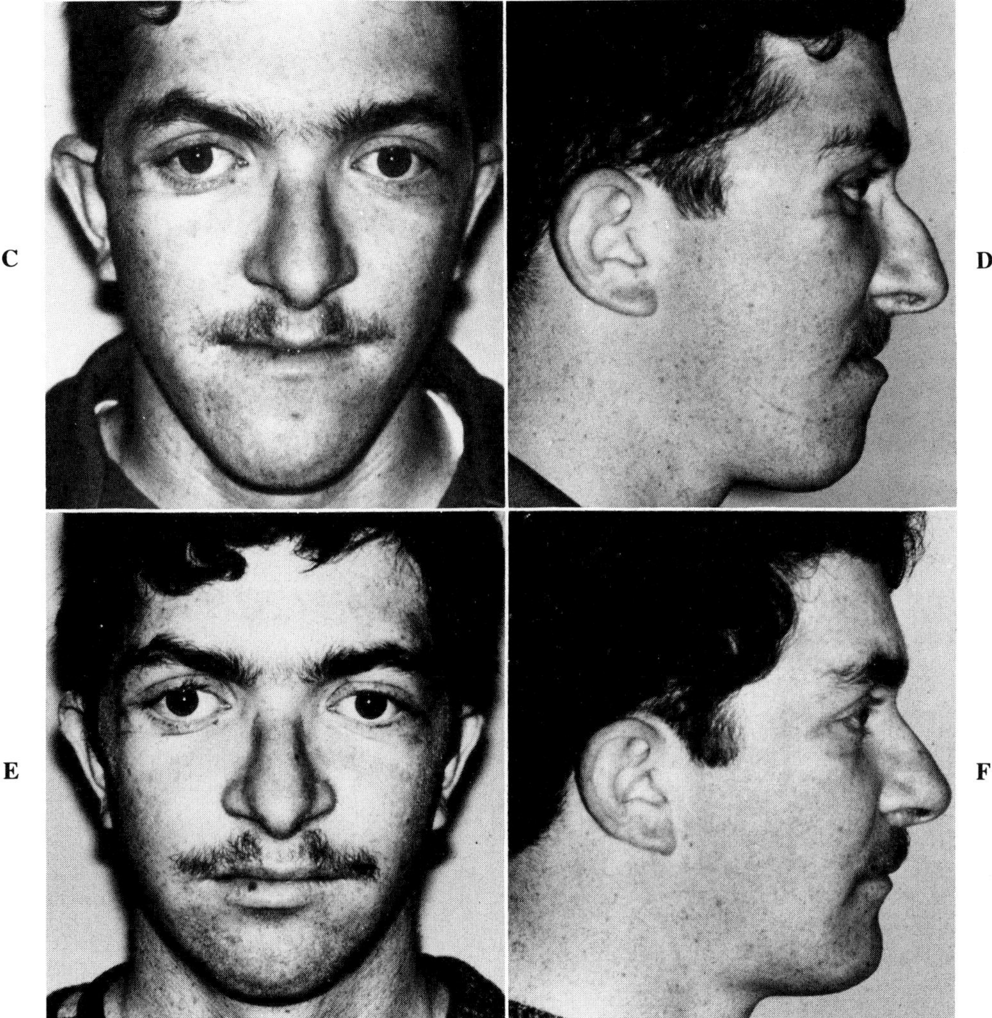

Fig. 9-15—cont'd.
C and **D**, Postoperative orbitomaxillary osteotomy and frontal augmentation. **E** and **F**, After mandibular osteotomies, LeFort I, and nasoseptal reconstruction.

SURGICAL OUTCOME

Reflecting the common prevalence of maxillomandibular deformity and orthognathic correction, the recent literature documents reasonably well the stability and complications for specific procedures as applied to defined diagnostic groups. This is not the case for subcranial high midface procedures, which are relatively less commonly performed. To date, reports of surgical outcome for high midface procedures reflect surgical experience with a multiplicity of techniques applied to heterogeneous patient populations.[9,21,33]

Published conclusions regarding surgical outcome therefore are quite individualized and not controlled for such factors as sites of surgical correction, techniques of osteotomy or stabilization, the outcome of a given surgical approach for specific diagnostic entities of similar severity, and the experience of the surgical team. In summary, assessment of the success of high midface procedures, to date, falls into the category of "in my experience" reporting. Several common conclusions emerge from these reports and represent a currently undocumented body of surgical principles for high midface surgery.

The *stability* of en bloc procedures in the high midface has been the subject of repeated comment.[9] To date, reports have not controlled the technique of osteotomy, the severity of deformity, the methods of stabilization, the types of grafts employed, or the role of growth in young patients. Certainly rigorous data, controlled for these factors, are lacking to substantiate clinical opinions.

In our experience several considerations are pertinent to the stabilty of orthognathic surgery in the high midface:

1. The ability to achieve passive mobilization, secure stabilization, and early osseous union appears to be paramount.
2. Sufficient soft tissue exposure and periosteal release incisions are needed for passive midface mobilization.
3. Stabilization of the particularly hypoplastic midface may present a problem, but with stepped interlocking malar osteotomy and directly wired interpositional grafts the majority of midface osteotomies achieve secure stabilization without the need to resort to rigid internal or external fixation schemes. I therefore do not hesitate to employ rigid fixation where graft-wire stabilization does not suffice.

Demonstrable clinical ability to achieve early osseous union with midface osteotomy remains a problematic issue. Animal studies to document the roles of different surgical techniques and their relation to healing are lacking. Early clinical union in maxillomandibular surgery appears to depend on the ability to provide a sufficient vascular pedicle to the mobilized bone and to secure adequate fixation. Autogenous cancellous onlays probably accelerate early union. With en bloc high midface procedures the surgeon is caught between mandates for passive mobilization through tissue relaxation and the need for a soft tissue pedicle. If not rendered as free grafts by surgery, the nasal and orbital elements of en bloc osteotomies are almost certainly less well perfused than the tissues with a LeFort I–level osteotomy. Finally, the biology of factors affecting the stability of high midface procedures is sketchy, at best. In our experience midface repositioning of 10 to 15 mm can be stable only as long as it provides for generous passive mobilization, secure stabilization, onlayed autogenous cancellous bone, and a stable postoperative occlusion. When these considerations cannot be adequately addressed, concomitant mandibular surgery is deferred.

One aspect of the relative stability of high midface procedures revolves around the question of surgery in the growing patient. Arguments for early surgery are derived from the psychosocial benefits that accrue and the hypothesis that end-stage deformity is ameliorated by early surgery. However, the following pertain:

Psychosocial indications for early surgery are predicated on an assessment of the severity of deformity and the adaptation of patient and family to the psychosocial consequences. Severe deformity in the child with poor adaptation is an undeniable surgical indication, regardless of the implications for stability or the subsequent growth and development.

With the exception of isolated entities such as craniosynostosis and hemifacial microsomia, even preliminary data are lacking to substantiate claims that early surgery aborts the expression of end-stage deformity.

Furthermore, data are lacking to document the prevalence of procedure-related *complications* for subcranial high midface osteotomy. It is probable that most complications are qualitatively similar to those of orthognathic surgery, with the addition of potentials for increased blood loss, intraorbital complications, and extended airway problems.[33] Our clinical experience, to date, would substantiate such conclusions.

Soft tissue prediction. The "state of the art" in planning high midface procedures does not approach that of suborbitonasal surgery in terms of the ability to predict soft tissue changes based on osseous movement. In our experience soft tissue–osseous change in the osseous naso-orbital region occurs in approximately a "one to one" ratio. Thre appears to exist a transition zone between the nasal osseous and nasal cartilaginous skeletons where one-to-one changes do not occur. These are the subject of current intensive study.

The prospect of simultaneous correction of nasal contour malformation with midface osteotomy has been explored in the literature.[16] Although such attempts are laudable, in my opinion contour deformity of the nasal cartiliginous skeleton will probably be best addressed by definitive second-stage procedures once overall soft tissue drape is adapted to gross osseous repositioning. We are, however, actively investigating the ability to identify those instances in which simultaneous definitive one-stage correction of specific nasal tip–cartilaginous and osseous malformation can be obtained.

ORTHODONTIC MANAGEMENT OF PATIENTS WITH HIGH MIDFACIAL DEFORMITY

In the majority of instances the coordination of orthodontic and surgical management for high midfacial deformities is quite similar to that for subnasoorbital deformities. Attention is directed to sequencing surgery and orthodontics in an attempt to avoid segmentalized maxillary surgery, thereby allowing a one-stage midface surgical procedure to be accomplished. The basic principle of attempting only stable orthodontic mechanics preoperatively applies in midfacial surgery. When stable orthodontic mechanics cannot circumvent the need for a second-stage operation, then a second procedure is planned from the outset.

FUTURE DEVELOPMENTS IN HIGH MIDFACE SURGERY

Predictably successful rehabilitation of individuals with high midfacial deformity will be predicated on the evolution of more sophisticated diagnostic techniques, the generation of a controlled data base to allow rational surgical planning based on anticipated surgical outcome, and the availability of more extensive data to assess the biologic compatibility of current surgical techniques.

Within the diagnostic realm, elucidation of specific criteria for high midfacial deformity represents a long-term horizon. More immediately advances in three-dimensional imaging should increase existing capabilities for anatomic evaluation.[19] In conjunction with these, controlled procedure-specific studies are needed to produce data that will allow a more rational timing and choice of procedure for the rehabilitation of patients with midfacial deformity.

SUMMARY

The evolution of high midface procedures parallels that of orthognathic surgery. However, to date, a lesser degree of sophistication has evolved regarding the application of the former. Similarly, lesser degrees of sophistication exist to allow quantitative prediction of concomitant soft tissue change associated with high midface osteotomies. Finally, the stability of high midface procedures is probably predicated on attention to basic orthognathic surgical principles; but this also has yet to be documented.

En bloc high midface osteotomies and various augmentation procedures allow the surgeon to address high midfacial malformations of varying severity. The functional disabilities associated with these deformities extend beyond the oral cavity and require that the surgeon and surgical team be familiar with aspects of neurologic, nasorespiratory, ocular, and oculoadnexal physiology and anatomy. In addition, the prevalence of multiple malformation syndromes associated with high midfacial deformities requires the capability to extend the diagnostic workup beyond anatomic assessment.

High midfacial deformity often involves the entire spectrum of osseous and soft tissue structures. Current capabilities for osseous reconstruction are, in general, limited by the soft tissue aspects of a given deformity. The composite management of soft tissue and osseous deformities is one of the greatest challenges in the field of craniomaxillofacial reconstruction and requires the creative collaboration of surgeons from multiple specialties.

ACKNOWLEDGMENTS

I would like to express my gratitude to the following clinicians for their roles in the management of patients presented: J. Bertoldi, R. Brown, P. Crump, K.Y. Kai, F. O'Ryan (my associate), N. Roth, K. Rotskoff, T. Rust, D. Stocking, and L. Wolford.

Recognition is also due C.W. Hoffman and K. Anderson, who undertook the responsibilities of illustration and photography.

Finally, my administrative assistant, A. Mazzuki, was instrumental in preparation of this manuscript.

REFERENCES

1. Converse, J.M., and Wood-Smith, D.: An atlas and classification of midfacial and craniofacial osteotomies. In Hueston, J., editor: Transactions of the Fifth International Congress on Plastic and Reconstructive Surgery, Melbourne, 1971, Butterworths.
2. Dann, J.J.: Suborbital ostectomy for simultaneous correction of sagittal orbitomaxillary hypoplasia and vertical maxillary excess. In preparation.
3. Dann, J.J., and O'Ryan, F.M.: Correction of macrogenia with rotational osteotomy. In preparation.
4. Dann, J.J., and Wolford, L.M.: Unpublished data, 1984.
5. DeMyer, W.: Median facial malformations and their implications for brain malformations. In Morphogenesis and malformation of face and brain, Birth Defects 9(7):155, 1975.
6. Epker, B.N., and Wolford, L.M.: Middle third facial osteotomies: their use in the correction of acquired and developmental dentofacial and craniofacial deformities. J. Oral Surg. **33**:491, 1975.
7. Epker, B.N., and Wolford, L.M.: Middle third facial osteotomies: their use in the correction of congenital dentofacial and craniofacial deformities, J. Oral Surg. **34**:324, 1976.
8. Epker, B.N., and Wolford, L.M.: Middle-third facial advancement: treatment considerations in atypical cases, J. Oral Surg. **37**:31, 1979.
9. Freihofer, H.P.M.: Results after midface osteotomies, J. Maxillofac. Surg. **1**:30, 1976.
10. Gillies, H., and Harrison, S.H.: Operative correction by osteotomy of recessed malar-maxillary compound in a case of oxycephaly, Br. J. Plast. Surg. **3**:123, 1950.
11. Grove, A.S.: Evaluation of exophthalmos, N. Engl. J. Med. **292**:1005, 1975.
12. Henderson, D., and Jackson, I.: Nasomaxillary hypoplasia—the LeFort II osteotomy, Br. J. Oral Surg. **11**:77, 1973.
13. Jackson, I.T.: Midface retrusion. In Whitaker, L.A., and Randall, P., editors: Symposium on reconstruction of jaw deformity, St. Louis, 1978, The C.V. Mosby Co.
14. Kawamoto, H.K.: The kaleidoscopic world of rare craniofacial clefts, Clin. Plast. Surg. **3**:529, 1976.
15. Kinnebrew, M.C., et al.: Rotational ostectomies of the midface and mandible to correct primary and compensatory abnormalities of midfacial hypoplasia. Platform paper, American Cleft Palate Association, Denver, 1982.
16. Kinnebrew, M.C., et al.: Modified LeFort II procedure for simultaneous corrections of maxillary and nasal deformities, J. Oral Maxillofac. Surg. **41**:295, 1983.
17. Kinnebrew, M.C., et al.: Enhancing the ease of performance of potential stability of midfacial surgery. In press, 1984.
18. Leonard, M., and Walker, G.F.: A cephalometric guide to the diagnosis of midface hypoplasia at the LeFort II level, J. Oral Surg. **35**:21, 1977.
19. Marsh, J.L., and Vannier, M.W.: The third dimension in craniofacial surgery, J. Plast. Reconstr. Surg. **71**:759, 1983.
20. Murray, J.E., and Swanson, L.T.: Midface osteotomy and advancement for craniosynostosis, J. Plast. Reconstr. Surg. **41**:299, 1968.
21. Murray, J.E., et al.: Twenty-year experience in maxillocraniofacial surgery, Ann. Surg. **190**:320, 1979.
22. Obwegeser, H.: Surgical correction of the small or retrodisplaced maxilla, J. Plast. Reconstr. Surg. **43**:351, 1969.
23. Ousterhout, D.K.: Orthognathic surgical treatment, West. J. Med. **136**:525, 1983.
24. Perrino, K.E., et al.: Late treatment of malunited malar fractures, J. Oral Maxillofac. Surg. **42**:20, 1984.
25. Popescu, V.C.: Advancement of the middle third of the face without bone grafting in a case of Crouzon's disease, J. Maxillofac. Surg. **2**:219, 1974.
26. Smith, D.W.: Recognizable patterns of human malformation, ed. 3, Philadelphia, 1982, W.B. Saunders Co.

27. Steinhauser, E.: Variations on LeFort II osteotomy for correction of midfacial deformities, J. Maxillofac. Surg. **8:**258, 1980.
28. Tessier, P.: The definitive plastic surgical treatment of severe facial deformities of craniofacial dysostosis, Crouzon's and Apert's disease, J. Plast. Reconstr. Surg. **48:**419, 1971.
29. Tessier, P.: Total osteotomy of the middle third face for faciostenosis or for sequellae of LeFort III fractures, J. Plast. Reconstr. Surg. **48:**553, 1971.
30. Warren, F., and Dann, J.J.: Diagnostic evaluation of nasal morphology: qualitative and quantitative assessment, J. Oral Maxillofac. Surg. In press.
31. Whitaker, L.A., et al.: The nasolacrimal apparatus in congenital facial anomalies, J. Maxillofac. Surg. **2:**59, 1974.
32. Whitaker, L.A., et al.: Structural goals in craniofacial surgery, Cleft Palate J. **12:**23, 1975.
33. Whitaker, L.A., et al.: Problems in craniofacial surgery, J. Maxillofac. Surg. **4:**131, 1976.

Index